ESSENTIALS OF MATERNITY NURSING

Family-Centered Care

Consultants

Jane Edmiston Buhr, RN, MHA, MBA
Editor
CRACOM Corporation
St. Louis, Missouri

Joea Bierchen, RN, EdD
Professor
Maternal-Newborn Nursing
St. Petersburg Junior College
St. Petersburg, Florida

Rita Tobler, RN, MSN
Assistant Professor
Coordinator, Level I
AD Nursing Program
Northern Kentucky University
Highland Heights, Kentucky

Donna Aldesperger, RN, MEd
Clinical Nurse Specialist
Maternal-Child Health
St. Elizabeth's Medical Center
Edgewood, Kentucky

ESSENTIALS OF MATERNITY NURSING

Family-Centered Care

Leonide L. Martin, *RN, MS, Dr PH*
Professor, Department of Nursing;
Director, Family Nurse Practitioner Program,
Sonoma State University,
Rohnert Park, California

Sharon J. Reeder, *RN, PhD, FAAN*
Professor of Nursing and Associate Dean,
School of Nursing,
University of California,
Los Angeles, California

J. B. Lippincott Company   PHILADELPHIA

NEW YORK   ST. LOUIS   LONDON

SIDNEY   TOKYO

Sponsoring Editor David P. Carroll
Developmental Editor Jane Edmiston Buhr, CRACOM Corp.
Senior Manuscript Editor Joy Moore, CRACOM Corp.
Indexer Nelle Garrecht
Art Director Maureen E. Arends, CRACOM Corp.
Design Coordinator Diane M. Beasley
Production CRACOM Corporation, St. Louis, MO
Compositor Graphic World
Printer/Binder Murray Printing

Library of Congress Cataloging-in-Publication Data

Martin, Leonide L.
    Essentials of maternity nursing : family-centered care / Leonide
L. Martin, Sharon J. Reeder.
        p.   cm.
    Includes bibliographical references.
    Includes index.
    ISBN 0-397-54791-9
    1. Obstetrical nursing.   2. Perinatology.   3. Family nursing.
I. Title.
    [DNLM: 1. Family—nurses' instruction.   2. Obstetrical Nursing.
3. Perinatology—nurses' instruction.   WY 157 M381e]
RG951.M3124   1991
610.73′678—dc20
DNLM/DLC
for Library of Congress   90-13239
                                                                  CIP

The authors and publishers have exerted every effort to ensure that drug selection
and dosage set forth in this text are in accord with current recommendations and
practice at the time of publication. However, in view of ongoing research, changes
in government regulations, and the constant flow of information relating to drug
therapy and drug reactions, the reader is urged to check the package insert for each
drug for any change in indications and dosage and for added warnings and precautions.
This is particularly important when the recommended agent is a new or infrequently
employed drug.

Preface

*T*he discipline of maternity nursing today is filled with challenges and opportunities for educators, students, and practitioners. Nursing educators are challenged by the need to assist students in learning how to provide safe and effective care for mothers, infants, and families. Students are challenged by the vast amount of material that must be understood and applied in the clinical setting in a relatively short period of time. They often need to balance their academic and personal lives with the demands of a full-time job. Practitioners are constantly challenged to keep current with legal and ethical issues and technologic advances, while at the same time controlling medical care costs and reducing the length of hospitalization for the client.

Yet, with these challenges come opportunities and rewards. Maternity nursing instructors are in the unique position of being able to guide students in their learning and share their joy at the miracle of birth. Maternity nursing students have the opportunity to see the impact they can have on the birth experience for mothers and their families and to see how their newly acquired knowledge and skill translate into practice. Practicing maternity nurses have an opportunity to use their skills in client teaching and the promotion of self-care.

From its inception the goal of this book has been to provide faculty and students with a primary resource for learning the art and science of maternity nursing. Based on the advice of instructors and students, the intent is to present information that is *essential* to the safe and effective delivery of nursing care. Because of the massive amount of information to be learned about maternity nursing, material covered in other courses is not repeated here. The pedagogic development of the content was carefully planned before writing began to present only material pertinent to maternity nursing from a clinical perspective. Towards this end the text was revised many times to ensure that important material is covered succinctly and completely. Moreover, important concepts are explained, why they are important is detailed and how they apply to the practice of maternity nursing is demonstrated.

The content, art, and pedagogy were developed in a manner consistent with how students reported they wanted to learn. With this in mind, a unique single-column design was established for this book that allowed placement of art and important information such as laboratory tests, legal and ethical considerations, emergency care, and drug guides as close to the appropriate content in the text as possible. This format enables the student to review all pertinent information in one area, minimizing the need to turn pages or look in other chapters. Thus, this unique design makes it easier to find information and is less confusing for the reader to follow.

Students reported that they needed a variety of pedagogic devices to help them learn the important concepts and how to apply them to clinical nursing. To satisfy their requests the following learning aids were carefully planned, written, and designed into the page layout.

ART/LABELS/LEGENDS

Special care was taken to closely integrate the art-legend-text material, enabling students to visualize a concept clearly. The text material first introduces students to the concept and provides the proper context. The art itself focuses on one point and was rendered to be straightforward and clear to the students. The art is labeled to direct students' attention to key points, while expanded legends clearly explain what is going on in the art. When students read the text, art, labels, and legend material, they will understand and visualize the concept completely.

ASSESSMENT TOOLS

Assessment tools contain complete and comprehensive guides that show students what to look for and what to ask the client. The assessment tools help assure that all pertinent areas have been covered in the assessment process. In most cases sample documentation is provided to show students what assessment information should be written in the client's chart.

CLIENT SELF-CARE EDUCATION GUIDELINES

With the trend toward earlier discharge of maternity clients, there is an increased emphasis on client education. Client self-care education guidelines are included to provide specific details on what information needs to be conveyed to clients, how the information can best be provided, and the rationale for its inclusion. Where appropriate, sample documentation is presented.

LEGAL AND ETHICAL CONSIDERATIONS

Because of the possibility of legal and ethical problems in maternity nursing, these areas are highlighted for students where appropriate. Rather than attempting to present specific facts about legal and ethical issues for the students to memorize, the text poses questions that challenge students' ethics and alerts them to potential legal pitfalls, court decisions related to specific areas of care or standards of care, and ethical dilemmas created by technologic advances. This approach is taken to prepare students for how they must think when practicing maternity nursing. If nurses are constantly thinking about what they are doing and asking appropriate questions as needed, perhaps they will be able to avoid problems for themselves and the hospitals.

CULTURAL CONSIDERATIONS

Since few people in a cultural group follow all practices attributed to the group, assessment emphasis is placed on identifying the cultural practices of individual clients. The text presents a cultural assessment tool that focuses on identifying individual, rather than group, pregnancy and delivery customs and practices, since these are areas where generalizations and assumptions might cause as many problems as a lack of understanding.

FOCUS ASSESSMENTS

Students' reported that one of the most difficult areas in learning how to deliver maternity care is differentiating between normal physiologic responses and the signs of pathology. Values that are normal in pregnant women often differ from normal values of nonpregnant women. Focus assessments help students understand the difference and recognize potential problems early. The focus assessments guide students in developing accurate, appropriate, goal directed nursing care plans for maternity clients.

NURSING CARE PLANS

The nursing care plans presented in this text provide students with comprehensive guidelines that can be used to formulate individualized care plans for their clients. Unique to this text is the inclusion of *rationales* for nursing interventions. Rationales explain the scientific reasons why interventions are performed.

LABORATORY VALUES, DRUG GUIDELINES, EMERGENCY NURSING PROCEDURES

Other relevant pedagogic devices provided to facilitate student learning include readily accessible marginal notes and text displays that contain pertinent laboratory values, pharmacology information, and emergency procedures. These are placed as close as possible to the appropriate material in the text to allow students quick and easy access to the information without disrupting the flow of the text or requiring the students to turn pages.

It is our hope that students will benefit from the current, accurate information that is presented in this unique format. All elements, including text, art, legends, labels, display material, and marginal notes have been designed to work together to make learning maternity nursing less of a challenge, and more of an opportunity.

Acknowledgments

As with any text of this size, it would be impossible to adequately acknowledge the contributions of all of the people who helped with this project. However, the following individuals have assisted greatly in a variety of ways to help complete this text.

A large debt of gratitude goes to the following individuals who provided guidance for the concept behind the book and contributed a great deal of the new and exciting ideas and information that can be found throughout: Joea Bierchen, RN, EdD, St. Petersburg Junior College, St. Petersburg, Fla., for contributions in the areas of legal and ethical issues and postpartum care; Carol Bear, RN, MEd, St. Louis Community College at Florissant Valley, St. Louis, Mo., for contributions on physiologic and psychosocial aspects of pregnancy; Donna Kiefer-Stephens, MSN Candidate, St. Elizabeth's Hospital, Belleville, Ill., for imput on prenatal education; Linda Whitenton, RN, MSN, St. Petersburg Junior College, St. Petersburg, Fla., for assistance with nutrition in pregnancy; and Betty Wajdowicz, RN, EdD, St. Petersburg Junior College, St. Petersburg, Fla., for assistance with antepartum maternal nursing care.

We are also indebted to the following individuals who conscientiously reviewed the manuscript in great detail through various drafts and provided expert guidance regarding the depth, breadth, and accuracy of content. They provided excellent critical comments, many of which have been incorporated throughout the text. They are Stuart Barger (Everett Community College), Susan Bodtke (Oklahoma State University), Genevieve Brace (Willmar Community College), Gail Jones (George Wallace State Community College), Sharon Murray (Golden West College), Carol Ottinger (Columbus State Community College), Marge Phillips (St. Louis Community College at Forest Park), Editha Sanchez (South Suburban College), and Julia Wiklof (Everett Community College).

Petra Allen and Stephanie Hoog, two competent, candid, and vocal students, helped enormously by providing insight into the needs and wants of student learners. Likewise, Susan Bodtke (Oklahoma State University), Mary Eimer (Jefferson College), Kathy Klepzig (East Central Junior College), and Editha Sanchez (South Suburban College) provided excellent sensitivity to student needs during the early stages of the book's development.

Every book needs one person with exceptional talent, skill, energy, and knowledge of the marketplace to make all the parts come together. Maureen E. Arends, Developmental Editor at CRACOM Corporation, fulfilled this role on this project. Without her exceptional efforts this book and the ancillaries would not have come to be.

We would also like to thank the following individuals from J.B. Lippincott for the roles they played. Nancy Mullins, former Nursing Editor, and Diana Intenzo, Editor-in-Chief of Nursing, showed daring and creativity in deciding to develop this unique book in a very different way; and Dave Carroll, Nursing Editor, was with us from the early stages, and we deeply appreciate his insights, support, and management of this project.

Creating an attractive book with a unique format is a very difficult undertaking in nursing and requires a team effort. We would like to thank the following individuals for their expertise: Diane Beasley, an exceptional designer; Kathy Dunn, Director of Production at J.B. Lippincott; Janet Greenwood, Production Manager at J.B. Lippincott; Joy Moore, Project Manager at CRACOM Corporation; Jeanne Gulledge, Production Designer at CRACOM Corporation; Jeanne Robertson, artist; Nadine Sokol, medical illustrator; and Donna Keifer-Stephens and Donna Adelsperger who provided numerous photographs.

Contents

II   *The Family and Reproduction*   29

III   The Family in the Antepartum Period   125

IV The Family in the Intrapartum Period 235

13   Second Stage of Labor   308

14   Operative Obstetrics   334

V   *The Family in the Postpartum Period*   *397*

VII   *Neonatal Disorders*   731

Nursing Procedures

Drug Guides

Nursing Care Plans

Contemporary Family-Centered Care

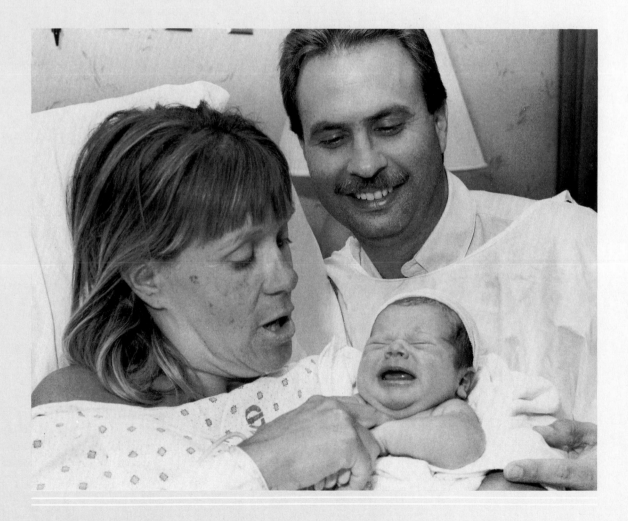

Family-Centered Care

IMPORTANT TERMINOLOGY

blended family Marriage of two divorced parents with children; "blends" two families into one

configuration Combination of members in a family

demographic Describing societal characteristics

matriarchy Family headed by mother

nuclear dyad Two-person family, e.g., husband and wife

reciprocal Mutual giving to each other

socialization Incorporation of social values and behaviors as one's own

values Important personal ideals

This chapter focuses on the various forms of family function that have evolved over the past 25 years reflecting the significant changes seen in American societal values. It also provides information about the birthing options available to a woman today and discusses how the nurse's role has changed in response to these choices.

Family Forms and Functions

Over the past several decades social changes have affected the structure and functions of the American family. Although a wide variety of family **configurations** exist in contemporary society, *family* can be defined as a group of kin united by blood, marriage, or adoption who (1) share a common residence for some part of their lives, (2) assume **reciprocal** rights and obligations with regard to one another, and (3) are the principal source of **socialization** of its members.[1] This definition encompasses both traditional and evolving family structures.

TABLE 1-1

Traditional Family Structures

Structure	Characteristics
Nuclear family	Husband, wife, and children live in a common household. One or both parents may be employed. Wife's career may be continuous or interrupted as the children are born.
Nuclear dyad	Husband and wife are alone. Couple may be childless or have no children living at home. Either or both may be employed; wife may enter labor force after children have left home.
Single-parent family	There is one head of household as a result of death, divorce, abandonment, or separation who often has preschool or school-age children. Head may or may not be employed; when financial aid is not received from absent spouse, parenting spouse usually pursues some form of occupation.
Three-generation family	This extended family may be formed by combinations of any of the above configurations.
Kin network	Nuclear households or unmarried members live in close geographic proximity and operate within a reciprocal system of exchange of goods and services.
Single adult	Man or woman, divorced or never married, lives alone.

Traditional Family Structures

Table 1-1 describes common characteristics of each of the acknowledged traditional configurations. Generally society has viewed traditional households (Fig. 1-1) with greater favor, considering them more stable and able to provide a legitimate anchorage for their children. Extended family forms can provide support and assistance during times of stress.

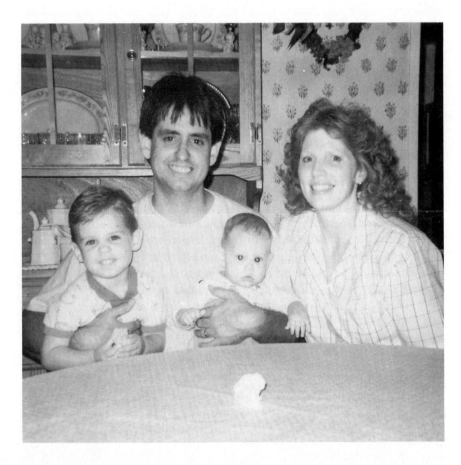

FIGURE 1-1

The Nuclear Family. Currently, career mobility often geographically separates nuclear families from their traditional support system, the extended family.

FIGURE 1-2
Male-Head, Single-Parent Family.
The male as head of a single-parent family represents 2.8% of all single-parent families.[2,3] Resources are available to assist single fathers in childrearing.[4] However, of those fathers who get custody of their children, more than 25% do not use any social network.[5]

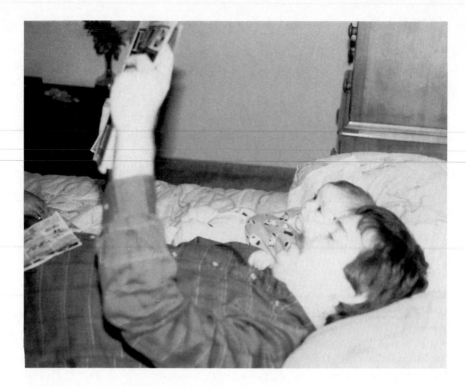

Evolving Family Structures

New family configurations that have evolved during the past quarter century reflect significant changes in American societal values (Fig. 1-2). Several interrelated factors have altered the role and status of women. They include (1) changes in the economy that affect women's participation in the labor force, (2) changes in the **demographic** structure of society resulting from the baby boom of the 1950s and the baby bust of the 1960s, (3) the feminist movement, (4) the development of effective contraceptive measures, and (5) legalization of abortion. Effective contraception and legalized abortion have allowed women greater control over their childbearing. Couples are marrying later, and families are having fewer children; contemporary women may elect to delay or avoid marriage, plan pregnancy, or opt not to have children at all. The majority of women with preschool children (51%) are employed outside the home, divorce rates have tripled, and there are more single-parent, **matriarchal** families.[6] Family roles and responsibilities have changed to accommodate the structural changes. Additional psychosocial stress also has been noted among nontraditional families. For example, **blended families** face problems if they fail to share a common family identity and form a single, cohesive unit.[7] Table 1-2 describes common characteristics of representative new family configurations.[3] The display on page 5 lists sociologic predictions for the American family of the 1990s.[2,8]

Functions of the Modern Family

The family has long been accepted as the basic unit of society. Aside from meeting basic needs for food, shelter, love, and security, families nurture the growth and development of each member, supporting and maintain-

TABLE 1-2

Evolving Family Structures

Structure	Characteristics
Blended family	A contemporary phenomenon, "yours, mine, and ours" families, formed when divorced parents remarry and bring children from previous marriages into the new relationship.[8]
Communal family	Household composed of more than one monogamous couple with children who share common facilities, resources and experiences; socialization of children is a group activity. Each member is a responsibility of the other members, and there is mutual concern for all aspects of the members' lives.
Unmarried parent with children	Often mother finds marriage is not feasible or desired. Children may be natural offspring or adopted.
Unmarried couple and child family	Social contract marriage: partners are committed to relationship without legal sanction. Couple shares common value system and emphasizes humanism and personal relationship. Father has prominent role in caretaking and socialization of the children. Both parents have intimate, continued, and sustained contact with their children. Common-law marriage: Children are either born to the partners or informally adopted. This structure is often found among poorer social strata in which members have experienced exceptional problems and constraints associated with legal marriage.[2]

ing the individual's morale and motivation. The World Health Organization has categorized the areas of family functions as (1) biologic, (2) economic, (3) educational, (4) psychologic, and (5) sociocultural.

Functions of the contemporary American family include generating affection, ensuring continuity of companionship, and providing personal security and acceptance. The family unit provides feelings of satisfaction and gives a sense of purpose. The functions of a family center around providing and ensuring safety and security for its members. For example, coping skills and problem solving mechanisms are taught and learned.

Initial socialization and social placement experiences occur within the family circle. For instance, birth order can indicate distinctive behavior expectation for each family member. Family interactions define status and role, rules, and behaviors. The family inculcates social controls and a sense of what is "right," i.e., socially acceptable behavior. The individual's later life-style and coping patterns often reflect the personal and cultural attitudes, values, and beliefs learned in and from the family.

The functioning of the family unit is not static. Roles may change and behavior expectations may alter. An example of change occurs when the family unit of two becomes a three-member family unit after the birth of a baby. Another example of role alteration occurs when the woman becomes the breadwinner and the man assumes the role of domesticity and of providing care for the other family members.

Predicted Changes in the Family of the 1990s

50% of first marriages will end in divorce.
60% of second marriages will end in divorce.
50% of children born in the 1980s will be living in single-parent homes.
25% of now-married mothers and fathers with children will be single-parenting.

Adapted from Skolnick A: The Intimate Environment: Explaining Marriage and the Family. Boston, Little, Brown, 1987, and Gelman D: The single parent's family albums. Newsweek, July 15, 1985.

TABLE 1-3

Developmental Tasks of the Childbearing Family

Stage of Family Life Cycle	Developmental Tasks
Beginning families	Forming a mutually satisfactory marital system
	Compromising individual priorities (financial expenditures, division of responsibilities, decision making, sexual relationship, communications)
	Realigning relationships (kin network, i.e., extended families, friends)
Childbearing families	Adjusting to pregnancy and impending/actual parenthood
	Assuming parenting role
	Adapting to alterations in life-style
	Reestablishing mutually satisfying relationships
	Realigning relationships with extended families to parenting/grandparenting roles

Adapted from Duvall E: Family Development. Philadelphia, JB Lippincott, 1977; Duvall E, Miller B: Marriage and Family Development. Philadelphia, JB Lippincott, 1985; and McGoldrick M, Carter E: The stages of family life cycle. In Henslin J (ed): Marriage and Family in a Changing Society. New York, The Free Press, 1985.

Developmental Tasks of the Childbearing Family

Developmental tasks arise from a family's need to adjust or modify previous patterns. Pregnancy and parenthood present major psychosocial challenges to the childbearing person or couple. Recognizing the need for alterations in self-concept, relationships, responsibilities, and life-style causes varying degrees of intrapersonal and interpersonal stress. Stress is increased when the family is required to consider a new developmental task, i.e., when pregnancy occurs while the couple has not yet reached a stable relationship and has not developed a shared concept of itself as a "family." Table 1-3 lists the developmental tasks of the childbearing family.[9-11]

Consumerism: Impact on Maternity Care
History of the Consumer Movement

The closing decades of the twentieth century have witnessed major changes in the American view of industry, social institutions, health, and health care. Consumers began ". . . to relearn the ability to take action on their own."[9] During the 1930s and 1940s consumers trusted physicians and hospitals implicitly, assuming a passive, "patient" role, and abdicated decision making to the professionals. By mid-century the attitudes of the health care consumer began to change. In the 1970s disillusion and dissatisfaction with the health care system provided impetus for self-care movements. Consumers began to take action to improve their own basic health status; emphasis shifted from medical remedies to illness prevention by incorporating nutrition, exercise, and a wellness–oriented life-style.[12,13] Further, an information explosion occurred; radio, television, newspapers, and magazines began to examine the strengths and flaws of the American health care system and to disseminate current medical knowledge in understandable terms. The assertive, more knowledgeable consumer emerged.[13]

The feminist movement emphasized the concept of women's rights to health care choices and control over their own bodies and experiences. Activists advocated natural methods of family planning, natural childbirth, alternative management of maternity health care, family participation in childbearing, shortened hospital stays, and birthing settings other than hospitals. The 1970s brought legalization of abortion.

Maternity clients were among the first to seek active participation in their health care. In the 1950s and 1960s the natural childbirth movement gained popularity as consumers found an alternative to standard obstetric practices. Viewing childbirth as a normal, health-oriented, and family-centered human event, clients began to reject the use of drugs in labor and delivery in isolation from their families.[12,13] They demanded the birth process be humanized and sought health care providers who taught and practiced the approaches developed by Dick-Read and Lamaze.

Childbearing women and their partners began to seek knowledge and demand a right to make choices in the conduct of their own pregnancies, labors, and deliveries. Women wanted to be awake and aware and to feel a central part of the birthing process. They sought to become equipped to cope with the stress of labor without heavy medication and to have their partners by their side to share the experience. Prenatal classes began to include education about the processes of labor and delivery; preparation for childbirth included instruction in techniques to reduce pain perception and enhance the sense of control over the process. Childbirth became a shared process with incorporation of the father as labor coach.

Maternity Client Expectations

Today's women expect to have a voice in the determination of their lives and well-being. Increasingly, they are demanding a larger role in determining the economic and social policies that affect their lives and the larger society in which they live.

More consumers are knowledgeable about their rights, potential options, and expected outcomes of health care. No longer passive dependents, many clients expect to take an active part in the management of their pregnancy-associated and childbirth experiences. Further, they expect health care providers to provide accurate and complete explanations of procedures, available options, and potential consequences of actions and decisions; they require informed consent and want to establish parameters for the type of care received. Clients also expect health care providers to honor their requests and decisions; high priority is placed on ambience and interpersonal relations during the pregnancy, delivery, and postpartum period. In essence, maternity clients expect competent, considerate, effective, and efficient care that meets their individual needs and desires.

New Directions and Dimensions

The concept of family-centered maternity care bagan to gain support in nursing circles during the 1960s. This approach recognized the pregnant woman as having social and emotional needs that deserved the nurse's attention and advocated consideration of other members of the family, particularly the father, during predelivery and postdelivery care. The concept of the "pregnant couple" began to evolve. Later this concept was expanded to the "pregnant family." The family unit, rather than the medical problem, became the focus for care. Nurses currently emphasize client teaching and plan care to meet the needs and desires of both participants in the childbearing experience.

Contemporary Options

Birthing Room

The first family-centered approach demanded by consumers was the birthing room. The traditional labor room was converted to a homelike environment.[14] Birthing beds were designed to look like home furniture but serve the purposes of the delivery table. Subdued lighting, pictures on the walls, rocking chairs, television, and carpeting were installed. The concept of the birthing room met with popularity, and its use continues in many geographic areas.

Mother-Baby Coupling

The first approach to achieving an early mother-infant relationship was postpartum "rooming-in." Mothers who elect this option have their babies in the room with them during hospitalization. A variation of this approach is "request coupling." Infants are transported from the nursery to the mother on request, and they remain together as long as desired. Mothers may request infants be observed in the nursery during the night or be returned to the mother for night feedings.

The increasing popularity of prepared childbirth, the birthing room, and rooming-in contributed to the development of contemporary LDRP (labor, deliver, recovery, postpartum) units. Mothers are admitted, labor, deliver, recover, and convalesce in the same hospital room. The infant remains with the mother from birth through discharge. The benefits of each mother-baby couple's having the same nurse responsible for their care include enhancement of family bonding and facilitation of development of the mother-infant relationship, immediate response to needs or problems, and elimination of the communication gap.

Early Discharge

The average length of hospital postpartum stay after vaginal birth is 2 to 3 days. In some areas healthy mothers whose prenatal, intrapartum, and immediate postpartum status meets specific health status criteria may be discharged within as few as 2 to 4 hours after delivery. These mothers and infants are seen in the physician's office 48 to 72 hours after discharge, or follow-up home visits to evaluate postpartum and neonatal status are made by nursing staff.[15-17]

Alternative Birthing Center

Two common themes in contemporary maternity care are an emphasis on client control and decision-making power and the desire for highly personalized health care. The alternative birthing center (ABC) is an outcome of these consumer demands. An ABC usually consists of one or more private birthing rooms in which a woman labors and gives birth.

The woman may be accompanied by her husband and, in some ABCs, by her children, other family members, and friends. Some ABCs may be only birthing rooms, and others may resemble motel-like hospital extensions. Mothers may have the option of remaining for postpartum care or having early discharge if they meet criteria. Usually nurse-midwife ABCs are separate from, but in close proximity to, hospitals to minimize time in transit should any complications arise unexpectedly. ABCs usually are available only to healthy women who have experienced uncomplicated pregnancies.

Home Birth

The desire for a more natural, family-centered approach to the child-bearing process and concern over increasing costs for hospital-based maternity care have resulted in increasing interest in alternative settings for childbirth.[11] Client mistrust of hospitals and negative feelings about the hospital environment are important factors in the decisions to give birth at home. Many women view labor as a vulnerable time and want their energies free to focus on this demanding process. They fear confrontations over the use of drugs for pain relief, stimulation of labor with oxytocins, and use of monitoring devices, amniotomies, forceps, or episiotomies. For a small but increasing number of women home birth is the alternative of choice.[12-14]

Concerns expressed by health professionals and consumers about home births center around the potential sudden complications that can occur during any normal birth. The lack of immediate access to needed medical or surgical assistance can be even more life threatening to mother, fetus, or both when complications arise outside of the medical setting. Criteria excluding clients from delivery in ABCs also should be applied to the selection of candidates for home birth.

Nursing Role in Family-Centered Care

Maternity nursing can be defined as the delivery of professional quality health care while recognizing, focusing on, and adapting to the physical and psychosocial needs of the childbearing woman, the family, and the newly born offspring. This definition views the family as a total unit within which each member is a distinct individual. The family-centered approach to care recognizes that childbearing is a unique human event that affects each member of the family; further, it recognizes that sharing the childbearing experience is both appropriate and beneficial to the family members.

Maternity nursing involves direct, personal care of the childbearing woman and her infant, as well as the related activities of teaching, counseling, and supervising throughout the various phases of the childbearing experience. A significant aspect of the nursing role in maternity care is that the clinical focus is primarily on the childbearing unit (mother, father, infant). Maternity nursing focuses on enabling childbearing families to achieve the highest possible level of physical, emotional, and social wellness. The nursing process provides the foundation for problem solving and effective, individualized, client-centered, goal-directed care. Figure 1-3 lists aspects of the multifaceted role of the contemporary maternity nurse.

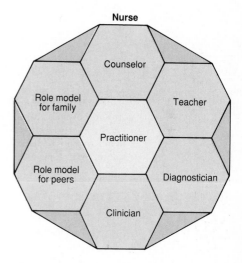

FIGURE 1-3

The Multifaceted Maternity Nursing Role. The dimensions of the contemporary maternity nursing role encompass assessing client health status and identifying client problems and needs (diagnostician), instituting therapeutic measures that protect or maximize client status (clinician), providing information needed for client decision making, e.g., referral or explanation of therapeutic regimen (counselor; teacher), and serving as a role model for both clients and peers.

Nursing care of the family unit involves purposeful, sustained interaction during which the nurse makes an assessment of the client's current status, problems, and resources and then takes action to relieve the problem, mobilizing and supporting family strengths. If the condition requires additional services from other members of the health team, clients are referred for consultation, service, or both.

REFERENCES

1. Eshelman J, Cashion B: Sociology: An Introduction. Boston, Little, Brown, 1985
2. Gelman D: The single parent's family albums. Newsweek, July 15, 1985
3. Greif G: Single fathers rearing children. J Marr Fam 47(1):185–191, February 1985
4. Riley D, Cochran M: Naturally occurring childrearing advice for fathers: Utilization of the personal social network. J Marr Fam 47(2):275–286, May 1985
5. Klinman D, Kohl D: Fatherhood U.S.A. New York, Garland, 1984
6. Cancellier P: The American family: Changes and challenges. Washington, DC, Population Reference Bureau, 1984
7. Alexander J, Kornfein M: Changes in family functioning amongst nonconventional families. Am J Orthopsychiatry 53(3):408–417, July 1983
8. Skolnick A: The Intimate Environment: Explaining Marriage and the Family. Boston, Little, Brown, 1987
9. Duvall E, Miller B: Marriage and Family Development. New York, Harper & Row, 1985
10. Duvall E: Family Development, ed 5. Philadelphia, JB Lippincott, 1977
11. McGoldrick M, Carter E: The stages of family life cycle. In Henslin J (ed). Marriage and Family in a Changing Society. New York, The Free Press, 1985
12. Naisbitt J: Megatrends. New York, Warner Books, 1984
13. Bierchen J: High tech, high touch nursing: Implications of megatrends for nursing education and practice in the '80s. Paper presented at the 72nd annual convention, Florida Nurses' Association, Orlando, Fla, September 1983
14. Birthing alternatives: A matter of choice and turf. Medical World News, May 18, 1984, pp 42–48
15. Norr K, Nacion K: Outcomes of postpartum early discharge, 1960–1986, a comparative review. Birth 14(3):135–141, September 1987
16. Jansson P: Early postpartum discharge. Am J Nurs 85(5):547–550, May 1985
17. Regan K: Early obstetrical discharge: A program that works. Can Nurse 80:32–35, October 1984

SUGGESTED READINGS

The development of family-centered maternity/newborn care in hospitals. A joint position statement prepared by the Interprofessional Task Force on Health Care of Women and Children. New York, The National Foundation/March of Dimes, June 1978

Romanzuk A: Helping the stepparent parent. Matern Child Nurs J 12:106, 1987

Standards for Obstetric, Gynecologic, and Neonatal Nursing, 2nd ed. Washington, DC, Nurses Association of the American College of Obstetricians & Gynecologists, 1986

Ethical and Legal Issues in Reproduction

IMPORTANT TERMINOLOGY

abortion Termination of pregnancy before fetal viability (22 weeks gestation)

accountability Held responsible for the effects of one's judgments and actions

artificial insemination Asexual reproduction technique whereby the husband's or donor's sperm is introduced directly into the woman's uterus by injection

bioethics Moral behaviors and dilemmas associated with the sanctity of human life

borrowed servant Legal term describing the hospital nurse as serving the physician under his or her direct order and supervision

breach of duty Occurs when the nurse performs an unauthorized act or carries out an authorized act improperly

defendant Person or institution charged with wrongdoing

in vitro fertilization Laboratory process that unites ovum and sperm and promotes embryo growth in a nutrient medium

liability Debt incurred through one's actions

litigation Legal actions taken to recover damages

malpractice Failure to provide care in compliance with established professional standards, resulting in harm

negligence Failure to perform legal duty, resulting in injury, loss, or damage

patient's rights Attitudes and services to which the health care consumer is entitled

plaintiff Person bringing suit, complaining of injury, loss, or damage

respondeat superior Legal term meaning "Let the master speak" or the employer is legally liable for the actions of the employee

standards of care Specific actions expected in the management of clinical practice; described in legal statutes and by professional organizations

surrogate mother Woman in whose body the product of artificial insemination is carried for gestation; infant is relinquished to adopting parents after delivery

tort Any wrongful act (intentional or unintentional) that results in injury, damage, or loss

Health care consumers are legally entitled to safe, competent medical and nursing care. In the eyes of the law poor judgment and careless or incompetent actions or both by health care providers endanger society by affecting life, health, or the ability to procreate. Health care errors can cause or contribute to the death or lifelong disability of clients, their unborn children, or both, resulting in the loss of present and future human resources. Society is stern regarding the loss of productive citizens and their potential contributions to its health, growth, and progress. This chapter discusses ethical and legal dimensions of contemporary maternity nursing, i.e., the climate for care, legal issues, and moral dilemmas that confront nurses providing care for childbearing clients. Emphasis is placed on the role and responsibilities of the nurse in protecting the clients' well-being and assuring safe, effective, client-centered, and goal-directed maternity care.

Legal Concepts and Historical Perspective

Before the mid-twentieth century, the public image of the physician as an almost-magical "healer" protected hospitals and nurses against lawsuits. Hospitals were perceived only as places in which the physician's treatments took place, and nurses were considered merely "handmaidens" who carried out the physician's orders. However, as health became identified as a fundamental civil right and consumers grew more knowledgeable about their rights as purchasers of health care, dissatisfied clients and their families sought legal satisfaction. Civil law was invoked, and penalties to health care providers for inappropriate and incompetent actions increased in frequency. Monetary compensation was awarded for injury, damage, or loss incurred while under medical supervision; legal penalties for jeopardizing client well-being included loss of license to practice and prison sentences for serious offenses.

Lawsuits involving physicians, hospitals, and other health care personnel have become commonplace. Increasingly, maternity care has been subjected to legal scrutiny. A substantial risk of litigation is associated with maternal-newborn health care. The ethical and legal dimensions of health care influence clinical practice profoundly and warrant serious consideration by physicians, nurses, and other health care providers.

Standards of Care

By mid-century, successful litigation had altered societal and legal perceptions of physician and hospital responsibility for client health and safety. Accrediting agencies such as the Joint Commission on Accreditation of Health Care Organizations (JCAHO) and medical specialty organizations such as the American College of Obstetricians and Gynecologists (ACOG) established written minimum **standards of care.** Hospitals and other health agencies also established standards of care, i.e., policies, procedures, and protocols that described acceptable, safe clinical practice in that agency. Together with state licensure regulations, such standards currently (1) describe responsible clinical practice, (2) provide recognized legal measures of the safety and quality of maternity care, and (3) govern hospitals and health provider practice.

The contemporary health care provider is required by law to exercise such reasonable care as the client's condition requires. The extent and

Facts That Must Be Established to Prove Guilt or Negligence

1. The defendant had a legal duty to protect the **plaintiff** from the injury, loss, or damage cited in the complaint.
2. That duty was not carried out, i.e., established standards of care were breached.
3. The plaintiff sustained injury, loss, or damage.
4. A causal relationship was found between the defendant's actions and the plaintiff's injury, loss, or damage, i.e., *proximate cause.*

type of care depend on the circumstances of the individual case. Civil **tort** law provides a legal avenue to compensation for **negligence** or harm or both. Medical or nursing negligence is termed *malpractice.* The display above lists the four conditions that must be present to demonstrate malpractice. In **litigation** care given is judged against accepted professional standards, and the caregiver is judged against his or her peers.

Commonly, expert testimony is used to establish negligence on the part of the **defendant.** The expertise of the witness must be established as equal to, or greater than, that of the defendant. When expert testimony identifies negligence in care or treatment, it becomes the responsibility of the jury (or court) to determine whether the injury, loss, or damage was caused by the defendant's actions or inactions. Judgment against health care providers who are found guilty of malpractice may include any or all of the following: loss of their license to practice, payment of financial penalties, or sentencing to prison.

Nursing Practice and Accountability

Nurse Practice Acts

The legal scope of nursing practice is legislated by each state. Nurse practice acts specify requirements for education, licensure, and standards of care for all levels of nursing. Since the boundaries of nursing practice vary among states, all nurses are held responsible for understanding, meeting, and maintaining his or her state's standards of practice.

Nursing Standards of Care

Standards of care also have been defined by the professional nursing organizations such as the American Nurses' Association (ANA) (see the material on p. 14) and the Organization for Obstetrical, Gynecologic and Neonatal Nurses (OOGN) (formerly the Nurses' Association of the American College of Obstetricians and Gynecologists). Nurses who provide care to maternity clients are expected to demonstrate the additional specialized knowledge and skills specified in the ANA and OOGN standards. Together with state licensure laws, these standards describe behaviors of the reasonably prudent nurse. Practicing nurses are held accountable under the law for demonstrating the application of current knowledge and skills in providing safe, responsible nursing care that is consistent with accepted standards and equal to that which, in a similar situation, would be demonstrated by the average nurse with the same education and experience.

Standards of Maternal and Child Health Nursing Practice

Standard I.   The nurse helps children and parents attain and maintain optimum health.

Standard II.   The nurse assists families to achieve and maintain a balance between the personal growth needs of individual family members and optimum family functioning.

Standard III.   The nurse intervenes with vulnerable clients and families at risk to prevent potential developmental and health problems.

Standard IV.   The nurse promotes an environment free of hazards to reproduction, growth and development, wellness, and recovery from illness.

Standard V.   The nurse detects changes in health status and deviations from optimum development.

Standard VI.   The nurse carries out appropriate interventions and treatment to facilitate survival and recovery from illness.

Standard VII.   The nurse assists clients and families to understand and cope with developmental and traumatic situations during illness, childbearing, childrearing, and childhood.

Standard VIII.   The nurse actively pursues strategies to enhance access to and utilization of adequate health care services.

Standard IX.   The nurse improves maternal and child health nursing practice through evaluation of practice, education, and research.

From American Nurses' Association: Standards of Maternal and Child Health Nursing Practice. Kansas City, Mo, The Association, 1983.

Status and Responsibilities

Increasing autonomy and independence in nursing has been accompanied by **accountability** to the client for nursing care and, to some degree, by responsibility for the client's well-being. The contemporary climate for nursing practice has been affected also by the changing (often expanding) legal concept of the nurse's role and responsibilities.

Respondeat Superior—"Let the Master Respond"

Until the recent expansion of professional credentials and roles, nurses have been viewed by the courts as subordinate employees of the physician or health agency or both, rather than as independent health practitioners. The physician or hospital, i.e., the employer, has been viewed as the "master" and held legally accountable for the actions of employees, e.g., nurses. However, the doctrine of **respondeat superior** does not release nurses from personal liability for tortious conduct (wrongful acts); legally, the employer may seek compensation from the nurse for any and all damages paid.[1]

Borrowed Servant

Early in the twentieth century hospitals also began to distinguish between the administrative and delegated medical functions of the nurse. While carrying out the orders of the physician, nurses were considered as acting as **"borrowed servants,"** and hospitals denied responsibility for torts arising from such actions. In a case during the 1950s, while acting under the orders of the physician, a delivery room nurse applied pressure to a client's chest, cracking her ribs. In the subsequent suit the obstetrician was found liable for the nurse's actions; the hospital was held blameless.[2] However, the borrowed servant variation of the doctrine of respondeat superior is applicable only in situations in which the nurse is acting under the direct supervision and control of the physician. Nurses remain liable for their own acts if injury, loss, or damage results.

Accountability extends beyond the nurse's individual sphere of care. If the nurse knows that the quality of care given by other members of the health team is inappropriate or inferior, he or she has a legal obligation to report such care to the appropriate authorities.[3] Nurses may be held negligent for failing to report deviations from established standards of client care management through appropriate channels. In a California case during the 1970s the concerns of maternity department nurses about an obstetrician's failure to practice in compliance with hospital rules and regulations resulted in an investigation and temporary loss of the physician's medical privileges.[4] The legal opinion identified the nurses' responsibility for protecting the client's well-being and found an absence of malice in the legal duty of nurses to report substandard or unsafe practice through appropriate clinical channels.

Legally nurses are held accountable for (1) performing within the scope of practice as defined by the state, professional organizations, and the employing agency and (2) providing and assuring safe, effective care that reflects the current established standards. In addition, they are responsible for reporting unsafe or inappropriate actions by other health professionals. Failure to meet the legal and professional criteria for safe, responsible practice constitutes a **breach of duty** (negligence). If the nurse is found guilty of breach of duty, license to practice may be suspended or revoked. Further, the nurse may become a defendant in a malpractice suit.

Avoiding Litigation and Liability

Nursing Documentation

The emphasis on professional accountability has resulted in an accompanying emphasis on clear, comprehensive documentation of nursing actions. Lawsuits may pend a number of years before reaching court. Written evidence of frequent nursing assessments of client status, administration of medications, treatments, nursing interventions, and client responses to care is not subject to the fallibility of human memory over time. The legal significance of accurate and complete charting is unquestioned.[5]

Continuing Education

As discussed previously, nurses are judged in comparison with their "reasonably prudent" peers. Nurses must maintain an adequate knowledge and skills base consistent with the current standards in their area of practice. Continuing education experiences provide one mechanism for maintaining competence to practice.[6] Thus nurses should seek opportunities to evaluate their own level of expertise and expand their knowledge of current advances in the area of practice through continuing education courses and in-service presentations and by reading current nursing literature, e.g., periodicals.

Assertiveness

Nurses need to become more assertive about the standard of care provided to their clients. As client (and nursing) advocates, they must address staff shortages, incompetent or unethical behavior, and the hazards to client safety that can result from inadequate or inappropriate staffing. If they are held accountable for their judgments and actions when required by hospital policy to "float," nurses should insist on an adequate orientation, supervision, and preparation for practice on other units.

Interpersonal Relations

The quality of the nurse–client relationship is an important factor in client satisfaction with nursing care. Awareness of and appropriate nursing management of the psychosocial needs of the client and family, e.g., prompt response to requests for information, effective nursing management of client needs, and considerate and courteous treatment of the client and family are important in reducing the threat of litigation to the nurse. Nurses who exhibit compassion and concern, as well as competence, are perceived favorably by clients and their families and seldom are involved in litigation.

Liability Insurance

Aside from being held legally **liable** for their own nursing judgments and actions, nurses also may be found negligent in a court of law for carrying out the orders of a physician or other health professional that their own education and experience identify as potentially jeopardizing their client. Further, they may be held liable for failing to report incompetent or unethical behavior promptly. The probability of legal judgments against the nurse is small when considered against the number of clients with whom the nurse interacts each day. However, the potential for litigation in maternal–newborn health care is growing; "shotgun lawsuits" involve all caregivers. Although rising, the cost of malpractice insurance for nurses in maternal–newborn care is small when considered against the cost of one settlement. Nurses who are covered by malpractice insurance are entitled to the services of an attorney who will represent their interests in any litigation. This option warrants careful consideration by those engaged in maternity nursing practice.

Moral Dilemmas in Maternity Nursing: Ethics and Bioethics

Nursing Ethics

Ethics may be defined as a philosophy of moral behavior.[7] One hallmark of a true profession is the development and public statement of a code of ethics, i.e., professional values, beliefs, and moral behaviors. All members of the profession are expected to share these beliefs and to demonstrate behaviors reflecting these values. The Nightingale Pledge, the International Council for Nurses (ICN) Pledge, and the ICN and ANA Codes for Nurses identify ethical nursing behaviors.

Early codes for nurses emphasized the nursing mandate to carry out the orders of the physician. As nursing grew and changed, later codes began to emphasize the nurse's obligation to the patient and the profession. The latest version of the ANA Code (1985) clearly identifies the nurse's ethical commitments to clients, the public, and the profession (see below).

Pledges and codes for nurses describe ethical professional behaviors and provide the foundation for nursing practice in maternity care. Additional ethical aspects of contemporary practice include ensuring informed consent and the client's right to self-determination and decision making. Curtin[8] has described nursing as "a moral art"; nursing knowledge and skills are directed toward safeguarding the holistic health and welfare of the human being. In maternity nursing practicing nurses often may be confronted with ethical dilemmas that arise from conflicts between their professional commitments and obligations to the physician, client, and profession and their personal values or religious beliefs.

Patient's Rights

The nurse's role as client advocate incorporates an ethical belief in the rights of the individual to safe, competent care, confidentiality, informed consent, and an active role in decision making. The concept of **patient's rights** was first discussed in a 1959 statement formulated by the National League for Nursing. More than a decade passed before those rights received major consideration by health care providers.[9] In 1973 the American Hospital Association (AHA) published that organization's official position entitled "A Patient's Bill of Rights." One purpose of the state-

---

American Nurses' Association Code of Ethics

1. The nurse provides services with respect for human dignity and the uniqueness of the client unrestricted by considerations of social or economic status, personal attributes, or the nature of health problems.
2. The nurse safeguards the client's right to privacy by judiciously protecting information of a confidential nature.
3. The nurse acts to safeguard the client and the public when health care and safety are affected by the incompetent, unethical, or illegal practice of any person.
4. The nurse assumes responsibility and accountability for individual nursing judgments and actions.
5. The nurse maintains competence in nursing.
6. The nurse exercises informed judgment and uses individual competence and qualifications as criteria in seeking consultation, accepting responsibilities, and delegating nursing activities to others.
7. The nurse participates in activities that contribute to the ongoing development of the profession's body of knowledge.
8. The nurse participates in the profession's efforts to implement and improve standards of nursing.
9. The nurse participates in the profession's efforts to establish and maintain conditions of employment conducive to high quality nursing care.
10. The nurse participates in the profession's effort to protect the public from misinformation and misrepresentation and to maintain the integrity of nursing.
11. The nurse collaborates with members of the health professions and other citizens in promoting community and national efforts to meet the health needs of the public.

From American Nurses' Association: Code for nurses with interpretative statements. Kansas City, Mo, The Association, 1985.

ment was to identify the ethical commitment to ensure the patient's right to safe, competent, considerate care and confidentiality. The document also placed additional emphasis on the patient's right to all relevant information in advance of decision making, i.e., informed consent.

In 1975 the International Childbirth Education Association (ICEA) elaborated on the AHA position in "The Pregnant Patient's Bill of Rights" (below). Inasmuch as decisions during pregnancy affect two patients rather than one, this document specifies that the pregnant woman has the right to all information regarding decisions that affect her own health, that of her unborn child, or both of them. Included also is her right to participate in decision making in all but the most serious medical emergencies.

Although these documents describe ethical behavior, they may also represent the client's legal rights. Maternity nurses acknowledge an ethical commitment to ensuring and protecting the rights of the childbearing client and fetus or newborn.

The Pregnant Patient's Bill of Rights

American parents are becoming increasingly aware that health professionals do not always have scientific data to support common American obstetrical practices and that many of these practices are carried out primarily because they are part of medical and hospital tradition. In the last 40 years many artificial practices have been introduced which have changed childbirth from a physiological event to a very complicated medical procedure in which all kinds of drugs are used and procedures carried out, sometimes unnecessarily, and many of them potentially damaging for the baby and even for the mother. A growing body of research makes it alarmingly clear that every aspect of traditional American hospital care during labor and delivery must now be questioned as to its possible effect on the future well-being of both the obstetric patient and her unborn child.

One in every 35 children born in the United States today will eventually be diagnosed as retarded; one in every 10 to 17 children has been found to have some form of brain dysfunction or learning disability requiring special treatment. Such statistics are not confined to the lower socioeconomic group but cut across all segments of American society.

New concerns are being raised by childbearing women because no one knows what degree of oxygen depletion, head compression, or traction by forceps the unborn or newborn infant can tolerate before that child sustains permanent brain damage or dysfunction. The recent findings regarding the cancer-related drug diethylstilbestrol have alerted the public to the fact that neither the approval of a drug by the U.S. Food and Drug Administration nor the fact that a drug is prescribed by a physician serves as a guarantee that a drug or medication is safe for the mother or her unborn child. In fact, the American Academy of Pediatrics Committee on Drugs has recently stated that there is no drug, whether prescription or over-the-counter remedy, which has been proven safe for the unborn child.

The Pregnant Patient has the right to participate in decisions involving her well-being and that of her unborn child, unless there is a clear-cut medical emergency that prevents her participation. In addition to the rights set forth in the American Hospital Association's "Patient's Bill of Rights" (which has also been adopted by the New York City Department of Health) the Pregnant Patient, because she represents TWO patients rather than one, should be recognized as having the additional rights listed below.

From International Childbirth Education Association's Committee on Patient's Rights. New York, The Association, 1975.

The Pregnant Patient's Bill of Rights—*continued*

1. *The Pregnant Patient has the right,* prior to the administration of any drug or procedure, to be informed by the health professional caring for her of any potential direct or indirect effects, risks or hazards to herself or her unborn or newborn infant which may result from the use of a drug or procedure prescribed for or administered to her during pregnancy, labor, birth, or lactation.

2. *The Pregnant Patient has the right,* prior to the proposed therapy, to be informed, not only of the benefits, risks, and hazards of the proposed therapy but also of known alternative therapy, such as available childbirth education classes which could help to prepare the Pregnant Patient physically and mentally to cope with the discomfort or stress of pregnancy and the experience of childbirth, thereby reducing or eliminating her need for drugs and obstetric intervention. She should be offered such information early in her pregnancy in order that she may make a reasoned decision.

3. *The Pregnant Patient has the right,* prior to the administration of any drug, to be informed by the health professional who is prescribing or administering the drug to her that any drug which she receives during pregnancy, labor and birth, no matter how or when the drug is taken or administered, may adversely affect her unborn baby, directly or indirectly, and that there is no drug or chemical which has been proven safe for the unborn child.

4. *The Pregnant Patient has the right,* if cesarean section is anticipated, to be informed prior to the administration of any drug, and preferably prior to the hospitalization, that minimizing her and, in turn, her baby's intake of nonessential preoperative medicine will benefit her baby.

5. *The Pregnant Patient has the right,* prior to the administration of a drug or procedure, to be informed if there is NO properly controlled follow-up research which has established the safety of the drug or procedure with regard to its direct and/or indirect effects on the physiological, mental and neurological development of the child exposed, via the mother, to the drug or procedure during pregnancy, labor, birth, or lactation (this would apply to virtually all drugs and the vast majority of obstetric procedures).

6. *The Pregnant Patient has the right,* prior to the administration of any drug, to be informed of the brand name and generic name of the drug in order that she may advise the health professional of any past adverse reaction to the drug.

7. *The Pregnant Patient has the right* to determine for herself, without pressure from her attendant, whether she will accept the risks inherent in the proposed therapy or refuse a drug or procedure.

8. *The Pregnant Patient has the right* to know the name and qualifications of the individual administering a medication or procedure to her during labor or birth.

9. *The Pregnant Patient has the right* to be informed, prior to the administration of any procedure, whether that procedure is being administered to her for her or her baby's benefit (medically indicated) or as an elective procedure (for convenience or teaching purposes).

10. *The Pregnant Patient has the right* to be accompanied during the stress of labor and birth by someone she cares for, and to whom she looks for emotional comfort and encouragement.

11. *The Pregnant Patient has the right* after appropriate medical consultation to choose a position for labor and for birth which is least stressful to her baby and to herself.

12. *The Obstetric Patient has the right* to have her baby cared for at her bedside if her baby is normal, and to feed her baby according to her baby's needs rather than according to the hospital regimen.

13. *The Obstetric Patient has the right* to be informed in writing of the name of the person who actually delivered her baby and the professional qualifications of that person. This information should also be on the birth certificate.

Continued

The Pregnant Patient's Bill of Rights—*continued*

14. *The Obstetric Patient has the right* to be informed if there is any known or indicated aspect of her or her baby's care or condition which may cause her or her baby later difficulty or problems.
15. *The Obstetric Patient has the right* to have her and her baby's hospital medical records complete, accurate, and legible and to have their records, including Nurses' Notes, retained by the hospital until the child reaches at least the age of majority, or, alternatively, to have the records offered to her before they are destroyed.
16. *The Obstetric Patient,* both during and after her hospital stay, *has the right* to have access to her completed hospital medical records, including Nurses' Notes, and to receive a copy upon payment of a reasonable fee and without incurring the expense of retaining an attorney.

It is the obstetric patient and her baby, not the health professional, who must sustain any trauma or injury resulting from the use of a drug or obstetric procedure. The observation of the rights listed above will not only permit the obstetric patient to participate in the decisions involving her and her baby's health care, but will help to protect the health professional and the hospital against litigation arising from resentment or misunderstanding on the part of the mother.

Bioethics

Bioethics is a modern term that refers to ethical conflicts and moral dilemmas about the sanctity of human life that result from biomedical research and technologic advances, e.g., the medical ability to terminate or preserve and extend life by artificial means vs. the ultimate quality of the life preserved.[8,9] Major bioethical issues that confront the professional nurse in maternal-newborn care include those related to eugenics and euthanasia.

Eugenics is defined as improvement of a race by selective control of human reproduction. *Positive eugenics* refers to selection in favor of genetic characteristics and traits perceived as having significant social value. *Negative eugenics* refers to minimizing or preventing procreation by those who carry genetic traits that have been perceived harmful or undesirable.[10] The discovery of successful methods of controlling conception, terminating undesired pregnancy, and sustaining life after birth has increased the complexity of decision making in reproductive health.

Eugenics-related issues in reproductive health include (1) assisted reproduction, i.e., **artificial insemination, in vitro fertilization,** embryo transplant, and **surrogate motherhood,** (2) sterilization, (3) amniocentesis to identify fetal genetic disorders in utero, and (4) **abortion.** See Legal and Ethical Considerations: Eugenics.

Preconceptual Ethical and Legal Considerations

Assisted Reproduction

An estimated 25% of couples are unable to achieve a pregnancy. Advances in biomedical technology enable many of these infertile couples to achieve a pregnancy through medically assisted reproduction techniques.[11] Methods include artificial insemination, in vitro fertilization, and embryo trans-

---

≡ LEGAL AND ETHICAL
≡ CONSIDERATIONS

Eugenics

1. Is it morally "right" to determine the human genetic pool by other than natural selection?
2. Who makes the decisions?
3. On what basis are decisions made?
4. What is the projected impact of the decision on the individual's quality of life? On the family? On society?
5. What are the emotional and economic consequences of the decision to the family? To society?

plant. Although limited success in assisted reproduction has occurred for decades, a storm of ethical and legal controversy has arisen in recent years. Supporters defend assisted reproduction techniques as life affirming; detractors denounce reproduction without sexual intercourse as unnatural.[12]

Concerns also have been expressed that assisted-reproduction techniques might be extended to include unmarried persons, e.g., surrogate mothers and third-party donors, and that in vitro fertilization might be used in eugenics research.[13-15] The recommendations of the national Ethics Advisory Board are listed below.

METHODS. The three techniques for medically assisted reproduction are described below.

Artificial insemination. **Homologous insemination (AIH)** is accomplished by injection of the husband's semen into the vagina, cervical os, or directly into the uterus. This method may be used to accomplish pregnancy when the prospective mother's cervical mucus is hostile to the husband's sperm. **Heterologous insemination (AID)** is accomplished by similar injection of donor semen and may be used in cases in which the husband is sterile or is a carrier of genetic disorder.[16] See Legal and Ethical Considerations: Donor-Assisted Reproduction.

In vitro fertilization. This type of fertilization is accomplished by inoculating nutrient media with ova extracted from the potential mother and sperm from the potential father; donor sperm may be used similarly. The "test tube baby," i.e., the fertilized egg/zygote, is incubated to the blastocyst stage, then placed in the uterus and attached to the uterine wall. In vitro fertilization with the husband's sperm can be used in cases in which the inability to conceive is related to the wife's nonpatent fal-

LEGAL AND ETHICAL CONSIDERATIONS

Donor-Assisted Reproduction

1. If either the woman or the donor is married, is this an act of adultery?
2. Is the child illegitimate?
3. What are the rights and obligations of the donor?
4. What are the rights of children so conceived to know the identity of the donor?
5. What are the children's rights to the donor's estate? What are their rights to the estate of the mother's spouse?
6. Should unmarried women be eligible to achieve pregnancy by this method?
7. What is the potential for accidental conception between close relatives in this pregnancy? In later conception by the child?
8. Should genetic screening be done on both the donor and potential mother?
9. What are the implications of the birth of a child with a congenital disorder?

Recommendations of the Ethics Advisory Board

1. The department should consider support of carefully designed research involving in vitro fertilization and embryo transfer in animals, including nonhuman primates, to obtain a better understanding of the process of fertilization, implantation, and embryo development, to assess the risks to both mother and offspring associated with such procedures, and to improve the efficacy of the procedure.
2. Research involving human in vitro fertilization and embryo transfer is ethically acceptable provided that if the research involves human in vitro fertilization without embryo transfer, these conditions must be satisfied:
   - The research complies with regulations governing research with human subjects.
   - The research is designed to establish the safety and efficacy of embryo transfer and to obtain important scientific information not reasonably attainable by other means.
   - Informed consent is obtained.
   - No embryos will be sustained in vitro beyond the stage normally associated with the completion of implantation (14 days after fertilization).
   - The public is advised of possible risk.
   In addition, if the research involves embryo transfer following human in vitro fertilization, embryo transfer will be attempted only with gametes obtained from lawfully married couples.

Adapted from Abramowitz S: The stalemate on (testtube) baby research. I. Test-tube. Hastings Cent Rep 14:7, February 1984.

LEGAL AND ETHICAL CONSIDERATIONS

Frozen Embryos

1. Who owns the embryo? The parents? The physician who performed the successful fertilization? The institution in which the assisted reproduction occurred? The State?
2. Who decides the fate, e.g., destruction, adoption by implantation, of the embryo?
3. What are the fetus'/infant's legal rights to State protection?
4. What are the fetus'/infant's/child's rights to inheritance?

lopian tubes; donor sperm can be used when the husband is sterile or carries a genetic defect. Modern technological advances permit embryos resulting from in vitro fertilization to be frozen for later implantation. See Legal and Ethical Considerations: Frozen Embryos.

In vivo fertilization. Embryo transplant is a recently developed technique in which the successful product of technologically assisted reproduction is surgically transplanted into the uterus of a woman who is unable to conceive. The infertile woman then carries the pregnancy through gestation to birth.

ETHICAL AND LEGAL ISSUES. Ethical and legal issues associated with the use of assisted-reproduction techniques focus primarily on the use of donor semen. Legal implications are presumed satisfied by written informed consent by all parties—wife, husband, and donor. Recommendations are that all parties remain anonymous and that the physician be given the right to select the donor. The consent usually includes a clause removing liability from the health professionals in the event the child is born with abnormalities. Any question of the child's legitimacy may be resolved by adoption.[12]

Surrogate mothers. The use of technologically assisted reproduction techniques with surrogate mothers has become very controversial. In such cases the surrogate donates an ovum and agrees to carry the pregnancy until birth and to relinquish the child to the biologic father and his spouse. Ethicolegal questions surround the payment of fees to the surrogate mother (equating with selling the child), the adopting parents' relationship with the surrogate, and the rights of the surrogate mother. Concern has been expressed about the potential problems in cases in which the child is born with impairments and is unwanted by either the adopting parents or the surrogate mother.[14] Gersz[15] argues that a well-drawn contract may avoid some of the difficulties of the three-way relationship. However, the 1987 Baby M case identified legal problems that can arise if the surrogate mother refuses to honor the agreement and takes legal action to keep the infant; in that case the court established a legal precedent by ruling against the surrogate mother.

Sterilization

Usually sterilization is an elective procedure initiated by the client. The most common procedure for women is tubal ligation; for men vasectomy is the method of choice. Inasmuch as these procedures are not consistently reversible at present, the decision to end fertility should involve both partners; ethical emphasis is placed on informed consent.

Legal and ethical issues associated with ending fertility prematurely include involuntary sterilization for eugenic reasons. Involuntary sterilization is compulsory in some states for inmates of state mental institutions, and legal guardians of severely mentally retarded persons have initiated such surgical intervention.[16] An additional ethical issue concerns sterilization as a method of birth control.

Postconceptual Ethical and Legal Considerations

Amniocentesis

With high frequency sound waves (ultrasonography), used to identify the location of the fetus and placenta, a sterile needle is inserted through the abdominal and uterine walls into the amniotic cavity. A small quantity of amniotic fluid is withdrawn, and the sample of exfoliated fetal cells is used for chromosome studies and genetic diagnosis. More than 40 genetically transmitted disorders can be identified while the fetus is yet in utero. Among these disorders are Down's syndrome and Tay-Sachs disease. Fetal sex can also be determined, allowing estimation of the risks of bearing a child with a familiar, sex-linked disorder. Most commonly amniocentesis is performed at or near the 16th gestational week. Findings enable the client to consider terminating the pregnancy before viability (22 weeks gestation). A relatively new procedure, chorionic villi sampling, may enable diagnosis of some congenital disorders at 8 to 10 weeks gestation and permit first trimester abortion.

Legal and ethical considerations demand that mothers at high risk for fetal disorders that can be identified by amniocentesis or chorionic villi sampling be informed that these diagnostic procedures are available. Risks and benefits of the procedure must be given the mother in the form of a written consent. Questions have been raised about possible physician liability in situations in which the client has been told the infant will be normal but it subsequently is defective.

Voluntary Abortion

In this context *abortion* is defined as the voluntary act of terminating pregnancy before viability. The ethical and legal aspects of this act have generated serious controversy in contemporary society. Issues include the mutually exclusive rights of the pregnant woman to terminate pregnancy and the right of the fetus to life. The gestational age at which the fetus is considered a person whose civil rights are violated by abortion has been a major point of contention. At issue also is parental notification in the case of pregnant minors. A related issue is whether abortion is an appropriate method of birth control.[16]

Pro-life advocates believe the fetus is human from the time of conception and that to destroy human life is murder and, hence, indefensible morally. Pro-choice advocates are not pro-abortion; they take the position that the mother has the ultimate responsibility and freedom of choice regarding her body. They uphold responsible use of contraception, amniocentesis to identify fetal defects, and adoption whenever possible, with abortion used only as a last resort.

The 1973 Supreme Court decision in *Roe v. Wade* was a landmark case in reproductive health litigation.[17] The court ruled that state laws prohibiting abortion were unconstitutional on the grounds of invasion of the woman's privacy. In addition, the court ruled that the fetus is ineligible for protection under the Fourteenth Amendment and that a pregnant woman has the exclusive right to decide to terminate pregnancy; neither her spouse nor the father of the fetus has a right to contest her decision. *Viability* was defined as the gestational point at which the fetus can survive extrauterine transition, i.e., 22 to 23 weeks after conception.

As a result of the *Roe v. Wade* decision, abortion has become legal throughout the United States. First trimester abortions are not subject to individual states' regulations; however, midtrimester abortions are subject to state regulation to protect the woman's health. States may regulate or prohibit or both last trimester abortions; in addition, states may impose protection for the fetus. Although parental notification about abortion services for pregnant adolescents can be required by the states, it can also be waived by a state court or administrative agency if the minor is judged mature enough to give informed consent.[18]

Legalization of abortion in 1973 did not end what has been termed a "holy war."[19] Both pro-life and pro-choice supporters have continued to exert political influence on legislators to gain their objectives. The Hyde Amendment of 1978 (see below) restricted use of federal funds for abortion; pro-choice supporters believe this restriction effectively discriminates against poor women since they tend to be dependent on general assistance for health care.[20] Pro-life supporters have encouraged enactment of state statutes that discourage easy access to legal abortion.[21]

Although a 1989 Supreme Court ruling *(Webster v. Reproductive Health Services)* did not overturn the previous decision, it did uphold the rights of individual states to impose legal restrictions on abortion to "further the State's interest in protecting potential human life." Important aspects of the 1989 ruling include the following: (1) although the Roe decision declared the fetus nonviable until the third trimester (after 24 weeks) and allowed states to prohibit or regulate abortion from that point in gestation, the court in the Webster case allowed that the state's interest in protecting potential citizens should not be limited by viability; (2) the court also found that Missouri law "creates . . . a presumption of viability at 20 weeks . . . " and upheld the Missouri statute requiring that a physician must rebut fetal viability with laboratory tests before performing an abortion. The court's ruling and comments by several justices generated strong speculation that the Roe decision would be altered or overturned during one of the cases scheduled for hearing in the court's next session. Observers also predict that the abortion issue will become a "political football" as pro-choice and pro-life supporters exert increased pressures on legislatures to expand, modify, or reverse current state statutes governing termination of pregnancy.[22,23]

IMPLICATIONS FOR PRACTICE. Most state laws contain "conscience clauses" that enable health professionals, i.e., nurses and physicians, to refuse to participate in or assist with abortions if such actions violate their individual ethical, moral, or religious principles. However, health professionals must recognize that, for some clients, abortion may represent a

---

1978 Hyde Amendment Stipulations for Use of Medicaid Funds for Abortion

The pregnancy is due to rape or incest and was reported promptly to a public-health agency or to the police.

The woman's life will be endangered by carrying the fetus to term (emotional well-being is not considered just cause).

Two or more physicians determine that the pregnancy will cause severe and long-term *physical* damage to the woman.

viable alternative to unwanted pregnancy. Further, the commitment to informed client consent may be construed legally as mandating referral to others who are able to meet the client's needs for information, counseling, or intervention.

Ethical and Legal Considerations for the Fetus and Sick Neonate

Rights of the Fetus

The fetus has rights from time of conception. He or she can be the beneficiary of a trust and inherit property. Although the fetus is not legally considered a person until born, the fetus' rights have been upheld in the courts. Ethical and legal controversies center around abortion and euthanasia (see Legal and Ethical Considerations: Fetal Rights). Recently a legal question has been raised about the legal liability of the substance-abusing mother for the consequences to the fetus; court rulings have convicted the mother of child abuse and forced pregnant mothers to enter rehabilitation programs during pregnancy.[24]

Fetal therapy has been another area of concern. Modern biomedical and surgical techniques make it possible to intervene surgically and treat some fetuses that previously would have died in utero or after birth. See Legal and Ethical Considerations: Treating the Fetus.

Euthanasia

Many define euthanasia as effecting a painless end to human life, i.e., "mercy killing." *Passive euthanasia* is failing to intervene to sustain life, e.g., acts of withholding life-supporting treatments from the newborn who is genetically or physiologically compromised to allow death as soon as possible. *Active euthanasia* is taking direct action to end the life of another, i.e., murder.[25]

Rights of the Newborn

As infant mortality rates continue to decline, approximately 250,000 babies are born with significant congenital defects or birth-associated injuries.[26] Modern biomedical technology enables health professionals to sustain or save the lives of many of these infants. See Legal and Ethical Considerations: Quality of Life.

Baby Doe Regulations

The controversy over the rights of handicapped newborns began in March 1983. Following a report that a newborn with Down's syndrome had died as the result of an uncorrected esophageal atresia, the Secretary of the Department of Health and Human Services (DHHS) issued the first Baby Doe regulation. The main thrust of the regulation was a threat to remove federal funding from hospitals that failed to comply with a notice that failure to feed or care for handicapped infants was against federal law; the intimation was that such actions could be considered child abuse.

Believing that the judiciary was interfering with decision making that rightfully was shared between the health professionals and the parents,

LEGAL AND ETHICAL CONSIDERATIONS

Fetal Rights

1. Does a mother who plans an abortion have the right to allow experimentation on the fetus in utero?
2. Can an aborted fetus be kept alive for experimental purposes?[12]
3. What are the rights of the fetus in terms of damages sustained in utero as the results of maternal substance abuse?

LEGAL AND ETHICAL CONSIDERATIONS

Treating the Fetus

1. What if the physician believes the fetus should be treated but the mother refuses consent?
2. Can the mother be charged with fetal abuse?
3. If the court orders the mother to permit fetal treatment, does this ruling invade her maternal rights to privacy and control over her own body?
4. Is the risk/benefit ratio of this therapy sufficiently favorable to justify the large financial expenditure if it is paid with public funds?

LEGAL AND ETHICAL CONSIDERATIONS

Quality of Life

1. How much should a person have to suffer for the sake of life?
2. What is the impact of the decision to sustain life on the family?
3. How much should society pay to support those individuals for whom the only prognosis is a lifelong need for continued expenditure of public funds without potential for their contribution to self or society?

the American Academy of Pediatrics sought an injunction against the regulation.[26] The injunction was denied. In September 1983 the regulation was reissued with little change. One change was that hotline notices for reporting "abuse" were posted only in nurse's stations. Murphy[27] found this attitude implied that nurses are not intelligent, participating members of the health team and intimated that they would not report abuse because of fear of reprisal.

One month after the regulation was reissued, a baby was born in New York state with multiple, severe, neural tube defects. After consulting with physicians and their own Roman Catholic priest, the parents chose conservative medical treatment to reduce the chance of infection rather than surgery to correct the defects. A lawyer in another state, unrelated to any of the participants, got a court order appointing a guardian for the infant. The guardian had a legal right to authorize the surgery (thus depriving the parents of their parental authority). The New York State Appeals Court eventually struck down the ruling, commenting on the often "offensive activities of those who sought to displace parental responsibility for management of medical care."[28]

Subsequent DHHS regulations were issued in 1984 (Nondiscrimination on the Basis of Handicap—required the rights of the fetus to be posted) and in 1985 (Child Abuse Prevention and Treatment Act, 1985). As shown below, the child abuse act explicitly defines medical neglect and permis-

---

Further Regulations Resulting From the Child Abuse Amendments of 1985 to Public Law 98—The Child Abuse Prevention and Treatment Act

Medical neglect: withholding of medically indicated treatment from a disabled infant with a life-threatening condition

Definition of "withholding medically indicated treatment":

> ". . . the failure to respond to the infant's life-threatening conditions by providing treatment (including appropriate nutrition, hydration, and medication) which, in the treating physician's (or physicians') reasonable medical judgment, will be most likely to be effective in ameliorating or correcting all such conditions."

Withholding medical treatment is not "medical neglect" under these conditions:

1. The infant is chronically and irreversibly comatose;

2. The provision of such treatment would merely prolong dying, not be effective in ameliorating or correcting all of the infant's life-threatening conditions, or otherwise be futile in terms of the survival of the infant; or

3. The provision of such treatment would be virtually futile in terms of the survival of the infant and the treatment itself under such circumstances would be inhumane.

Definition of "reasonable medical judgment": "medical judgment that would be made by a reasonably prudent physician knowledgeable about the case and the treatment possibilities with respect to the medical condition involved."

Adapted from Murray TH: The final anticlimactic rule on Baby Doe. Hastings Cent Rep 15(3):5-7, June 1985.

sible exceptions to the rule. Murray[29] calls the regulation anticlimactic and believes it will have a minimum impact on medical and ethical decision making; the contemporary trend is toward aggressive treatment of non-lethal conditions and a narrowing of parental and physician discretion on treatment decisions.

Yearly several cases are reported that illustrate the bioethical and legal conflicts between the sanctity and the quality of life, e.g., the body functions of a pregnant woman with profound and irreversible brain damage incompatible with life are maintained mechanically to increase fetal chances of survival; an abortion is sought by a husband to increase his comatose pregnant wife's chance of survival and recovery. Strangers then bring suit to block these actions, and the life-or-death decisions are made by other than the family or physician.

The contemporary biomedical ability to choose who will be born, live, or die has generated continuing, serious, ethical debate in contemporary society. Nurses considering positions in reproductive health settings should identify their own feelings and values about bioethical issues. They should anticipate the eventuality of serving as advocates or providing care for clients who must consider or have chosen for them options that conflict with the nurse's own personal beliefs.[30,31] In providing client care nurses must often separate personal from professional values.[32] Confronting, examining, and resolving ethical conflicts between personal and professional values enables nurses to ensure the rights of all clients to safe, competent, and considerate care.

REFERENCES

1. Chaska N: The Nursing Profession: A Time to Speak. New York, McGraw-Hill, 1983, p 55
2. Trandel-Korenchuk D: Borrowed Servant and Captain-of-the-Ship Doctrines. Nurse Pract: 7(2):33-34, February 1982
3. *Darling v. Charleston Community Hospital.* In Kelly L: The Nursing Experience, Trends, Challenges, and Transitions. New York, Macmillan, 1987
4. *Applebaum M.D. v. Board of Directors of Barton Memorial Hospital.* In The Regan Report on Nursing Law, Vol 21, No 6. November 1980
5. Kelly L: The Nursing Experience, Trends, Challenges and Transitions. New York, Macmillan, 1987
6. Kristjanson L, Scanlan J: Assessment of continuing nursing education needs: A literature review. J Contin Educ Nurs 20(3):118-123, May/June 1989
7. Mappes T, Zembaty JS: Biomedical Ethics, 2nd ed. New York, McGraw-Hill, 1986
8. Curtin L: Ethical Issues in Nursing Practice and Education in Ethical Issues in Nursing and Nursing Education. New York, National League for Nursing, 1980, pp 19-28
9. Ellis J, Hartley C: Nursing in Today's World, Challenges, Issues, and Trends, 3rd ed. Philadelphia, JB Lippincott, 1989
10. Lewis M, Warden C: Law and Ethics in the Medical Office Including Bioethical Issues. Philadelphia, FA Davis, 1983, p 142
11. Physicians' Update, Obstetrics/Gynecology. Society for Assisted Reproduction Technology, October 1, 1989
12. Annas G: Redefining parenthood and protecting embryos: Why we need new laws. Hastings Cent Rep 14(5):50-52, October 1984
13. Abramowitz S: A stalemate on test-tube baby research. Hastings Cent Rep 14(1):5-9, February 1984
14. Furrow B: Surrogate motherhood: A new option for parenting? Law Med Health Care 12(3):106, 1984
15. Gersz G: The contract in surrogate motherhood: A review of the issues. Law Med Health Care 12(3):107-113, 1984
16. Lewis M, Warden C: Law and Ethics in the Medical Office Including Bioethical Issues. Philadelphia, FA Davis, 1983, pp 158, 172-173
17. *Jane Roe et al. v. Henry Wade.* Supreme Court of the United States, Opinion No 70-40, January 1973
18. Hatcher R et al: Contraceptive Technology 1986-1987, 15th ed. New York, Irvington Publishers, 1989, p 264
19. Donovan P: The holy war. Fam Plann Perspect 17(1):5-9, January/February 1985
20. Annas G: *Roe v. Wade* reaffirmed. Hastings Cent Rep 13(4):21-23, 1983
21. APHA high court brief to oppose rules restricting abortions. Nation's Health 8:1-8, August 1985
22. The battle over abortion. Time, pp 62-63, July 17, 1989
23. New limits on abortion rights are upheld by 5-4 majority. Social Policy, pp 1698-1700, July 8, 1989
24. St. Petersburg Times, August 23, 1989

25. Lewis M, Warden C: Law and Ethics in the Medical Office Including Bioethical Issues. Philadelphia, FA Davis, 1983, p 184
26. Lyon J: New treatments, new choices. Nurs Life 4(2):48–52, 1984
27. Murphy C: The changing role of the nurse in making ethical decisions. Law Med Health Care 12(4):173–175, 184, September 1984
28. Fleishman A, Murray T: Ethics committees for Infant Doe? Hastings Cent Rep 13(6):5–9, 1984
29. Murray T: The first anticlimactic rule on Baby Doe. Hastings Cent Rep 15(3):5–7, June 1985

30. Bushy A, et al: Ethical principles: Application to an obstetric case. JOGN Nurs 18(3):207–212, May/June 1988
31. McClosky J, Grace J (eds): Current Issues in Nursing. Boston, Blackwell Scientific Publications, 1985
32. Cushing M: Euthanasia: A legal perspective. In McClosky J, Grace H (eds): Current Issues in Nursing. Boston, Blackwell Scientific Publications, 1985, pp 1044–1071

SUGGESTED READINGS

Chervenak F, et al: When is termination of pregnancy during the third trimester morally justifiable? N Engl J Med 310(8):501–503, February 23, 1984

Drane J: The defective child: Ethical guidelines for painful dilemmas. JOGN Nurs 13(1):42–48, January/February 1984

Infants' Bioethics Task Force and Consultants: Guidelines for infants bioethics committees. Pediatrics 72(2):306–310, August 1984

Yarling R, McElmurry BJ: Moral foundation of nursing. Adv Nurs Sci 8(2):63–73, 1986

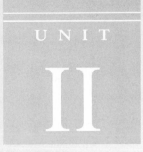

UNIT II

The Family and Reproduction

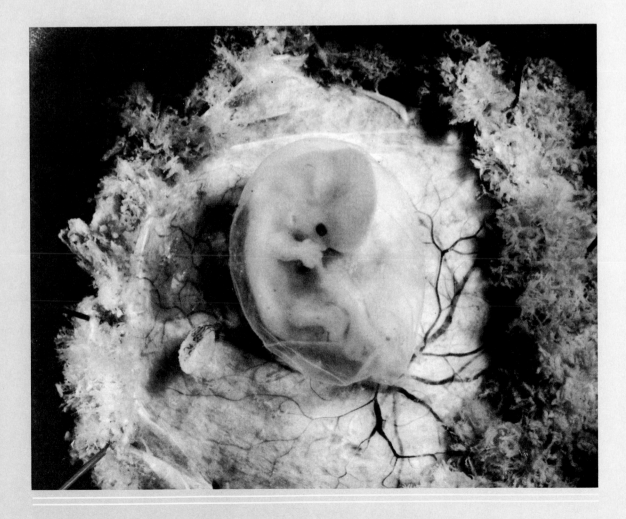

CHAPTER 3

Reproductive Anatomy and Physiology and Sexual Response

IMPORTANT TERMINOLOGY

androgen Male hormone responsible for development of secondary sex characteristics

estrogen Female hormone responsible for development of secondary sex characteristics

false pelvis Upper part of the pelvis; supports the uterus during late pregnancy.

gonad Generic term describing ovaries, testes, or both

gonadotropin Gonad-stimulating hormone; generates gonadal secretory activities

hypertrophy Increase in size or bulk

menarche Onset of initial menstruation

orgasm Pleasurable climax of sexual excitement

proliferative phase Estrogen-dominated initial phase of menstrual cycle; characterized by endometrial hypertrophy

secretory phase Progesterone-dominated, postovulation second phase of menstrual cycle; characterized by secretory endometrium

semen Thick, opalescent fluid ejaculated at peak of sexual excitement; contains spermatozoa and glandular secretions

sexual response cycle Physiologic responses to erotic stimuli; four phases: excitement, plateau, orgasmic, resolution

true pelvis Birth canal; divided into inlet, midplane, and outlet

This chapter presents male and female anatomy and physiology as they relate to the reproduction process. It also discusses the physiology of menses and the four stages of the sexual response cycle.

Female Pelvis
Bony Structure

The pelvis has three important functions: (1) it bears the weight of the upper body and distributes that weight to the legs; (2) it contains the female reproductive organs; and (3) it serves as the birth canal. The bony structure of the pelvis is shown in Figure 3-1. When full body growth has occurred (between 20 to 25 years of age) the ilium, ischium, and pubis are joined firmly and form a cup-shaped cavity.[1]

The *ilium,* the largest of the innominate bones, forms the upper and back parts of the pelvis. The flaring upper border forms the hip prominence, i.e., the iliac crest.

The *ischium* is the lower part below the hip joint. In the seated position the body rests on bony projections from the iscium, i.e., the ischial tuberosities.

The *pubis* is the front part of the pelvis. The two pubic bones extend from the hip joints to the anterior articulation (symphysis pubis) and turn down toward the ischial tuberosities to form the pubic arch.

The *sacrum* and *coccyx* form the lowest portion of the spinal column. The sacrum is a triangular wedge-shaped bone formed from the fusion of five vertebrae. It serves as the back part of the pelvis. The coccyx, also formed by the fusion of four vertebrae, forms a tail end to the spine.[2] The coccyx usually is movable at the sacrococcygeal articulation. It may be pressed back during labor to allow more room for the passage of the fetus.

The marked projection formed by the junction of the last lumbar vertebra and the sacrum is the *sacral promontory,* an important obstetric landmark.

FIGURE 3-1

Front and Lateral Views of the Female Pelvis. The bony pelvis consists of the two hipbones (innominates), the sacrum, and the coccyx. Each hipbone is divided into three parts: ilium, ischium, and pubis. There are four pelvic articulations: between the two pubic bones (symphysis pubis), between each ilium and the sacrum (sacroiliac), and between the sacrum and the coccyx (sacrococcygeal).

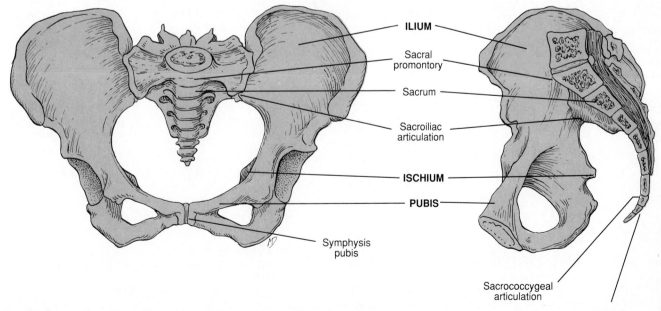

ILIUM

Sacral promontory

Sacrum

Sacroiliac articulation

ISCHIUM

PUBIS

Symphysis pubis

Sacrococcygeal articulation

Coccyx

Articulations

The four pelvic articulations (Fig. 3-1) are lined with fibrocartilage. During pregnancy hormonal actions cause thickening and softening of the articulations. Joint mobility increases, producing a slight pelvic "wobbliness" and placing additional strain on the surrounding muscles and ligaments, thus contributing to the backache and leg aches of late pregnancy. This mobility allows limited movement of the sacrum and coccyx during labor to permit fetal descent.

True and False Pelves

The pelvis may be regarded as a two-story basin divided into two parts by the linea terminalis.[3] The greater or *false pelvis* supports the uterus during late pregnancy and directs the fetus into the true pelvis for delivery.

The lesser or *true pelvis* is the birth canal. It is divided into three parts: an inlet or brim, a cavity, and an outlet. During labor the descending fetus must accommodate to the changing diameters of the true pelvis.

Female Reproductive System

Table 3-1 summarizes the structures and functions of the female reproductive organs. Figures 3-2 through 3-7 illustrate important aspects of the reproductive organs.

TABLE 3-1

Female Reproductive System

Organ	Function
External Genitalia (Vulva)	
Mons veneris	Cushions symphysis pubis; contributes to sexual arousal
Labia majora	Cover and protect the labia minora and the vaginal os
Labia minora	Cover and protect vestibule, urethra, and nulliparous vaginal os; upper folds enclose clitoris
Clitoris	Sexual arousal and orgasm; secretes smegma
Internal Organs	
Ovaries	Release ovum monthly during reproductive years; secrete estrogen and progesterone
Fallopian tubes	Transport ovum, sperm, and zygote; site of fertilization
Uterus	Usual site of implantation; supports and protects the pregnancy; contractions expel products of conception
Cornua	Provide sperm access to fallopian tubes for fertilization and zygote entry into uterus for implantation
Fundus	Domed top of uterus; highly contractile in labor to expel products of conception; postpartum contractions necessary for uterine involution
Corpus	Body of the uterus; usual site of implantation is upper segment
Cervix	Protective functions; cervical secretions contribute to vaginal lubrication, are bacteriostatic, and surrounding ovulation enhance sperm survival and motility
Vagina	Conveys menstrual flow to outside of body; secretions moisten and lubricate tissue, facilitating coitus; receives penile ejaculation during coitus; transports fetus during birth
Accessory Organs	
Breasts	Contribute to sexual arousal; secrete colostrum and milk for infant
Bartholin's (vestibular) glands	During sexual stimulation secrete alkaline mucus, which moistens and lubricates the vestibule and lower vagina; facilitates coitus; enhances sperm motility and viability
Skene's glands	Produce secretions that lubricate vestibule

External Structures

The collective external female reproductive organs are called the *vulva*.[3] They include (1) the mons veneris, (2) the labia majora, (3) the labia minora, (4) the clitoris, (5) the vestibule, (6) the hymen, (7) the urethral meatus, and (8) the various glandular and vascular structures (Fig. 3-2).

The *mons veneris* (mound of Venus) is a rounded, fatty mound over the symphysis pubis that is covered with crinkly hair. The mons serves to cushion and protect the anterior surface of the symphysis from pressure and friction.

The *labia majora* are two prominent longitudinal folds of adipose tissue covered with skin and extending downward and backward from the mons veneris. They cover and protect the labia minora and the vaginal os. They join at the bottom to form the anterior border of the perineal body. The inner surfaces are smooth and moist. After puberty the external surfaces are covered with hair.

The *labia minora* are two thin folds situated between the labia majora, extending down and backward from the clitoris. At their upper limits the minora separate. The upper fold forms the clitoral prepuce (hood); the lower fold forms the clitoral frenulum. At their lower limits they unite with the labia majora to form the fourchette (anterior border of the perineal body). The function of the labia minora is to protect and obscure the vestibule, urethral meatus, and vaginal os.

The *clitoris* is a small, highly sensitive projection composed of erectile tissue, nerves, and blood vessels covered by thin epidermis. The clitoris is analogous to the male penis and is considered the chief area of erotic sensation in the female.

The *vestibule* is the almond-shaped area between the labia minora that extends from the clitoris to the fourchette. It is perforated by the (1) urethral meatus, (2) vaginal os, (3) ducts of Bartholin's glands, and (4) ducts of Skene's glands. The *Bartholin glands* are two small glands located beneath the vestibule on either side of the vaginal opening. *Skene's glands* open on the vestibule on either side of the urethra.

The *hymen,* a thin sheath of mucous membrane at the vaginal orifice, marks the division between the internal and external organs. All of the following hymenal assessment findings are within normal parameters: (1) a small circular or crescent-shaped opening admits one or two fingers; (2) the hymen forms a complete septum across the lower end of the vagina; and (3) the hymen is absent.

The *perineum* is the area between the lower portion of the vulva and the anus. It is formed by the muscles and fascia of the pelvic floor and is covered with skin. Figure 3-3 illustrates the muscles of the pelvic floor.

Classes preparing clients or couples for childbirth include exercises that help the pregnant woman develop awareness of perineal tension and relaxation; client-induced perineal relaxation is helpful during childbirth. Surgical incision of the perineum, i.e., episiotomy, may be performed to shorten labor by reducing the perineal resistance to the oncoming head and to facilitate vaginal delivery.[4] Damage to the pubococcygeus muscle during childbirth may result in herniation of the bladder (cystocele) or the rectum (rectocele) or uterine prolapse (descent of cervix and uterine into the vagina) or both.[5]

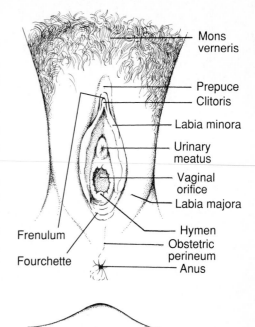

FIGURE 3-2

External Genitalia of the Female. The external female genitalia are called the vulva. The vulvar area begins at the lower margin of the pubis and ends at the perineum. The vulva protects the internal organs and is important in sexual arousal.

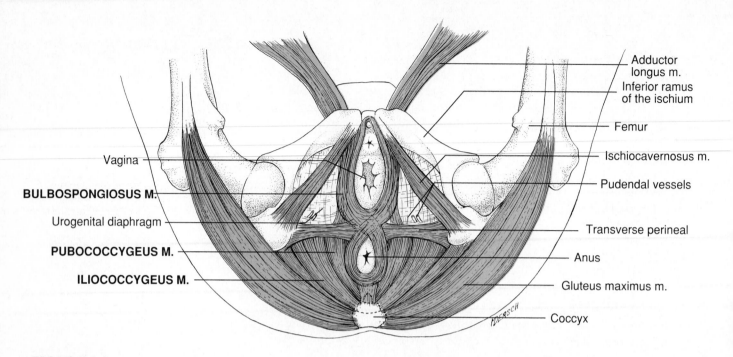

Adductor longus m.
Inferior ramus of the ischium
Femur
Ischiocavernosus m.
Pudendal vessels
Transverse perineal
Anus
Gluteus maximus m.
Coccyx

Vagina
BULBOSPONGIOSUS M.
Urogenital diaphragm
PUBOCOCCYGEUS M.
ILIOCOCCYGEUS M.

FIGURE 3-3
Muscles of the Pelvic Floor (Female Perineum). The muscles of the pelvic floor include the pubococcygeus, iliococcygeus (levator ani), transverse perineal, and bulbospongiosus muscles. Together these muscles stabilize and support the pelvic structures.

Internal Organs and Structures

The female internal organs of reproduction include the ovaries, fallopian tubes, uterus, and vagina. These organs have an abundant blood supply.

Ovaries

The ovaries are two almond-shaped organs situated in the upper part of the pelvic cavity on either side of the uterus. They are embedded in the posterior fold of the broad ligament and are supported by the suspensory, ovarian, and mesovarium ligaments (Fig. 3-4). Their chief functions are the development and expulsion of ova and the secretion of estrogen and progesterone. Estrogen and progesterone effect cyclic changes in the uterine endometrium. Table 3-2 lists selected functions of estrogen and progesterone.

Fallopian Tubes

The two thin, flexible, muscular, trumpet-shaped fallopian tubes extend from the uterine cornua along the upper margin of the broad ligaments to the ovaries. The tubes are responsible for the capture and transport of the mature ovum after its expulsion from the ruptured follicle. Three tubal features serve to accomplish these tasks: (1) the distal ends of the tubes are fimbriated; (2) the tubes are lined with ciliated and secretory epithelium; and (3) longitudinal and circular muscle fibers provide peristaltic action. Fertilization usually occurs in a fallopian tube.

Uterus

The uterus is a hollow, thick-walled, muscular organ. It serves three important functions: (1) menstruation, (2) support the protection of the

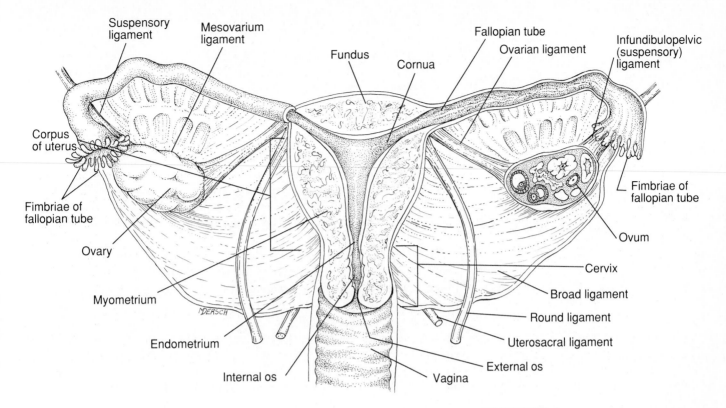

FIGURE 3-4

Anterior View of the Internal Female Reproductive Organs. The internal reproductive organs of the female are supported in the pelvic cavity by suspensory ligaments. Round ligament pain is a common complaint in late pregnancy as the ligaments stretch as a result of uterine growth.

TABLE 3-2

Functions of Estrogen and Progesterone

Estrogen	Progesterone
Dominates proliferative phase of menstrual cycle; stimulates hypertrophy of uterine endometrium in preparation for implantation	Dominates during secretory phase of menstrual cycle; completes preparation of uterine endometrium for implantation
Affects regulation of carbohydrate, water, sodium, and calcium metabolism	Reduces smooth muscle motility; enhances opportunity for embryo implantation
Affects skin texture and fat distribution, body temperature and metabolic rate, protein synthesis in the liver, blood clotting, and erythropoiesis	Induces ovulation-associated rise in body temperature
Increases acidity of vaginal secretions; protects against infection	Stimulates postovulation production of thick cervical mucus that is hostile to sperm
Immediately before ovulation, stimulates cervical mucus changes (thin, watery mucus favorable to sperm passage; characteristics: ferning, spinnbarkheit)	Acts on estrogen-stimulated mammary tissue to complete preparation for lactation
Helps prepare breasts for lactation	

growing embryo and fetus during pregnancy, and (3) muscular contractions to expel the fetus during labor and delivery.

The uterus varies in size and shape according to the age of the woman and whether or not she has borne children. It resembles a flattened pear in appearance and has two primary divisions. The upper triangular portion is the *corpus,* and the lower, constricted, cylindric portion that projects into the vagina is the *cervix* (Fig. 3-4). The fallopian tubes extend from the uterine cornua (horns) at the upper outer margin on either side. The upper rounded portion between the tubal insertion points is the fundus.

The nonpregnant uterus is suspended in the pelvic cavity between the bladder and the rectum. The lower portion of the anterior wall is united with the bladder wall by a layer of loose connective tissue. The lower posterior wall and the upper portion of the vagina are separated from the rectum by the cul-de-sac of Douglas (Fig. 3-5).

The thick uterine wall is composed of three layers: (1) endometrium, the inner mucosal layer that lines the uterine cavity; (2) myometrium, the muscular layer; and (3) perimetrium, or serosa, the outer layer. Endometrial responses to estrogen and progesterone levels are reflected in the phases of the menstrual cycle.

Because of its unique muscular structure, the uterus is capable of enlarging to accommodate the growing products of conception (Fig. 3-6). The muscle arrangement also enables expulsion of the fetus at the end of a normal labor. The uterine cavity is somewhat triangular. It is widest at the fundus and narrowest at the internal os of the cervix. In the nonpregnant woman the cavity is little more than a slit.

FIGURE 3-5

Female Reproductive Organs as Seen in Sagittal Section. This view of the female reproductive organs shows the position of the nonpregnant uterus in relation to other pelvic structures, e.g., symphysis pubis and bladder. Introducing an endoscope through the posterior fornix (culdoscopy) allows the physician to visualize the internal pelvic structures.

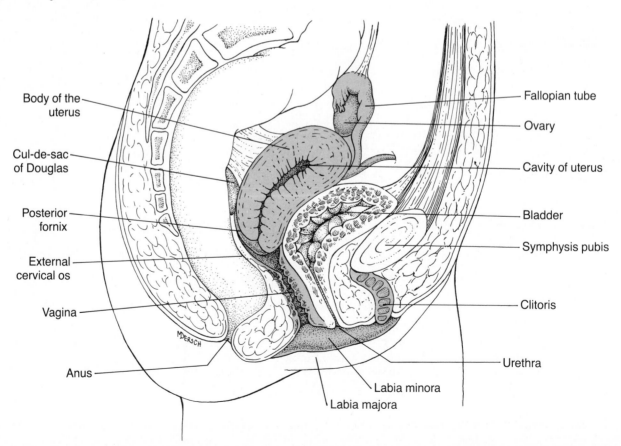

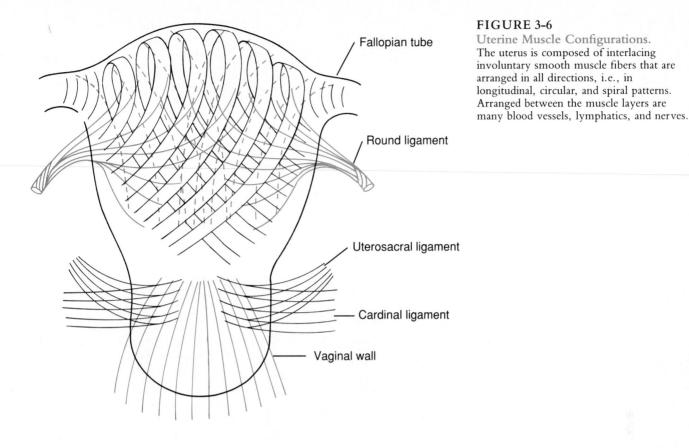

Fallopian tube

Round ligament

Uterosacral ligament

Cardinal ligament

Vaginal wall

FIGURE 3-6
Uterine Muscle Configurations.
The uterus is composed of interlacing involuntary smooth muscle fibers that are arranged in all directions, i.e., in longitudinal, circular, and spiral patterns. Arranged between the muscle layers are many blood vessels, lymphatics, and nerves.

UTERINE BLOOD SUPPLY. The uterus receives its blood supply from the ovarian and uterine arteries (Fig. 3-7).

Blood returns through the uterovaginal plexus to the venous circulation. Both the arteries and the veins traverse the broad ligament to provide circulation for the reproductive organs.

LIGAMENTS. The uterus is supported by three sets of ligaments and by the muscles of the pelvic floor. The three paired ligaments are known as the (1) broad ligaments, (2) round ligaments, and (3) uterosacral ligaments (Fig. 3-3).

The *broad ligaments* are winglike folds of peritoneum that extend from the lateral uterine margins to the pelvic walls, creating a septum that divides the pelvic cavity into anterior and posterior compartments. They enfold the fallopian tubes, the ovaries, and the round and ovarian ligaments. The lower portion, the *cardinal ligament*, is composed of dense connective tissue that is firmly joined to the cervix. The median margin connects with the sides of the uterus and encloses the uterine vessels.

The *round ligaments* are two fibrous cords attached on either side of the fundus just below the fallopian tubes. They extend forward through the inguinal canal, ending in the upper portion of the labia majora. These ligaments aid in holding the fundus forward.

The *uterosacral ligaments* are two cordlike structures that extend from the posterior cervical portion of the uterus to the sacrum. They help support the cervix. The uterovesical ligament is merely a fold of peritoneum that passes over the fundus and extends over the bladder. The rectovaginal ligament is a fold of peritoneum that passes over the posterior surface of the uterus and encircles the rectum.

FIGURE 3-7

Blood Supply of the Uterus and Adnexa. The uterine artery, the principal source of blood, is a main branch of the hypogastric artery and divides into two branches; the main branch includes fundal, tubal, and ovarian divisions. The lower branch supplies the lower portion of the cervix and the upper vagina. Four or five arteries supply the ovaries; they arise from the anastomosis of the ovarian artery, a branch of the aorta, with the ovarian branch of the uterine artery.

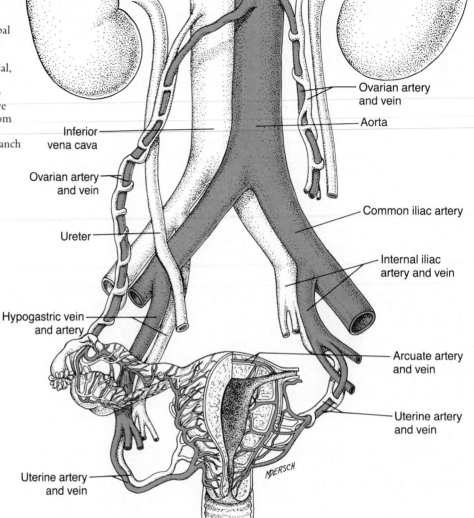

Inferior vena cava

Ovarian artery and vein

Ureter

Hypogastric vein and artery

Uterine artery and vein

Ovarian artery and vein

Aorta

Common iliac artery

Internal iliac artery and vein

Arcuate artery and vein

Uterine artery and vein

POSITION OF THE UTERUS. Since the uterus is a freely movable organ that is suspended in the pelvic cavity between the bladder and the rectum, its position can be influenced by a full bladder or rectum. The uterus can be pushed forward or backward. It also changes position when the woman stands, lies supine, or turns on her side.

CERVIX. Because the cervix is anchored securely in place by the uterosacral ligaments, it is less movable than the body of the uterus. Its muscular wall is not as thick as the rest of the uterus; the lining is folded and contains crypts that produce mucus. There are two openings to the cervical canal. The *internal os* leads from the uterine cavity into the cervical canal, and the *external os* opens into the vagina. In the nonpregnant woman the cervical canal is narrow, barely admitting a probe. However, during labor the cervix dilates to a size sufficient to permit the passage of the fetus.

Vagina

The vagina is a dilatable passage located between the bladder and the rectum. It is 8 to 12 cm long and is lined with mucus membrane (Fig.

3-3). The cervix projects into the *fornix* (a blind vault at upper end of the vagina). For descriptive purposes the fornix is divided into four parts: the lateral fornices are the spaces between the vaginal wall and either side of the cervix; the anterior fornix is the area between the cervix and the front vaginal wall; and the posterior fornix extends behind the cervix to the back vaginal wall. If the woman is in a supine position after coitus, semen pools in the posterior fornix, facilitating entry to the cervix.

The vagina serves several important functions: (1) excretion of menstrual flow, (2) receptacle for deposit of sperm, (3) copulation, and (4) as the birth canal. In the nulliparous woman vaginal rugae (ridges) give the vagina a corrugated appearance. Normally the anterior and posterior walls of the vagina are in contact: however, they are capable of great stretching to permit childbirth.

The vagina receives an abundant blood supply from branches of the uterine, inferior vesical, median hemorrhoidal, and internal pudendal arteries. The passage is surrounded by a venous plexus; the vessels follow the course of the arteries and eventually empty into the hypogastric veins.

Accessory Structures: Mammary Glands

Because of their importance as accessory glands and their functions associated with reproduction, the mammary glands are discussed in this section. Breast development at puberty and lactation occur in response to high levels of female hormones. The breasts are abundant with nerves and are sensitive to pressure.

The breasts of a woman who has never borne a child are conic or hemispheric in form; shape and size vary among women and at different ages. The breasts of women who have nursed one or more babies tend to become pendulous. Certain exercises can aid in restoring the tone of breast tissue after lactation has been terminated.

External Structure

The external surface of each breast is divided into (1) the soft, smooth skin surface surrounding the circumference of the gland to the areola (pigmented area surrounding the nipple); (2) the areola; and (3) the nipple.

AREOLAE. Pigmentation of the areolae varies from pink to brown. The surface of each areola is roughed by small, fine lumps of papillae known as Montgomery's glands. These enlarged sebaceous glands are scattered over the areola. Hormonal influences in pregnancy cause the areolae to darken; often this darkening is a presumptive sign of pregnancy in the primigravida.

NIPPLES. The nipples are composed of sensitive erectile tissue. They form large, conic papilla projecting from the center of the areolae. The openings of the milk ducts are at the summit of each nipple.

Internal Structure

The breasts are composed of glandular tissue and fat. Each organ is divided into 15 to 20 lobes, which are separated by fibrous and fatty walls (Fig.

FIGURE 3-8
**Glandular Tissue and Ducts of the
Mammary Gland.** The mammary glands
(breasts) are two highly specialized
cutaneous glands located on either side of
the anterior wall of the chest between the
third and sixth ribs. After childbirth
prolactin stimulates secretion of milk by
the acini glands in the tubular alveoli.

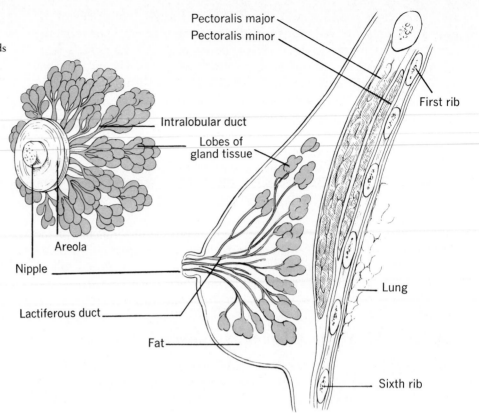

3-8). Each lobe is subdivided into many lobules (alveolar glands), which contain numerous acini cells.

The acini cells comprise a single layer of epithelium, beneath which is a small amount of connective tissue richly supplied with capillaries. Milk secretion begins in the acini cells of the tubular alveoli. The products necessary for the milk filter from the blood by osmosis. As the lactiferous (milk) ducts leading from the alveoli approach the nipple, they dilate to form little reservoirs in which milk is stored; they narrow again as they pass into the nipple. The size of the breast is determined by the amount of fatty tissue. Size is not predictive of a woman's ability to produce adequate amounts of milk to nurse her infant successfully.

BLOOD SUPPLY. The internal mammary and intercostal arteries supply the breast glands; the mammary veins follow these arteries. In addition, there are many cutaneous veins that become dilated during lactation.

CHANGES DURING PREGNANCY. Under the influence of estrogen, progesterone, chorionic gonadotropin, and placental lactogen, several changes occur in the breasts: (1) blood vessels become dilated and engorged; (2) the connective tissue between the lobules becomes edematous; and (3) both the acini and the lactiferous ducts dilate. True alveoli are formed during the first pregnancy in response to the high levels of estrogen and progesterone. However, milk is not produced by the acini cells until after delivery when estrogen and progesterone levels drop and prolactin is secreted.

TABLE 3-3

Male Reproductive System

Organ	Function
External Genitalia	
Penis	Organ of copulation and urination
Shaft	During sexual stimulation the corpora cavernosum and corpus spongiosum distend with blood (erection)
Glans	Sexual arousal; contains urethra
Prepuce	Retractable foreskin covers the glans and urethral os in the uncircumcised male
Scrotum	Suspends testes in optimal environment; contracts on exposure to cold to bring testes closer to body
Internal Organs	
Testes	Male gonads
Leydig's cells	Produce testosterone
Seminiferous tubules	Spermatogenesis
Sertoli cells	Supply nutrients, hormones, enzymes for spermatozoal maturation
Accessory Organs	
Epididymis	Secretes glycogen that nourishes and supports spermatozoa during their maturation
Vas deferens	Stores sperm; under autonomic nervous system stimulation contractions propel semen into ejaculatory duct
Ejaculatory duct	Conducts sperm into urethra for ejaculation
Prostate	Secretes seminal fluid component that neutralizes acidic seminal fluid and enhances sperm motility
Seminal vesicles	Secrete both slightly alkaline nutrient fluid that regulates semen pH and prostaglandins that stimulate fallopian tube motility and expedite sperm progress toward the ovum
Cowper's (bulbourethral) glands	During sexual stimulation secretions lubricate end of the penis for sexual intercourse (coitus)

Male Reproductive System

Table 3-3 lists structures and functions of the male reproductive organs. The male reproductive system comprises the penis, the testes, and an excretory duct system with their accessory structures (Fig. 3-9).

External Structures

Penis

The penis, the male organ of copulation, consists of two lateral cavernous bodies (two corpora cavernosa) and a central core of erectile tissue (corpus spongiosum) that encloses the urethra. The enlarged conic structure at the distal end of the penis, an extension of the corpus spongiosum, is called the *glans penis.* The glans contains the external orifice of the urethra and, in uncircumcised males, is covered by a fold of thin, retractable skin called the prepuce (foreskin).

Scrotum

The scrotum is a saclike structure suspended between the penis and the anus. It contains the testes and the epididymides. Its purpose is to protect the temperature-sensitive testes from heat and cold. If the testes do not

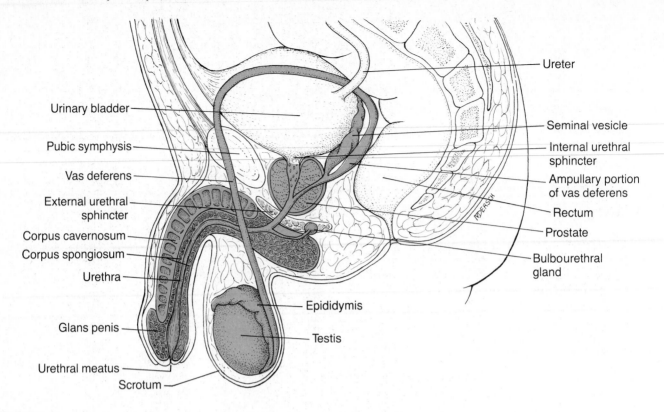

FIGURE 3-9

Organs of the Male Reproductive System. The organs of the male reproductive system include the penis, testes, epididymides, vas deferens, accessory glands, and various ducts. The testes and epididymides are suspended outside the pelvic cavity in the scrotum.

descend into the scrotum before puberty, the male will be sterile (unable to produce sperm).

The scrotal sac is composed of loose, wrinkled skin and fascial connective tissue and is covered with sparse hair. The skin is somewhat darker than that of the rest of the body and contains many sebaceous glands. A layer of smooth muscle fibers forms the *dartos fascia*. An extension of the dartos muscle forms a septum that separates the testes from each other; its location is marked by the central ridge on the scrotal surface. The dartos fascia is sensitive to environmental temperature; it responds to cold by contracting, drawing the scrotum closer to the body wall.

Internal Organs

Testes

The male ability to reproduce is govered principally by the testes; the testes are the site of spermatogenesis and testosterone production (Fig. 3-10). A protective fibrous capsule, the tunica albuginea, encloses each testicle and subdivides it into approximately 250 lobules. Each lobule contains *seminiferous tubules,* the coiled ducts in which spermatogenesis occurs. The testes also contain two other specialized types of cells: Leydig's cells and Sertoli's cells.

Leydig's (interstitial) *cells* are located in the connective tissue that surrounds and supports the seminiferous tubules. Interstitial cell-stimulating hormone (ICSH), released by the anterior pituitary gland, stimulates the Leydig cells to produce testosterone. ICSH is identical to the female luteinizing hormone (LH) that triggers ovulation; however, ICSH does not display the same marked cyclic variation.

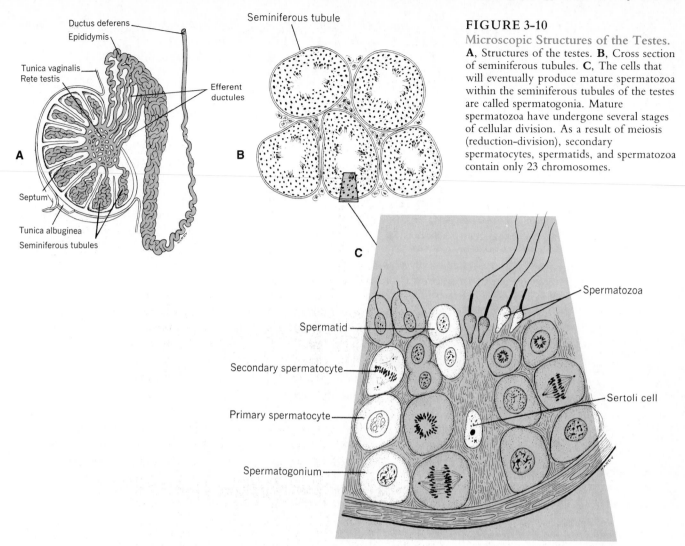

FIGURE 3-10
Microscopic Structures of the Testes.
A, Structures of the testes. **B,** Cross section of seminiferous tubules. **C,** The cells that will eventually produce mature spermatozoa within the seminiferous tubules of the testes are called spermatogonia. Mature spermatozoa have undergone several stages of cellular division. As a result of meiosis (reduction-division), secondary spermatocytes, spermatids, and spermatozoa contain only 23 chromosomes.

Sertoli's cells support and nourish the spermatogenic cells and are important for sperm transport within the seminiferous tubules.

Duct System

EPIDIDYMIS. The seminiferous tubules join at the rete testes (Fig. 3-10) and enter the epididymis. Immature sperm cells enter, are stored, undergo maturation, and acquire motility in the epididymis. Epididymal cells secrete glycogen to nourish and sustain the sperm cells during their maturation.

VAS DEFERENS. The ducts of the epididymis empty into the vas deferens, a thin, muscular tube that passes upward out of the scrotum, becoming part of the spermatic cord. The vas deferens stores mature sperm until ejaculation.

EJACULATORY DUCT. Just outside the prostate gland, the vas deferens unites with the ducts of the seminal vesicles to form the ejaculatory duct.

The ejaculatory duct passes through the prostate gland; during orgasm, spermatozoa are ejected into the urethra for exit.

Accessory Structures

Seminal Vesicles

Seminal vesicles are convoluted saclike structures attached to the vas deferens behind the bladder and anterior to the rectum. Glandular tissue lining the seminal vesicles secretes a slightly alkaline fluid that helps regulate the pH of the seminal fluid. The seminal fluid also contains fructose, an energy source for the sperm, and prostaglandins. Prostaglandins are believed to facilitate sperm and egg passage by causing smooth muscle contractions of the fallopian tubes.

Prostate Gland

The prostate gland is shaped like a chestnut. It surrounds the base of the urethra and the ejaculatory ducts. It secretes an alkaline fluid that empties into the urethra, enhancing sperm motility and helping to neutralize the slightly acidic secretions of the vagina.

Cowper's (Bulbourethral) Glands

The Cowper's glands are tiny structures that lie at the base of the prostate on either side of the urethra. In response to sexual stimulation these glands secrete a mucinous substance that lubricates the urethra and the end of the penis.

Seminal Fluid

Spermatozoa are produced in the seminiferous tubules of the testes, undergo meiosis, and mature in the epididymis and then are stored in the vas deferens. Although immobile while in the epididymis, sperm become activated when mixed with accessory gland secretions. They are highly motile after ejaculation.

Seminal fluid consists of spermatozoa and secretions of the seminal vesicles, prostate, and Cowper's glands. It contains a variety of nutrients and prostaglandins that support sperm survival and movement through the female reproductive tract. Sperm can survive 2 to 3 days after ejaculation into the female reproductive tract. See Laboratory Values for characteristics of normal seminal fluid when examined within 2 hours of ejaculation. Vasectomy, an elective procedure for male sterilization, prevents semen from passing into the ejaculatory duct for expulsion.

Sexual Maturity
Conception to Puberty

Although the sex of a fetus is determined at conception, anatomic male/female differentiation is not evident in an early embryo. Approximately 7 to 10 weeks after conception, testes or ovaries begin to form and are distinguishable. At birth primitive sex cells (spermatogonia) are found in

▍▍LABORATORY VALUES

Characteristics of Normal Sperm Specimen

Quantity: 2 to 6 ml emitted per ejaculation
pH: slightly alkaline (7.35 to 7.50)
Appearance: milky
Normal count: 45 to 200 million spermatozoa
Morphology: >70% normal
Motility: >60%

> = greater than; < = less than.

the male. The female ovary contains a lifetime supply of primitive egg cells (oogonia); no evidence exists that any more are ever formed. Maturation of the sex cells begins with puberty.

Puberty

Puberty is the transition period between childhood and sexual maturity.[6] Hypothalamic secretion of gonadotropin-releasing hormone (GRH) initiates puberty in both males and females. GRH stimulates release of pituitary gonadotrophic hormones that in turn generate production of ovarian estrogen and testicular testosterone. Estrogen and testosterone stimulate sexual maturation of the reproductive organs and are responsible for the development of female or male secondary sex characteristics.

Female Sexual Maturation

Female puberty usually occurs between 9 and 16 years of age; the average age at onset is 12 to 13 years old.[6] Heredity, race, nutritional status, climate, and environment influence initiation of sexual maturity. For example, puberty tends to occur earlier in warmer climates.

Alterations in neuroendocrine activity are associated with puberty and sexual maturation (Fig. 3-11). In the female ovarian responses to gonadotrophic pituitary hormones include production of estrogen and

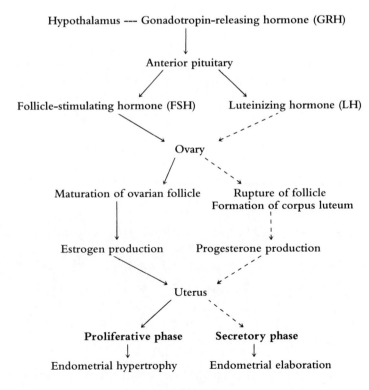

FIGURE 3-11

Neuroendocrine Relationships and the Menstrual Cycle. Hypothalamic release of gonadotropin-releasing hormone (GRH) stimulates the anterior pituitary gland to secrete follicle-stimulating hormone (FSH) and luteinizing hormone (LH). FSH causes maturation of the ovarian follicles; the follicular cells secrete estrogen. Estrogen causes increased pituitary secretion of LH and inhibits further secretion of FSH. LH, in turn, stimulates rupture of the ripe follicle, expelling the ovum and forming the corpus luteum, which secretes progesterone. The menstrual cycle reflects uterine responses to the changing levels of estrogen and progesterone.

Hypothalamus --- Gonadotropin-releasing hormone (GRH)

Anterior pituitary

Follicle-stimulating hormone (FSH)   Luteinizing hormone (LH)

Ovary

Maturation of ovarian follicle   Rupture of follicle
Formation of corpus luteum

Estrogen production   Progesterone production

Uterus

Proliferative phase   **Secretory phase**

Endometrial hypertrophy   Endometrial elaboration

Ischemic phase
In the absence of conception, the corpus luteum degenerates. Falling estrogen/progesterone levels initiate the ischemic phase, and menstruation results.

progesterone. Estrogen is responsible for initiation and maintenance of the female secondary sex characteristics, e.g., enlargement of the structures of the female reproductive system, breast development, hair and fat distribution, skeletal structure, and vocal range. Uterine responses to the levels of estrogen and progesterone result in **menarche** (initial menstruation). These cyclic monthly events continue throughout a woman's reproductive life.

Oogenesis

The female capacity to reproduce is dependent on successful maturation and expulsion of an ovum. Estimates suggest as many as 6,800,000 potential ova are present in primordial follicles by the fifth month of gestation. Although the majority degenerate, approximately 2,000,000 remain at birth.[3] These germ cells develop and undergo mitotic transformation to primary oocytes during intrauterine life. Cellular replication ceases, and the oocytes lie dormant until puberty.[2] Once each month, from puberty until menopause, approximately 20 follicles will be activated; only one will ripen and eject an ovum.

Menstrual Cycle

Hormonal control of the menstrual cycle involves interactions between the endocrine and reproductive systems. Figure 3-12 illustrates the cyclic monthly events associated with menstruation.[6] For convenience the menstrual cycle may be divided into three phases: (1) proliferative, (2) secretory, and (3) menstrual.

FIGURE 3-12

Physiologic Changes Characteristic of Menstrual Cycle Phases. Physiologic responses accompany the cyclic alterations in circulating levels of pituitary gonadotropins and ovarian hormones (menstrual cycle phases). Endometrial hypertrophy, elaboration, and sloughing represent uterine responses to the changing estrogen/progesterone levels. Body temperature and cervical mucus changes also reflect responses to the circulating levels of ovarian hormones; these characteristic changes enable clients to identify the cyclic fertile period and to plan avoiding or achieving pregnancy.

Adapted from Bierchen J: Nursing care of the childbearing family. In Lagerquist S (ed): Addison-Wesley's Nursing Examination Review, 3rd ed. Menlo Park, Calif, Addison-Wesley, 1987.

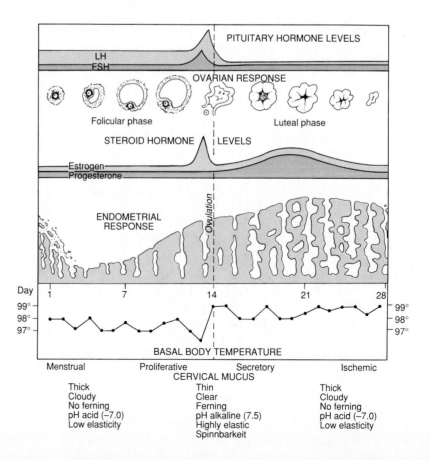

Proliferative Phase and Associated Events

The first days of the new menstrual cycle are called the follicular, estrogenic, or proliferative phase. These terms describe the interrelated events that occur between the 5th and 14th days. Immediately after menstruation, the uterine endometrium is very thin. Release of the anterior pituitary hormone FSH stimulates graafian follicle maturation, initiating the new cycle. Follicular cells secrete estrogen. Estrogen stimulates endometrial cells in the uterus to proliferate, and the uterine lining hypertrophies (thickens); the endometrial cells become taller, and the glands that dip into the endometrium become longer and wider.[7]

CERVICAL MUCUS. Increased levels of preovulatory estrogen also prepare the genital tract for sperm migration. Cervical secretions are scant and viscous early in the cycle. Near the time for ovulation the mucus becomes more receptive to spermatozoa, i.e., thin, watery, and it exhibits *spinnbarkheit* (is stretchy); on microscopic examination it displays a fernlike pattern.[8] Daily examination of cervical mucus enables clients to identify signs of impending ovulation and to act appropriately to either achieve or avoid pregnancy.

BASAL BODY TEMPERATURE. Body temperature is affected by activity, environment, and other factors, e.g., infection. Basal body temperature is the lowest temperature of an awake, healthy person.[8] In the ovulating woman physiologic variations in basal body temperature accompany hormonal changes of the menstrual cycle. The basal temperature is lower during the proliferation phase of the cycle; ovulation is immediately preceded by a slight, sudden drop (0.4° to 0.8° F) in basal body temperature, immediately followed by a rise (0.5° to 1.0° F) that is sustained over 24 to 72 hours.[8] Because the temperature variation is so small, a special thermometer is required to ensure accuracy if the client chooses to add this personal assessment component for her family planning.

Secretory Phase and Associated Events

Immediately preceding ovulation, the pituitary gland secretes large amounts of LH. The sudden surge in LH concentration triggers rupture of the mature follicle and expulsion of the egg and follicular fluid. Ovulation begins the secretory phase of the cycle. Follicular cells in the follicular remnant form the corpus luteum. The corpus luteum secretes large amounts of estrogen and progesterone. Progesterone augments estrogenic effects on the uterine endometrium, causing it to become more vascular and glandular. Progesterone also stimulates the uterine glands to secrete large quantities of glycogen and lipids. The glands become greatly dilated and tortuous (resembling a corkscrew); the endometrium becomes more succulent and hospitable to implantation of the fertilized egg. In addition, progesterone inhibits smooth muscle motility, facilitating uterine implantation and protecting the embryo from expulsion.

CERVICAL MUCUS. Under progesterone stimulation the cervical mucus thickens and is scant after ovulation. The thick mucus is hostile to penetration by sperm.

BASAL BODY TEMPERATURE. The rise in basal body temperature accompanying ovulation is attributed to the thermogenic effect of progesterone on the central nervous system. If pregnancy occurs, the basal temperature remains elevated past the expected time of menstruation. If the egg cell is not fertilized, the corpus luteum begins to degenerate on or about the 24th day of the cycle, and basal body temperature returns to normal.

Menstrual Phase

As the corpus luteum degenerates, estrogen and progesterone production rapidly declines. In response to the lowered hormone levels, blood vessels in the endometrium become constricted and ischemic. As endometrial tissues are deprived of oxygen and nutrients, the lining begins to disintegrate and slough. On or near the 14th postovulatory day, menstruation begins.

Male Sexual Maturation

Puberty occurs approximately 2 years later in the male than in the female and lasts approximately 4 years. In the male GRH stimulates pituitary secretion of FSH, which initiates sperm production. The male analogue of LH, ICSH, generates testosterone production. Testosterone, an androgen, is responsible for the male secondary sex characteristics, e.g., development and maturation of the genitalia and larynx, hair distribution, and characteristic male skeletal structure. Testosterone production can occur independently of spermatogenesis; however, spermatogenesis cannot occur in the absence of testosterone. Unless testosterone is present in adequate amounts, fertility is impaired.

Spermatogenesis

The male primordial germ cells, i.e., spermatogonia, are formed during fetal life but lie dormant until hormonal changes associated with puberty stimulate multiplication and maturation. Unlike the cyclic oogenesis, once spermatogenesis begins, multiple germinal cells continuously undergo the mitotic/meiotic processes that transform spermatogonia to spermatozoa (Fig. 3-10). Spermatogenesis continues throughout the male reproductive life.

Sexual Response Cycle

The most widely accepted theory of sexual response was proposed by Masters and Johnson.[9] Their theory identifies four sequential phases of male and female sexual response: (1) excitement, (2) plateau, (3) orgasmic, and (4) resolution. These phases are discussed in terms of physiologic vasocongestion and myotonia (Table 3-4). Vasocongestion causes genital engorgement and distention. Myotonia begins as increasing muscle tension and ends with rhythmic, involuntary contractions.

The *excitement phase* begins with the onset of erotic feelings and sensations and produces intense vasocongestion and increasing myotonia. With continued excitement and stimulation the *plateau phase* is reached; this phase immediately precedes orgasm. When vasocongestion reaches a critical point and a muscle contraction reflex is initiated in the pelvic muscles, the *orgasmic phase* occurs. The final phase, *resolution,* occurs when

TABLE 3-4

Phases of Sexual Response

Phase	Female Response	Male Response
Excitement	Vaginal lubrication; vagina lengthens and distends. Cervix and fundus elevate. External genitalia become congested. Clitoral size increases	Penis becomes erect. Scrotal sac thickens. Testes move upward.
Plateau	Labia minora and lower one-third of vagina become engorged. Clitoris retracts under prepuce.	Testes continue upward. Penile engorgement continues.
Orgasmic	Rhythmic muscle contraction occurs.	Muscles contract rhythmically, followed by ejaculation of semen.
Resolution	Engorgement dissipates. Clitoris recedes to normal size and position. Uterus descends.	Penile engorgement dissipates. Scrotal sac thins. Testes descend.

the genitals and other organs have returned to their usual states. If orgasm is not achieved, resolution does occur but at a much slower rate.

Other physiologic responses to sexual stimulation include (1) increased blood pressure, respiratory rate, and heart rate, (2) genital engorgement, (3) changes in genital skin color, (4) increased muscle tension, and (5) involuntary reflexive muscle contractions.[10]

Female Sexual Response

Sexual arousal in the female results from a complex interaction of physiologic and psychologic stimuli. The breasts and other nongenital areas are involved in sexual response. During sexual excitement the breasts enlarge, and the nipples become erect as a result of congestion. These are erotic areas for women.

Sexual arousal in the female elicits physiologic responses similar to those of the male. Parasympathetic nerve impulses from the sacral area of the spinal cord are activated, causing (1) dilation of the blood vessels supplying the clitoris and vestibular bulbs, (2) stimulation of vestibular gland secretions that moisten the vestibule and lower end of the vagina, and (3) vaginal expansion and elongation. Distended with blood, the clitoris and vestibular bulbs become erect. The clitoris is an erotic center, abundantly endowed with sensory nerves that respond to local stimulation.

Immediately before orgasm, pelvic congestion and venous dilation cause vaginal edema. Local distention narrows the vaginal canal, increasing penile friction and eliciting orgasm. Orgasm immediately activates sacral and lumbar reflexes that cause the muscles of the uterus, tubes, and perineum to contract rhythmically, aiding sperm transport upward through the tract. Muscular contractions also expel the blood and fluid trapped in the tissues. Because of the extent of pelvic congestion and the capacity for distention of pelvic structures, much of the blood and edema cannot be removed rapidly and may flow back into the distended structures. As a result, many women are capable of restimulation seconds after orgasm. These women may have repeated orgasms before the blood flow to erectile tissues diminishes and the organs and muscles return to their usual state. Sexual arousal and orgasm are not necessary to achieve pregnancy.

Male Sexual Response

Male sexual arousal results from a complex interaction of physical and psychologic stimuli that activate the autonomic nervous system (ANS). Erection, orgasm, and ejaculation occur under ANS stimulation.

The penis comprises three long cylinders of erectile tissue that are surrounded by an elastic sheath. Each cylinder contains blood vessels and spaces that distend with blood during sexual arousal. The two upper cylinders, the corpora cavernosa, are responsible for penile rigidity and increase in length and width with erection. The distal end of the corpus spongiosum terminates in the glans; during sexual excitement the glans enlarges to provide a soft protective cushion for the rigid corpus cavernosa. The glans is rich in nerve endings and is the male area of maximum erotic sensation.

At the peak of sexual excitement, orgasm, a sudden, pleasurable feeling of release, occurs. Ejaculation occurs as a result of several simultaneous physiologic events: (1) a stretch reflex transmits sympathetic impulses to smooth muscles in the walls of the testicular ducts, epididymides, vas deferens, and ejaculatory ducts, causing peristalsis; (2) the impulses stimulate rhythmic contractions, releasing secretions of the Cowper's glands, prostate, and seminal vesicles; (3) other impulses stimulate pulsating contractions of skeletal muscles at the base of the penile erectile columns; and (4) seminal fluid is expelled. After orgasm and ejaculation, the blood flow diminishes, and the penis returns to a normal, flaccid state.

REFERENCES

1. Stern J: Essentials of Gross Anatomy. Essentials of Medical Education Series. Philadelphia, FA Davis, 1988
2. Seeley R, Stephens T, Tate P: Anatomy and Physiology. St. Louis, Times Mirror/Mosby College Publishing, 1989
3. Pritchard J, MacDonald P, Gant N: Williams Obstetrics, 17th ed. Norwalk, Conn, Appleton-Century Crofts, 1985
4. Creasy R: Preterm labor and delivery. In Creasy R, Resnick R: Maternal-Fetal Medicine: Principles and Practice. 2nd ed Philadelphia, WB Saunders, 1989
5. Willson J: Immediate and remote effects of childbirth injury. In Willson J, Carrington E (eds): Obstetrics and Gynecology. 8th ed. St. Louis, CV Mosby, 1987
6. Bierchen J: Nursing care of the childbearing family. In Lagerquist S (ed): Addison-Wesley's Nursing Examination Review, 3rd ed. Menlo Park, Calif, Addison-Wesley, 1987
7. Cunningham FG, MacDonald PC, Gant NF: Williams Obstetrics. 18th ed. Norwalk, Conn, Appleton & Lange, 1989
8. Hatcher R et al: Contraceptive Technology 1988-1989, 15th ed. New York, Irvington Press, 1988
9. Masters W, Johnson V: Human Sexual Response. Boston, Little, Brown, 1966
10. Vick R: Contemporary Medical Physiology. Menlo Park, Calif, Addison-Wesley, 1984

SUGGESTED READINGS

Goss C: Gray's Anatomy of the Human Body, 30th ed. Philadelphia, Lea & Febiger, 1984
Hatcher R et al: Contraceptive Technology 1988-1989, 15th ed. New York, Irvington Press, 1988
Speroff L et al: Clinical Gynecology, Endocrinology, and Infertility, 3rd ed. Baltimore, Williams & Wilkins, 1984

Stewart F et al: Understanding Your Body, Every Woman's Guide to Gynecology and Health. New York, Bantam Books, 1987
Yen S, Jaffe R: Reproductive Endocrinology: Physiology, Pathophysiology and Clinical Management, 2nd ed. Philadelphia, WB Saunders, 1985

Placental and Fetal Development

IMPORTANT TERMINOLOGY

amnion Inner membrane that encloses the growing fetus

amniotic fluid Liquid contained within the amniotic cavity in which the fetus floats during intrauterine life

autosome Any chromosome other than the sex chromosomes

chorion Outer fetal membrane in contact with the maternal decidua basalis

chromosome Linear thread in cell nucleus that contains the DNA, which transmits genetic information

conception Union of sperm and ovum

decidua basalis That part of the uterine endometrium that unites with the chorionic villi to form the placenta

diploid number Normal complement of chromosomes in body cells (46)

dizygotic twins Two fetuses develop from two fertilized ova

ductus arteriosus Channel that carries blood between the fetal pulmonary artery and the aorta

ductus venosus Channel that carries blood between the umbilical vein and the inferior vena cava

embryo The developing human from the second to the eighth week after conception

fetus The growing human from weeks 9 to 40

foramen ovale Opening between the atria of the fetal heart

gamete The mature reproductive cell, either ovum or spermatozoon

gametogenesis Development of the reproductive cell; oogenesis or spermatogenesis

haploid number One-half the normal total chromosome number, i.e., 23; occurs only in sex cells

mitosis Cellular replication process resulting in formation of two daughter cells that are identical to the parent cell

meiosis Cellular replication process of reduction division; occurs in sex cells, resulting in haploid number of chromosomes

monozygotic twins Production of two fetuses from one fertilized ovum; occurs as a result of division of the inner cell mass

oogenesis Formation and development of the female gamete (ovum)

oogonium Primordial cell from which an oocyte originates

somatic Pertains to nonreproductive (body) cells

spermatogenesis Formation and development of the male gamete (sperm)

spermatogonium Primordial cell from which the spermatocyte originates

teratogen Agent that causes abnormal development of embryo

zygote Fertilized ovum; formed by union of male and female gametes

This chapter focuses on the physical process of fertilization and development of the utero/placental/fetal unit. Also discussed is the relationship between maternal and fetal circulation.

Gametogenesis

With the exception of mature sex cells, all human cells contain 46 **chromosomes. Somatic** (body) cells contain 22 paired autosomes and one sex-specific pair of chromosomes (XX or XY). Each parent provides one of the chromosomes in each pair. Somatic cells replicate by **mitosis,** i.e., cellular division that produces two daughter cells that are identical to the parent cell in both character and chromosome number.

Sex cells, however, undergo a unique reduction-division process called **meiosis.** The mature **gamete,** either ovum or spermatozoon, has received one of each pair of chromosomes in the original parent cell (**oogonium** or **spermatogonium**). Thus it contains the **haploid number** of chromosomes and carries 22 **autosomes** and one sex chromosome (X or Y) in its nucleus.[1]

Oogenesis

At birth each ovary contains a vast number of germ cells (primordial ova). This huge supply of follicles is more than adequate for the (approximately) 35 years of a woman's reproductive life. There is no evidence that any new germ cells are formed.[2] The majority of primordial ova apparently degenerate spontaneously, and only 400 to 500 ova will actually mature and be expelled during the years of sexual maturity (Fig. 4-1). Each month during the reproductive years, shortly before ovulation occurs, the primary oocyte undergoes meiosis, forming the secondary oocyte and the first polar body.[3]

Only after fertilization does the secondary oocyte divide, producing the second polar body and the zygote. If fertilization does not occur, the ovum begins to degenerate; the life of the ovum is believed to be less than 24 hours.[2]

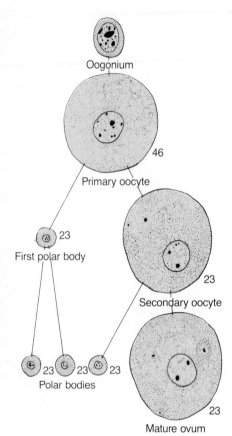

Oogonium

46
Primary oocyte

23
First polar body

23
Secondary oocyte

23   23   23
Polar bodies

23
Mature ovum

FIGURE 4-1

Oogenesis. Each month, beginning at puberty and ending with completion of menopause, one of the follicles that contain primary oocytes enlarges and ruptures, expelling the female gamete, i.e., ovum.

Spermatogenesis

In the sexually mature male spermatogonia continuously multiply by mitosis to form primary spermatocytes,[4] which contain 44 autosomes and one X and one Y sex chromosome (Fig. 4-2). The mitotic/meiotic transformation from spermatogonium to spermatozoon continues throughout a man's reproductive life.

Transport of Ovum and Sperm

Ovum Transport

The fallopian tube is responsible for (1) capturing the ovum on its expulsion from the ruptured follicle, (2) transferring the ovum into its lumen, (3) providing a temporary environment for the ovum and the spermatozoon, and (4) transporting the ovum or zygote into the uterus. The fallopian tube is the usual site of fertilization.

The fimbriated ends of the fallopian tubes are lined with hairlike projections called cilia. Immediately before and after ovulation high estrogen levels enhance tubal motility. During ovulation contractions of the tubal muscle pull the ovary in the direction of the tubal opening.[5,6] The fimbriae completely cover the ovary at the site of ovulation.[2] When the follicle ruptures, the cilia vibrate to sweep the follicular fluid and ovum into and through the fallopian tube toward the uterine cavity (Fig. 4-3).

Sperm Transport

Ejaculation deposits seminal fluid containing highly motile spermatozoa in the vagina near the cervix. The whipping motion of their tails enables spermatozoa to swim with a quick vibratory motion, perhaps as fast as 3 mm a minute. Some spermatozoa reach the cervix almost immediately after ejaculation.[2] Their transport is aided by the muscular contractions of the uterus and tubes. Spermatozoa have been observed in the fallopian tube within minutes of insemination. Those spermatozoa residing in cervical secretions can survive and remain motile and capable of fertilization for as long as 72 hours.

Fertilization

Fertilization occurs in the ampulla (distal one-third of the fallopian tube). When the spermatozoon encounters the egg, enzymes in the sperm head are released that allow it to penetrate the membrane surrounding the ovum.[7] Once penetration is complete, both sperm and ovum (gametes) are enclosed by the same membrane. A physiologic barrier prevents penetration by other spermatozoa. Rarely does more than one spermatozoon penetrate the ovum.[7]

The nuclear membranes of the sperm and ovum disappear soon after penetration. The nuclei fuse and their chromosomes combine to form the **zygote** (Fig. 4-3). The sex of the **fetus** is determined at fertilization by the combination of the sex chromosomes from the two gametes. The zygote contains the full complement, or **diploid number** (46), of chro-

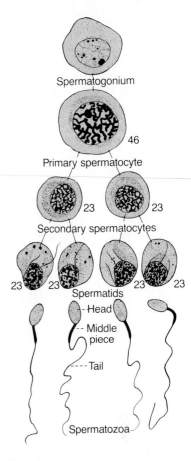

FIGURE 4-2

Spermatogenesis. The first (meiotic) division of the primary spermatocyte produces 2 secondary spermatocytes. Each of them contains the haploid number of chromosomes (23), i.e., secondary spermatocytes contain 22 autosomes and an X or a Y sex chromosome. The mitotic second maturation division produces 4 haploid spermatids. Each of the 4 spermatids carry 22 autosomes and 1 sex chromosome (2 spermatids carry an X and two carry a Y sex chromosome. Each spermatid develops a tail and eventually becomes a mature spermatozoon.

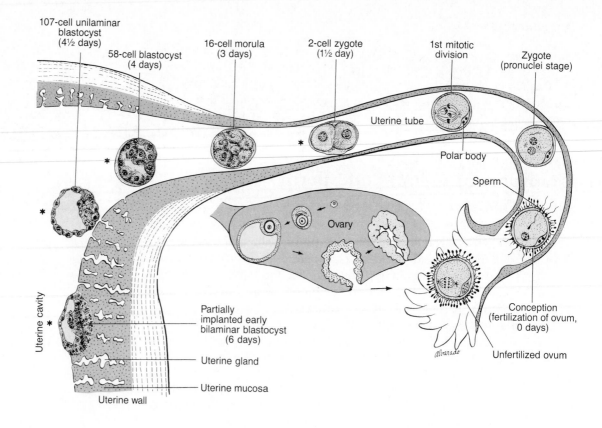

107-cell unilaminar blastocyst (4½ days)

58-cell blastocyst (4 days)

16-cell morula (3 days)

2-cell zygote (1½ day)

1st mitotic division

Zygote (pronuclei stage)

Uterine tube

Polar body

Sperm

Ovary

Uterine cavity

Partially implanted early bilaminar blastocyst (6 days)

Uterine gland

Uterine mucosa

Uterine wall

Conception (fertilization of ovum, 0 days)

Unfertilized ovum

Alvarado

FIGURE 4-3

Ovum Transport and Fertilization.
Transport of the ovum into the fallopian tube and fertilization within the tube, followed by cleavage (cell division) to the 8- to 16-cell stage. The product, referred to as a morula, is delivered into the uterus where it develops into a blastocyst and implants in the endometrium on the sixth or seventh postfertilization day.

Adapted from Gasser RF: Atlas of Human Embryos. Hagerstown, Md, Harper & Row, 1975.

mosomes. Mitotic cellular replication begins with each cell dividing rapidly into two identical new cells. The early cell divisions produce a solid mass of cells, the morula.

Implantation occurs about 7 days after fertilization. The fertilized ovum remains in the fallopian tube for approximately 3 days before entering the uterine cavity. Actual implantation occurs 3 to 4 days later. Figure 4-3 also illustrates the sequence of events occurring during transport of the ovum/zygote/morula/blastocyst. Figure 4-4 describes the periods of intrauterine development.

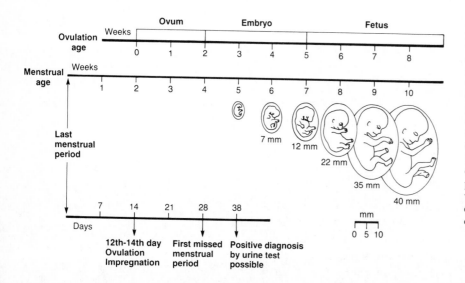

FIGURE 4-4

Periods of Prenatal Development.
Although conception does not occur until approximately mid-cycle, pregnancy is divided into 10 lunar months (40 weeks) from the first day of the last menstrual period; lunar months always encompass four calendar weeks (28 days × 10 weeks = 280 days gestation). The gestation of the embryo/fetus is approximately 2 weeks less (38 weeks = 266 days). The first 14 days are designated as the period of the ovum. The period of the embryo encompasses lunar weeks 4 through 10. The period of the fetus extends from the end of week 10 to the time of birth.

Multiple Pregnancy

Multiple fetuses arise from two different processes. Twins are either dizygotic or monozygotic. Most commonly twins result from the fertilization of two separate ova by different spermatozoa and are called **dizygotic** (Fig. 4-5). Dizygotic twins are not true twins because they are produced by the union of two separate ova and spermatozoa.

Approximately one-third as often, **monozygotic,** or identical, twins are conceived (Fig. 4-6). Several theories have been developed to explain monozygotic twinning. However most authorities believe it is the result of the spontaneous division of the fertilized ovum at an early stage of development.[2,8]

Either or both processes may be involved in the production of larger numbers of fetuses at one birth. Quadruplets, for example, may arise from one to four ova.

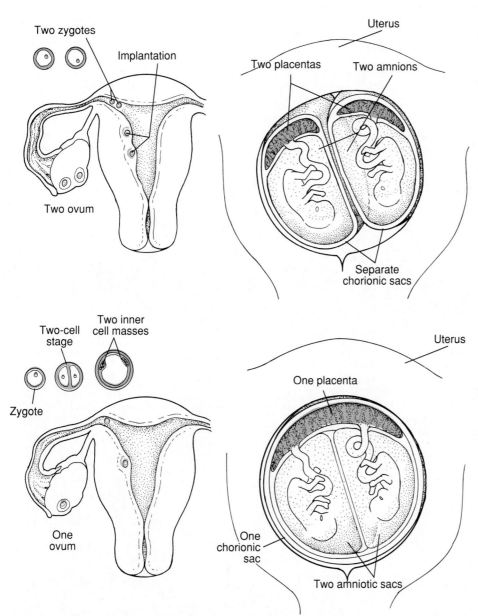

FIGURE 4-5
Dizygotic Twinning. Dizygotic (fraternal) twins may be of the same or opposite sexes. Each fetus has its own amnion, chorion and placenta. If the implantation sites are very close, the placentas may be fused.

FIGURE 4-6
Monozygotic Twinning. This type of twinning occurs when two embryos develop from the same zygote by division of the inner cell mass. Two identical embryos develop, each within its own amniotic sac, but sharing one chorionic sac and a single placenta.

Implantation

The trophoblast, the peripheral cell layer of the fertilized ovum, is responsible for implantation. These cells release enzymes that enable them to burrow into the uterine endometrium, erode the walls of endometrial blood vessels, and tap into the maternal bloodstream. Fingerlike projections, the chorionic villi, develop out of the trophoblastic layer and extend into blood-filled spaces of the uterine endometrium. These villi contain blood vessels that are connected to the fetus and are the means by which oxygen and nutrients are received from the mother.

Cells in the chorionic villi also produce human chorionic gonadotropin (hCG). This hormone maintains the corpus luteum, which in turn continues progesterone production.[7] Progesterone assists with implantation by inhibiting uterine motility. Progesterone also stimulates further endometrial growth, which provides a supportive environment for the developing embryo.

Development of Utero/Placental/Fetal Unit
Decidua

During the secretory phase of the menstrual cycle progesterone stimulates the endometrium to become very vascular. This very vascular endometrium is called the *decidua*. For descriptive purposes the decidua is divided into three portions (Fig. 4-7). The union of the chorionic villi and the **decidua basalis** forms the placenta.

FIGURE 4-7

Decidua and Developing Embryo/Fetus. The decidua basalis directly underlies the implanted ovum; the union of the chorionic villi with the decidua basalis forms the placenta. The decidua vera is not in contact with the ovum. The decidua capsularis is the portion of the endometrium that is pushed out by the growing embryo. **A,** The decidua capularis expands over the embryo and by gestational week 16 lies in contact with the decidua vera; **B,** The growing embryo progressively obliterates the uterine cavity.

Adapted from Fitzgerald MJT: Human Embryology: A Regional Approach. Hagerstown, Md, Harper & Row, 1978.

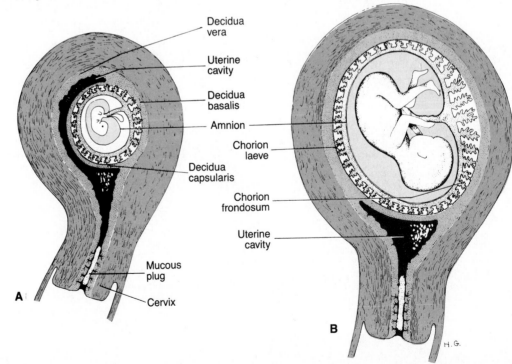

Decidua vera
Uterine cavity
Decidua basalis
Amnion
Chorion laeve
Decidua capsularis
Chorion frondosum
Uterine cavity
Mucous plug
Cervix
A
B
H.G.

Amnion and Chorion

Amnion

During the second week an inner membrane (amnion) begins to develop and surround the embryo. The amniotic cavity is filled with fluid. **Amniotic fluid** is formed from filtrates from the maternal bloodstream and fetal urine. It maintains the fetus at an even temperature, cushions it against possible injury, and allows free fetal movement. In addition, the fetus drinks amniotic fluid. Cells shed by the fetus are found in amniotic fluid. By the 16th gestational week, amniocentesis can be performed for chromosomal studies on the shed cells.[9]

Chorion

The trophoblast layer of the fertilized ovum forms the outer membrane (chorion) that surrounds the fetus (Fig. 4-7). The chorion lies against the decidua basalis and overlies the amnion. The chorionic villi not in contact with the decidua degenerate and almost disappear, leaving a slightly roughened membrane. Together with the amnion, these two membranes form the "bag of waters" that encloses the growing embryo and fetus.

Placenta

The placenta is formed by the union of the chorionic villi and the decidua basalis. By the eighth week a sample of chorionic villi can be obtained by aspiration biopsy.[10] Since villi are fetal tissue, analysis of their chromosomes can identify genetic abnormalities and may be used as an alternative to amniocentesis.

Placental structure is complete by the 12th week of gestation. The full-term placenta weighs approximately 500 g and is approximately 20 cm in diameter and 2 cm thick[11] (Fig. 4-8).

FIGURE 4-8

Full-Term Placenta. **A,** Fetal surface; **B,** maternal surface. The fetal surface is smooth, glistening, and covered by amnion. Beneath this membrane a number of large blood vessels may be seen. The maternal surface is red and fleshlike and is divided into approximately 20 segments called cotyledons. The cotyledons are further divided into approximately 200 lobules, each of which is a circulatory unit containing a single spiral artery. Nutrient-rich and well-oxygenated maternal blood enters the intervillous space by way of the spiral arteries.

From Fitzgerald MJT: Human Embryology: A Regional Approach. Hagerstown, Md, Harper & Row, 1978.

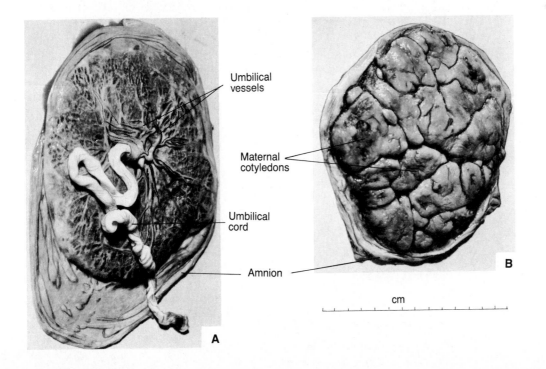

Umbilical vessels

Maternal cotyledons

Umbilical cord

Amnion

cm

A

B

TABLE 4-1

Placental Functions

Function	Effect
Gas exchange	By diffusion, exchanges oxygen from maternal bloodstream for fetal carbon dioxide
Transport of nutrients	Makes sodium, chloride, fat-soluble vitamins, glucose, amino acids, iron, calcium, iodine, water-soluble vitamins, and water available to meet fetal growth needs
Antibody transport	Confers transient passive immunity to fetus and newborn from maternal immunoglobulins
Excretion of fetal metabolic wastes	Maintains favorable acid-base and electrolyte balances
Heat transfer	Maintains optimum environment
Hormone production	
Human chorionic gonadotropin (hCG)	Maintains corpus luteum until establishment of placenta
Human placental lactogen (hPL)	Regulates maternal metabolism to maintain supply of needed nutrients for fetus; facilitates glucose transport across the placenta; stimulates breast development and preparation for lactation
Estrogen	Stimulates uterine growth and uteroplacental blood flow, myometrial contractility, and growth of mammary tissue; affects regulation of maternal metabolism, blood clotting, and red blood cell production (see also Table 3-2)
Progesterone	Maintains endometrium; inhibits uterine motility; stimulates development of breast alveoli; affects maternal metabolism

Placental Functions

Table 4-1 lists placental functions and identifies the method of transfer of key substances. Maternal and fetal circulations are completely separate. Exchange of oxygen and nutrients from the maternal bloodstream and wastes from the fetus occurs in the intervillous spaces (Fig. 4-9). However, if breaks occur in the membrane surrounding the villi, fetal blood cells may enter the maternal bloodstream (Fig. 4-10).

FIGURE 4-9

Placental Circulation. Maternal blood in the placental venous sinuses surrounds the villi that contain fetal blood. Fetal blood, depleted of both nutrients and oxygen and carrying metabolic wastes, enters the villous capillaries from the umbilical arteries. Oxygen and nutrients from the maternal blood in the intervillous spaces are absorbed into the villous capillaries. The oxygenated and nutrient-rich blood is returned to the fetus through the umbilical vein.

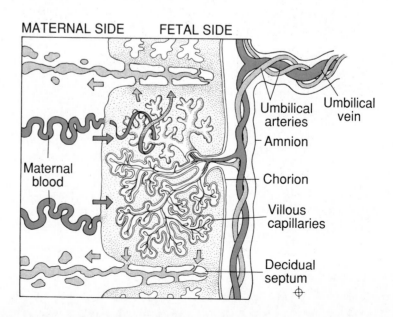

MATERNAL SIDE   FETAL SIDE

Maternal blood

Umbilical arteries

Umbilical vein

Amnion

Chorion

Villous capillaries

Decidual septum

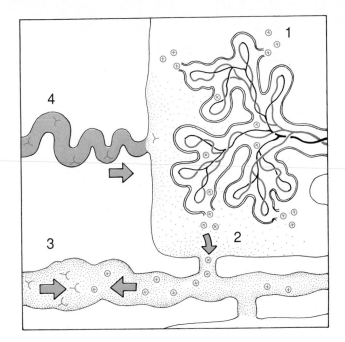

FIGURE 4-10

Transplacental Fetal and Maternal Transfusion. *1,* Transfusion of fetal red blood cells through membrane breaks is responsible for sensitization of the Rh-negative woman carrying an Rh-positive fetus. *2,* On entry to the maternal circulation, Rh-positive fetal red blood cells stimulate formation of maternal antibodies, *3.* Transplacental fetal/maternal transfusion occurs most frequently at delivery, placing subsequent pregnancies at risk, *4.*

Placental Permeability

Diffusion is the most important mechanism regulating transfer of maternal/fetal substances.[7] Gases, electrolytes, water, and drugs move across the placenta from the area of higher concentration (maternal bloodstream) to the area of lesser concentration (fetal circulation). Facilitated transport, active transport, and pinocytosis also move substances such as glucose, amino acids, and immunoglobulins across the placenta. Bulk flow of water results from differences in hydrostatic and osmotic pressures.

Umbilical Cord

The placenta is connected to the fetus by the umbilical cord. Although cords may vary, the average cord is approximately 45 to 60 cm long and 1.5 cm in diameter.[11] The cord contains two arteries and one vein that are twisted on each other; they are protected from pressure by a transparent, bluish-white, gelatinous substance called Wharton's jelly.

Blood Circulation

Uteroplacental Circulation

Key substances, i.e., oxygen and nutrients, are transported to the intervillous spaces by the maternal uterine circulation. Uterine blood flow is approximately 600 to 700 ml/min, which at term constitutes 10% of the total maternal cardiac output.[7] Nearly 90% of the total uterine blood flow enters the intervillous spaces; 10% supplies the myometrium.

Uterine blood flow is diminished by (1) vasoconstriction associated with chronic hypertension, pregnancy-induced hypertension, or vasopressor medications; (2) decreased maternal blood pressure and cardiac output related to supine hypotensive syndrome (compression of the inferior vena cava by the large term uterus interferes with return circulation to the right atrium); or (3) vigorous maternal exercise that may divert blood to the muscles from the uteroplacental circulation. Uterine blood flow is enhanced only by bed rest. At rest blood flow to other organs and tissues is diminished, and the blood supply to the placenta and fetus increases.

Uterine contractions also interrupt blood flow to the intervillous spaces. A contraction that lasts 45 seconds interrupts blood flow for approximately 30 seconds. During the interruption the fetus must exist on the supplies of oxygen and nutrients remaining in the intervillous spaces. Usually enough oxygen is contained in the spaces to meet fetal needs for 90 seconds. However, vasoconstriction, prolonged contractions, too short intervals between contractions, or high uterine resting tone between contractions (sustained muscle tension) reduces the total amount of oxygen available to the fetus at any given time.

Umbilical Cord Circulation

The umbilical cord is the other vulnerable link in the system for maternal-fetal exchange of oxygen, nutrients, and wastes. Should the cord become compressed between fetal head and pelvis, twisted around the neck, or entangled, the interference with cord circulation can seriously affect fetal oxygenation.

Fetal Circulation

The fetal circulation is presented in Figure 4-11. While in utero, the fetal lungs do not function as organs of respiration. Oxygenated blood enters the fetal circulation through the umbilical vein. Although a portion of the oxygenated blood goes through the liver, most of it goes through the **ductus venosus** to the inferior vena cava.

Oxygenated blood enters the right atrium from the inferior vena cava and passes directly through the **foramen ovale** to the left atrium. It then passes into the left ventricle and exits through the aorta.

The blood that circulates into the arms and the head returns through the superior vena cava to the right atrium. However, instead of circulating through the foramen ovale as before, the blood is directed downward through the right ventricle into the pulmonary arteries. Although a portion circulates through the lungs to provide tissue perfusion, the majority flows through the **ductus arteriosus** to the aorta.

The blood in the aorta, with the exception of that going to the head and upper extremities, passes downward to supply the trunk and lower extremities. Blood returns through the internal iliac and hypogastric arteries and through the umbilical arteries to the placenta for discharge of wastes and fresh oxygenation.

CHARACTERISTICS OF FETAL BLOOD. Three unique characteristics enhance oxygen transport from maternal to fetal blood: (1) fetal hemoglobin has a unique affinity for oxygen and accepts significantly more oxygen than does adult hemoglobin; (2) the concentration of hemoglobin in fetal blood is 25% higher than that in adult blood; and (3) the more alkaline pH of blood in the umbilical vein further increases its capacity to accept oxygen.

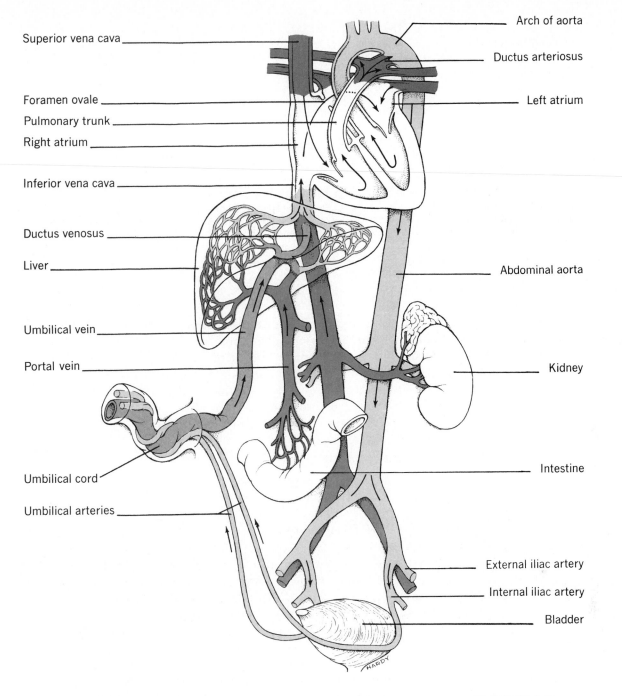

Superior vena cava

Foramen ovale

Pulmonary trunk

Right atrium

Inferior vena cava

Ductus venosus

Liver

Umbilical vein

Portal vein

Umbilical cord

Umbilical arteries

Arch of aorta

Ductus arteriosus

Left atrium

Abdominal aorta

Kidney

Intestine

External iliac artery

Internal iliac artery

Bladder

FIGURE 4-11

Diagram of the Fetal Circulation.
The fetal circulation contains three unique structures. The ductus venosus connects the umbilical vein with the inferior vena cava. The foramen ovale permits passage of blood between the two atria. The ductus arteriosus connects the pulmonary arteries with the aorta. The majority of the blood bypasses the lungs since they do not function during intrauterine life. Blood returns to the placenta for gas exchange by way of the umbilical arteries.

Circulation Path After Birth

As soon as the baby is born and breathes, several alterations in structure and function occur: (1) the lungs fill with air and begin to function, (2) intrathoracic pressure increases, (3) placental circulation ceases, and (4) fetal structures close. The physiologic changes not only alter the character of the blood in many vessels but make the special fetal structures unnecessary. In fact, persistence of the fetal circulation complicates successful transition to independent extrauterine life.

After the umbilical cord is clamped, the large amount of blood returned to the heart and lungs equalizes the pressure in both atria, causing the

TABLE 4-2

Changes in Fetal Circulation After Birth

Structure	Before Birth	After Birth
Umbilical vein	Brings arterial blood to liver and heart	Obliterated; becomes round ligament of liver
Umbilical arteries	Brings arteriovenous blood to placenta	Obliterated; become vesical ligaments on anterior abdominal wall
Ductus venosus	Shunts arterial blood into inferior vena cava	Obliterated; becomes ligamentum venosum
Ductus arteriosus	Shunts arterial and some venous blood from pulmonary artery to aorta	Obliterated; becomes ligamentum arteriosum
Foramen ovale	Connects right and left auricles (atria)	Obliterated usually; at times open
Lungs	Contain no air and very little blood	Filled with air and well supplied with blood
Pulmonary arteries	Bring little blood to lungs	Bring much blood to lungs
Aorta	Receives blood from both ventricles	Receives blood only from left ventricle
Inferior vena cava	Brings venous blood from body and arterial blood from placenta	Brings venous blood only to right auricle

From Guyton AC: Medical Physiology, 7th ed. Philadelphia, WB Saunders, 1986.

foramen ovale to close. The instantaneous closure of the foramen ovale changes the entire course of the blood flow and converts the fetal circulation to that of the adult. The ductus arteriosus and ductus venosus eventually shrivel and in 2 to 3 months are converted to ligaments.

The umbilical cord vessels become filled with clotted blood; ultimately, they are converted to fibrous cords. The umbilical vein becomes the round ligament of the liver. Table 4-2 compares fetal and newborn/adult circulation.

Fetal Development
Duration of Pregnancy

The estimated length of pregnancy can be calculated in several ways. Pregnancy is considered as encompassing (1) 10 lunar months from the first day of the last menstrual period (each lunar month contains 4 lunar weeks of 7 days, i.e., 280 days), (2) 40 weeks of gestation, or (3) 9 calendar months divided into 3 trimesters (each with 3 months). In 10% of pregnancies birth occurs 1 week or more before the estimated date; in another 10% it occurs approximately 2 weeks later than expected.

Intrauterine development is divided into three periods, i.e., that of the ovum, the **embryo,** and the fetus. They may be described in terms of menstrual age (lunar weeks since the first day of the last menstrual period) or ovulation age (weeks after fertilization/conception). Figure 4-4 compares ovulation and menstrual ages for the weeks beginning each of these prenatal periods. The following section correlates embryonic and fetal development by ovulation age and lunar month.

Stage of the Ovum: The First 4 Weeks

Events during the first week after fertilization are depicted in Figures 4-3 and 4-4. During the second week the yolk sac appears. It forms blood cells during the embryonic stage of development and gives rise to cells that later become sex cells. Portions of the yolk sac form the embryonic digestive system and may play an important part in transfer of nutrients to the developing embryo.

During the first weeks after implantation and early placental development, the amnion and the embryonic disk are formed from the inner cell mass. Differentiation into primitive germ layers occurs as early as 7½ days after fertilization.

Embryonic Development

Second Lunar Month (Lunar Weeks 4 to 10)

The stage of the embryo generally is identified as beginning by the third week after **conception** and ending on completion of week 8. This is the most critical stage of intrauterine development as all organ systems develop during these few weeks.

The embryo is most susceptible to the effects of tetratogenic agents during this period of intense cellular differentiation. The malformation that results seems to depend on the organ that is in the critical early stages of differentiation at the time of exposure.

Third Lunar Month

By the start of week 8 (lunar week 10) the embryo is recognizable as human, and trunk movements can be observed. By the end of that week all essential structures are present.

Fetal Development

The fetal period begins with the start of postconception week 9.[12] The weeks 9 to 20 are characterized by particularly rapid growth. Table 4-3 summarizes important characteristics of fetal development by lunar month. Sonographic techniques have contributed much to understanding intrauterine behavior.[9] As pregnancy progresses, the fetus becomes capable of performing increasingly complex movements.

Week 9

At the beginning of the fetal stage of development, the head is disproportionately larger than the body, and the extremities are very short. Limb movement has been observed during postconception week 9. Urine formation begins during weeks 9 to 12.

Week 10

By the 10th week after conception cephalic features are clearly evident, centers of ossification are present, fingers and toes have become differentiated, buds for the "baby" teeth are present, and sockets for these develop in the jawbone.

TABLE 4-3

Fetal Development

First Lunar Month

Fetus is 0.75 cm to 1 cm in length.
Trophoblasts embed in decidua.
Chorionic villi form.
Foundations for nervous system,
   genitourinary system, skin, bones, and
   lungs are formed.
Buds of arms and legs begin to form.
Rudiments of eyes, ears, and nose appear.

4   weeks

Second Lunar Month

Fetus is 2.5 cm in length and weighs 4 g.
Fetus is markedly bent.
Head is disproportionately large,
   owing to brain development.
Sex differentiation begins.
Centers of bone begin to ossify.

8   weeks

Third Lunar Month

Fetus is 7 cm to 9 cm in length and
   weighs 28 g.
Fingers and toes are distinct.
Placenta is complete.
Fetal circulation is complete.
Rudimentary kidneys secrete small
   amounts of urine.

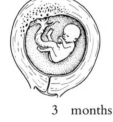

3   months

Fourth Lunar Month

Fetus is 10 cm to 17 cm in length
   and weighs 55 g to 120 g.
Sex is differentiated.
Heartbeat is present.
Nasal septum and palate close.

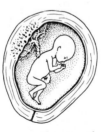

4   months

Fifth Lunar Month

Fetus is 25 cm in length and
   weighs 223 g.
Lanugo covers entire body.
Fetal movements are felt by mother.
Heart sounds are perceptible by
   auscultation.

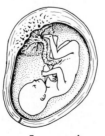

5   months

Sixth Lunar Month

Fetus is 28 cm to 36 cm in length and
   weighs 680 g.
Skin appears wrinkled.
Vernix caseosa appears.
Eyebrows and fingernails develop.

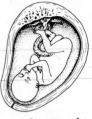

6   months

Seventh Lunar Month

Fetus is 35 cm to 38 cm in length and
   weighs 1200 g.
Skin is red.
Pupillary membrane disappears from eyes.
Fetus has an excellent chance of survival.

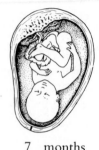

7   months

Eighth Lunar Month

Fetus is 38 cm to 43 cm in length and
   weighs 2.7 kg.
Fetus is viable.
Eyelids open.
Fingerprints are set.
Vigorous fetal movement occurs.

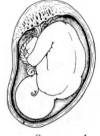

8   months

Ninth Lunar Month

Fetus is 42 cm to 49 cm in length and
   weighs 1900 g to 2700 g.
Face and body have a loose wrinkled
   appearance because of subcutaneous
   fat deposit.
Lanugo disappears.
Amniotic fluid decreases.

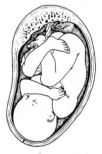

9   months

Tenth Lunar Month

Fetus is 48 cm to 52 cm in length and weighs 3000 g.
Skin is smooth.
Eyes are uniformly slate colored.
Bones of skull are ossified and nearly together at sutures.

Week 11

By the 11th week there is movement of the fetal chest. The fetus becomes capable of intrauterine fetal "breathing" (moving amniotic fluid in and out of the respiratory tract). During the fetal stage of development, all body structures grow and mature; body proportions change as the arms and legs lengthen.

By the end of the first trimester (lunar week 12; postconception week 10), all major organ systems have begun development. The fetal heart rate may be audible by Doppler (electronic augmentation).

Fourth Lunar Month

During weeks 11-14 (lunar weeks 13-16) tissue and organ growth continue. By the close of the fourth lunar month, gender is clearly evident. Very rapid fetal growth begins with week 13.

Fifth Lunar Month

The fifth lunar month (lunar weeks 17-20) is significant clinically because it is the midpoint in gestation. Brown fat begins to form during the 15th week. Fetal growth slows by week 18. During weeks 15-18, skeletal muscles become active and the mother is aware of fetal movement (quickening). By the end of the fifth lunar month (lunar week 20), lanugo, fine, downy hair, covers the entire body. The fetal heart rate usually is audible by fetoscope. Confirmation of the estimated date of confinement (EDC) is supported further by finding the uterine fundus at the level of the umbilicus.

Sixth Lunar Month

By the end of the second trimester (24 lunar weeks; 22 weeks after conception) the head is still quite large, and eyebrows and lashes can be seen. The internal and middle ears are well developed, and the fetus is capable of reacting to sudden noise with active movements. The lack of much subcutaneous fat gives the skin a red, wrinkled appearance. Vernix caseosa, a protective coat of fatty, cheesy substance, covers the skin.

Seventh Lunar Month

Pulmonary surfactant begins to form during postconception week 24. By the end of the 28th lunar week (26 weeks after conception) the pupillary membrane has disappeared from the fetal eyes, and the eyes are partly open. Fetal taste buds are developed, and the fetus can react to the taste of substances injected into the amniotic fluid. During weeks 26 to 29 the pulmonary vasculature becomes capable of gas exchange and the central nervous system capable of controlling respiration.

Eighth Lunar Month

At the end of the eighth lunar month (32 lunar weeks; 30 weeks after conception) deposition of subcutaneous fat begins; substantial weight gain occurs, and the fetus has a more rounded appearance. In the male fetus the testes are descending.

Ninth Lunar Month

During the final 2 months of gestation the fetus completes the tasks that enable transition to independent life and survival following birth. By the 36th lunar week the skin is pink, and the body is rounded. Lanugo generally disappears. The fetus exhibits definite sleep-wake patterns.

Tenth Lunar Month

Term is reached ten lunar months or 40 weeks after the first day of the last menstrual period. During the last weeks of gestation the fetus gains significant subcutaneous fat and weight. Small amounts of lanugo may be present on the shoulders and upper body, but most has disappeared from body surfaces. Myelination of the brain begins. The fetus is fully developed and moves actively within the uterus. Adequate pulmonary surfactant is present to enable independent gas exchange after birth.

Teratogenesis

Susceptibility to **teratogens** declines rapidly during the fetal phase. Development during this phase consists primarily of growth and maturation of the structures formed in the preceding embryonic phase. Deformations are less likely to occur; however, teratogenic agents may interfere with the development of normal function.[13] The fetal brain is particularly vulnerable.

In recent years the long-term teratogenic effects of substance abuse, e.g., alcohol, tobacco, heroin, cocaine, in pregnancy have become a matter of major national concern. Maternal substance abuse has been associated with fetal intrauterine growth retardation and postnatal growth deficiencies.[14] The irreversible effects of alcohol abuse long have been documented and include (1) malformations of the head and face, (2)

TABLE 4-4

Criteria for Estimation of Gestational Age

Lunar Month	Biparietal Diameter* (cm)	Crown-Rump Length† (cm)	Weight† (g)	Fundal Height (normal findings)
Fourth	3.2	12	110	Midway between pubis and umbilicus
Fifth	4.5	16	300	Fetal heart tone (FHT) audible with Doppler At umbilicus Quickening FHT audible with fetoscope
Sixth	5.8	21	650	Fundus 18 cm above symphysis
Seventh	6.9	25	1100	Fundus 24.5 cm above symphysis
Eighth	7.9	28	1800	Fundus 28 cm above symphysis
Ninth	8.8	32	2600	Fundus 31.5 cm above symphysis
Tenth	9.7	36	3400	Fundus 35 cm above symphysis

*Adapted from Scammon R, Calkins L: Growth in the Fetal Period. Minneapolis, University of Minnesota Press, 1929, as adapted by Reid D, Ryan K, and Benirschke K: Principles and Management of Human Reproduction. Philadelphia, WB Saunders, 1972, p 786.
†Adapted from Pritchard J, MacDonald P, Gant N: Williams Obstetrics, 17th ed. New York, Appleton-Century-Crofts, 1985, p 143.

growth retardation, (3) damage to the central nervous system, (4) poor ability to focus attention, (5) delayed motor development, (6) irritability, and (7) hyperactivity.[15]

Serious concern has arisen about similar long-term effects from maternal cocaine abuse during pregnancy. Studies have demonstrated teratogenic effects on animals, and strong suspicion has been raised about the impact of maternal cocaine use on human fetuses.[16] Researchers have documented an increased incidence of the following pregnancy/newborn complications: (1) preterm birth, (2) low birthweight, (3) smaller head circumferences, (4) hypertonicity, and (5) neurologic impairment[17-21]; permanent behavioral and learning disabilities have been predicted.[18,19]

Assessment of Intrauterine Fetal Age

Sonography enables estimation of fetal age, growth, and development. Table 4-4 presents average criteria for estimating normal growth and development of the fetus.

REFERENCES

1. Sadler R: Langman's Medical Embryology, 5th ed. Baltimore, Williams & Wilkins, 1985
2. Cunningham F, MacDonald P, Gant N: Williams Obstetrics, 18th ed. Norwalk, Conn, Appleton & Lange, 1989
3. Moore K. The Developing Human, Clinically Oriented Embryology, 3rd ed. Philadelphia, WB Saunders, 1982
4. Spence A, Mason E: Human Anatomy and Physiology, 3rd ed. Menlo Park, Calif, Benjamin/Cummings, 1987
5. Glass R: Sperm and egg transport, fertilization, and implantation. In Creasy R, Resnik R (eds): Maternal-Fetal Medicine: Principles and Practice, 2nd ed. Philadelphia, WB Saunders, 1989
6. Laros R: Fertilization, development, physiology and disorders of the placenta: Fetal development. In Willson J, Carrington E: Obstetrics and Gynecology, 8th ed. St. Louis, CV Mosby, 1987
7. Guyton A: Textbook of Medical Physiology, 7th ed. Philadelphia, WB Saunders, 1986
8. Moore K: Before We Are Born, Basic Embryology and Birth Defects. Philadelphia, WB Saunders, 1977
9. Willson J: Diagnostic methods in obstetrics and gynecology. In Willson J, Carrington E: Obstetrics and Gynecology, 8th ed. St. Louis, CV Mosby, 1987
10. Simpson J, Elias S: Prenatal diagnosis of genetic disorders. In Creasy R, Resnik R (eds): Maternal-Fetal Medicine: Principles and Practice, 2nd ed. Philadelphia, WB Saunders, 1989
11. Benirschke K: Normal Development. In Creasy R, Resnick R: Maternal-Fetal Medicine: Principles and Practice, 2nd ed. Philadelphia, WB Saunders, 1989
12. Korones S: Anatomic and functional aspects of fetal development. In Sciarra J et al (eds): Gynecology and Obstetrics, Vol. 2. Hagerstown, Md, Harper & Row, 1988
13. Langman J: Medical Embryology, 5th ed. Baltimore, Williams & Wilkins, 1985
14. Jones K: Effects of chemical and environmental agents. In Creasy R, Resnik R (eds): Maternal-Fetal Medicine: Principles and Practice, 2nd ed. Philadelphia, WB Saunders, 1989
15. US Department of Health and Human Services (USDHHS): Alcohol and birth defects: The fetal alcohol syndrome and related disorders. Pub No ADM 87-1531. Rockville, Md, USDHHS, 1987
16. American Society for Pharmacology and Experimental Therapeutics (ASPET) and Committee on Problems of Drug Dependence: Scientific perspectives on cocaine abuse. The Pharmacologist 29(1):20-27, 1987
17. Ryan L, Ehrlich S, Finnegan L: Cocaine abuse in pregnancy: effects on the fetus and newborn. Neurotoxicology and Teratology 9:315-319, 1988
18. Finnegan L: Influence of maternal drug dependence on the newborn. In Kacew S, Lock S (eds): Toxicologic and Pharmacologic Principles in Pediatrics. New York, Hemisphere Publishing, 1988, pp 183-198
19. Chasnoff I: Perinatal effects of cocaine. Contemporary Ob-Gyn, pp 163-179, May 1987
20. Chasnoff I: Cocaine use in pregnancy. New Engl J Med 313(11):666-669, 1985
21. Bingol N et al: Teratogenicity of cocaine in humans. Amer J Human Genetics 2(10):45, 1985

SUGGESTED READINGS

Bernhardt J: Sensory capabilities of the fetus. MCN 12(1):44, 1987

Brackhill Y: Medication in maternity. Childbirth Educator, p 28, Winter 1986/1987

Ericson A: What is a teratogen? Childbirth Education, p 44, Winter 1986/1987

Ramsay J: Prenatal influences on fetal development. Nursing 1986, 3(December):432, 1986

Reproductive Genetics

allele One of two or more genes that occupy corresponding positions on paired chromosomes; alleles carry specific hereditary characteristics

aneuploidy Abnormal number of chromosomes; may involve either autosomes or sex chromosomes; responsible for many congenital disorders (e.g., Down's syndrome, Turner's syndrome)

amniocentesis Transabdominal aspiration of amniotic fluid for chemical or cytologic examination

autosomal inheritance Hereditary trait(s) carried by chromosomes other than the sex chromosomes

dominant Hereditary characteristic expressed even when carried on only one of the paired chromosomes

euploidy State of having complete sets of chromosomes

gene Self-producing unit of chromosomal DNA; directs protein synthesis; transmits hereditary traits

genotype Basic combination of genes in an organism, i.e., "gene type"

hemizygous Possessing only one of a gene pair that determines a trait

heterozygous Paired chromosomes carrying different genes in the same position on each chromosome

homologous chromosome Genetically similar in essential structure

homozygous Identical genes occupying the same position on two paired chromosomes

karyotype Genetic composition of body cells, i.e., "cell type"; photomicrograph of a single cell in metaphase arranged to show the chromosomes in descending order of size

mosaicism Possessing cells of two different genetic patterns

mutation Permanent alteration in gene structure

pedigree Diagram of an individual's ancestors; used in analysis of genetically transmitted traits

phenotype Physical appearance of an individual; determined by the combination of dominant and recessive traits received from the parents, i.e., "show type"

recessive No expression of transmitted trait unless carried by both alleles on the paired chromosomes, i.e., received from both parents

sex-linked inheritance Transmission of the hereditary characteristic by genes carried on the sex chromosome(s)

trait Distinguishing genetic characteristic

translocation Transfer of one part of a chromosome to (1) another location on the same chromosome or (2) to another chromosome

This chapter presents basic information on the most commonly seen genetic disorders and their causes. The nurse's role is initially one of counselor, providing a couple with the needed information to make an informed decision before becoming pregnant. The nurse then assesses the couple for referral for extended counseling or explains and clarifies the diagnostic procedures recommended. Her primary role, though, is to serve as the client advocate.

Biologic Determinants of Inheritance

Chromosomes are the biologic links between parent and child. These threads of deoxyribonucleic acid (DNA) in the cell nucleus contain the **genes,** i.e., the hereditary units that transmit familial traits from generation to generation. Each gene carries coded information that determines the structure and production of specific proteins. In humans most genes occur in allelic pairs. Each member of the pair is found at the same location on the homologous parental chromosomes and controls the same function. The genes may be identical or they may code for alternate expressions of the same trait.[1]

Some genes are **dominant.** Traits carried on dominant genes are expressed in all offspring. Other genes are **recessive.** The traits they transmit are expressed only when an identical gene is present on both **homologous chromosomes.** At fertilization the unique combination of dominant and recessive **alleles** received from his or her ancestors **(genotype)** determines each person's (1) cell characteristics **(karyotype),** (2) physical appearance **(phenotype),** and (3) predisposition to certain disorders.

Some disorders occur more frequently among people of certain cultures or among some families. Disorders may result from abnormalities in chromosome number or from the actions of specific genes. Research and advances in contemporary biomedical technology have enabled geneticists to identify specific chromosomes or genes or both that are responsible for the development of certain hereditary disorders. Client history and contemporary diagnostic procedures (1) permit prenatal identification of parental genetic characteristics that are associated with the transmission of some inherited disorders; (2) facilitate estimation of the statistical risk of transmission; and (3) allow couples to make informed decisions about reproduction.

Patterns of Inheritance: Common Hereditary Disorders

Normal mitosis and meiosis are shown in Figure 5-1. Errors that occur during either process of cellular division result in chromosomal abnormalities. Errors in chromosome number or structure may occur in au-

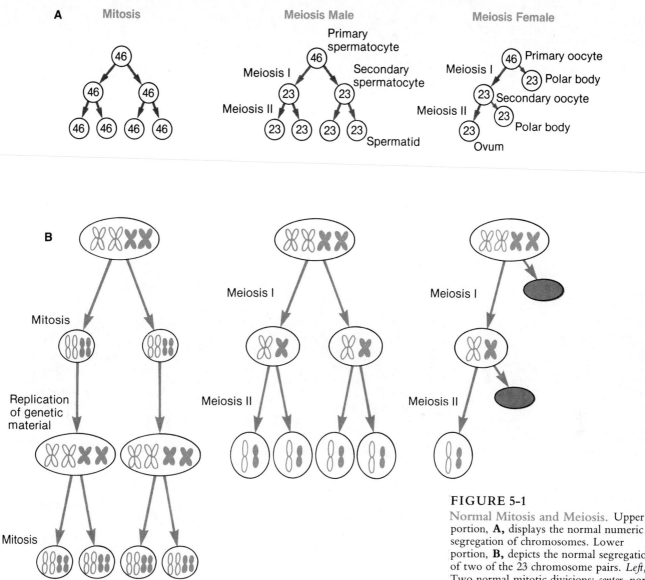

A Mitosis Meiosis Male Meiosis Female

Primary spermatocyte

Meiosis I Secondary spermatocyte

Meiosis I Primary oocyte

Polar body

Secondary oocyte

Meiosis II Polar body

Meiosis II Spermatid

Ovum

B Mitosis

Replication of genetic material

Mitosis

Meiosis I

Meiosis II

Meiosis I

Meiosis II

FIGURE 5-1

Normal Mitosis and Meiosis. Upper portion, **A,** displays the normal numeric segregation of chromosomes. Lower portion, **B,** depicts the normal segregation of two of the 23 chromosome pairs. *Left,* Two normal mitotic divisions; *center,* normal meiosis in the male; *right,* normal meiosis in the female. The nucleus of a normal human cell contains 46 chromosomes (22 pairs of autosomes and one pair of sex chromosomes [XX in females and XY in males]. Each chromosome is composed of DNA strands containing thousands of genes. As a result of meiosis, a mature gamete contains 23 chromosomes (one member of each chromosome pair) and one sex chromosome (an X in the ova; either an X or a Y in the sperm). At fertilization one member of each chromosome pair is inherited from each parent, restoring the normal number of 46 chromosomes.

tosomes or sex chromosomes or both and are responsible for many congenital disorders. Table 5-1 presents characteristic findings and health problems commonly associated with selected chromosomal abnormalities.

Numeric Chromosomal Errors: Aneuploidy

Aneuploidy, an abnormal number of chromosomes, is probably the most common chromosomal abnormality seen in clinical practice.[2] When there is an extra chromosome in each cell, the disorder is known as a **trisomy.** When a chromosome is missing in each cell, the disorder is termed a **monosomy.** These disorders may originate at conception because the egg or the sperm had an abnormal chromosome number, or they may occur after fertilization as the result of misdivision of the chromosomes during mitosis. Numeric abnormalities occur as results of nondisjunction, anaphase lag, and polyploidy.

TABLE 5-1

Selected Chromosomal Abnormalities

Genotype	Synonym	Assessment Findings	Associated Health Problems
Autosomal Aneuploidy			
Trisomy 21	Down's syndrome	Broad, short skull Flat facial profile Slanted, palpebral fissures	Varying degrees of mental retardation (average IQ: 25-50; may be higher in some)
		Brushfield spots in iris Flat, low-set ears Protruding tongue Broad, short neck Short, broad hands with transverse mid-palmar simian crease Hypotonia Poor Moro reflex Joint hyperflexibility	Higher incidence of congenital heart disease At high risk for infectious diseases At high risk for acute childhood leukemia
Mosaicism 21	Down's syndrome	Same as above	Normal intelligence Other problems as described above
Trisomy 18	Edwards' syndrome	Ears: low set, malformed Jaw: micrognathia (underdeveloped) Hand: clenched fist with fingers 2 and 5 overlapping fingers 3 and 4 Congenital heart defects Feet: rocker-bottom	Profound mental retardation Death usually within 2 to 3 months of birth
Trisomy 13	Patau's syndrome	Head: microcephalic (small; closed suture lines; closed fontanels) Microphthalmia (very small eyeballs) Cleft lip Malformed ears Polydactyly (extra digits) Congenital heart defects Urogenital defects Polycystic kidneys	Profound mental retardation Early demise (50% die within first year)
Sex Chromosome Aneuploidy			
45,XO monosomy	Turner's syndrome	Congenital lymphedema Webbed neck Short stature beginning in childhood Cubitus valgus (short carrying angle at elbow) Low hairline Streak ovaries Normal intelligence	Amenorrhea Always infertile
47,XXY	Klinefelter's syndrome	Long limbs with longer lower extremities Tall, slim stature Gynecomastia Small, soft testes or cryptorchidism Small penis	Diagnosis less likely until puberty Lack of virilization at puberty Sterile Tendency to mental retardation
Chromosomal Structure Abnormality			
Deletion of short arm of chromosome 5	Cri-du-chat (cat's-cry) syndrome	Mewing cry caused by laryngeal maldevelopment Microcephaly Eyes: Hypertelorism (abnormal width between the eyes); prominent epicanthal folds Jaw: micrognathia Low birthweight Hypotonia	Mental retardation Failure to thrive Early demise

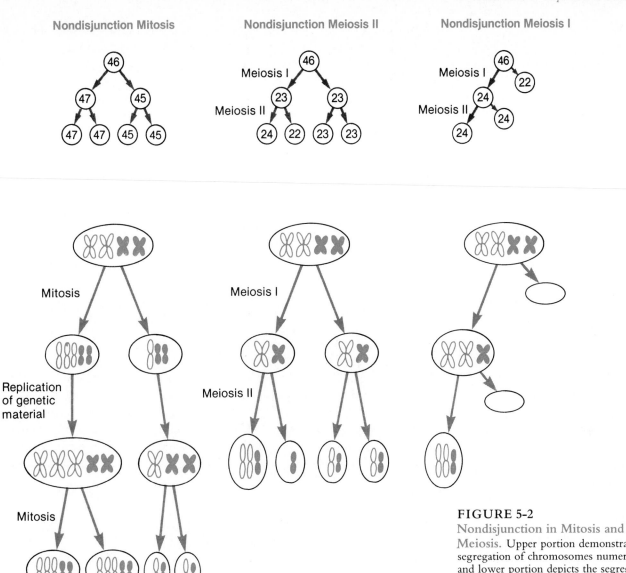

FIGURE 5-2

Nondisjunction in Mitosis and Meiosis. Upper portion demonstrates the segregation of chromosomes numerically, and lower portion depicts the segregation of two of the 23 chromosome pairs. *Left,* Mitosis, two mitotic divisions, with nondisjunction occurring in the first and the error passed through the subsequent division; *center,* meiosis in the male, with nondisjunction occurring in the second division of meiosis, resulting in normal and abnormal spermatids; *right,* meiosis in the female, with nondisjunction occurring in the first division of meiosis, resulting in an abnormal ovum.

NONDISJUNCTION. Nondisjunction is responsible for the majority of chromosomal number abnormalities. If during cellular division a pair of chromosomes fails to separate, one daughter cell will contain both chromosomes, whereas the other has none. Although it is more common during meiosis, nondisjunction also may occur during mitosis. Figures 5-1 and 5-2 allow comparison of normal mitotic and meiotic cellular division with that which occurs in nondisjunction.

ANAPHASE LAG. During anaphase one chromosome of a pair fails to move as rapidly as its sister chromosome and is lost. Often this loss results in a mosaic cell population. In **mosaicism** one cell may have a normal chromosomal complement, i.e., be **euploid**, and one may be monosomic, e.g., 45XO/46XX mosaicism.[3] Mosaicism occurs frequently in a disorder known as Turner's syndrome.[4]

POLYPLOIDY. In polyploidy the cells contain two or more times the normal number of chromosomes, e.g., the triploid number of chromosomes (69). Polyploidy is rare and most commonly results in spontaneous abortion.

Frequency of Occurrence

The frequency of numeric chromosomal errors in human conceptions is high; however, the vast majority of these pregnancies end in spontaneous abortion. In an estimated 61.5% of first trimester spontaneous abortions, there is an abnormal number of chromosomes.[2] Autosomal trisomies and polyploidy are the most common numeric abnormalities detected in abortuses. Trisomies have been found in 52% of abortuses.[5]

Numerous studies have found that trisomy 21 (Down's syndrome) is the most common chromosomal aneuploidy among liveborn humans. However, balanced reciprocal **translocations** occur with approximately the same frequency.[2] Table 5-2 presents data describing the incidence of selected chromosomal abnormalities in newborns.

DOWN'S SYNDROME. An extra chromosome 21 is present in 94% of Down's syndrome infants. Approximately 4% have translocations involving chromosomes 21 and 14 (most common), 15 (less common), or 13 (rare); (2) chromosomes 21 and 22; or (3) the homologous chromosome 21. Approximately 25% of translocations are familial. The distal portions of the long arm on chromosome 21 appear responsible for the syndrome.[6]

AGE FACTOR. The frequency of meiotic nondisjunction resulting in trisomic conceptions increases with maternal age. Table 5-3 illustrates the significant increase in risk of giving birth to a Down's syndrome (trisomy 21) infant with advancing maternal age. **Amniocentesis** to detect Down's syndrome is recommended strongly for women more than 30 years of age.[7]

In addition, in 25% of cases the male parent is the source of the additional chromosome. This suggests that by the fourth decade of life paternal age also may be a significant factor in the conception of a Down's syndrome child.[2]

TABLE 5-2

Incidence of Selected Chromosomal Abnormalities in Newborns

Type	Incidence: Live Births
Sex Chromosome	
Females	
45,XO (Turner's syndrome)	1:10,000
47,XXX	1:950
Males	
47,XXY (Klinefelter's syndrome)	1:1000
47,XYY	1:1000
Autosome	
Trisomies	
Trisomy 13 (Patau's syndrome)	1:20,000
Trisomy 18 (Edwards' syndrome)	1:8000
Trisomy 21 (Down's syndrome)	1:8000 = 1000

Adapted from Jones O: Basic genetics and patterns of inheritance. In Creasy R, Resnik R (eds): Maternal-Fetal Medicine: Principles and Practice, 2nd ed. Philadelphia, WB Saunders, 1989.

TABLE 5-3

*Incidence of Down's Syndrome Births
Related to Maternal Age*

Age	Ratio	Age	Ratio
30	1:885	38	1:176
31	1:826	39	1:139
32	1:725	40	1:109
33	1:592	41	1:85
34	1:465	42	1:67
35	1:365	43	1:53
36	1:287	44	1:41
37	1:225	45	1:32

Adapted from Hook E, Lindsje A: Down syndrome in live births by single year maternal age interval in a Swedish study: Comparison with results from a New York State study. In Creasy R, Resnik R (eds): Maternal-Fetal Medicine: Principles and Practice, 2nd ed. Philadelphia, WB Saunders, 1989.

Sex Chromosome Aneuploidy

The presence or absence of a Y chromosome determines the sex of humans. An increased number of either the X or the Y chromosome increases the probability of anatomic anomalies and mental retardation. Turner's and Klinefelter's syndromes are due to an abnormal number of sex chromosomes (see Table 5-1).

Chromosomal Structure Abnormalities

Abnormalities of chromosomal structure occur as a result of breakage and reunion of chromosomes. The exchange of material between chromosomes of different pairs is known as **reciprocal translocation** (Fig. 5-3). If all genetic material is retained, the individual is unaffected but is a **balanced carrier** of the rearrangement. The majority of balanced structural rearrangements are familial.

Balanced carriers may experience reproductive problems caused by the conception of pregnancies with an unbalanced chromosomal complement (Fig. 5-4). The particular combination of deleted or duplicated chromosomal segments in the zygote may result in either spontaneous abortion or the birth of an infant with serious physical or mental defects or both. For example, deletion of the short arm of chromosome 5 results in an infant born with cri-du-chat (cat's cry) syndrome (see Table 5-1).

Inversions form another chromosomal structure alteration. Inversions reduce pairing between homologous chromosomes. Gametes formed with abnormal chromosomes may be monosomic for one portion of the chromosome and trisomic for another portion.[2]

Mendelian Disorders

A large number of genetic disorders follow the inheritance patterns described by Mendel (i.e., dominant gene, recessive gene, X-linked gene).

FIGURE 5-3

Mechanism of Reciprocal Translocation. *I*, Two normal chromosome pairs. *II*, Breakage of one member of each pair. *III*, Exchange of broken segments. *IV*, Reunion to form a balanced rearrangement (translocation). The majority of balanced structural rearrangements are familial. Translocations involving chromosome 21 may result in children born with Down's syndrome. Because a balanced translocation can be transmitted from one generation to another, a family history of Down's syndrome should be investigated. Chromosomal analysis of the affected child will indicate whether the abnormality is due to nondisjunction or is secondary to a familial translocation.

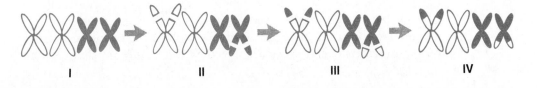

I II III IV

Chromosomes
of translocation
carrier parent

Possible
gametes

Chromosome
constitution of
resulting conception

Normal
gametes

Normal parental
chromosomes

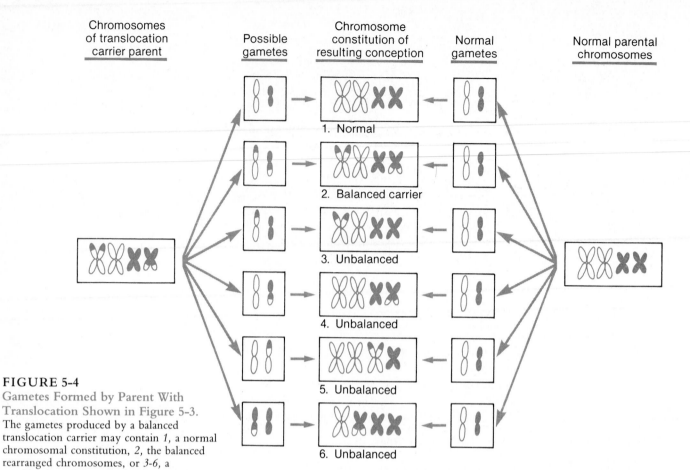

1. Normal

2. Balanced carrier

3. Unbalanced

4. Unbalanced

5. Unbalanced

6. Unbalanced

FIGURE 5-4
Gametes Formed by Parent With Translocation Shown in Figure 5-3. The gametes produced by a balanced translocation carrier may contain *1,* a normal chromosomal constitution, *2,* the balanced rearranged chromosomes, or *3-6,* a combination of the two chromosome pairs. The conceptions formed by union with the gamete of a normal parent are depicted in the center column.

The mathematical probabilities for the offspring of various matings can be calculated by use of the Punnett square (Fig. 5-5).

Dominant disorders are those in which the presence of a single abnormal gene causes important phenotypic changes or disease, even when the other member of the pair is normal. When a **heterozygous** (Aa) parent has a dominant disorder, the probability that he or she will contribute the abnormal member of the gene pair to a fetus is 1:2, or 50%.

Because the **penetrance** and **expressivity** of some dominant genes vary greatly, the diagnosis of a parental disorder often is made only after the birth of an affected child. If a gene is fully penetrant, the phenotype is always expressed. However, in some disorders penetrance may be only 80%, and there is a 20% chance that the gene will not be expressed in the usual identifiable manner. **Variable expressivity** frequently is seen in families with autosomal dominant traits; the range of abnormality expressed may vary from minor to severe.

Recessive disorders are those in which both members of the gene pair are abnormal. When only one member of the pair is abnormal, the individual is unaffected but is heterozygous for the gene. Figure 5-6 illustrates the estimated probabilities for transmission to the offspring as 1:2:1.

Anyone may carry recessive genes for several rare disorders. Although these genes may be passed from generation to generation, the likelihood that a carrier will reproduce with another carrier of the same rare gene is quite low. In some instances both members of the couple are carriers of the same abnormal gene because they are closely related (consanguinity).

Autosomal probabilities

FIGURE 5-5
Mendelian Genotypes: Punnet Square Probabilities

Sex-Linked Probabilities

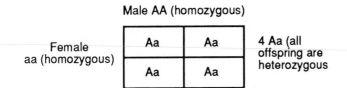

Male AA (homozygous)

Female aa (homozygous)

Aa	Aa
Aa	Aa

4 Aa (all offspring are heterozygous

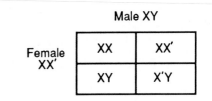

Male XY

Female XX'

XX	XX'
XY	X'Y

All offspring of this union (1) are heterozygous, (2) display the characteristics of the dominant gene (A), and (3) carry the recessive gene (a).

Two offspring are female; one will be normal (XX), and one is a carrier of the X-linked trait like her mother (XX'). Two offspring are male; one is normal (XY), and one is afflicted with the X-linked disorder (X'Y).

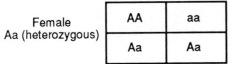

Male Aa (heterozygous)

Female Aa (heterozygous)

AA	aa
Aa	Aa

One child of this union is homozygous (AA) for the dominant gene. One child is homozygous (aa) and displays the recessive gene trait. Two children are carriers (Aa), and three of the four offspring display the characteristics of the dominant gene (A).

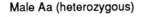

Male AA (homozygous)

Female Aa (heterozygous)

AA	AA
Aa	Aa

Male X'Y

Female XX

X'X	X'X
XY	XY

Two offspring are female; both carry the recessive gene (X') but are unaffected. Both male offspring are normal. Carrier males transmit X-linked traits to their daughters but not to their sons.

Two offspring of this union are homozygous dominant (AA). Two are heterozygous (Aa) and carry the recessive gene. All four display the traits of the dominant gene (A).

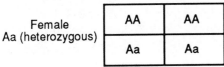

Male Aa (heterozygous)

Female aa (homozygous)

Aa	aa
Aa	aa

Male X'Y

Female X'X

X'X'	X'X
X'Y	XY

Two offspring of this union are female; both carry the recessive gene (X'), but only one is afflicted (X'X'). Only one of the two males is afflicted.

Two offspring of this union (1) are heterozygous (Aa), (2) display the dominant trait (A), and (3) are carriers of the recessive gene (a). Two offspring are homozygous (aa) and display the recessive trait.

FIGURE 5-6

Recessive Inheritance. (*A*, normal gene; *a*, abnormal gene; *AA*, normal genotype; *Aa*, carrier; *aa*, disease.) Note that the frequency of *aa* children when both parents are *Aa* carriers is 1:4, or 25%.

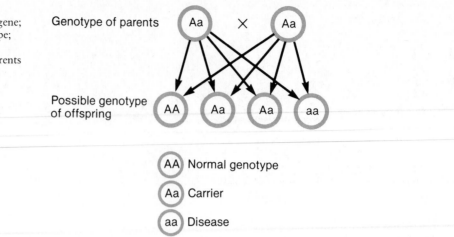

AUTOSOMAL DOMINANT DISORDERS. Traits controlled by dominant genes are expressed in both **homozygous** and heterozygous individuals; both exhibit the same characteristic, and all offspring share that same characteristic. Principal characteristics and examples of congenital disorders resulting from autosomal dominant traits are listed in the display below.

Codominance. Individuals who are heterozygous for two dominant traits express both traits. An example of codominance is the blood type AB. In this instance the expression of blood type is controlled by a single gene; therefore, if the gene for type A has been received from one parent and the gene for type B from the other, the offspring shows both parental traits.

AUTOSOMAL RECESSIVE DISORDERS. Traits controlled by recessive genes are expressed only when the person is homozygous for that characteristic, i.e., inherited the identical gene from both parents. Inborn errors of metabolism are inherited most commonly as autosomal recessive disorders; often they threaten survival and are associated with a high risk for

---

Principal Characteristics of Autosomal Dominant Traits

Every affected child (except mutations) has at least one affected parent.
An affected person need only be heterozygous for the given allele.
There is a 50% probability of transmission to each offspring.
There is father-to-son transmission.
Male and female offspring are affected equally.
Expression of the gene rarely skips a generation; there are affected individuals
    in several generations.
Examples of autosomal dominant inherited disorders:
    Achondroplastic dwarfism
    Apert's syndrome
    Crouzon's disease
    Hereditary spherocytosis
    Huntington's chorea
    Marfan's syndrome
    Osteogenesis imperfecta
    Treacher Collins' syndrome

Adapted from Jones O: Basic genetics and patterns of inheritance. In Creasy R, Resnik R (eds): Maternal-Fetal Medicine: Principles and Practice, 2nd ed. Philadelphia, WB Saunders, 1989.

Principal Characteristics of Autosomal Recessive Traits

Both parents must carry at least one mutant gene (phenotypically normal parents are carriers).

Trait is more common in consanguinous couples (parents are close blood relatives, e.g., first cousins).

Every affected individual is homozygous.

Trait is not expressed in persons possessing a single mutant gene.

Both males and females may be affected.

There is a 25% risk of involvement of the siblings of an affected individual.

The disease tends to be more severe than those resulting from autosomal dominant disorders.

Examples of autosomal recessive disorders:
Albinism
Cystic fibrosis
Galactosemia
Microcephaly
Phenylketonuria
Sickle cell anemia
Tay-Sachs disease
Thalassemia

Adapted from Jones O: Basic genetics and patterns of inheritance. In Creasy R, Resnik R (eds): Maternal-Fetal Medicine: Principles and Practice, 2nd ed. Philadelphia, WB Saunders, 1989; and Waechter E et al: Nursing Care of Children, 10th ed. Philadelphia, JB Lippincott, 1985.

permanent brain damage.[7] Principal characteristics of and examples of congenital disorders caused by autosomal recessive traits are listed in the display above.

X-LINKED DISORDERS. Because genes located on the sex chromosomes are not distributed equally to males and females, some inherited traits are unique to one gender, i.e., common either to males or to females. Most commonly, sex-linked traits are carried on the X chromosome. Males are considered **hemizygous** (possessing only one of the abnormal gene pair). Females may be either heterozygous or homozygous for the abnormal gene.[3]

  X-linked dominant disorders are nearly twice as common as in males. However, because heterozygous females also have a normal gene, the effects of X-linked dominant traits are more severe in males. Principal characteristics and representative examples of X-linked dominant disorders are listed below.

Principal Characteristics of X-Linked Dominant Traits

Affected individuals are more commonly female.

Heterozygous females will transmit the abnormal gene to 50% of both daughters and sons.

Homozygous females will transmit the abnormal gene to all offspring.

All males with the affected gene will manifest the disorder.

Affected males transmit the abnormal gene to all daughters but not to their sons.

Examples of X-linked dominant disorders:
Vitamin D-resistant rickets (hypophosphatemia)
Blood group X

From Creasy R, Resnik R (eds): Maternal-Fetal Medicine: Principles and Practice, 2nd ed. Philadelphia, WB Saunders, 1989.

Principal Characteristics of X-Linked Recessive Traits

Affected individuals are most commonly male.

An affected male transmits the abnormal gene to all daughters but not to his sons.

The trait is transmitted through carrier females to 50% of their sons.

Examples of X-linked recessive disorders:

Color blindness

Duchenne's muscular dystrophy

Glucose-6-phosphate dehydrogenase deficiency

Hemophilia A and B

Kinky-hair syndrome

Adapted from Polin R, Mennuti M: Genetic disease and chromosome abnormalities. In Fanaroff A, Martin R: Neonatal-Perinatal Medicine, 4th ed. St. Louis, CV Mosby Co, 1987; and Waechter E, et al: Nursing Care of Children, 10th ed. Philadelphia, JB Lippincott, 1985.

Among **X-linked recessive disorders** hemophilia is the most well-known. All daughters of affected fathers will be carriers of the trait but are phenotypically normal; there is a 50% probability that their sons will receive the abnormal gene. Principal characteristics and examples of X-linked recessive disorders are listed above.

Fragile-X syndrome is a relatively recent discovery.[8] It is one of the most common causes of mental retardation in males.[4]

LETHAL ALLELES. Lethal alleles cause fetal death during the prenatal period; dominant lethal alleles theoretically result in spontaneous abortion. **Sublethal alleles** have a late onset (disease occurs in infancy or childhood). Tay-Sachs disease, Duchenne's muscular dystrophy, and cystic fibrosis reflect the late-onset impact of sublethal genes.[1]

Multifactorial Disorders

Many of the most common congenital abnormalities are multifactorial in origin, i.e., due to a combination of genetic and environmental factors. Most often they are single defects such as cleft lip, cleft palate, pyloric stenosis, congenital heart disease, or neural tube defects, e.g., anencephaly, myelomeningocele. The first trimester is the period of greatest hazard to the developing embryo/fetus. Each organ system has a critical period of development, and congenital malformations often reflect the gestational week of exposure to teratogenic agents (Table 5-4). Teratogenic agents include drugs, toxic chemicals, radiation, and viral infections.[9]

TABLE 5-4

Selected Congenital Malformations Associated With Gestational Week of Environmental Insult

Malformation	Gestational Week
Anencephaly	3-4
Myelomeningocele	4
Esophageal atresia and tracheoesophageal fistula	4
Transposition of the great vessels	5
Ventricular septal defect	5-6
Cleft lip	5-7
Cleft palate	8-12
Omphalocele	10
Hypospadias	12

Adapted from Polin R, Mennutti M: Genetic disease and chromosomal abnormalities. In Fanaroff A, Martin R (eds): Neonatal-Perinatal Medicine. St. Louis: CV Mosby, 1987.

TABLE 5-5

Common Multifactorial Defects

Cleft Lip	Cleft Palate	Neural Tube Defects
Incidence: varies among ethnic groups 　Caucasians　　　　1:1000 　Blacks　　　　　　0.4:1000 　Japanese　　　　　1.7:1000 60%–80% occur in males	Incidence: 1:2500 　Little variation among ethnic 　　groups 　More common in females	Incidence: varies geographically and 　among ethnic groups 　British Isles　　　4.5–5:1000 　Ireland, Scotland,　7–7.8:1000 　　Wales 　United States　　　1.5–2:1000 Lower incidence in blacks and 　Orientals

Adapted from Creasy R, Resnik R (eds): Maternal-Fetal Medicine: Principles and Practice, 2nd ed. Philadelphia, WB Saunders, 1989, pp 57-58.

The occurrence risks in close relatives are based on studies of families in which the defect has occurred. The risk for siblings is 2% to 7% and increases with each affected child.[2] The risk to other close relatives, e.g., nieces, nephews, first cousins, although low, often is higher than that for the general population.[10]

SINGLE DEFECTS. Cleft lip or cleft palate or both may be (1) caused by a single gene, (2) associated with a numeric chromosomal abnormality, e.g., trisomy 13, or (3) related to a teratogenic agent such as thalidomide. Table 5-5 compares the incidence of cleft lip, cleft palate, and neural tube defects.

NEURAL TUBE DEFECTS. Neural tube defects (NTDs) occur during early fetal development because of a failure of fusion or a disruption of the neural tube that later forms the central nervous system. Although they may be associated with chromosomal abnormalities or certain recessive disorders, the majority of NTDs are multifactorial in origin. NTDs and cardiac abnormalities are the major congenital malformations occurring in the United States.

NTDs are described according to their location and anatomic structure. Considerable variability in expression occurs. NTDs may range from a lumbar meningocele with little or no neurologic impairment to anencephaly.[7] **Anencephaly,** a failure of development of the brain and skull, is the most severe NTD and is incompatible with survival. **Myelomeningocele** (spina bifida), a defect in formation of the spinal cord, surrounding tissues, and spinal column, is another common NTD.

Genetic Counseling

Genetic counseling is a communication process that deals with the human problems associated with either the occurrence or the risk of a genetic disorder. Counseling enables clients to make informed decisions about the possibility of genetic disease in the present family or the probability of genetic disease in future descendants. These decisions may involve selecting from reproductive options, e.g., sterilization or childless marriage, adoption or donor insemination, or termination of an existing pregnancy, i.e., abortion of an affected fetus.

Reasons for Seeking Genetic Counseling

A genetic problem has affected more than one individual in the family.

A child with a previously diagnosed congenital defect or group of malformations has been born in the family.

A child with a suspected genetic condition has been diagnosed within a family.

A family has one or more children who are mentally retarded.

A child has delayed physical or mental developmental milestones.

An individual has a birth defect that has been previously undiagnosed.

The individual or family is concerned that some environmental agent, e.g., drugs, pesticides, x-ray treatment, may cause abnormalities in the offspring.

Closely related couples want to know their risk of having a child with a birth defect.

Adapted from Waechter E, et al: Nursing Care of Children, 10th ed. Philadelphia, JB Lippincott, 1985.

Under ideal circumstances potential parents would seek the information needed for informed decision making before pregnancy. Often, however, affected couples are unaware of their potential for transmitting genetic defects. Most commonly they seek genetic counseling only after the birth of a child with congenital anomalies. Common reasons that couples seek genetic counseling are listed above.

Any pregnancy has a 2% to 3% chance of resulting in a child born with a defect or congenital malformation[6]; however, the vast majority of these defects will not be detected by contemporary methods of prenatal diagnosis.

Nursing Role

The nursing role in caring for clients at risk for producing offspring with genetic disorders includes (1) identifying at-risk clients, (2) referring clients for genetic screening and counseling, (3) enabling clients to make informed decisions about reproductive options, (4) assisting clients to cope effectively with the diagnosis of a genetic disorder in themselves or their children or both, and (5) safeguarding the client's right to privacy.

Frequently nurses are involved in the initial client contact, assessing clients for referral and taking family histories. Nurses provide preliminary counseling and coordinate appointments with physicians for evaluation and extended counseling. Often nurses are responsible for explaining or clarifying the diagnostic actions recommended, e.g., testing procedures or the results and implications of the findings. Nurses are able to evaluate the clients' understanding of information presented and their responses. They work with the client during the decision-making process and identify resources for implementation of their decisions. Throughout the counseling process the nurse-client rapport and relationship allow the nurse to serve as a client advocate.

Assessment

Identification of At-Risk Clients

All potential childbearing families are assessed for a history of risk of common genetic disorders because (1) some disorders occur more frequently among people of certain ethnic ancestry (see Cultural Implications); (2) other disorders tend to be familial; and (3) maternal age is a factor in Down's syndrome. A brief screening questionnaire may be used effectively to identify clients or couples who might benefit from more extensive genetic screening and counseling. The assessment tool presents a sample of important questions.

HISTORY. During the inital interview with clients seeking genetic counseling, any factors that may alter the approach to counseling should be identified. Questions regarding how and by whom the referral was made, e.g., physician, nurse, friend, family member, or self-referral because of knowledge available to the public, may elicit information that assists the nurse in assessing the client's current level of knowledge and anxiety. The client's response to the referral and her perception of prenatal diagnosis also are assessed.

FACTORS SURROUNDING A CURRENT PREGNANCY. The current gestational status, i.e., number of weeks elapsed since conception, is estimated,

---

CULTURAL IMPLICATIONS

Some ethnic groups are at higher risk for the transmission of certain congenital disorders than are other members of the general population.

Hereditary Disorder	Ethnic Group At Risk
Tay-Sachs disease: a fatal, autosomal recessive disorder with late onset (infancy or early childhood); causes blindness, mental retardation, and death by age 3 or 4	Eastern European (Ashkenazi) Jews; if Jewish clients are uncertain whether or not they are of Ashkenazic or Sephardic descent, genetic screening should be offered
Hemoglobinopathies	
Thalassemias: a group of hereditary anemias of varying severity α-Thalassemia: caused by mutation or deletion of gene controlling α-hemoglobin production; one form causes fatal fetal hydrops syndrome	Occur in all ethnic groups, but some subtypes are more common among some cultures Highest risk: people of Southeast Asian descent, e.g., Vietnamese, Cambodians, Laotians; also common in Africans and Filipinos
β-Thalassemia major: causes severe, transfusion-dependent anemia, marked disturbances of growth and development, and early death from congestive heart failure	Individuals whose ancestors came from lands bordering the Mediterranean sea, e.g., Greece, Italy Note: Recently this disorder has been recognized in persons of African origin and from parts of India and Pakistan, the Middle East (e.g., Iran), mainland China, and Southeast Asia.
β-Thalassemia minor: characterized by mild, microcytic anemia that may become more severe during pregnancy	Same populations as above
Sickle cell anemia: an autosomal co-dominant disorder; causes painful crises; requires close supervision of client during pregnancy and may require transfusions; carriers have one normal gene for HbA and one gene for HbS	Persons of African descent
Hereditary spherocytosis: an autosomal dominant disorder; chronic hemolysis-related anemia; may cause occasional crisis similar to that of sickle cell anemia during pregnancy; causes neonatal jaundice that may require transfusion or splenectomy or both	Uncommon but occurs in all ethnic groups; most common genetic hemolytic disorder in Caucasian descendants of Northern Europeans

Adapted from Creasy R, Resnik R, (eds): Maternal-Fetal Medicine: Principles and Practice, 2nd ed. Philadelphia, WB Saunders, 1989.

ASSESSMENT
TOOL

Screening Questionnaire to Identify Candidates for Prenatal Diagnosis

	YES	NO
1. Will you be age 35 or older when this baby is due?	___	___

2. Have you, the baby's father, or anyone in either of your
   families ever had:

	YES	NO
a. Down's syndrome or mongolism?	___	___
b. Spina bifida or myelomeningocele (open spine)?	___	___
c. Hemophilia?	___	___
d. Muscular dystrophy?	___	___
e. Cystic fibrosis?	___	___
3. Do you or the baby's father have a birth defect?	___	___

  If yes, who? Please describe. _____
  _____
  _____

4. Have you or the baby's father had a child born dead or   ___   ___
   alive with a birth defect not listed in question 2?
   If yes, please describe. _____
   _____
   _____

5. Do you or the baby's father have any close relatives who   ___   ___
   are mentally retarded?
   If yes, list cause if known. _____
   _____
   _____

6. Do you or the baby's father or any close relatives in   ___   ___
   either of your families have any known inherited genetic
   or chromosomal disease or birth defect not listed above?
   If yes, please describe. _____
   _____
   _____

7. Have you or the baby's father in a previous marriage had   ___   ___
   three or more spontaneous pregnancy losses?

8. Do you or the baby's father have any close relatives who   ___   ___
   are descended from Jewish people who lived in Eastern
   Europe (Ashkenazic Jews)?
   If yes, have you or the baby's father ever been   ___   ___
   screened for Tay-Sachs disease?
   If yes, please indicate who was screened and the
   results. _____
   _____
   _____

9. If the client or the baby's father is black:
   Have you or the baby's father or any close relative ever   ___   ___
   been screened for sickle cell trait and found to be
   positive?

10. If the client or the baby's father is of Mediterranean
    ancestry:
    Have you or the baby's father or any close relative ever   ___   ___
    been screened for or found to have a trait for thalassemia
    or Cooley's anemia?

11. Have you taken any medications (other than iron or   ___   ___
    multivitamins) or recreational drugs since your last
    menstrual period? (Please include prescription drugs.)
    If yes, please give name of drug and how often taken
    during this pregnancy. _____
    _____
    _____

Adapted from American College of Obstetricians and Gynecologists (ACOG): Antenatal Diagnosis of Genetic Disorders. Questionnaire for identifying couples at increased risk for offspring with genetic disorders. ACOG Tech Bull No 108. Washington, DC, ACOG, 1987, p 3.

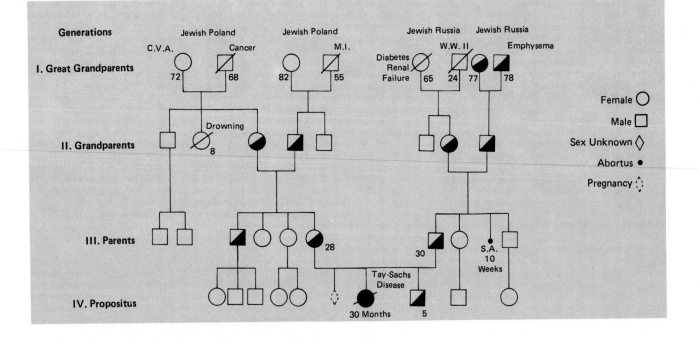

FIGURE 5-7
Sample Pedigree Demonstrating
Recessive Inheritance of Tay-Sachs
Disease and the Carrier State. Slanted
line (/) through symbol represents deceased
individual. Carriers are depicted by partially
blackened symbol. Affected individual is
depicted by totally blackened symbol.

and the couple's feelings about the pregnancy are explored. The nurse
should determine if the pregnancy was planned or if there is ambivalence
about continuing the pregnancy. Emphasis is placed on encouraging the
client or couple to verbalize their ideas and anxieties before beginning the
counseling. The clients' statements and interactions enable the nurse to
assess the accuracy of their knowledge and their expectations regarding
the counselor.

PEDIGREE. Obtaining a detailed family history enables the nurse to con-
struct a linear **(pedigree)** picture of the occurrence of the genetic defect
(Fig. 5-7). The outcome of all previous pregnancies and the health and
development of liveborn children are reviewed. A history of repeated
spontaneous abortions should be explored and any known cause noted.
The health and reproductive histories of the couple's parents, their siblings, and both sets of grandparents are explored. In addition, their ethnic
origins and any possibility of consanguinity (intrafamily parentage) are
noted.

CAUSE OF DEATH OF FAMILY MEMBERS. If a family member is deceased,
the cause and approximate age at which death occurred should be noted.
A history of a birth defect or mental retardation should alert the nurse
to explore the possibility of retrieving items such as medical records,
autopsy reports, and pictures for review.

MEDICAL RECORDS. A review of medical records may enable the nurse
or physician to determine that the health problems in previous pregnancies
or of other family members do not indicate an increased risk for the fetus.

Methods of Prenatal Diagnosis

Advantages of contemporary techniques used for intrauterine diagnosis
of fetal genetic defects are described in Table 5-6. The estimated risk of
pregnancy complications or loss is identified.

TABLE 5-6

Prenatal Diagnosis of Fetal Genetic Defects

Procedure	Advantages
Serum α-fetoprotein	High levels may indicate a fetal neural tube defect Low levels may indicate aneuploidy (e.g., Down's syndrome) Risk: essentially none
Ultrasonography (midtrimester): high-frequency sound waves are reflected off maternal and fetal organs and create characteristic echos that are translated into pictures	Determines placental site, number of fetuses and fetal location, amount and location of amniotic fluid for aspiration Identifies fetal organs, cardiac movement, renal agenesis, polycystic kidneys; dilation of cerbral ventricles (hydrocephalus); neural tube defects Permits diagnosis of multiple malformation syndromes Risk: no known risks to mother or fetus have as yet been identified
Amniocentesis (midtrimester): a 22-gauge spinal needle is used to penetrate the abdominal wall and amniotic sac to withdraw a sample of amniotic fluid for analysis	Fetal sex—cytologic examination of uncultured cells for Barr body and fluorescent Y body (the Barr body displays one less X than the fetus, i.e., a female fetus has one X in the Barr body, a male fetus has none): aids in identifying sex-related disorders Fetal karyotype: identifies abnormal chromosome number, e.g., missing or extra chromosomes, and structural abnormalities, e.g., deletions, inversions, translocations Microassays and ultramicroassays: includes the amount of α-fetoprotein for diagnosis of neural tube defects; assays enzymes, measures stored chemicals, identifies surface antigens Risk: amniocentesis-related loss is rare; most common problem is transient, self-limited spotting or minimal leakage of amniotic fluid (Simpson and Elias[6] estimate loss at <0.5%).
Chorionic villous sampling (CVS) (first trimester)	Potential for detection of the same defects as amniocentesis with the exception of neural tube defects Risk: transcervical—2%-4%; transabdominal—2%-3%
DNA analysis	Uncultured or cultured cells from amniotic fluid allow identification of α-thalassemia, β-thalassemia, and sickle cell disease
Percutaneous umbilical blood sampling: with patient viewed through use of ultrasound, a 23- or 25-gauge spinal needle is directed into the umbilical vein to withdraw a sample of fetal blood	Similar to amniocentesis but allows direct withdrawal of fetal blood samples for rapid chromosomal analysis Risk: estimated at 2%-3%

Adapted from Simpson J, Elias S: Prenatal diagnosis of genetic disorders. In Creasy R, Resnick R: Maternal-Fetal Medicine: Principles and Practice, 2nd ed. Philadelphia, WB Saunders, 1989.

MATERNAL SERUM α-FETOPROTEIN. For clients whose history indicates a risk for NTD, the peak level of serum α-fetoprotein (AFP) should be measured at 16 to 18 weeks. If the level exceeds 25 ng/ml, the physician may order ultrasonography or amniocentesis to document an open NTD.[11] Low levels of AFP may indicate fetal Down's syndrome. Amniocentesis or chorionic villous sampling is necessary to confirm the diagnosis.[12]

ULTRASONOGRAPHY. Midtrimester ultrasonography is used to visualize the fetus and contents of the amniotic sac or to enable amniocentesis, fetal skin biopsy, and fetal blood sampling (Fig. 5-8). Ultrasonography also can identify fetal structural defects.

AMNIOCENTESIS. Prenatal genetic diagnosis is most often performed when the fetus is at risk for a disorder that may be diagnosed by studying cell samples obtained by amniocentesis (Fig. 5-9). This relatively simple and safe outpatient procedure may be performed at 14 to 16 weeks of pregnancy. Centrifuging the sample of amniotic fluid separates the cells shed by the fetus. The supernatant fluid contains a number of hormones,

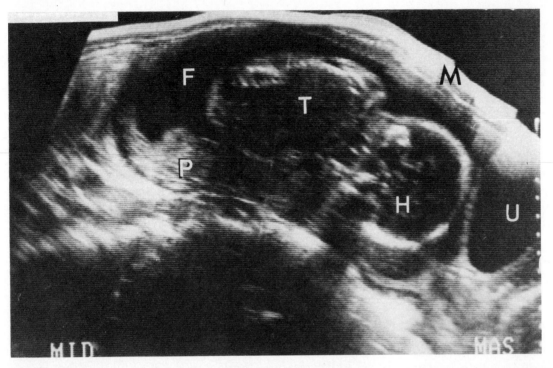

A

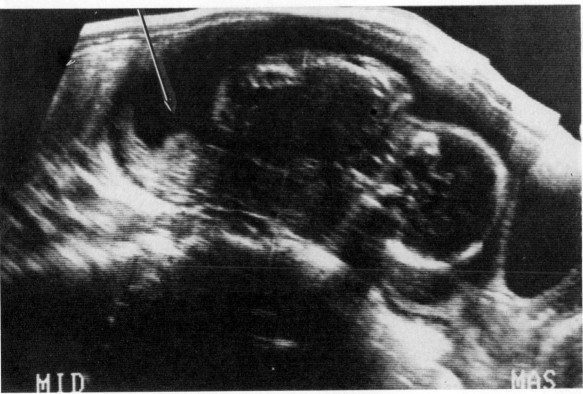

B

FIGURE 5-8

Ultrasound of Intrauterine Pregnancy. **A,** B-mode gray-scale ultrasound of intrauterine pregnancy. (*M,* Maternal abdominal wall; *H,* fetal head; *T,* fetal trunk; *P,* posterior placenta; *F,* amniotic fluid; *U,* maternal urinary bladder.) **B,** Same ultrasound. Arrow shows site selected for amniocentesis.

FIGURE 5-9
Amniocentesis. Amniotic fluid is
withdrawn for analysis by transabdominal
needle aspiration.

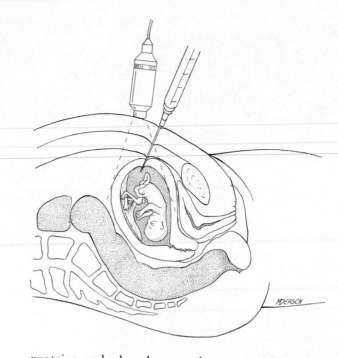

proteins, and other elements that are useful for the diagnosis of fetal status.
For example, AFP is measured for the prenatal diagnosis of NTDs. Nursing actions associated with amniocentesis are discussed in Chapter 22.

CELL CULTURE. Viable fetal cells are placed in plastic flasks or dishes
containing a nutrient medium. The temperature, pH, and atmospheric
conditions of the culture are adjusted and controlled in specially designed
incubators. After a period of time viable cells attach to the flask and begin
to multiply by mitosis. Chromosome analysis, detection of enzyme defects, and DNA isolation procedures can be performed after adequate cell
growth. The absence of a gene or the presence of a **mutant** gene may be
detected by sophisticated molecular genetic techniques.

FIGURE 5-10
Transcervical Chorionic Villous
Sampling. With the client in a lithotomy
position and under ultrasound visualization,
a small sampling catheter is introduced
through the cervix and into the placenta.
The catheter is connected to a 20- to 30-ml
syringe containing 5 ml of tissue culture
media. By negative pressure 10 to 25 mg of
chorionic villi are aspirated for analyses.

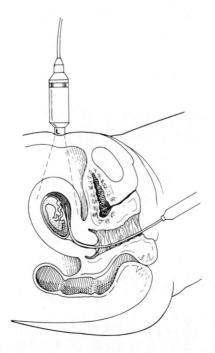

CHORIONIC VILLOUS SAMPLING. Chorionic villous sampling (CVS) is a relatively new method of prenatal diagnosis. CVS usually is performed from gestational weeks 9 to 12. Two techniques have been developed to obtain small fragments of the developing placenta for study, i.e., transcervical and transabdominal sampling (Figs. 5-10 and 5-11). The process of cell culturing is performed as described previously. With the exception of neural tube defects CVS has the potential for diagnosing the same disorders detected by amniocentesis but at an earlier point in gestation. This enables early elective termination of pregnancy; abortion at 12 to 16 weeks is safer, more rapid, and less expensive than one performed later.[13]

Nursing Diagnosis

Nursing diagnoses are used to define the focus for individualized client and family teaching and counseling. They are derived from the total data base. Representative potential nursing diagnoses for the client or a couple with a diagnosis of a genetic disorder are listed in the Potential Nursing Diagnoses below. Integrating knowledge of the implications of specific genetic disorders with an understanding of the psychosocial impact of such a diagnosis enables the nurse to (1) identify actual present nursing diagnoses, (2) project potential nursing diagnoses, (3) establish client-centered goals, (4) plan appropriate goal-directed nursing care, i.e., provide anticipatory guidance and client teaching, and (5) evaluate the effects of nursing interventions and goal attainment.

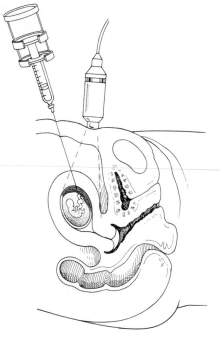

FIGURE 5-11

Transabdominal Chorionic Villous Sampling. With the patient visualized through ultrasound, a spinal needle is inserted lengthwise into the long axis of the placenta, connected to a 20- to 30-ml syringe containing culture media and heparin, and a similar sample of chorionic villi is aspirated by negative pressure. There are several variations of this technique. The transabdominal approach is indicated for women who have herpes or chronic cervicitis.

POTENTIAL NURSING DIAGNOSES

Anxiety—related to diagnostic procedures or potential findings
Knowledge Deficit—regarding diagnostic procedures, the implications of the diagnosis, options, special infant/child care, available community resources
Potential for Injury—related to testing procedures
Ineffective Individual Coping—related to the implications of diagnostic findings and personal perception of inability to parent effectively
Ineffective Family Coping: Compromised (Scapegoating)—related to the response of a significant other to the diagnosis
Decisional Conflict—related to personal values vs. the available options
Anticipatory Grieving—related to loss of the "healthy" baby
Dysfunctional Grieving—related to perceived inability to produce a "normal" child
Injury—related to testing procedures
Altered Family Processes—related to the emotional and/or financial impact of the birth of a child with a genetic defect
Family Coping: Potential for Growth—related to bonding, acceptance of the child's defect, and integration of newborn into the developing family unit.
Situational Low Self-Esteem—related to personal perception of the event, e.g., diagnosis of personal genetic disorder, birth of affected child
Parenting, Altered—related to impaired parental-infant bonding secondary to obvious congenital defects and/or feelings of inadequacy
Powerlessness—related to perceived lack of personal control over events

Focus Assessment

Examine client history, family history for risk factors associated with specific disorders (e.g., maternal age, ethnic background, previous reproductive history).

Observe for nonverbal indicators of emotional stress, e.g., irritability, inability to concentrate, withdrawal.

Determine individual teaching, learning, or referral needs regarding:
 Prognosis and implications of the specific genetic disorder.
 Methods of diagnosis.
 Advantages and disadvantages of specific diagnostic procedures, e.g., chorionic villi sampling.
 Available options and resources.

Observe family interaction.

Establish the personal meaning of the diagnosis.

Identify previous patterns of coping with crisis.

Determine current support system.

Observe response to and interaction with infant, e.g., eye contact, talking to infant, cuddling.

Note acceptance of parenting role, e.g., interest in or avoidance of infant contact, care.

Planning and Intervention

Period Before Diagnosis

Nursing interventions during the prediagnosis period are designed to reduce client anxiety, minimize client knowledge deficits, and maximize client and family potential for effective problem solving and decision making. All interviews and client teaching should be planned carefully to minimize psychologic stress and maximize nurse-client communication. An adequate amount of uninterrupted time and privacy should be provided to establish rapport and trust and to allow the client or the couple to explore and express their feelings, fears, and concerns.

Anticipatory guidance. At the time a client makes an initial appointment, the nurse may suggest that the couple attend the first session together. If a form requesting a family history will be sent in advance of the visit, the nurse should explain the purpose of the form and the information needed. Clients should be encouraged to telephone the nurse if they need further guidance in completing the form or have any questions about the interview. If a child is to be examined for evidence of a genetic defect, the nurse also should inform the family about the physical examination and any tests that will be performed during that visit.

Client teaching. In most cases prenatal counseling can be done by the nurse-counselor. Teaching content and the nursing approach are individualized to the client and the disorder, i.e., (1) instruction is based on the client's or couple's current level of knowledge, and (2) relevant information is presented in terms the client or the couple can understand. Major emphasis is placed on the fact that screening may not detect all affected individuals or all birth defects. In the most common case, i.e., advanced maternal age without significant family history, effective client counseling assists the couple to make informed decisions about prenatal testing (see Client Self-Care Education: Down's Syndrome).

During counseling it is not unusual for clients to ask for the nurse-counselor's opinion or advice about testing. Care must be taken to provide

Down's Syndrome

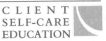

Intervention	Rationale
1. Explain basic functions of genes and chromosomes.	1. Enables client to understand subsequent teaching specific to Down's syndrome.
2. In simple terms discuss trisomy and translocation as causes of Down's syndrome.	2. Permits understanding that the underlying causes are beyond personal or professional control.
3. Describe the variation in type and degree of health problems associated with Down's syndrome.	3. Increases understanding of the personal implications.
4. Compare the risk of having a child with Down's syndrome at the client's age; contrast with the risk at other ages (see Table 5-3).	4. Personalizes the risk of conceiving a child with the defect(s).
5. Describe medical procedures involved in prenatal diagnosis (ultrasonography, amniocentesis, chorionic villous sampling).	5. Reduces anxiety about the diagnostic procedures.
6. Explain rationale, advantages, limitations, risks.	6. Enables informed decision making.
7. Discuss options available if tests identify fetal Down's syndrome, e.g., termination of pregnancy.	7. Allows client or couple to explore their own feelings before decision making.
8. If client is at risk for Rh isoimmunization, discuss RhoGam administration following anmiocentesis.	8. Minimizes risk of sensitization that might result from accidental escape of Rh-positive fetal cells into the maternal circulation.

accurate information and avoid directing a course of action. The decision to pursue prenatal diagnosis rests only with the couple; the same information may be viewed differently by each couple based on personal and cultural factors.

A minimum of several days should elapse before the couple is contacted to determine their decision. After counseling the couple needs time to discuss all the information presented, to explore their feelings about the diagnostic procedure, and to consider the potential consequences of each of the alternatives. Many factors influence the decision-making process: (1) personal and cultural values, (2) religious beliefs, (3) self-image, (4) the marital relationship, (5) individual concepts of parenthood, (6) presence and needs of other children, (7) attitudes of other family members, (8) career aspirations, (9) financial costs, and (10) other individual considerations. Both parents must be comfortable with their decision.

Evaluation of Counseling

Period Before Diagnosis

The nurse contacts the clients, answers any questions that have arisen since the interview, and requests information about their decision. If the discussion reveals a great deal of ambivalence, difficulty, or disagreement about the decision, additional counseling is offered.

PREPARATION FOR DIAGNOSTIC PROCEDURES. Before the diagnostic procedure the nurse evaluates the effects of the previous client teaching. He or she reviews and reinforces previous discussions, describes the steps in the procedure, explains sensations that the client may experience, and answers any additional questions. The nurse determines the client's or couple's understanding of the anticipated procedure and any associated risks and confirms and documents informed consent. Representative outcome criteria are listed below.

Period After Diagnosis

ASSESSMENT. When the diagnosis of a genetic disorder has been confirmed, nursing assessments are directed toward identifying the couple's response to and understanding of the diagnosis and the implications of the disorder. When the disorder is confirmed in a child, additional assessments focus on the couple's response to the diagnosis, their coping abilities, their knowledge about any special care needs, and their awareness of community resources for support and assistance.

PLANNING INTERVENTION. The nurse must anticipate the psychologic trauma to clients and families who receive a diagnosis of a genetic disorder in a current pregnancy or in a newborn or to those who must accept the probability of transmitting a genetic defect to their children. The client or couple should be encouraged to express and explore their feelings and to communicate openly with each other and with members of their support system. Providing emotional support, assistance with the grieving process, and information needed for effective problem solving are essential components of the nursing approach to helping clients cope with their personal crises.

When the diagnosis of a congenital disorder is established for a newborn, additional immediate nursing efforts are directed toward encouraging bonding and involving the parents in caring for their child. The nurse should help the client and family focus on the child rather than on the disorder.

Client teaching. The nursing objectives are to (1) minimize client anxiety, fear, and depression, (2) facilitate acceptance of the infant, (3) enable positive coping and problem solving, and (4) support a positive self-

---

Prediagnostic Nursing Evaluation: Representative Outcome Criteria

The client or couple will do the following:
1. Verbalize understanding of the personal indications for the diagnostic procedure(s).
2. Accurately identify the advantages, limitations, and risks associated with the specific diagnostic procedure(s).
3. Acknowledge awareness of the option to refuse the procedure(s).
4. Identify potential consequences of refusing the procedure(s).
5. Express her or their decision to have the procedure(s) performed.
6. Sign the permit authorizing the physician to perform the procedure.

Postdiagnostic Nursing Evaluation: Representative Outcome Criteria

The client or couple will do the following:
1. Demonstrate positive bonding behaviors (e.g., eye contact, stroking, cuddling, calling the infant by name).
2. Accurately answer questions about the disorder and its implications for care.
3. Verbalize confidence in their abilities to parent successfully.
4. Demonstrate comfort and competence in providing safe, basic, and special care for their infant.
5. Explore additional resources for support and assistance.

image. The nurse encourages the parents to participate actively in the infant's care. Discussions, demonstrations, and guided practice in performing basic and special care procedures safely and accurately assist the parents in developing competence and confidence in their abilities to meet their infant's special needs.

Anticipatory guidance. The nurse discusses expected infant behaviors and growth and developmental needs to assist parents in planning for the future. Referral to appropriate parent-support groups and special services available in the community allows the parents to gain needed assistance.

Evaluation

When the diagnosis of a genetic defect has been confirmed, nursing evaluation focuses on determining the parental response to client teaching and anticipatory guidance. Representative outcome criteria are listed above.

Legal and Ethical Issues

The ability to identify fetal genetic defects during pregnancy can provide some parents with a choice of reproductive options. However, controversy surrounds the right to decide the life of the fetus. Contemporary bioethical and legal issues associated with genetic screening and reproductive options include questions about negative eugenics and fetal rights. The quality of the child's life may be a central issue in a painful personal dilemna. For example, the potential abilities of any given child born with Down's syndrome are unknown; a child with Tay-Sachs disease faces a short life filled with pain and rapidly diminishing mental abilities. The parents' decision affects the total family and its future.

Nurses who provide care for these clients will have examined these issues also and resolved any personal and professional value conflicts that might interfere with an ethical therapeutic, nurse-client relationship. Respect and advocacy for the client's rights to make decisions based on accurate information and without coercion are central to maternity nursing practice.

REFERENCES

1. Jenkins J: Human Genetics. Menlo Park, Calif, Benjamin/Cummings, 1983
2. Jones O: Basic genetics and patterns of inheritance. In Creasy R, Resnik R (eds): Maternal-Fetal Medicine: Principles and Practice, 2nd ed. Philadelphia, WB Saunders, 1989
3. Sarto G: Genetic considerations. In Danforth D, Scott J (eds): Obstetrics and Gynecology, 5th ed. Philadelphia, JB Lippincott, 1986
4. Feingold M: Evaluating the malformed infant. In Avery G: Neonatology. Philadelphia, JB Lippincott, 1987
5. Thompson J, Thompson M: Genetics in Medicine, 4th ed. Philadelphia, WB Saunders, 1986
6. Simpson J, Elias E: Prenatal diagnosis of genetic disorders. In Creasy R, Resnik R (eds): Maternal-Fetal Medicine: Principles and Practice, 2nd ed. Philadelphia, WB Saunders, 1989
7. Cunningham F et al: William's Obstetrics, 18th ed. Norwalk, Conn, Appleton & Lange, 1989
8. Shapiro L et al: Prenatal diagnosis of fragile X chromosome. Lancet 1:99, 1982
9. Polin R, Mennutti M: Genetic disease and chromosomal abnormalities. In Fanaroff A, Martin R (eds): Neonatal-Perinatal Medicine. St. Louis, CV Mosby, 1987
10. Milunsky A: The prenatal diagnosis of neural tube and other congenital defects. In Milunsky A (ed): Genetic Disorders and the Fetus, 2nd ed. New York, Plenum Press, 1986
11. Pagana K, Pagana T: Diagnostic Testing and Nursing Implications, 2nd ed. St. Louis, CV Mosby, 1986
12. Palomaki G, Haddow J: Maternal serum alpha-fetoprotein, age, and Down's syndrome risk. Am J Obstet Gynecol 156:450, 1987
13. Mishell D: Control of human reproduction: Contraception, sterilization, and pregnancy termination. In Danforth D, Scott J (eds): Obstetrics and Gynecology, 5th ed. Philadelphia, WB Saunders, 1986

SUGGESTED READINGS

Asimov I: The genetic code. Signet Science Library. New York, New American Library, Times-Mirror, 1962

Beck F et al: Human embryology, 2nd ed. St. Louis, CV Mosby, 1985

Brock D et al: Prospective prenatal diagnosis of cystic fibrosis. Lancet 1:1175, 1985

Cohen F: Clinical genetics in nursing practice. Philadelphia, JB Lippincott, 1984

Creasy R, Resnik R (eds): Maternal-Fetal Medicine: Principles and Practice, 2nd ed. Philadelphia, WB Saunders, 1989

Cuckle H, Wald N: Maternal serum alpha-fetoprotein measurement: A screening tool for Down's syndrome. Lancet 1:926, 1984

Davis R et al: Decreased levels of amniotic fluid alpha-fetoprotein associated with Down syndrome. Am J Obstet Gynecol 185:541, November 1985

Embury S et al: Rapid prenatal diagnosis of sickle cell anemia by a new method of DNA analysis. N Engl J Med 316:656, March 12, 1987

Fibision W: The nursing role in the delivery of genetic services. Issues Health Care Women 4(1):1-15, 1983

Hodges L et al: Preventing congenital tragedy: An opportunity for nursing. Health Care Women Inf 5(4):211, 1984

Hoffman H: Anomalies of the developing central nervous system. St. Louis, CV Mosby, 1986

Hogge W, Golbus M: Antenatal diagnosis of mendelian disorders. In Sciarra J et al (eds): Gynecology and Obstetrics, Vol 3. Hagerstown, Md, Harper & Row, 1984

Jacson L: Chorionic villi sampling. Registry Newsletter, December 10, 1984

Lange I: Congenital anomalies: Detection and strategies for management. Semin Perinatol 11:151, October 1985

LaRochelle D: Prenatal genetic counseling: Ethical and legal interfaces with the nurse's role. Issues Health Care Women 4(1):77-92, 1983

Main D, Mennuti M: Neural tube defects: Issues in prenatal diagnosis and counseling. Obstet Gynecol 67:1-16, January 1986

Merkatz I et al: An association between low maternal serum alpha-fetoprotein and fetal chromosome abnormalities. Am J Obstet Gynecol 148:866, 1984

Policy statement for maternal serum alpha-fetoprotein screening program. Am J Obstet Gynecol 156:269, February 1987

Sciarra J et al (eds): Gynecology and Obstetrics, Vol 3. Hagerstown, Md, Harper & Row, 1984

Tishler C: The psychological aspects of genetic counseling. Am J Nurs 81:732, 1981

Verp M: Antenatal diagnosis of chromosome abnormalities. In Sciarra J et al (eds): Gynecology and Obstetrics, Vol 3. Hagerstown, Md, Harper & Row, 1984

Warshaw J, Hobbins J (eds): Principles and Practice of Perinatal Medicine. Maternal-Fetal and Newborn Care. Menlo Park, Calif, Addison-Wesley, 1983

Watson JD: The double helix. A personal account of the discovery of the structure of DNA. New York, New American Library, Times Mirror, 1968

Worthington S: Genetic screening. JOGN 13 (suppl):32s, March/April 1984

Infertility

IMPORTANT TERMINOLOGY

azoospermia Absence of spermatozoa in semen

anovulation Failure to produce and expel a mature ovum

coitus Vaginal intercourse

endometriosis Disorder in which ectopic endometrial tissue is found in various sites; monthly bleeding from ectopic pelvic implants can cause dense adhesions

hydrocele Accumulation of serous fluid in a saclike cavity in the testes

infertility Inability to conceive during 1 year of unprotected intercourse

luteal phase Postovulation phase of the menstrual cycle; uterine lining responds to progesterone stimulation; endometrial biopsy reveals secretory endometrium

luteal phase deficiency Inadequate production of progesterone during postovulation phase of cycle

oligospermia Sperm count of less than 20 million mature spermatozoa per milliliter

sterility Inability to achieve pregnancy because of factor(s) that cannot be altered

varicocele Enlargement of the veins in the spermatic cord

Considering the complexity of reproductive processes, it is not surprising that unprotected **coitus** during the monthly "fertile" period does not always result in a pregnancy. However, only 15% of couples experience interference with their ability to conceive.[1] Instruction about conception-promoting coital techniques, timing for coitus, or correction of minor abnormalities will enable many of these couples to conceive.

In general, after 1 year's exposure without contraception, the possibility of **infertility** should be explored. However, for some couples investigation should be initiated earlier. Because fertility declines with age, couples in their thirties would be justified in seeking advice somewhat sooner. Early evaluation also is indicated when anxiety about failure to conceive is high or when there is a history of events associated with an increased risk of infertility, e.g., amenorrhea, acute salpingitis, repeated episodes of pelvic inflammatory disease. A reassuring consultation is helpful if only to dispel fears and reduce anxiety concerning the existence of major abnormalities.

Nursing Role

The nursing role in caring for clients or couples who are concerned about inability to achieve a pregnancy includes (1) identifying clients who may benefit from counseling or infertility investigation; (2) referring clients for evaluation; (3) assisting clients to cope effectively with their fears and anxiety or with the shock, denial, anger, and depression arising from a diagnosis of infertility or **sterility;** (4) enabling clients to make informed decisions about reproductive options; and (5) protecting the client's right to privacy.

Nurses are responsible for assisting clients to become active participants in the diagnostic or treatment process and to make informed decisions. The nurse works with clients during the decision-making process and identifies resources for implementation of their decisions. Throughout the infertility investigation the nurse-client rapport and relationship allow the nurse to serve as client advocate.

Effective management of interactions with infertile couples is facilitated by clearly communicating understanding and empathy, desire, willingness, and ability to help. Nurses who provide care, emotional support, or counseling to infertile couples must be comfortable with their own sexuality. They must be able to discuss sexual behaviors and controversial treatment options objectively without embarrassment or value judgments.

Biologic Determinants of Fertility

Normal male fertility depends on the ability to produce, transport, and ejaculate a sufficient quantity of normal, mature, motile spermatozoa that are capable of penetrating and surviving in the cervical mucus, ascending through the uterine cavity into the fallopian tube, and entering the ovum. The normal process of spermatogenesis takes approximately 3 months.

Female fertility depends on the ability to produce and ovulate a healthy ovum that is captured by the tubal fimbriae and transported promptly through a patent fallopian tube. After fertilization the zygote must be transported through the fallopian tube to the uterine cavity, implanted into the uterine endometrium, and grown and developed normally.

The normal processes of gametogenesis depend on effective interaction of specific endocrine and reproductive system hormones. Infertility and sterility result from anatomic or physiologic factors or both that interfere with gametogenesis or the transport of mature gametes. In rare instances psychologic factors also may interfere with an individual's ability to achieve pregnancy. The infertile couple is considered one biologic reproductive unit; interference with normal reproductive function in either or both may cause inability to conceive. Table 6-1 summarizes common causes of infertility.

Male Factors

FAULTY SPERMATOGENESIS. Either congenital or acquired conditions may interfere with the successful production of sufficient numbers of healthy, mature, motile spermatozoa that are capable of fertilizing an ovum. **Oligospermia** is present in 25% of infertile males.[2]

TABLE 6-1

Causes of Infertility

Male Factors (%)	Female Factors (%)
Faulty spermatogenesis or transmission (30-40)	Ovulatory disorders (faulty oogenesis) (20-25) Tubal factors (25) Cervical factors (obstruction, hostile cervical mucus) (15) Other (chronic infections, debilitating diseases, severe nutritional deficiencies, age, psychologic factors) (5) Unknown (5)

Adapted from Mattox J: Infertility. In Wilson J, Carrington E: Obstetrics and Gynecology, 8th ed. St. Louis, CV Mosby, 1987.

Congenital conditions. Oligospermia may be related to the effects of a congenital **varicocele.** The dilated veins may increase local heat, decrease spermatogenesis, and reduce sperm motility. **Azoospermia** may result from (1) genetic abnormalities such as Klinefelter's syndrome, (2) undescended or hypoplastic testes, or (3) severe hypothyroidism.

Acquired conditions. Significant trauma can result in injury to testicular structures or in autoimmune formation of sperm-immobilizing antibodies.[3,4] Infection such as postpubescent orchitis, nonspecific urethritis, or chronic prostatitis can result in testicular atrophy. Previous genital surgery, e.g., herniorrhaphy, **hydrocelectomy,** may result in impaired blood supply to the testes. Excessive use of alcohol, marijuana, or nicotine can alter sperm production significantly.[2]

Inadequate sperm penetrance. Some infertile men produce sperm specimens that meet the criteria for normal fertility; however, their sperm are unable to successfully penetrate an ovum.[5]

INTERFERENCE WITH SPERM TRANSMISSION. The tubular transport system may be occluded by severe congenital hypospadias, structural abnormalities of the ejaculatory system as the result of maternal use of diethylstilbestrol (DES) during the pregnancy, or postinfection scarring of the epididymis, vas deferens, or urethra.[2] The organism most commonly implicated in tubal scarring and occlusion is *Neisseria gonorrhoeae.*

Female Factors

OVULATORY DISORDERS. Faulty oogenesis, or ovarian failure, may be due to congenital defects, endocrine disorders and tumors, and acquired conditions.

Congenital conditions. Chromosomal abnormalities associated with congenital primary ovarian failure include Turner's syndrome (karyotype 45,XO) and mosaicism (karyotype 45,XO/XX or 46,XO/XXX).

Endocrine disorders and tumors. Any disorder that affects the hypothalamic-pituitary-ovarian feedback cycle also causes anovulatory infertility.[6] Ovarian function also may be affected by hyperplasia or tumors of the adrenal cortex, hypothyroidism, tumors of the pituitary gland or hypothalamus.

Acquired conditions. Intense athletic activities have been associated with secondary amenorrhea. A high incidence of exercise-related amenorrhea has been identified among long-distance runners, joggers, and ballet dancers. Chronic infection, debilitating diseases, and severe nutritional deficiencies also may affect the feedback cycle that stimulates ovulation. A weight loss greater than 15% of total ideal body weight has been implicated in development of secondary amenorrhea, e.g., clients with severe anorexia nervosa often experience menstrual irregularities or cessation of menses.

TUBAL FACTORS. Approximately 25% of infertile women are unable to conceive a pregnancy because of partial or complete occlusion of the fallopian tubes.[2] Although congenital anomalies may affect the female tubal transport system, the most common cause of tubal occlusion is gonococcal, chlamydial, or polymicrobial salpingitis. Damage to the tubal mucosa or fimbriae and kinking or immobilization of the fallopian tubes can occur following infection. Acute appendicitis, infection related to an intrauterine device, or pelvic surgery also may increase the potential for tubal-factor infertility. Adhesions may reduce or prevent tubal motility. **Endometriosis** may result in scarring or fixation of the fallopian tubes, and ectopic endometrial implants may occlude the tubal lumen.[2]

UTERINE FACTORS. Although uterine malformations, malposition, and tumors occasionally are implicated in faulty implantation or early abortion, they rarely interfere with conception.[2] However, uterine and cervical abnormalities that interfere with conception or contribute to spontaneous abortion or premature labor have been found in women whose mothers received DES therapy during the pregnancy.

CERVICAL FACTORS. Large cervical polyps, pedunculated uterine fibroids, or cervical stenosis can interfere with the passage and ascent of spermatozoa. Alterations in cervical mucus patterns can result from hormonal deficiencies, chronic infection, or medications. Antisperm antibodies in cervical secretions have been suggested as a possible cause of infertility in some women.[2,4,7]

Assessment

Because multiple factors can impair fertility, assessment of the infertile couple must be systematic and comprehensive. The past and present health status of both partners should be explored carefully. The nurse should also assess the couple's current level of knowledge, concerns, response to referral, perception of and attitude toward infertility assessment, and any cultural or religious considerations that may influence the therapeutic relationship or compliance with recommendations. Because extensive infertility investigations involve considerable time, emotional stress, and financial expense, both partners should display interest in identification and resolution of the problem. Table 6-2 describes normal findings of selected tests commonly used for the assessment of fertility.

History

The medical and social history of both partners is explored carefully. Samples of assessment tools used in gathering historical data are presented on pages 100-104. During the initial interview the nurse validates, clarifies, and, when necessary, expands on the information provided.

TABLE 6-2

Common Tests for Assessment of Fertility

Test	Procedure	Normal Findings
Male		
Semen analysis	Fresh ejaculate is examined to determine the quantity, quality, morphology, and motility of spermatozoa.	Volume: 2-6 ml *pH:* 7-8 Viscosity: liquefaction within 30 min Sperm count: 20-250 million/ml Motility: >60% within 1 hr of collection Mobility: 3 to 4 + (quality of motility) Morphology: >60% normal sperm
Female		
Sims-Huhner (postcoital) test	Within 6 to 12 hours after intercourse a sample of mucus is aspirated from the client's endocervix and examined to identify the quality of the mucus and its ability to sustain spermatozoal life. Microscopic examination notes the presence, numbers, and motility of viable spermatozoa.	Abundant, thin, clear, spinnbarkheit; more than 12 highly motile sperm per high-power field[8]
Rubin's test	Transcervical insufflation of CO_2	Tubal patency identified by (1) kymographic reading of CO_2 pressure <150 mm Hg; (2) auscultation of the characteristic swishing sound caused by gas passing through a patent tube; (3) referred pain in the shoulder caused by gas irritation of the phrenic nerve
Endometrial biopsy	Usually the biopsy is scheduled 5 to 7 days before the expected onset of the next menses or on days 21 to 24 of a 28-day cycle. The cervix is stabilized with a surgical tenaculum, and a uterine sound inserted to determine the size of the uterus. Samples are taken from the anterior, posterior, and lateral walls by suction curette.	Ovulation confirmed by finding secretory endometrium[8]
Hysterosalpingography	Transcervical instillation of contrast media outlines and fills the uterus and the fallopian tubes.	No abnormality noted; media flows into pelvis through fimbriated ends of patent tubes
Pelvic ultrasonography	High-frequency sound waves bounce off the anatomic structures and are converted electronically into an image of the uterus and adnexa (may be abdominal or vaginal).	Reveals no abnormality
Laparoscopy	With client under general anesthesia, a sterile needle is introduced through the abdominal wall just below the umbilicus, and CO_2 under controlled pressure is passed into the abdominal cavity. The gas causes the abdominal wall to balloon out and away from the abdominal contents. The needle is removed and a trocar is inserted through the incision to aid introduction of the laparoscope.	No abnormality noted visually.

Physical Examination

Both partners should have a complete, general physical examination. Often deviations from the normal physical profile of childbearing-age clients are evident on gross inspection, e.g., excessive or low weight for height, abnormal body configuration or hair distribution. Deviations such as these suggest a need for additional exploration of the client's history and focused physical assessment.

Male Examination

Careful physical examination of the male genitalia by the primary health provider may reveal abnormalities that would explain the infertility, e.g.,

Text continued on page 104.

A S S E S S M E N T   T O O L

Husband's Medical History Form, Infertility Clinic

Name: Date:
Address: Tel.:
Occupation: Age: Religion:
Employer: Ins.:
Bus. Tel.:   Cert. No.:
Referred by: Gr. No.:
Birth Place: Name Rel./Friend:
Birth Date: Address:

All previous occupations: | List all states or countries in which you have lived:

Education: Please encircle the last   Grade   5   High School   1 2 3 4   Post Grad. _____ yrs.
             grade you completed   6   7   8   College   1 2 3 4   Degrees

CHIEF COMPLAINTS   P. I. Please do not write in this space.
Please list all symptoms you have NOW.
1. _____
2. _____
3. _____
Routine checkup—no symptoms [ ]

FAMILY HISTORY	Age	If Living Health	Age at death	If Deceased Cause	Please Encircle — Has any blood relative had		Who
Father					Cancer	no yes	
Mother					Tuberculosis	no yes	
Brother or sister 1.					Diabetes	no yes	
2.					Heart trouble	no yes	
3.					High blood pressure	no yes	
4.					Stroke	no yes	
5.					Epilepsy	no yes	
Husband or wife					Mental illness	no yes	
Son or daughter 1.					Suicide	no yes	
2.					Congenital deformities	no yes	
3.					NOTE:		
4.					This is a confidential record of your medical history and		
5.					will be kept in this office. Information contained here		
6.					will not be released to any person except when you		
7.					have authorized us to do so.		

PERSONAL HISTORY
ILLNESS: Have you had
(Please Encircle all Answers no or yes)

Measles or German measles .... no   yes
Chickenpox or mumps .... no   yes
Whooping cough .... no   yes
Scarlet fever or scarlatina .... no   yes
Pneumonia or pleurisy .... no   yes
Diphtheria or smallpox .... no   yes
Influenza .... no   yes
Rheumatic fever or heart disease   no   yes
Arthritis or rheumatism .... no   yes
Any bone or joint disease .... no   yes
Neuritis or neuralgia .... no   yes
Bursitis, sciatica or lumbago .... no   yes
Polio or meningitis .... no   yes
Bright's disease or kidney infection   no   yes

Gonorrhea or syphilis .... no   yes
Anemia or jaundice .... no   yes
Epilepsy .... no   yes
Migraine headaches .... no   yes
Tuberculosis .... no   yes
Diabetes or cancer .... no   yes
High or low blood pressure .... no   yes
Nervous breakdown .... no   yes
Food, chemical or drug poisoning   no   yes
Hay fever or asthma .... no   yes
Hives or eczema .... no   yes
Frequent colds or sore throat .... no   yes
Frequent infections or boils .... no   yes
Any other disease .... no   yes
ALLERGIES: Are you allergic to
Penicillin or sulfa .... no   yes
Aspirin, codeine or morphine .... no   yes

Mycins or other antibiotics .... no   yes
Merthiolate or mercurochrome ..... no   yes
Any other drug .... no   yes
Any foods .... no   yes
Adhesive tape .... no   yes
Nail polish or other cosmetics ...... no   yes
Tetanus antitoxin or serums .... no   yes
INJURIES: Have you had any
Broken bones .... no   yes
Sprains or dislocations .... no   yes
Lacerations (extensive) .... no   yes
Concussion or head injury .... no   yes
Ever been knocked out .... no   yes
TRANSFUSIONS: Have you ever had
Blood or plasma transfusion .... no   yes
Weight: now _____ one year ago _____
Max _____ when _____ Height _____

Please review the section you have just completed and wherever you answered "yes" fill in the year (guess if necessary) and also where there is more than one illness to a line encircle the ones you have had. Example: Chickenpox or mumps .... 1961 .... no (yes)

A S S E S S M E N T   T O O L   *(continued)*

SURGERY: Have you had

Tonsillectomy .... no   yes
Appendectomy .... no   yes
Any other operation (give details)   no   yes

Give DETAILS below of all hospitalizations for surgery or illness including name and address of Doctor and Hospital . . . .

Have you ever been advised to have any surgical operation which has not been done? [1] no   [2] yes   what ....

Systems: Please check those you have had.

Eye disease [ ], Eye injury [ ], Impaired sight [ ], Ear disease [ ], Ear injury [ ], Impaired hearing [ ],
Trouble with: Nose [ ], Sinuses [ ], Mouth [ ], Throat [ ], Have you checked any in this group? ....   no   yes
Fainting spells [ ], Loss of consciousness [ ], Convulsions [ ], Paralysis [ ], Frequent or severe headaches [ ], Dizziness [ ], Depression
or anxiety [ ], Hallucinations [ ], Have you checked any in this group? ....   no   yes
Enlarged glands [ ], Goiter or enlarged thyroid [ ], Skin disease [ ], Have you checked any in this group? ....   no   yes
Chronic or frequent cough [ ], Chest pain or angina pectoris [ ], Spitting up of blood [ ], Night sweats [ ], Shortness of breath [ ],
Palpitation or fluttering heart [ ], Swelling of hands, feet, or ankles [ ], Varicose veins [ ], Extreme tiredness or weakness [ ], Have you
checked any in this group? ....   no   yes
Kidney disease or stones [ ], Bladder disease [ ], Albumin, sugar, pus, etc. in urine [ ], Difficulty in urinating [ ], Awake to urinate
nightly [ ], Have you checked any in this group? ....   no   yes
Stomach trouble or ulcers [ ], Indigestion [ ], Liver or gallbladder disease [ ], Colitis or other bowel disease [ ] Appendicitis [ ],
Hemorrhoids or rectal bleeding [ ], Constipation or diarrhea [ ], Recent change in bowel action or stools [ ], Recent change in appetite
or eating habits [ ], Have you checked any in this group? ....   no   yes

HABITS: Do you

Sleep well? .... no   yes
Use alcoholic beverages .... no   yes
    Every day? .... no   yes
Smoke? .... no   yes
    How much? ....
Exercise enough .... no   yes
Is your diet well balanced? .... no   yes

List any drugs or medications you take regularly or frequently:

_____
_____
_____
_____
_____
_____
_____

MARITAL HISTORY

Prior marriage? ....
Was pregnancy achieved? ....

When? (Dates) ....
Any other proof of fertility? ....
....
....

Is sex entirely satisfactory? ....
Reaction of wife: ....

Estimated frequency of coitus (intercourse) per month: ....
Remarks: ....
....
....
....
....
....

INFERTILITY STUDIES

	Result	Date	Where Done
Semen analysis			
Thyroid tests:			
Hormone tests:			
Medicines given:			
Other tests:			

(Courtesy of Division of Human Reproduction, Hospital of the University of Pennsylvania, Philadelphia, PA)

A S S E S S M E N T   T O O L

Wife's Medical History Form, Infertility Clinic

Name:	Date:	Unit No.:
(Nee):	Tel.:	Husb.:
Address: Age:	Ins.:	Occupation: Age:
Occupation:	Cert. No.:	Employer
Employer:	Gr. No.:	Bus. Address:
Bus. Tel.:	Name Rel./Friend:	Bus. Tel.:
Referred by:	Address:	Religion: Husb. Wife:
Birth Place:		[ ] Single [ ] Divorced
Birth Date:		[ ] Married [ ] Widow (er)

All previous occupations: List all states or countries in which you have lived:

Education: Please encircle the last   Grade   5   High School   1 2 3 4   Post Grad. _____ yrs.
                      grade you completed   6   7   8   College   1 2 3 4   Degrees

Date of last physical exam.

P. I. Please do not write in this space.

Chief Complaints: Please list all symptoms you have NOW.
1. _____
2. _____
3. _____

Routine checkup—no symptoms [ ]

FAMILY HISTORY	Age	If Living Health	Age at death	If Deceased Cause	Please Encircle Has any blood relative had		Who
Father					Cancer	no yes	
Mother					Tuberculosis	no yes	
Brother or sister 1.					Diabetes	no yes	
2.					Heart trouble	no yes	
3.					High blood pressure	no yes	
4.					Stroke	no yes	
5.					Epilepsy	no yes	
Husband or wife					Mental illness	no yes	
Son or daughter 1.					Suicide	no yes	
2.					Congenital deformities	no yes	
3.					NOTE: This is a confidential record of your medical		
4.					history and will be kept in this office. Information contained		
5.					here will not be released to any person except when		
6.					you have authorized us to do so.		

PERSONAL HISTORY
ILLNESS: Have you had
(Please Encircle all Answers no or yes)

Measles or German measles	no	yes	Gonorrhea or syphilis	no	yes	Mycins or other antibiotics	no	yes
Chickenpox or mumps	no	yes	Anemia or jaundice	no	yes	Merthiolate or mercurochrome	no	yes
Whooping cough	no	yes	Epilepsy	no	yes	Any other drug	no	yes
Scarlet fever or scarlatina	no	yes	Migraine headaches	no	yes	Any foods	no	yes
Pneumonia or pleurisy	no	yes	Tuberculosis	no	yes	Adhesive tape	no	yes
Diphtheria or smallpox	no	yes	Diabetes or cancer	no	yes	Nail polish or other cosmetics	no	yes
Influenza	no	yes	High or low blood pressure	no	yes	Tetanus antitoxin or serums	no	yes
Rheumatic fever or heart disease	no	yes	Nervous breakdown	no	yes	INJURIES: Have you had any		
Arthritis or rheumatism	no	yes	Food, chemical or drug poisoning	no	yes	Broken bones	no	yes
Any bone or joint disease	no	yes	Hay fever or asthma	no	yes	Sprains or dislocations	no	yes
Neuritis or neuralgia	no	yes	Hives or eczema	no	yes	Lacerations (extensive)	no	yes
Bursitis, sciatica or lumbago	no	yes	Frequent colds or sore throat	no	yes	Concussion or head injury	no	yes
Polio or meningitis	no	yes	Frequent infections or boils	no	yes	Ever been knocked out	no	yes
Bright's disease or kidney infection	no	yes	Any other disease	no	yes	TRANSFUSIONS: Have you ever had		
			ALLERGIES: Are you allergic to			Blood or plasma transfusion	no	yes
			Penicillin or sulfa	no	yes	Weight: now _____ one year ago _____		
			Aspirin, codeine or morphine	no	yes	Max _____ when _____ Height _____		

Please review the section you have just completed and wherever you answered "yes" fill in the year (guess if necessary) and also where there is more than one illness to a line encircle the ones you have had.   Example: Chickenpox or mumps ....1961 .... no (yes)

(continued)

A S S E S S M E N T   T O O L   *(continued)*

SURGERY: Have you had   no   yes   Give DETAILS below of all hospitalizations for surgery or illness including name and address of
Tonsillectomy ....   Doctor and Hospital . . . .
Appendectomy ....   no   yes
Any other operation (give details)   no   yes

Have you ever been advised to have any surgical operation which has not been done? [1] no [2] yes what ....

Systems: Please check those you have had.
Eye disease [ ], Eye injury [ ], Impaired sight [ ], Ear disease [ ], Ear injury [ ], Impaired hearing [ ],
Trouble with: Nose [ ], Sinuses [ ], Mouth [ ], Throat [ ], Have you checked any in this group? ....   no   yes
Fainting spells [ ], Loss of consciousness [ ], Convulsions [ ], Paralysis [ ], Frequent or severe headaches [ ], Dizziness [ ], Depression
or anxiety [ ], Hallucinations [ ], Have you checked any in this group? ....   no   yes
Enlarged glands [ ], Goiter or enlarged thyroid [ ], Skin disease [ ], Have you checked any in this group? ....   no   yes
Chronic or frequent cough [ ], Chest pain or angina pectoris [ ], Spitting up of blood [ ], Night sweats [ ], Shortness of breath [ ],
Palpitation or fluttering heart [ ], Swelling of hands, feet, or ankles [ ], Varicose veins [ ], Extreme tiredness or weakness [ ], Have you
checked any in this group? ....   no   yes
Kidney disease or stones [ ], Bladder disease [ ], Albumin, sugar, pus, etc. in urine [ ], Difficulty in urinating [ ], Awake to urinate
nightly [ ], Have you checked any in this group? ....   no   yes
Stomach trouble or ulcers [ ], Indigestion [ ], Liver or gallbladder disease [ ], Colitis or other bowel disease [ ], Appendicitis [ ],
Hemorrhoids or rectal bleeding [ ], Constipation or diarrhea [ ], Recent change in bowel action or stools [ ], Recent change in appetite
or eating habits [ ], Have you checked any in this group? ....   no   yes

HABITS: Do you

Sleep well?	no	yes	
Use alcoholic beverages	no	yes	
Every day?	no	yes	
Smoke?	no	yes	
How much?			
Exercise enough	no	yes	
Is your diet well balanced?	no	yes	

List any drugs or medications you
take regularly or frequently:

_____
_____
_____
_____
_____

OBSTETRICAL-GYNECOLOGICAL REVIEW

Age at first menstruation _____ Age at first coital
experience ____ Number of living children (at present) _____
Number of pregnancies _____
Number of live births _____ Number of multiple
pregnancies _____
Number of stillbirths (more than 20 weeks) _____
Number of abortions, miscarriages (20 weeks or less) _____
Number of children dead _____ Age of oldest child _____
Number of births with deformities _____

GYNECOLOGICAL HISTORY

Are menstrual cycles regular? .... Are your periods similar? ....
Interval between periods ....
Length of flow .... Date of last menstrual cycle ....
Amount of flow ....[1] Light [2] Moderate [3] Heavy
Was the quality, quantity, and duration of flow for this last cycle similar in
comparison with previous cycles? ....
   [1] No (specify how it differed) ....
.... [2] Yes
Has there been any bleeding in between periods? ....
   [1] No   [2] Yes (specify) ....

Were any medications taken during cycle? ....
   [1] No   [2] Yes (specify) ....
Dysmenorrhea (menstrual discomfort) ....
   [1] None   [2] Intermittent   [3] Constant
Type of menstrual discomfort experienced
   [1] None   [3] Dull   [5] Cramp
   [2] Sharp   [4] Ache   [6] Backache

PREMENSTRUAL SYMPTOMS

Bloating	no	yes
Breast tenderness	no	yes
Pelvic pain	no	yes
Backache	no	yes
Headache	no	yes
Irritability	no	yes
Edema	no	yes
Acne	no	yes

INTERMENSTRUAL DISCHARGE

Type [1] None [3] Yellow [5] White
     [2] Tan   [4] Bloody [6] Other (specify)
Amount .... Scant Heavy

Itching	no	yes
Odorless	no	yes
Frequent	no	yes
Regular pattern	no	yes

MARITAL HISTORY

Prior marriage? .... when? (Dates) ....   Was pregnancy achieved? ....
Is sex entirely satisfactory? ....   Dyspareunia (discomfort during coitus): no .... yes ....
Estimate frequency of coitus (sexual   Does coitus occur during menses? Yes .... No ....
intercourse) per month: ....
Reaction of husband: ....   On which days of flow? ....
Remarks: ....   Is this consistent? ....
....
....

(continued)

A S S E S S M E N T   T O O L   *(continued)*

INDICATE THE INFORMATION FOR ANY OF THE FOLLOWING STUDIES WHICH YOU HAVE HAD.

	Date	Result	Doctor
Basal body temperature record:			
Biopsy test:			
Thyroid test:			
Gas (Rubin) test:			
X-ray of uterus and tubes:			
Postcoital test: (survival of seed in your secretions)			
Cautery of cervix:			
Hormone test:			
Inseminations:			
Medicines given:			
Other:			

(Courtesy of Division of Human Reproduction, Hospital of the University of Pennsylvania, Philadelphia, PA)

congenital anomalies of the penis, varicocele, undescended or hypoplastic testes, testicular atrophy. Accurate measurement of testicular size and volume with an orchidometer is an important component of the initial infertility examination.[2]

SEMEN EVALUATION. Semen analysis to determine the quantity and quality of the male partner's semen is an important component of the initial investigation. The quality of a man's semen is influenced by physical and emotional factors and by sexual activity. Thus the sperm count varies from day to day. Accurate evaluation of male fertility requires the examination of three semen specimens gathered at monthly intervals. Standards established by the World Health Organization for normal male semen analysis are listed in Table 6-2. Diminished fertility is associated with findings below the lower limits of these norms. If the specimens repeatedly demonstrate abnormalities, the male partner may be referred to a urologist for further evaluation.

Female Examination

Careful pelvic examination may identify structural abnormalities that can influence fertility, e.g., ovarian cysts, thickened adnexa from past pelvic inflammatory disease (PID), nodules along the uterosacral ligaments resulting from endometriosis, fixed retroverted uterus. If the client is a DES daughter, particular attention must be given the cervix for any signs of abnormalities. Signs of chronic cervicitis and vaginal infection are noted also. Cervical and vaginal smears may be taken and examined for signs of sexually transmitted organisms, e.g., *Chlamydia trachomatis, Trichomonas vaginalis, N. gonorrhoeae.*

Ovarian Factor Assessment

Basal Body Temperature

Determining the presence and time of ovulation is important to increasing the chances of successful fertilization. Determining the basal body temperature (BBT) is helpful, particularly in determining the time of ovulation in women who experience frequent menstrual irregularities and in identifying anovulatory menses in women who are otherwise without evidence of abnormality (Fig. 6-1).

Laboratory Tests

Assessment of reproductive status includes laboratory tests to determine body response to expected endocrine activity (see Laboratory Values for normal laboratory findings.)

Cervical Mucus Examination

The maximum effect of estrogen occurs immediately near the time of ovulation. Cervial mucus responses include decreased viscosity, ferning (Fig. 6-2), and increased alkalinity.[2] Abundant alkaline, clear, watery, elastic mucus facilitates sperm penetration and survival.

Plasma Progesterone

Plasma levels of progesterone increase significantly after ovulation following formation of the corpus luteum. Serum progesterone assays are drawn between the second day after ovulation and the onset of menses. Usually three monthly assays are drawn and evaluated to determine post-ovulation progesterone levels.

Endometrial Biopsy

The response of the uterine endometrium to progesterone can be evaluated by examining tissue samples taken during the **luteal** (postovulation) **phase** of the menstrual cycle (Fig. 6-3). Characteristic time-related cellular changes reflect normal endometrial responses to progesterone. Findings of tissue changes that are more than 2 days behind those expected suggest possible **luteal phase deficiency**.[2]

LABORATORY VALUES

Cervical mucus	Demonstrates "ferning" at time of ovulation; pH: 7.6 to 8.0
Plasma progesterone	Normal luteal phase level: >2 ng/ml
Endometrial biopsy	Histology identifies presence of "secretory endometrium"

FIGURE 6-1
Basal Body Temperature (BBT) Curves. Ovulation is indicated if the BBT curve reveals a drop of 0.4° F followed by an elevation of 0.4° to 0.8° F above the baseline that is sustained during the last 2 weeks of the cycle; the biphasic temperature curve reveals the thermogenic effects of progesterone. If the thermal rise is present for less than 10 days, luteal phase deficiency (inadequate progesterone secretion) is suspected.[9]

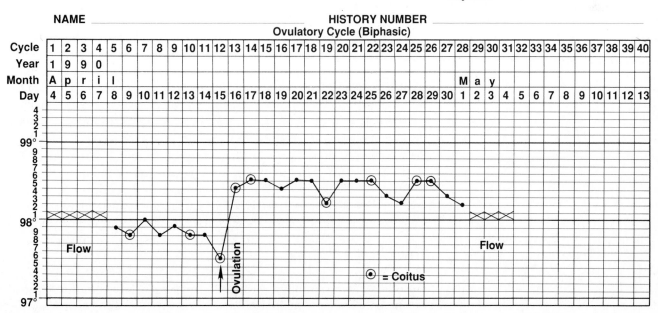

FIGURE 6-2
Cervical Mucus Ferning. Arborization, i.e., ferning, is caused by the effects of estrogen on the concentration of sodium chloride and other electrolytes in the mucus; high estrogen levels produce more complete arborization.[9] When the mucus is spread on a glass slide and allowed to dry, the pattern it forms resembles a fern leaf.[10] Ferning is absent in anovulatory women.

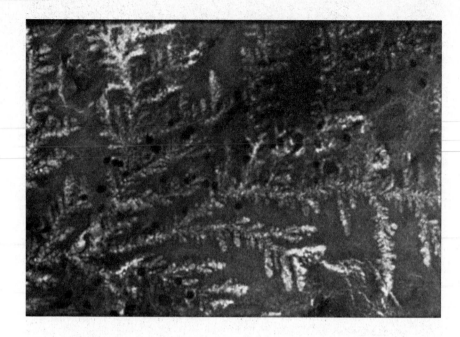

FIGURE 6-3
Endometrial Biopsy. A curette is gently introduced through the cervical canal to the level of the uterine fundus, and one or two samples of tissue are removed for examination by the pathologist. Endometrial biopsy identifies estrogen/progesterone-induced endometrial changes and is helpful in ruling out a chronic inflammatory condition of the endometrium.

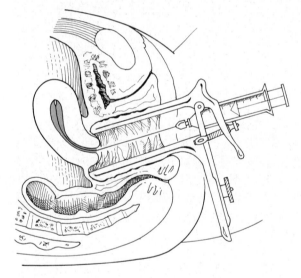

Uterine and Tubal Factor Assessment

Tubal Patency Determination (Rubin's Test)

The patency of the fallopian tubes can be assessed by introducing CO_2 gas under pressure through the uterine cavity. With the client in the lithotomy position, CO_2 is insufflated transcervically. Characteristic findings accompany passage of the gas through patent fallopian tubes (see Table 6-2). Although this test was used extensively in the past, it is being replaced by other tests that allow more definitive assessment of the uterine cavity and the tubes, e.g., hysterosalpingography, ultrasonography.

Hysterosalpingography

Instilling radiopaque dye through a small tube into the uterus permits roentgenographic visualization of the uterus and fallopian tubes. Hys-

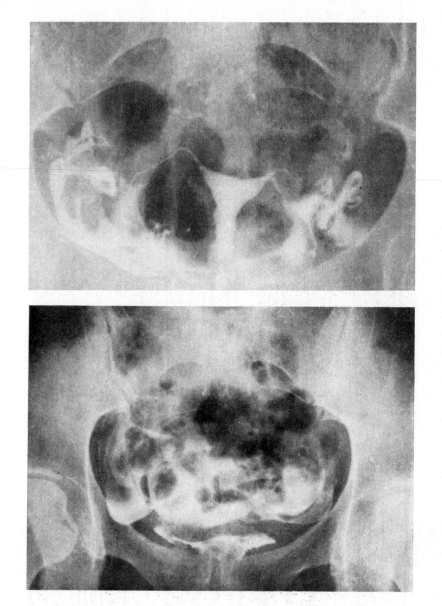

FIGURE 6-4

Hysterosalpingography. Transcervical instillation of 1 to 2 ml of contrast medium is performed under fluoroscopy; the small amount of radiopaque dye may outline small abnormalities that would be obscured by a larger amount of medium. Larger amounts of medium are then instilled to distend the uterus, and they flow upward through the fallopian tubes. Serial x-ray films are taken to record the progress of the flow through the reproductive cavities as the media is instilled.

From Mastroianni L Jr: Variations of Fertility. In Romney Sl, Gray MJ, Little AB (eds): Gynecology and Obstetrics: The Health Care of Women. New York, McGraw-Hill, 1975.

terosalpingography has become the method of choice for evaluating the structure and patency of the uterus and fallopian tubes (Fig. 6-4). Visualization of the anatomic structures on x-ray film can identify uterine and tubal abnormalities, sites of tubal obstruction, tubal fixation caused by adhesions, and uterine leiomyomas (fibroid tumors).

Pelvic Ultrasonography

Ultrasonography is a biomedical adaptation of marine sonar technology. Sound wave echos create a picture of the pelvic structures.[11] Abdominal or vaginal ultrasonography may be used to visualize the reproductive structures. Ultrasonography can identify anatomic abnormalities and often is used to determine follicular development and maturation in planning for therapeutic interventions, e.g., surgical removal of an ovum for use in in vitro fertilization.

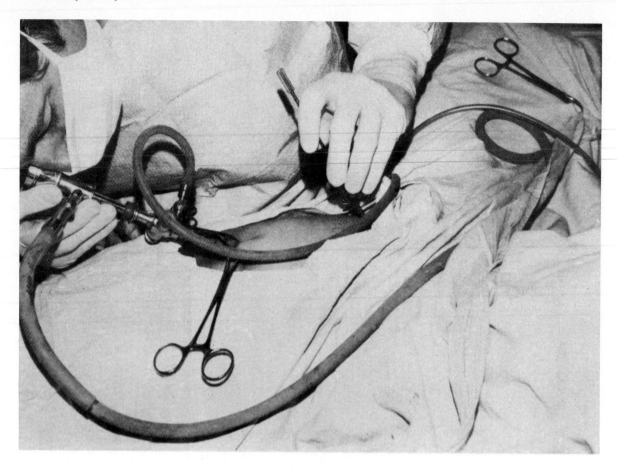

FIGURE 6-5

Double-Puncture Laparoscopy. The double-puncture technique allows the surgeon to use a probe to move the ovaries and tubes for optimum visualization, to explore the fimbriated ends of the fallopian tubes, and to view the undersurface of the broad ligaments and ovaries. Unsuspected pelvic disease, adhesions, and endometriosis have been discovered through use of this technique.

From Seitz HM Jr, Rosenfeld RL: Endoscopy in the management of infertility. Clin Obstet Gynecol 17:86, 1974.

Laparoscopy

Insertion of an endoscope through a small abdominal incision permits direct visualization of pelvic structures. Laparoscopy is essential in the study of infertile women when there is no obvious cause for failure to achieve pregnancy.[2] Immediately before the laparoscopy, a cannula is placed at the cervix. A thin solution of methylene blue dye is introduced through the cannula. The double-puncture technique (Fig. 6-5) allows the surgeon to manipulate the reproductive organs for optimum inspection. If the tubes are patent, dye can be seen spilling from the ends.

Cervical Factor Assessment

The Sims-Huhner (postcoital) test is used to identify the quality of the cervical mucus and its effects on sperm survival and motility.[13] The test is another component of the initial investigation into possible infertility. To maximize the potential for concurrent achievement of pregnancy, the test usually is timed for 1 or 2 days before expected ovulation, e.g., the 12th or 13th day of the 28-day menstrual cycle. At that time the influence of estrogen increases the cervical mucus' hospitality to spermatozoa.

Anxiety—related to anticipated diagnosis of infertility/sterility
Anticipatory Grieving—related to potential diagnosis of infertility or sterility
Knowledge Deficit—regarding infertility assessment procedures, reproductive options
Pain—related to diagnostic procedures
Dysfunctional Grieving—related to diagnosis of infertility or sterility
Powerlessness—related to lack of control over reproductive processes
Ineffective Individual Coping—related to depression associated with diagnosis of infertility or sterility
Situational Low Self-Esteem—related to individual perception of infertility
Ineffective Family Coping: Compromised—related to diagnosis of infertility or sterility
Altered Family Processes—related to scapegoating associated with diagnosis or cause of partner's infertility or sterility
Spiritual Distress—related to conflict between religious beliefs and prescribed health regimen
Decisional Conflict—related to conflict between religious beliefs and choices or treatment for infertility or sterility
Noncompliance—related to cultural mores, value conflicts
Sexual Dysfunction—related to grieving

□ POTENTIAL
NURSING DIAGNOSES

Infertility

Nursing Diagnosis

Nursing diagnoses are used to define the focus for individualized client or couple teaching and counseling and are derived from the total data base. To establish accurate nursing diagnoses the nurse integrates knowledge of the implications of diagnostic findings with an understanding of the psychosocial impact of a diagnosis of infertility or sterility. See Potential Nursing Diagnoses for representative potential nursing diagnoses for the client or couple with a diagnosis of infertility/sterility.

Focus Assessment

Establish length of time the couple has engaged in unprotected intercourse, frequency of intercourse.
Identify accuracy of current knowledge regarding fertile period of menstrual cycle, timing of intercourse to coincide.
Examine client history for contributing factors (e.g., irregular menses, prior use of contraceptives, pelvic infections, surgery).
Determine knowledge regarding common diagnostic procedures (e.g., basal body temperature, postcoital test, microscopic examination of sperm specimen).
Note response to discussion of subject and procedure.
Observe for nonverbal indicators of emotional stress (e.g., irritability, inability to concentrate, withdrawal).
Observe family interaction. Establish mutual desire to pursue diagnosis.
Elicity information describing perception of self.
Establish the personal meaning of infertility of sterility.
Identify indvidual teaching, learning, or referral needs regarding:
    Methods of diagnosis, specific procedures.
    Advantages and disadvantages of specific diagnostic procedures (e.g., hysterosalpingography).
    Findings of diagnositc tests.
    Available treatment options and resources.
    Emotional and financial costs of selected procedures (e.g., drug therapy, in vitro fertilization).

Planning and Implementation
Before Diagnosis

Clients or couples who suspect and fear a diagnosis of infertility or sterility often are sensitive and emotionally vulnerable. The nurse must consider the psychosocial aspects of infertility during all client contacts. Establishing and maintaining rapport and mutual trust with the couple is essential to effective nursing interventions. During the prediagnostic period nursing actions focus on enabling effective client coping and cooperation. Nursing interventions are designed to (1) reduce client anxiety, (2) minimize client knowledge deficits, (3) maximize client or couple potential for active participation in the diagnostic process, and (4) enable effective, shared problem solving and decision making.

All interviews and client teaching should be planned carefully to minimize psychologic stress and maximize nurse-client communication. An adequate amount of uninterrupted time and privacy should be provided to encourage the client or couple to explore and express their feelings, fears, and concerns. Open communication between the partners, e.g., sharing feelings and fears, also encourages mutual understanding and support.

Anticipatory Guidance

Objectives for the initial consultation are to enable effective assessment of the couple as a biologic reproductive unit and to ensure their shared understanding of the pattern, processes, and expense of a comprehensive infertility investigation. At the time a client makes an initial appointment the nurse suggests that the couple attend the sessions together.

Client Teaching

Client teaching is vital to ensuring the accuracy of the infertility investigation. Many findings of the initial investigation will be questionable if the client does not understand and comply fully with the recommendations, e.g., inaccurate or inconsistent measurement or recording of BBT. Further, the nurse should be prepared to answer questions about common investigative procedures (see Table 6-2). Because of the potential for client embarassment, the nurse must provide information in a matter-of-fact manner. (See Client Self-Care Education: Infertility Tests.)

Semen Analysis

If the man will cooperate, he may be encouraged to provide a fresh semen specimen for analysis while at the clinic. For clients who will not comply with this method for specimen collection, a special condom that is not coated with spermicidal powder can be provided to collect the specimen.

Ovarian Factor Tests

The timing for several of the tests in the infertility investigation is related to ovulation. Methods used to enable the client to identify ovulation also are used in fertility awareness family planning (see Chapter 19).

Infertility Tests

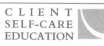

Action	Rationale
Semen analysis	
1. Collect three specimens at monthly intervals.	1. Increases accuracy of findings.
2. Abstain from intercourse for 2 to 3 days before specimen gathering.	2. Encourages accumulation of sufficient spermatozoa for analysis; prolonged abstinence is discouraged because spermatozoal motility diminishes.
3. Masturbate and ejaculate into a clean, wide-mouthed, screw-top glass or plastic container. Cap it tightly.	3. Protects specimen from contamination or loss from spillage.
4. Clients who will not comply with this method may use a specialized condom.	4. Both the sheath and the powder of an over-the-counter condom may be spermicidal.
5. Avoid exposure of specimen to excessive heat or cold.	5. Excessive heat or cold may destroy sperm cells or alter motility.
6. Examine specimen within 1 hour after collection.	6. Reduces potential for damage to spermatozoa; assures more accurate findings.
Sims-Huhner (postcoital) test	
1. Time test to coincide with ovulation as determined by the BBT record.	1. Enables examination of hospitable cervical mucus; maximizes the potential for coincidental conception.
2. Abstain from intercourse for 2 to 3 days before specimen gathering.	2. Encourages accumulation of sufficient sperm for analysis; prolonged abstinence is discouraged because spermatozoal motility diminishes.
3. Avoid douching or vaginal lubrication before coitus.	3. Alters cervical mucus.
4. After intercourse, remain in bed with hips elevated for 10 to 15 minutes.	4. Encourages ascent of spermatozoa; reduces semen loss resulting from gravitational drainage.
5. Report for examination within 2 hours.	5. Increases accuracy of findings.
Rubin's (tubal patency) test	
1. Schedule test for 4 to 5 days after end of menstrual period.	1. Avoids ovulation and displacement of a fertilized ovum.
2. Take a laxative on the night before the test and an enema or bisacodyl (Dulcolax) suppository on the morning of the test.	2. Cleanses lower bowel.
3. Void immediately before the insufflation.	3. Empties bladder; reduces discomfort.
4. Relax as much as possible during the test.	4. Tension and apprehension may contribute to tubal spasm.
5. Describe the experienced sensations.	5. Enables diagnosis; identifies symptoms of subdiaphragmatic irritation by gas passing through a patent fallopian tube.
6. Rest with hips elevated for 2 to 3 hours after the test.	6. Encourages exit of gas into abdominal cavity; reduces dizziness, pain, and cramping.

Continued

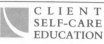

Infertility Tests (Continued)

Action	Rationale
Endometrial biopsy	
1. Time test approximately 1 week before the expected onset of the next menses.	1. Biopsy identifies endometrial response to ovarian hormone levels.
2. Some brief minor cramping may be experienced.	2. Uterine response to surgical insult.
3. Wear a perineal pad for 1 or 2 days after the biopsy; do not use tampons.	3. May experience some minor vaginal bleeding; pads are less irritating and enable more accurate estimate of bleeding.
4. Notify physician if bleeding requires the use of more than one pad per hour.	4. Excessive bleeding should be evaluated by the primary health care provider.
5. Take oral temperature every 4 hours while awake for 48 hours after procedure. Report any elevation promptly.	5. Identifies sign of infection.
6. Rest as much as possible during the next 24 hours.	6. Facilitates healing; reduces stress.
7. Avoid heavy lifting.	7. Minimizes risk of increased intra-abdominal pressure.
8. Avoid douching and intercourse for 72 hours after the biopsy.	8. Reduces potential for infection.
Hysterosalpingography	
1. Schedule test 4 to 5 days after completion of menstruation.	1. Avoids possibility of inducing abortion if unknown pregnancy is present.
2. Take a laxative on the night before the test and an enema or bisacodyl suppository on the morning of the test.	2. Cleanses lower bowel and improves visualization of pelvic structures.
3. Void immediately before the insufflation.	3. Empties bladder; reduces discomfort.
4. Relax as much as possible during the test.	4. Tension and apprehension may contribute to tubal spasm.
5. Describe experienced sensations.	5. Enables diagnosis; identifies symptoms of subdiaphragmatic irritation from dye passing through a patent fallopian tube.
6. Wear a perineal pad after the test.	6. Absorbs draining contrast media.
7. Promptly report any elevated temperature, malaise, or abdominal pain.	7. Allows early identification and treatment of infection.

BASAL BODY TEMPERATURE. BBT may be taken orally or rectally.[10,11] However, the client must use the same method consistently. A special thermometer is used to measure the BBT. It measures a smaller range of degrees of temperature and has a larger space between each number, thus increasing the ease of accurately identifying minimum changes in temperature. The nurse should confirm that the client understands (1) how to shake down the thermometer each night; (2) that she must insert the thermometer immediately upon awakening and before any physical activity; (3) the importance of leaving the thermometer in place for 5 minutes; (4) how to read and record the temperature; and (5) signs of ovulation and artifacts that may confuse the reading.

CERVICAL MUCUS EXAMINATION. Client teaching focuses on the changes associated with ovulation: (1) the volume of mucus increases (the woman must interpret the amount she feels with her fingers at the entrance and inside her vagina); (2) a slippery, clear cervical mucus the consistency of an egg white surrounds ovulation; and (3) the mucus can be stretched between her fingers into a thin strand that measures 3 inches or more.[10]

SIMS-HUHNER (POSTCOITAL) TEST. Examining the cervical mucus shortly after intercourse reveals the character of the mucus and the number and characteristics of the sperm deposit. Under ideal circumstances the test should be timed to coincide with ovulation as identified by the client's BBT record.

ENDOMETRIAL BIOPSY. The procedure is scheduled approximately 1 week before the onset of the next expected menstrual period. No preparation is required, and no anesthesia is necessary. The only discomfort experienced is momentary minor cramping.

Uterine and Tubal Factor Tests

RUBIN'S (TUBAL PATENCY) TEST. Blowing CO_2 gas through the uterine cavity into the fallopian tubes may cause some minor discomfort. The client may be aware of the placement of the rubber-tipped cannula in the cervix or may feel a "pinch" from the tenaculum used to hold the catheter in place. She may be aware of the gas entering and passing through her uterus or may experience sudden abdominal pain caused by tubal spasm. Clients who have at least one patent fallopian tube complain of shoulder pain resulting from subdiaphragmatic irritation caused by the gas.

PELVIC ULTRASONOGRAPHY. If abdominal ultrasonography is to be used, the client must drink freely and avoid urinating for 2 hours before the test. The full bladder enhances visualization of the uterus and adnexa.[8] This instruction may be omitted if vaginal ultrasonography is used.

HYSTEROSALPINGOGRAPHY. Roentgenographic visualization of the uterus and fallopian tubes requires approximately 15 minutes. The procedure may cause some minor discomfort (see Client Self-Care Education: Infertility Tests). The client may experience shoulder pain or transient minor cramping and dizziness.[11]

LAPAROSCOPY. Preoperative teaching is the same as for any abdominal surgical procedure and should include a discussion of the following: (1) nothing by mouth after midnight on the day of the procedure; (2) abdominal preparation and povidone-iodine scrub; (3) Foley catheter insertion; (4) intravenous fluid infusion; (5) use of either general or regional anesthesia; (6) preoperative medication; and (7) the procedure itself as necessary (see Table 6-2). Postoperative instructions include the following: (1) the client may return home within 2 to 6 hours after surgery; (2) she will need someone to drive her home, and she should not drive for at least 24 hours after the procedure; (3) any muscle soreness or shoulder pain caused by gas irritation should subside within 24 to 36 hours; (4) any abdominal pain should be relieved by analgesics, and the physician should be notified if the pain persists longer than 12 hours or is not relieved by the medication; (4) she may experience some vaginal spotting for a

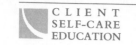

Improving Potential for Conception

Action	Rationale
1. Combine information derived from BBT and cervical mucus testing (self-examination).	1. Identifies fertile period.
2. Avoid douching or the use of vaginal lubricants.	2. Minimizes risk of altering vaginal pH or cervical mucus.
3. Abstain from intercourse for 2 to 3 days before the week of estimated ovulation.	3. Allows accumulation of mature sperm.
4. Beginning 3 days before the earliest day of ovulation, have intercourse every 24 to 36 hours until the rise in temperature indicates ovulation has occurred.	4. Exposure occurs during the fertile period.
5. Elevate hips on pillow during and after intercourse.	5. Pool of semen is deposited at the cervical os.
6. Use "missionary" (male superior) position. Knee-chest or prone position is suggested if uterus has been identified as retroverted.	6. Same as above.
7. Male should stop thrusting and penetrate as deeply as possible when he is about to ejaculate.	7. The majority of the sperm are in the first drops of ejaculate; they should be deposited as close to the cervical os as possible.
8. After intercourse, maintain position and remain quiet for a minimum of 20 minutes.	8. Retains semen pool at cervical os.

Adapted from Stewart F et al: Understanding Your Body. New York, Bantam Books, 1987.

few days; and (5) any signs of infection, chest pain, cough, or shortness of breath, dizziness, or faintness should be reported promptly.[11]

Improving the Potential for Conception

A significant percentage of couples experiences spontaneous resolution of primary infertility after either the initial infertility consultation or after assessment of tubal patency.[2] This effect may be due to the fact that many couples who presume they are infertile are, in actuality, not having intercourse often enough or are not having intercourse at the time of ovulation.[11] In some cases insufflation may clear the tubes of thin adhesions.[2] Before or during the preliminary investigation, i.e., during the 3 months of semen analysis and ovulation graphing, the couple may improve their potential for conception by following some simple recommendations (see Client Self-Care Education: Improving Potential for Conception).

Assessment After Diagnosis

When the diagnosis of infertility or sterility has been confirmed, nursing assessments focus on identifying the couple's response to the diagnosis; coping abilities, mechanisms, and support systems; understanding of the underlying problem, the implications of the disorder, and their reproductive options; and their awareness of community resources for support and assistance.

Planning and Implementation

The nurse must anticipate the psychologic trauma to couples who receive a diagnosis of infertility or sterility. Psychosocial and cultural values individualize the personal meaning of inability to conceive; the intrapersonal or interpersonal aspects of the diagnosis may be overwhelming. Often the nurse is called on to act as counselor in what is an emotionally charged situation. Facing the prospect of a barren marriage involves many feelings that must be recognized and resolved. Enabling or supporting effective individual and family coping is a major focus of the nursing role.

The couple should be encouraged to express and explore their feelings and reactions and to communicate openly with each other and the members of their support system. The partners' mutual perception of infertility as a shared problem and their use of family support systems are vital in supporting and strengthening the coping abilities of the family unit. To help clients cope with their personal crises, the nurse provides emotional support, assistance with the grieving process, and information needed for effective problem solving.

Client Teaching

Adequate and accurate information is essential to achieving effective problem solving and making informed decisions when selecting among reproductive options. Teaching is directed toward ensuring the couple's understanding of the problem and enabling their selection of an option appropriate to their individual needs and desires.

Male Infertility Management

Artificial Insemination

In selected cases artificial placement of semen is an effective therapeutic modality. This method involves depositing the semen directly around the cervix by injection (Fig. 6-6) or by use of a sperm-containing cervical cap placed at the cervical os. Artificial insemination may be accomplished using either the husband's sperm or donor sperm.

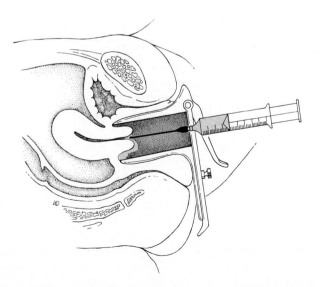

FIGURE 6-6
Artificial Insemination. One technique for artificial insemination involves placing fresh semen at the cervical os with a cannula and syringe. The timing is based on the ovulatory phase of the female.

AIH. Homologous artificial insemination with the husband's semen (AIH) is useful in cases in which the Sims-Huhner (postcoital) test consistently reveals few or no spermatozoa of good quality present in the cervical mucus. In selected cases the use of a "split ejaculate" is recommended. This technique requires that the husband ejaculate into two containers. The initial ejaculate, i.e., first specimen, is used for insemination (see Client Self-Care Education: Infertility Tests for semen analysis).

AID. In cases of azoospermia (absence of spermatozoa in the ejaculate) or severe oligospermia (markedly decreased numbers of spermatozoa in the ejaculate), donor semen (AID) may be used for insemination. AID is used in cases when the husband suffers from a genetic defect or in cases of Rh sensitization when an Rh-negative donor is used. Selection must consider the donor's general health status, genetic background, Rh type, and, under ideal circumstances, physical characteristics that resemble those of the husband. Donors also should be screened for the human immunodeficiency virus, HIV.

Fresh ejaculate can be frozen and stored for future use. The use of frozen semen for AID offers several distinct advantages: (1) the specimen is readily available; (2) the client's visits need not be timed to coincide with delivery of a fresh specimen; (3) a wider selection of donor specimens is possible; (4) repeated insemination may be accomplished within a given cycle; and (5) if several specimens have been stored, the same donor can be used for a subsequent pregnancy. Although the incidence of successful achievement of pregnancy appears somewhat less with frozen sperm, there is no evidence of greater risk of genetic abnormalities or of spontaneous abortion (see Legal and Ethical Considerations).

Gamete Intrafallopian Transfer (GIFT)

When infertility is related to male semen inadequacy or for couples with unexplained infertility, surgical retrieval of a woman's eggs for laboratory fertilization with her partner's sperm and immediate placement of the egg-sperm mixture in the distal end of the client's fallopian tube may result in successful conception. Fertilization and early embryonic development would proceed as in spontaneous pregnancy during transit of the fallopian tube.[14]

Client teaching includes review of normal ovulatory processes; discussion of daily ultrasound monitoring of follicular development and maturation and of serum hormone measurements; description of laparoscopic removal of the ovum just before ovulation; and preoperative teaching for laparoscopy.

Female Infertility Management

Ovarian Factors

PHARMACOLOGIC MANAGEMENT. Pharmacologic agents have been used successfully in the management of **anovulation,** sporadic ovulation, luteal phase deficiency, and infertility problems associated with cervical mucus. Agents used in management of functional anovulation include clomiphene citrate (Clomid), human menopausal gonadotropin (menotropins [Per-

---

≡ LEGAL AND ETHICAL
≡ CONSIDERATIONS

In February 1988 both the Food and Drug Administration and the Centers for Disease Control recommended that all donated semen be frozen and quarantined for at least 6 months so the semen donors can be tested for antibodies to the AIDS virus.

gonal]), gonadotropin-releasing hormone (GnRH), and bromocriptine mesylate (Parlodel). Clomiphene citrate has been the drug of choice for initial management of ovarian infertility (see Drug Guide: Clomiphene Citrate).

If clomiphene therapy is unsuccessful, menotropins may be used alone or in combination with clomiphene. Combination treatment with clomiphene, menotropins, and human chorionic gonadotropin (hCG) to induce final egg maturation and ovulation has been used effectively. Menotropins therapy has been successful in 90% of anovulatory women; there are, however, many disadvantages. See Drug Guide: Menotropins for information about client teaching.

GnRH treatment requires the use of an intradermal catheter and a portable hormone pump; for 2 to 4 weeks every 90 minutes throughout the day, small bursts of GnRH automatically are administered.[17] When ovulation suppression is due to hyperprolactinemia, bromocriptine mesylate may be used to inhibit pituitary secretion of prolactin.[11]

Luteal phase deficiencies are associated with inadequate progesterone levels. Because natural progesterone is destroyed by gastric acids, supplemental progesterone is administered either by injection or by means of vaginal suppositories. Treatment begins 3 days after ovulation and is continued daily until the next menstrual period; if pregnancy occurs, treatment is continued until gestational week 6 or 7.[2,11]

Tubal Factors

PHARMACOLOGIC MANAGEMENT. When ectopic endometrial implants occlude the fallopian tubes, a synthetic androgen danazol (Danocrine) may be used to suppress ovulation and menstruation and cause implant atrophy. Therapy is begun during menstruation to ensure the client is not pregnant. In clinets with moderate-to-severe endometriosis the recommended therapy is 400 mg twice daily; dosage is adjusted on the basis of client response. Elimination of endometrial nodules usually requires 4 to 6 months of continuous therapy.[16]

Client teaching. Client teaching includes management of common side effects of danazol therapy: (1) depilatories may be used to treat the transient overgrowth of facial hair (hirsutism); (2) fluid retention, edema, and weight gain can be minimized by controlling salt intake; (3) excessive skin oiliness or acne can be controlled by scrupulous skin hygiene; (4) low estrogen-induced atrophic vaginitis can be managed with vaginal lubricants; and (5) muscle cramps can be avoided by adding potassium-rich foods to the diet, e.g., orange juice, bananas. The need for close medical supervision throughout the therapy should be emphasized; clients should be monitored for signs of adverse effects, e.g., liver dysfunction.

SURGICAL TREATMENT. Surgical techniques have been developed for treatment of pelvic adhesions and tubal occlusion. The postoperative prognosis depends on the extent of previous damage to adnexal structures. When the tubes are patent, excision of pelvic adhesions may enable successful capture and transport of the ovum. Microsurgery and laser technology have enhanced potential for treatment of tubal occlusions.[18] However, as yet tuboplasty has been most successful in restoring tubal function after sterilization; tubal reversal pregnancy rates have been as high as 65%.[2,19]

Clomiphene citrate (Clomid or Serophene): Nonsteroidal compound; similar in structure to estrogen; binds to estrogen-receptor sites.

Indications: Hypothalamic-suppression anovulation; oligo-ovulation; luteal phase deficiency; before in vitro fertilization.[15]

Gynecologic Action: Induces ovulation by transmitting false feedback signals of low estrogen levels to the hypothalamus and pituitary; results in release of follicle-stimulating hormone (FSH) and gonadotropins. They, in turn, stimulate ovulation.

Administration and Dosage: Oral administration.
   Initial dosage: 50 mg/day for 5 days on days 5 through 9 of menstrual cycle.
   Subsequent dosage: If ovulation has not occurred after the first course, a second course of 100 mg/day for 5 days is begun 30 days later.
Although most clients respond with ovulation after the first or second course of medication, a third course of 100 mg/day for 5 days may be administered for those who have not demonstrated ovulation.[11] Dosage may be increased to as much as 250 mg/day in some women; supplemental estrogen may be required if cervical mucus diminishes.[15]

Maternal Contraindications: Allergy, ovarian cysts, liver disease, visual problems, premature menopause, hyperstimulation syndrome, i.e., ovarian tenderness and enlargement.[11,15]

Potential Side Effects and Complications: Side effects usually are mild and are dose related: vasomotor flushing similar to menopausal "hot flashes"; symptoms resembling premenstrual syndrome (breast tenderness, abdominal bloating, weight gain, Mittelschmerz, headache, irritability, insomnia); visual symptoms (blurring, spots, flashes); hair loss; nausea and vomiting; multiple gestation.

Nursing Implications:
1. Assess client's medical history to identify contraindications for administration.
2. Assess for signs of side effects and pregnancy during follow-up visits.

Client Teaching:
1. Discuss the significant financial expense of this treatment: cost of medication possibly exceeding $100 per month; monthly office visits; laboratory tests for serum progesterone levels.
2. Emphasize that clomiphene can restore normal fertility by inducing ovulation but that successful ovulation may not necessarily result in immediate achievement of pregnancy.
   As many as 55% to 75% of couples conceive during the first 3 months of successful treatment.
   For others, treatment may be continued for as long as 6 to 9 months to increase the potential for conception.
   If failure to ovulate is the only fertility problem and couples persist in their treatment, pregnancy rates may be as high as 80%.
For amenorrheic clients, clomiphene therapy may be preceded by medroxyprogesterone (Provera) treatment, 10 mg/day for 5 days. Withdrawal bleeding should occur within a few days of the last dose. The first day of bleeding is counted as cycle day 1, and clomiphene is begun on day 5.
Instruct about self-measurement of BBT and cervical mucus examination.
Explain need for close monitoring of response to therapy.
   Follow-up visits are scheduled monthly to check for hyperstimulation syndrome and pregnancy.
   Serum progesterone levels may be ordered monthly 1 week after ovulation if BBT records are unclear.
   If BBT and serum progesterone levels show ovulation has not occurred, dosage will be increased, e.g., 100 mg/day, 150 mg/day, 200 mg/day.
   Medroxyprogesterone treatment may be needed between courses of clomiphene until ovulation occurs.
   Report any signs of side effects promptly; dosage may require reduction or discontinuance.
Discuss timing of intercourse. Ovulation should occur 5 to 10 days after the last clomiphene tablet. Couple should begin having intercourse every 24 to 36 hours on day 11 and continue until BBT demonstrates ovulation.

Menotropins (Pergonal): Gonadotropin; contains equal amounts of FSH and luteinizing hormone (LH).

Indications:
Female: Hypogonadotropic anovulation not caused by primary ovarian failure.
Male: For hypogonatropic azoospermia it is administered concurrently with human chorionic gonadotropin (hCG).

Gynecologic Action: Stimulates follicular growth and maturation.

Administration and Dosage: Injectable only; reconstitute with sodium chloride; use immediately. Discard any solution remaining in vial.
Initial dosage: 75 international units (IU) of FSH/LH daily for 7 to 12 days, followed 1 day after last dose by 5000 to 10,000 U of hCG. If there is evidence of ovulation, in the absence of pregnancy this dosage should be repeated for two more cycles.
Subsequent dosage: If pregnancy has not occurred during the initial three cycles, in the absence of complications dosage is increased to 150 IU of FSH/LH daily for 7 to 12 days, followed 1 day later by 5000 to 10,000 U of hCG. This dosage is repeated for two more cycles.

Maternal Contraindications: Primary ovarian failure (high levels of both FSH and LH), any cause of infertility other than anovulation, thyroid and adrenal dysfunction, abnormal bleeding of unknown origin, ovarian cysts.

Potential Side Effects and Complications: Hyperstimulation syndrome (ovarian enlargement and tenderness, ascites, pleural effusion), hemoconcentration or arterial thromboembolism, nausea, vomiting, and diarrhea, ectopic pregnancy, multiple gestation.[11,15,16]

Nursing Implications:
1. Assess client's medical history to identify contraindications for administration.
2. Assess for signs of side effects and pregnancy during follow-up visits.

Client Teaching:
1. Discuss the significant financial expense of this medication; costs may exceed $2000 per cycle. Treatment may require 3 to 8 months or cycles.
2. Explain need for close monitoring of response to therapy.
    Emphasize need for daily ultrasonography and blood tests during each treatment cycle. Client must be monitored closely for signs of adverse effects, e.g., hyperstimulation syndrome.
    Report any signs of side effects promptly; may require immediate discontinuance.
Explain the incidence of both multiple gestation (twins, triplets, quadruplets) and the very high rate of pregnancy loss related to premature birth.
If client is to self-administer injections, discuss and demonstrate correct technique for reconstituting drug, aspirating proper dosage, selecting sites, and injecting intramuscularly. Have client return-demonstrate techniques.
Discuss timing of intercourse. Encourage daily intercourse from last day of personal administration through ovulation.

In Vitro Fertilization and Embryonic Transfer

In vitro fertilization and embryonic transfer provide an option for couples whose infertility is due to irreversible tubal damage, endometriosis, DES exposure, or other factors.[20] In this approach follicular fluid and the mature oocyte are removed surgically from the woman's ovary (Fig. 6-7). Under controlled laboratory conditions, the ova are placed in a tissue culture and are incubated for several hours; then they are mixed with the client's partner's sperm to encourage fertilization and initial incubation of the embryo. Embryonic transfer is scheduled for 48 hours after the laparoscopy. The tiny embryo is inserted through a catheter into the woman's cervix for implantation.[21,22] Success rates approximate 15% to 25%; however, spontaneous abortion in the first weeks of pregnancy is common in approximately 30% of pregnancies achieved by in vitro fertilization

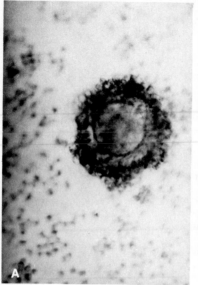
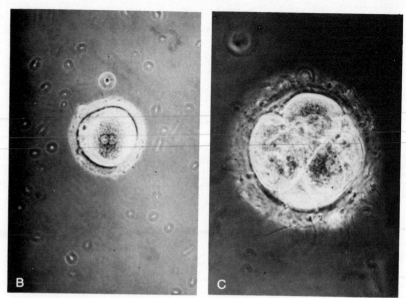

FIGURE 6-7

In Vitro Fertilization. In vitro fertilization involves obtaining an oocyte, fertilizing it, and transferring it to the uterus. **A,** Mature egg just aspirated. **B,** Fertilized egg (two pronuclei seen) 16 hours after insemination. **C,** Four-cell embryo shortly before embryonic transfer.

From Pace-Owens S: In vitro fertilization and embryo transfer. JOGN Nurs Suppl 14:44s-48s, November/December 1985.

(see Client Self-Care Education: In Vitro Fertilization and Embryonic Transfer).

SURROGATE EMBRYONIC TRANSFER. Surrogate embryonic transfer involves five steps: (1) synchronization of the ovulation times between donor and recipient women; (2) artificial insemination of the donor woman with sperm from the husband of the infertile recipient; (3) washing out of the donor's uterus approximately 5 days after fertilization; (4) successful recovery of the embryo from the lavage fluid; and (5) transfer of the embryo to the recipient's uterus. This has not proved to be a highly successful method of infertility treatment but remains one option for couples who are infertile due to the female's untreatable ovarian failure.

Referral

Often, because of the severe psychosocial and psychosexual stress associated with the threat to self-concept, couples with infertility problems are anxious, depressed, angry, or hostile. In addition to providing strong emotional support during client contacts, the nurse may suggest the couple contact a national lay group called RESOLVE. This organization provides information and support to couples who are experiencing infertility or sterility problems. Contact with other couples who have shared the same anxieties and concerns and who have resolved their problems and feelings may be invaluable.

Client Teaching

During the postdiagnostic period client teaching is directed toward ensuring that the couple understands their particular infertility problem and the reproductive options available for resolution.

In Vitro Fertilization and Embryonic Transfer

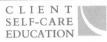

CLIENT
SELF-CARE
EDUCATION

Intervention	Rationale
Review of normal ovulatory processes	Ensures client understanding of treatment goals
Administration of menotropins	Stimulates the simultaneous maturation of several follicles; more eggs are available for fertilization
Daily ultrasonography beginning 1 week before anticipated removal of eggs	Monitors follicular development and maturation
Drawing of daily serum hormone levels at each ultrasonography visit	Enables determination of optimum hormonal doses and identifies time eggs are mature
Injection of hCG	Induces final phase of egg maturation
Scheduling of laparoscopy	Eggs must be abstracted exactly 36 hours after the hCG injection just before ovulation
Preoperative teaching for laparoscopy: describe procedures	Enables informed consent; reduces anxiety
Postoperative teaching:	Provides anticipatory guidance; enables client compliance
May return home 2 to 3 hours after eggs are abstracted	
Must return 48 hours later	Optimum time for embryonic transfer
Must remain lying down for first 6 to 8 hours after the embryonic transfer; may then return home but must rest in bed for 2 days	Increases potential for successful implantation

Evaluation

Before Diagnosis

Nursing evaluation focuses on determining the couple's response to anticipatory guidance and client teaching. See the display on page 122 for representative outcome criteria.

Before Diagnostic Procedures

Before the diagnostic procedure the nurse evaluates the effects of the previous client teaching. The nurse reviews and reinforces previous discussions, determines compliance with recommended prediagnostic behaviors, describes the steps in the procedure, explains sensations that the client may experience, and answers any additional questions. The nurse determines the client's or couple's understanding of the anticipated procedure and any potential risks and confirms and documents informed consent.

After Diagnosis

When the diagnosis of anatomic or physiologic interference with the ability to conceive has been established, nursing evaluation focuses on the

Prediagnosis Nursing Evaluation: Representative Outcome Criteria

The couple will do the following:
1. Attend diagnostic and counseling sessions together.
2. Express willingness to do the following:
   a. Expend the considerable time and money required for a comprehensive infertility investigation.
   b. Comply with recommended behaviors during testing.
3. Verbalize understanding of the emotional stresses engendered by the infertility investigation.
4. Perform behaviors required to ensure provision of accurate data and samples required for the initial investigative procedures.
   a. Abstain from intercourse before semen analysis and cervical mucus tests as directed.
   b. Provide semen samples for analysis as directed.
   c. Monitor and record BBT readings accurately and consistently.
5. Return for follow-up visits as scheduled.

couple's response to client teaching and anticipatory guidance and on informed consent to specific treatment modalities (see below for representative outcome criteria).

LEGAL AND ETHICAL CONSIDERATIONS

Current issues center on delineating parameters for technologically assisted reproduction—issues such as the following:
  Use of donor semen for artificial insemination
  Surrogate motherhood
  Rights of frozen embryos

Legal and Ethical Considerations

Advances in biomedical technology have created new options for many infertile couples—and new legal and ethical dilemmas in reproductive health practice. A majority of the ethicolegal questions are concerned with technologically assisted reproduction (see margin). In particular, recent litigation has focused national attention on in vitro fertilization, the rights of the parents to frozen embryos (*York v. Georgeanna Jones Institute for Reproductive Medicine,* 1989), the legal rights of the embryo, and conflicting applicable statutes in some states. For example, under Louisiana law a frozen embryo has legal status and the right to representation in court; however, under another Louisiana law a woman has a legal right to abort an implanted embryo through the first trimester.[23]

Postdiagnostic Nursing Evaluation: Representative Outcome Criteria

The couple will do the following:
1. Accurately answer questions regarding the disorder and its interference with the ability to conceive.
2. Verbalize understanding of the management options available.
   a. Identify appropriate medical or surgical procedures specific to the management of the underlying disorder.
   b. Identify the risks and benefits of each option.
3. Select the reproductive option that best suits their needs, abilities, and desires.
4. Explore additional resources for support and assistance.
5. Experience resolution of the underlying physical or psychosocial problem(s).

A strong commitment to legal and ethical resolution of the client's problems underlies effective nursing care in infertility management. Often nurses must confront their own personal and professional values regarding the causes and treatments of congenital and acquired interference with the ability to conceive. Ensuring the client's rights to effective, compassionate care and access to resolution of underlying problems when possible are important aspects of the nursing role in the management of infertility.

REFERENCES

1. Diamond M: Surgical aspects of infertility. In Sciarra J et al (eds): Gynecology and Obstetrics, Vol 5. Hagerstown, Md, Harper & Row, 1988
2. Mattox J: Infertility. In Willson J, Carrington E: Obstetrics and Gynecology, 8th ed. St. Louis, CV Mosby, 1987
3. Bronson R et al: Sperm antibodies: Their role in infertility. Fertil Steril 42(2):171, 1984
4. Sogor L: Immune aspects of infertility. In Sciarra J et al (eds): Gynecology and Obstetrics, Vol 5. Hagerstown, Md, Harper & Row, 1986
5. Yanagimachi R, Yanagimachi H, Rogers B: The use of zona-free animal ova as a test system for the assessment of the fertilizing capacity of human spermatozoa. Biol Reprod 15:471, 1976
6. Mattox J: Amenorrhea. In Willson J, Carrington E: Obstetrics and Gynecology, 8th ed. St. Louis, CV Mosby, 1987
7. McShane P et al: Cellular immunity to sperm in infertile women. JAMA 253(24):3555, 1985
8. Pagana K, Pagana T: Diagnostic Testing and Nursing Implications, 2nd ed. St. Louis, CV Mosby, 1986
9. Wilson R: Diagnostic methods in obstetrics and gynecology. In Willson J, Carrington E: Obstetrics and Gynecology, 8th ed. St. Louis, CV Mosby, 1987
10. Hatcher R et al: Contraceptive Technology, 1988-1989, 14th ed. New York, Irvington Press, 1988
11. Stewart F et al: Understanding your body. New York, Bantam Books, 1987
12. Siegler A: Gynecologic endoscopy in infertility. Obstet Gynecol Clin North Am 14(4):831-864, December 1987
13. Hammond M: Evaluation of the infertile couple. In Kemper R (ed): Obstetrics and Gynecologic Clinics of North America. Philadelphia, WB Saunders, 1987
14. Asch R et al: Preliminary experiences with gamete intrafallopian transfer (GIFT). Fertil Steril 45:366-371, 1986
15. Kennedy J, Adashi E: Ovulation induction. Obstet Gynecol Clin North Am 14(4):831-864, December 1987
16. Physician's Desk Reference, 43rd ed. Oradell NJ, Medical Economics, 1989
17. Hurley D et al: Induction of ovulation and fertility in amenorrheic women by pulsatile low-dose gonadotropin-releasing hormone. N Engl J Med 310:1069-1074, 1984
18. Williams T: Surgical procedures for inflammatory tubal disease. Obstet Gynecol Clin North Am 14(4):831-864, December 1987
19. Moghissi K, Evans T: Infertility. In Danforth D, Scott J (eds): Obstetrics and Gynecology, 5th ed. Philadelphia, JB Lippincott, 1986
20. Diamond M, DeCherney A: In-vitro fertilization (IVF) and gamete intrafallopian transfer (GIFT). In Kemper R (ed): Obstetrics and Gynecologic Clinics of North America. Philadelphia, WB Saunders, 1987
21. Holmes H: In vitro fertilization: Reflections on the state of the art. Birth, issues in perinatal care and education 15(3):134-144, September 1988
22. Pace-Owens S: In vitro fertilization and embryo transfer. JOGN Nurs Suppl: 44s-48s, November/December 1985
23. Cronin M, Feldinger F: Ethics: The Rights of Frozen Embryos. Time, July 24, 1989

SUGGESTED READINGS

Bernstein J et al: Assessment of psychological dysfunction associated with infertility. JOGN Suppl 63s-66s, November/December 1985

Clapp D: Emotional responses to infertility: Nursing interventions. JOGN 13:32, November/December 1985

Christianson C: Support groups for infertile patients. JOGN 15:293, July/August 1986

Creighton H: In vitro fertilization. Nurs Manage 16:12, April 1985

Cunningham F et al: William's Obstetrics, 18th ed. Norwalk, Conn, Appleton & Lange, 1989

Daly M, Hotteling K: Psychology and life stages of women. In Willson J, Carrington E: Obstetrics and Gynecology, 8th ed. St. Louis, CV Mosby, 1987

Darland N: Infertility associated with luteal phase defect. JOGN 14:212, May/June 1985

Davis M, Hotelling K: Psychology and life stages of women. In Willson J, Carrington E: Obstetrics and Gynecology, 8th ed. St. Louis, CV Mosby, 1987

Freeman E et al: Psychological evaluation and support in a program of in vitro fertilization and embryo transfer. Fertil Steril 43:48-53, 1985

Grimes E, Richardson M: Management of the infertile couple. In Sciarra J et al (eds): Gynecology and Obstetrics, Vol 5. Hagerstown, Md, Harper & Row, 1988

Nunley W et al: Homologous insemination—revisited. Am J Obstet Gynecol 153:201-206, 1985

Ritchie W: Ultrasound in the evaluation of normal and induced ovulation. Fertil Steril 43:167-181, 1985

Schlaff W: Transmission of disease during artificial insemination. N Engl J Med 315:1289, 1986

Smith P: Ovulation induction. JOGN Suppl 37s-43s, November/December, 1985

Soules M: The in vitro fertilization pregnancy rate: Let's be honest with one another. Fertil Steril 43:511, 1985

Stenchever M: How to use the sperm penetration assay. Contemp Ob/Gyn 23:219, 1984

Tripp-Reimer T: Cultural assessment. In Bellack J, Bamford P: Nursing Assessment. Belmont, Calif, Wadsworth, 1984

Wallach E et al: Ethical considerations in treating infertility. Contemp Ob/Gyn 23:226, 1984

Wallach E et al: Ethical dilemmas of infertility. Contemp Ob/Gyn 29:170, March 1987

Wilkes C et al: Pregnancy related to infertility diagnosis, number of attempts, and age in a program of in vitro fertilization. Obstet Gynecol 55:350-352, 1985

Vick R: Contemporary Medical Physiology. Menlo Park, Calif, Addison-Wesley, 1984

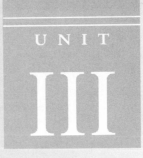

The Family in the Antepartum Period

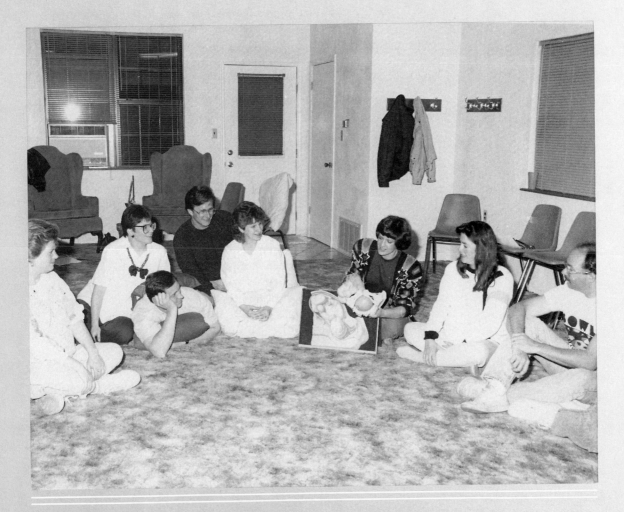

Physiologic and Psychosocial Aspects of Pregnancy

IMPORTANT TERMINOLOGY

ballottement Rebound of a fetus; felt after administering a light tap to the abdominal wall or cervix

Braxton Hicks contractions Intermittent, irregular, usually painless uterine contractions that begin after the third month of pregnancy and continue throughout pregnancy

Chadwick's sign Blue-violet color of the cervix, vagina, and vulva; present after the fourth week of pregnancy

chloasma Brownish facial pigmentation that appears over the nose and cheeks during pregnancy; also called the "mask of pregnancy"

colostrum Thin yellowish fluid secreted by the breasts before true breast milk arrives

epulis Hypertrophy of the gingival papillae around the gums

Goodell's sign Softening of the cervix; present as early as 1 or 2 months gestation

Hegar's sign Softening of the lower uterine segments; present after sixth to eighth week of pregnancy

lightening Descent of the fetal presenting part into the pelvic cavity; occurs 2 to 3 weeks before onset of labor

linea nigra Pigmented line extending from the pubic symphysis toward the umbilicus

products of conception Includes fetus, fetal membrane, amniotic fluid, and placenta

quickening Mother's first perception of fetal movement; usually occurs between 16 and 20 weeks

striae gravidarum Shining, reddish lines on the abdomen, thighs, or breasts caused by over stretching the skin

This chapter presents the anatomic and physiologic changes seen in the pregnant female. It also discusses the psychologic effects the pregnancy has on the couple and their immediate family.

Symptoms and Signs of Pregnancy

Physiologic adaptations to pregnancy result in anatomic and physiologic changes that can be categorized as subjective symptoms or objective signs of pregnancy. These symptoms and signs of pregnancy are divided into three groups: presumptive (pregnancy is suspected), probable (pregnancy is likely), and positive (pregnancy is certain) (Table 7-1).

Presumptive Symptoms

As the woman's body begins adapting to the altered hormonal levels that occur with pregnancy, she may experience physical changes and discomforts. Several subjective symptoms, e.g., nausea, breast changes, urinary frequency, lassitude, and quickening, are common in early pregnancy and result from normal anatomic and physiologic responses. However, because these complaints also accompany many other disorders, they are considered only presumptive symptoms of pregnancy.

TABLE 7-1

Symptoms and Signs of Pregnancy

Symptoms	Signs
Presumptive	
Nausea, vomiting, morning sickness	Amenorrhea (menstrual suppression)
Breast tenderness and fullness	Skin changes
Frequent urination	Striae gravidarum
Lassitude, easy fatigability	Pigment changes (chloasma, linea nigra)
Quickening	Increased perspiration
	Epulis (bleeding gums)
	Breast changes
	Enlargement
	Areolar darkening
	Changes in internal genitalia
	Goodell's sign
	Chadwick's sign
Probable	
None	Uterine enlargement
	Fetal outline identified by abdominal palpation and detected vaginally by ballottement
	Braxton Hicks contractions
	Positive pregnancy test
	Cervical changes: Hegar's sign
Positive	
None	Fetal heart sounds
	Fetal movements felt by examiner
	Ultrasonographic verification of presence of a fetus

Nausea and Vomiting

Approximately 50% of all pregnant women have no nausea during the early part of pregnancy. Approximately one-third of the women who do experience nausea report episodes of vomiting. The nausea often occurs in the early part of the day and is called "morning sickness." However, it can occur at any time of the day. Nausea and vomiting may result from increased human chorionic gonadotropin (hCG) levels, altered carbohydrate metabolism, or gastroesophageal reflux. Since nausea and vomiting occur in many other conditions, these symptoms are of no diagnostic value unless associated with other evidence of pregnancy.

Breast Changes

The purpose of hormone-stimulated breast changes during pregnancy is to prepare for lactation and breast-feeding. The breasts become larger, firmer, and more tender after the second month of pregnancy (Fig. 7-1). As the breasts increase in size, the blood vessels supplying the area enlarge, and the veins beneath the skin become more prominent and visible. In the latter months of pregnancy colostrum may leak spontaneously or be expressed from the nipples by gentle massage. **Colostrum** is a thick yellowish fluid and is a precursor of breast milk.

Frequent Urination

Bladder irritability resulting in frequent urination is an early symptom of pregnancy. The irritability results from pressure exerted on the bladder

FIGURE 7-1

Pregnancy- and Lactation-Induced Breast Changes. Breast enlargement during pregnancy is due to estrogen/progesterone-stimulated growth of the secretory ductal system. As pregnancy progresses, the nipple and its surrounding areola (pigmented area) become darker in color. The areola tends to become puffy. Its diameter, which rarely exceeds 3 cm (1½ inches) in the nulligravida, gradually widens to reach 5 or 6 cm (2 to 3 inches) by the end of pregnancy. Sebaceous glands enlarge and appear as small darkened protuberances or follicles on the areola.

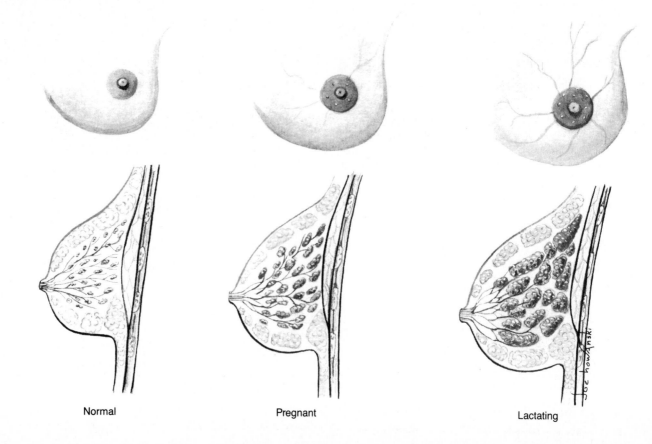

Normal   Pregnant   Lactating

by the enlarging uterus, creating the same sensation felt when the bladder is stretched by urinary volume. Increased vascularization and pelvic congestion also contribute to urinary frequency and urgency. During the second trimester the uterus rises upward out of the pelvis, and urinary frequency subsides. Urinary frequency may recur, particularly during the last weeks of pregnancy. At that time the fetal presenting part settles into the pelvis and presses against the bladder.

Lassitude and Fatigue

The pregnant woman may experience periods of lassitude and drowsiness early in pregnancy, sometimes even before the first missed menstrual period. These periods of fatigue are due to the increased metabolic needs of the developing fetus, which cause a lowered maternal blood sugar level.

Quickening

Quickening refers to the first fetal movements perceived by the mother. Women occasionally misinterpret movement of gas in the intestines as motions of a baby and, on this basis, imagine themselves to be pregnant. Therefore the woman's statement that she feels the baby move cannot be regarded as absolute proof of pregnancy. Quickening usually occurs between 16 and 20 weeks gestation.

Presumptive Signs

Altered hormonal levels cause identifiable changes in body structure and function, but physical signs in early pregnancy can also be caused by other conditions, e.g., tumors. Presumptive signs of pregnancy include physical assessment findings such as breast changes and vaginal mucosa color changes. The most common presumptive sign of pregnancy is amenorrhea.

Amenorrhea

Amenorrhea (menstrual suppression) is the earliest occurring sign of pregnancy. Absence of menstruation only suggests pregnancy since it can also result from a number of other conditions.

Skin Changes

Observable skin changes result from increased estrogen and progesterone production, metabolic changes, and breast and abdominal enlargement. The nurse must recognize these signs and educate the client about their cause and duration.

PIGMENT CHANGES. Pigmentation is caused by the anterior pituitary hormone melanotropin. Pigmentary deposits in the skin vary greatly in size, shape, and distribution. They are usually more pronounced in brunettes than in blondes. Certain pigmentary changes are common in pregnancy. The **linea nigra,** a dark, pigmented line extending from the umbilicus to the mons veneris, is a common pigmentary change (Fig. 7-2). The linea nigra never disappears entirely, although it usually becomes

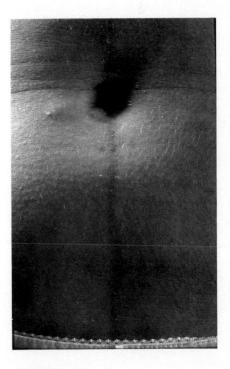

FIGURE 7-2

Linea Nigra. The skin in the abdominal midline may become pigmented during pregnancy. The color change is induced by the anterior pituitary hormone melanotropin. The linea nigra usually appears during the third month of pregnancy in primagravidas. In multiparas the entire line may appear before the third month.

much less pronounced after delivery. The external genitalia and any existing pigmented nevi also may darken.

Some pregnant women develop irregular, muddy brown-colored spots or blotches over the nose and cheeks. This condition is **chloasma,** or the "mask of pregnancy." Chloasma often causes considerable mental distress but usually disappears after delivery. Oral contraceptives can cause chloasma in nonpregnant women.

STRIAE GRAVIDARUM. The abdominal wall distends in the later months of pregnancy to accommodate the increasing size of the uterus. This distention causes streaks, or striations **(striae gravidarium),** in the skin at the outer edges of the abdomen and the anterior and outer aspects of the thighs (Fig. 7-3). Striae may also develop on the breasts and the buttocks. The striations are pink or slightly reddish on a white woman's skin and are golden on darker skin. The streaks, commonly called stretch marks, are caused by the stretching, rupture, and atrophy of the deep connective tissue in the skin. Striae result whenever the skin's capacity to stretch (elasticity) is exceeded. After delivery striae gradually fade to the silvery whiteness of scar tissue. Striae also can occur in other conditions that cause great abdominal distention such as accumulation of fat in the abdominal wall or the development of large, rapidly growing abdominal tumors.

VASCULAR MARKINGS. Vascular "spiders" are minute, fiery-red skin blemishes with branching lengths extending from a central body. They develop more often in white women but also occur (but are less noticeable) in black and Oriental women. Vascular spiders are of no clinical significance and will usually disappear after delivery. Palmar erythema (redness in palm of hand) and spider nevi (branched dilated capillaries) also are common. They are thought to be caused by a dramatic increase in circulating estrogens and will disappear after delivery.

Sweat Glands

There is increased activity of sebaceous and sweat glands and hair follicles during pregnancy as a result of the increased basal metabolic rate (BMR). The accelerated sweat gland activity produces increased perspiration, which is useful in elimination of waste material. This increased activity results from the progesterone-induced increased basal body temperature and the increased metabolic rate during pregnancy.

Epulis

Epulis (gingival granuloma gravidarum), hypertrophy of the gingival papillae around the gums, causes nodules to form and the gums to bleed easily. The nodules may be treated by excision if they become large, are painful, or bleed excessively. Epulis can occur during the last two trimesters, and clients may complain of bleeding gums when brushing their teeth.

Breast Changes

Enlargement and engorgement of the breasts and darkening of the pigment of the nipple and areola are observable presumptive signs. The nipple and areolar pigmentation never completely disappear after delivery.

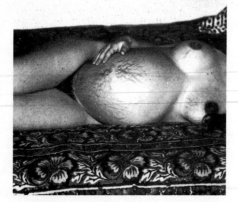

FIGURE 7-3
Striae Gravidarum. Striae gravidarum, commonly called "stretch marks," appear during the second half of pregnancy in 90% of gravidas. They tend to appear on the abdomen, thighs, and breasts. This condition occurs because the skin is stretched beyond capacity and represents a change in skin connective tissue. Striae fade after delivery but never completely disappear.

Internal Genitalia Changes

Changes in the internal genitalia are caused by vascular congestion. They are the only physical signs detectable within the first 3 months of pregnancy. Health professionals view **Chadwick's sign** and **Goodell's sign** as presumptive signs of pregnancy.

CHADWICK'S SIGN. As vascular congestion increases, the mucous membranes of the cervix, vagina, and vulva become a deep red to purple or bluish color. This coloration change is first seen during the fourth to sixth week of pregnancy. Since this sign can also be caused by any condition resulting in congestion of the pelvic organs, it is considered a presumptive sign of pregnancy.

GOODELL'S SIGN. Softening of the cervix usually occurs near the time of the second missed menstrual period but may be apparent as early as 1 month after conception. On digital examination the nonpregnant cervix has a consistency similar to the cartilaginous tip of the nose. The pregnant cervix' consistency feels like that of the lips or an earlobe. This change is due to increased vascularity, edema, and hyperplasia of the cervical glands.

Probable Signs of Pregnancy

Probable signs are more indicative of pregnancy than the presumptive signs. However, they still do not confirm pregnancy because they all can be caused by other conditions.

Hegar's Sign

After the sixth week of pregnancy **Hegar's sign** is perceptible. At this time the lower uterine segment (isthmus), or lower part of the body of the uterus, becomes much softer than the cervix. On bimanual examination it can be compressed almost to the thinness of paper because the growing embryo has not yet enfringed on it. This is one of the most valuable probable signs of pregnancy.

Uterine Enlargement

The uterus expands as it adapts to the increasing size of the fetus. Uterine enlargement, which is progressive and accompanied by amenorrhea, is a probable sign of pregnancy and results from estrogen and progesterone stimulation (Fig. 7-4). The fundus is palpable at the pubic symphysis at 12 weeks gestation. Fundal height is an important assessment component in confirming gestational progress and identifying abnormalities such as hydatidiform mole (degenerative process in chronic villi) and intrauterine growth retardation as pregnancy progresses.

Fetal Ballottement and Outline

A valuable sign suggesting the presence of a fetus is **ballottement** (from the French *balloter,* to toss up like a ball). During the fourth and fifth months of pregnancy the fetus is small in relation to the amount of amniotic fluid present. During vaginal examination a sudden finger tap on the cervix causes the fetus to rise in the amniotic fluid and then rebound

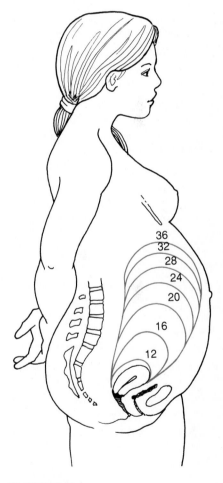

FIGURE 7-4

Uterine Enlargement During Pregnancy. Uterine enlargement is the result of (1) increased vascularity and dilation of blood vessels, (2) growth (hyperplasia) of new muscle fibers and fibroelastic tissue, (3) increased size of existing muscle fibers and fibroelastic tissue (hypertrophy), and (4) development of the lining of the uterus (decidua) for pregnancy.

FIGURE 7-5

Ballottement. The principle of ballottement is that an object floating in fluid can be made to move upward by a tap and its rebound can be felt. The examiner gently taps the bottom of the cervix, causing the fetus to rise in the amniotic fluid sac. When the fetus sinks back to the bottom of the amniotic sac, a gentle tap can be felt on the examiner's finger. This response is a probable sign of pregnancy.

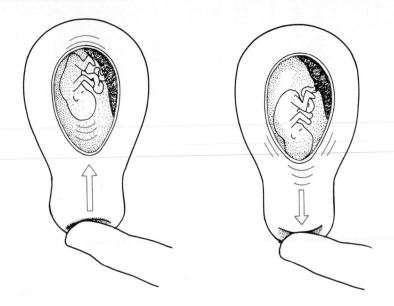

to its original position, tapping the examiner's finger (Fig. 7-5). When the tap is done by an experienced examiner, this response is the most certain of the probable signs of pregnancy.

After the sixth month of pregnancy the outline of the fetus (e.g., head, back, knees, elbows) can be easily identified by abdominal palpation. As pregnancy progresses, the outline of the fetus becomes more clearly defined. The ability to outline the fetus makes pregnancy extremely probable. In rare instances, however, tumors of the uterus may also mimic the fetal outline, making this sign fallible.

Braxton Hicks Contractions

Braxton Hicks contractions are uterine contractions that are generally painless and begin during the early weeks of pregnancy. They occur at intervals of 5 to 10 minutes throughout pregnancy. The client may or may not be conscious of them. These contractions become stronger during later pregnancy and may be palpated during bimanual examination or by placing the hand on the abdomen. This consistent contraction and relaxation of uterine muscles assists in expanding the uterus to accommodate the growing fetus. When near term, clients often mistake Braxton Hicks contractions for labor contractions because they become stronger.

Pregnancy Tests

Since the dawn of civilization efforts have been made to devise a satisfactory test for pregnancy. Currently, urine is the specimen used in most pregnancy tests. Pregnancy testing confirms or refutes the presence of hCG, which is secreted by the early chorionic villi of the implanted ovum. hCG appears in the maternal blood and is excreted in the urine. Pregnancy tests are not yet considered positive signs of pregnancy because too many factors influence the accuracy of the tests and false negatives or false positives are common. Categories of currently used pregnancy tests (Table 7-2) are (1) immunologic (antibody) tests used in both laboratory and home pregnancy tests; (2) radioimmunoassay tests; and (3) radioreceptor assay.

TABLE 7-2

Comparison of Pregnancy Tests

Category	Specimen	Time Required	Earliest Detection	Accuracy
Immunologic laboratory	First-voided morning urine	Slide: 2 min Tube: 2 hr	1 to 2 weeks after last missed menstrual period (42 days after conception)	Slide: 95% to 98% Tube: 98%
Home	First-voided morning urine	45 min to 2 hr	2 weeks after last missed menstrual period	97%
Radioimmunoassay (RIA)	Serum	1 to 3 hr	6 to 9 days after ovulation	Almost 100%
Radioreceptor assay (RRA)	Serum	1 hr	8 days after conception	90% to 95%

Positive Signs of Pregnancy

Although some of the previously mentioned signs, particularly the hormone tests, ballottement, and palpating the fetal outline, are rather conclusive evidences of pregnancy, they are not 100% certain. Errors in technique can invalidate the hormone tests, whereas other conditions can produce a high positive hCG value; on rare occasions the other pregnancy signs can be simulated by nonpregnant conditions.

Positive signs of pregnancy usually are not present until after the fourth month of gestation, with the exception of ultrasonography, which detects fetal cardiac activity as early as 8 weeks gestation. These signs are completely objective, cannot be confused with pathologic states, and offer absolute proof of pregnancy. If the term *positive* is used in the strictest sense, i.e., physical evidence, there are only four positive signs of pregnancy: (1) the presence of fetal heart sounds, (2) fetal movements felt by an examiner, (3) roentgenographic outline of the fetal skeleton, and (4) visualization of cardiac activity and fetal movement by ultrasonography. Fetal skeletal roentgenography is not performed nowadays; however, it is positive proof of pregnancy.

Fetal Heart Sounds

Pregnancy is validated when distinct fetal heart sounds are heard by an experienced examiner. Doppler ultrasonography is used to hear fetal heart sounds. Some facilities may still use a fetoscope for detecting fetal heart sounds, but Doppler ultrasonography requires less skill to use and can amplify the fetal heart sounds so they are audible to the human ear (Fig. 7-6). It detects heartbeats by the 10th to the 12th week of pregnancy, and the fetoscope does so at the 20th week. The fetal heart rate may vary from 110 to 160 beats per minute, with 140 beats per minute the average at term.

Fetal Movements Felt by Examiner

Client perception of fetal movements can vary remarkably and be misleading in the diagnosis of pregnancy. An experienced examiner's feeling the characteristic thrust or kick of the fetus is positive evidence of pregnancy. Often this occurs after the fifth month of pregnancy.

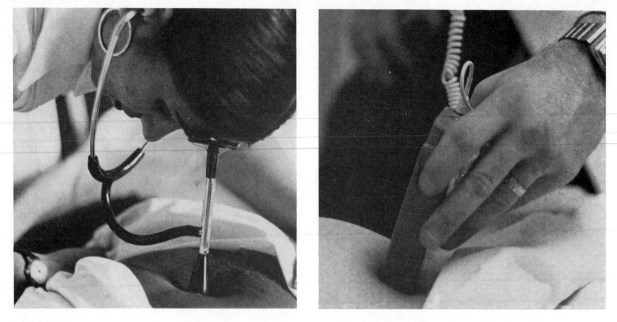

FIGURE 7-6
Detecting Fetal Heartbeat. Both the fetoscope, **A,** and Doppler ultrasonography, **B,** can be used to detect fetal heartbeat. Use of the fetoscope frees the hands for other activities. The Doppler device is hand-held but is more sensitive to the fetal heartbeat sounds. In many instances the heartbeat is heard earlier using the Doppler method.

Ultrasonographic Verification

The presence of an early embryo can be detected using real-time ultrasonography (ultrasound examination). The fetal sac in the uterus provides a uniquely identifiable pattern. The test becomes increasingly accurate as pregnancy advances and fetal cardiac activity and movements of the extremities can be observed. Ultrasonography is most useful clinically when the diagnosis of uterine pregnancy is questionable, such as when tubal ectopic pregnancy is suspected.

Systems Adaptation

During pregnancy the woman's body adapts to meet both the oxygen and nutrient needs of the developing fetus and her own increased metabolic needs. These systems changes are normal, inevitable, and temporary. The systems revert to the prepregnant state when postpartal convalescence is complete.

Metabolic Changes

Demands created by a rapidly growing fetus cause significant metabolic changes. This metabolic increase occurs in response to oxygen needs of the fetus and additional cardiac demands of the pregnant woman. The BMR begins to increase near the fourth month of pregnancy. At term it has increased 15% to 20%, and it returns to the prepregnancy level 5 to 6 days after delivery if breast feeding does not occur.

Pregnancy also affects carbohydrate metabolism. The fasting blood sugar level is lower during pregnancy. It is suspected that insulin production is increased. The metabolic stress of pregnancy and antagonistic effects of hormones can cause subclinical (gestational) diabetes, which may be detected for the first time during routine prenatal care.

Circulatory Changes

Circulatory changes occur to meet the demands of the growing uterus, placenta, and fetus. Blood flow increases to the organs that have additional workload, including the uterus (placenta and fetus) and the kidneys.

Specific benefits of the marked increase in circulating blood volume include (1) meeting the demands of the hypertrophied vascular system of the uterus, (2) protecting mother and fetus against effects of impaired venous return in supine and erect positions, and (3) safeguarding against adverse effects of blood loss associated with parturition.

Blood

During pregnancy the total volume of blood in the body increases approximately 30% to 50%. The pattern of increase begins in the first trimester, expands most rapidly during the second trimester, and plateaus during the last weeks of pregnancy. The minimum hematologic values for both healthy nonpregnant and pregnant women are 12 g hemoglobin, 3.75 million erythrocytes, and 35% hematocrit. Those values apply to both because the pregnant woman is producing red blood cells and increasing plasma volume simultaneously. Thus her actual concentration of red blood cells is approximately the same as under normal conditions. If adequate iron reserves are in the body and if sufficient iron is supplied by the diet, these hemotologic values will remain within expected limits during pregnancy. During pregnancy approximately 800 mg/day of iron is required to provide increased red blood cell production and to meet the increased needs of the fetus. Since the body's iron reserves are usually less than 500 mg, pregnant women need an iron supplement. Taking an iron supplement may be deferred until the second trimester to reduce the aggravation of nausea and vomiting.

Heart

The pregnancy-induced increase in blood volume in turn increases the cardiac workload. During pregnancy the heart needs to pump approximately 50% more blood per minute. If there is a preexisting cardiac condition, this increased workload can precipitate heart failure. Increased cardiac output peaks at the end of the second trimester and returns to the nonpregnant level during the last weeks of pregnancy. Immediately after delivery cardiac output rises again.

Blood Pressure

The arterial blood pressure of the pregnant woman is affected by her posture; it is highest when she is sitting and lowest in the lateral recumbent position. Arterial blood pressure falls during the late second or early third trimester of pregnancy and rises slowly thereafter as a result of increased volume circulating through flaccid blood vessels, causing vasodilation. Two separate factors affect the pregnant woman's blood pressure: diminished venous return from the lower extremities and compression of the inferior vena cava.

Decreased venous return from the lower extremities is due to pressure of the gravid uterus on the pelvic veins. This is a normal occurrence in pregnancy that occurs when the woman is erect. It contributes to de-

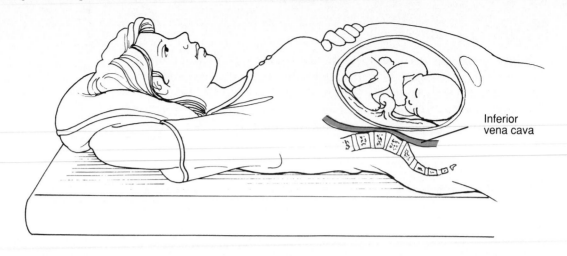

FIGURE 7-7
Vena Caval Compression and Vena Caval Syndrome. When the pregnant woman is supine, the uterus can compress the vena cava. Compression of the vena cava reduces the blood flow returning to the heart and results in hypotension or vena caval syndrome.

pendent edema, to the development of hemorrhoids and varicose veins of the legs and vulva, and to orthostatic (postural) hypotension.

Compression of the inferior vena cava (Fig. 7-7) reduces blood return to the heart and can reduce cardiac filling and cardiac output. The result is supine hypotension (vena caval syndrome) and produces feelings of light-headedness, drowsiness, nausea, and clamminess while in the supine position. Supine hypotension also decreases blood perfusion through the placenta. An immediate intervention to alleviate this undesirable state is to turn the woman on her side, thus relieving pressure on the vessels and restoring adequate circulation.

Uterine Blood Flow

Blood flow to the uterus increases by 80% during pregnancy to provide a sufficient supply to the placenta and to the myometrium and endometrium. By term, one-sixth of the total maternal blood volume is in the uterine vascular system. Complications that could result in uterine hemorrhage must be identified, diagnosed, and treated promptly.

Coagulation Value Changes

During pregnancy increases in various clotting mechanism factors increase the tendency for blood to coagulate. Concentration of fibrinogen increases approximately 50%, and fibrinolytic activity (the splitting or dissolving of a clot) is depressed. Fibrinolytic activity remains depressed through the postpartum period, and the woman continues at risk for thrombosis.

Respiratory Changes

Progesterone acts directly on the respiratory center of the brain, causing changes to occur. Pregnancy increases oxygen requirements 15% to 20% because both maternal and fetal blood must be oxygenated. One effect of progesterone is decreased airway resistance, which results in a 30% to 40% increase in the volume of air breathed per minute.

In the later months of pregnancy the uterus exerts a great deal of upward pressure on the diaphragm, causing temporary displacement. This crowding of the chest cavity produces a feeling of shortness of breath, which is relieved when the uterus descends into the pelvic cavity **(lightening)** 2 to 3 weeks before labor begins.

Respiratory tract response to elevated estrogen levels is to increase vascularization, resulting in congestion of the nasopharynx. Women may mistake this congestion for a cold and take over-the-counter medications for relief. During each prenatal visit the nurse should inquire if any non-prescription medications are being taken and if the client has experienced nasal congestion.

Gastrointestinal Changes

Anatomic Changes

The intestines and stomach are displaced upward by the enlarging uterus during pregnancy. The appendix is often displaced laterally and upward, even as high as the right flank. This anatomic shift can alter the physical findings in a client with appendicitis as well as the pregnant client's perception of the pain's location.

Physiologic Changes

The functioning of the digestive system may be altered during pregnancy. Increased progesterone levels result in a generalized relaxation of smooth muscle. Gastrointestinal tract motility is decreased, resulting in prolonged gastric emptying time, slower peristalsis, and longer intestinal transit time. The pressure changes created by smooth muscle relaxation, combined with slower esophageal peristalsis, contribute to gastroesophageal reflux. Reflux of acidic stomach secretions into the lower esophagus results in client complaints of heartburn.

Decreased peristalsis also causes the constipation and flatulence that are common during pregnancy; at least one-half of all gravid women suffer from these disorders. The entire gastrointestinal tract is affected by diminished motility, decreased smooth muscle tone, and pressure from the expanding uterus during pregnancy.

Liver and Gallbladder Changes

Some hepatic function laboratory test results are altered by pregnancy. Test results that could erroneously suggest hepatic disease include increases in serum alkaline phosphatase and leucine aminopeptidase and a decrease in serum cholinesterase. Although palmar erythema and spider nevi are characteristically seen in clients with liver disease, they also can occur in healthy pregnant women.

Gallbladder function is also altered by pregnancy. Increased progesterone levels cause bile to become thick and slightly hypercholesterolemic. A tendency toward decreased tone and distention results in an extended emptying time. These changes during pregnancy predispose the client for gallstone formation.

Urinary and Renal Changes

The kidneys must excrete both the pregnant woman's waste products and those of the growing fetus. Physiologic adaptations of the urinary system during pregnancy include (1) a slight increase in the size of the kidneys, (2) a 50% increase in glomerular filtration rate, (3) impaired reabsorption of glucose, (4) dilation of the ureters, and (5) diminished ureteral peristalsis. The nocturnal urinary output during pregnancy increases approximately 60% to 90% and has a lower specific gravity.

Ureteral Changes

The ureters become markedly dilated during pregnancy because of the pressure of the gravid uterus on the ureters as they cross the pelvic brim and because of ureteral wall softening. This wall softening is caused by the action of progesterone on smooth muscle. Because dilated ureters are unable to propel urine efficiently, urinary stasis occurs and in turn increases the risk for infection. Dilation does not impair the ureter permanently unless infection has developed or pregnancy occurs again before the ureters return to normal, i.e., 4 to 6 weeks after delivery.

Alteration in Laboratory Results

Many blood and urinary laboratory values are altered by pregnancy (Table 7-3) because of changes in renal and metabolic function. Since ureteral dilation results in retention of urine, results from some commonly used dye-excretion kidney function tests will be altered. Plasma creatinine and urea concentrations decrease. Results of urinary concentration tests can be altered since it is normal for the pregnant woman to fail to concentrate urine after fluids are withheld. In this instance the kidneys simply mobilize extracellular fluid.

TABLE 7-3

Laboratory Values Altered During Pregnancy

Value	Alteration
Urine	
Glomerular filtration rate	Increases 30% to 50%
Urea concentration	Decreases
Urinary electrolytes	Increases
Urinary concentration after withholding of fluids	May not occur
Urinary glucose	Present
Urinary protein	Increases
Urinary sodium	Increases
Urinary uric acid	Increases
Blood	
Butanol-extractable iodine (BEI)	Increases
Fasting blood sugar	Decreases
Lactosuria	Present
Plasma creatinine	Decreases
Protein-bound iodine (PBI)	Increases
Sedimentation rate	Increases
Thyroxine (T_4)	Increases
Triiodothyronine (T_3)	Decreases
Urea	Decreases

Kidney Changes

Pregnant women tend to excrete glucose in the urine because of their increased glomerular filtration rate and the decreased capacity of the tubules to reabsorb glucose during pregnancy. Although a reduced renal threshold for glucose is often associated with pregnancy, the presence of any sugar in the urine should always be reported to the physician. Lactosuria (milk sugar in urine) may be present, particularly during the latter part of pregnancy and the postpartum period, and is an expected finding.

Bladder Changes

The bladder functions efficiently during pregnancy. The urinary frequency experienced during the first few months of pregnancy is caused by pressure exerted on the bladder by the enlarging uterus. Frequency occurs again with lightening before the onset of labor.

Endocrine Changes

The mother's endocrine system adapts to meet the needs of both the mother and fetus. The displays on pages 140 and 141 present the effects of estrogen and progesterone in pregnancy.

Pituitary Body

ANTERIOR LOBE. During pregnancy gonadotropins are no longer cyclically released. The estrogen and progesterone produced by the placenta inhibit their release from the pituitary gland.

POSTERIOR LOBE. The posterior lobe of the pituitary secretes the hormone oxytocin, which stimulates uterine muscle contraction. The effects of endogenous oxytocin are not apparent until the onset of labor. The action of oxytocin is suppressed by progesterone until the blood levels of oxytocin exceeds that of progesterone. Exogenous oxytocin is used to initiate labor, to increase contraction quality during labor, to enhance uterine contraction after delivery to decrease postpartal bleeding, and to initiate the let-down reflex for the breast-feeding mother.

Thyroid Gland

Thyroid function is also altered by pregnancy. The following thyroid-function measurements increase during pregnancy: serum protein-bound iodine (PBI) level, butanol-extractable iodine (BEI) level, and thyroxine (T_4) level. These increases occur because an elevated level of thyroid-binding protein is present in the blood.

The triiodothyronine (T_3) uptake level decreases during pregnancy, indicating an increase in the binding of circulating triiodothyronine. This increased value is a reflection of the high level of circulating estrogen during pregnancy.

Adrenal Glands

The adrenal cortex hypertrophies during pregnancy, but it is believed that its activity increases. Increased production of aldosterone, the hormone

Estrogen's Effects in Pregnancy

Gastrointestinal System

Causes epulis (bleeding gums)
Decreases gastric hydrochloric acid and pepsin secretion

Genitourinary System

Encourages renal retention of sodium and water
   Increases plasma volume
   Shifts fluid balance
Dilates ureters and renal pelvis
Hypertrophies bladder wall
Relaxes bladder and trigone

Reproductive System

Increases breast size
   Promotes development of ducts, alveoli, and nipples
   Encourages fat storage
Increases uterine size and weight
   Promotes myometrium growth
   Increases blood supply
   Increases endometrium proliferation
   Vascularizes and congests cervix
Enlarges external genitalia
Thickens vaginal wall and increases pliability
   Causes vaginal secretions to thicken and become white and acidic
   Thickens vaginal epithelium

Musculoskeletal System

Increases connective tissue's pliability
   Relaxes pelvic joints and ligaments
   Increases stretching capacity of cervix
   Decreases pulmonary resistance

Cardiovascular System

Increases ureteroplacental blood flow

Hematology

Binds with and decreases T_3
Increases blood clotting potential
   Decreases fibrinolytic activity

Skin

Increases pigmentation (chloasma, linea nigra)
Causes vascular changes (spider nevi, palmar erythema)

responsible for renal reabsorption of sodium, counteracts the tendency to excrete sodium as the result of the influence of progesterone. This increased activity begins early in pregnancy and continues throughout, resulting in decreased ability of the kidneys to handle sodium. Often fluid retention and either occult or overt edema results.

Ovaries

The ovaries are inactive during pregnancy except for the activity of the corpus luteum. Follicular activity is suspended after fertilization of the ovum, and there is no further ovulation until after delivery.

Progesterone's Effects in Pregnancy

Respiratory System

Causes vocal cords to increase in size (voice becomes deeper)

Gastrointestinal System

Thickens gallbladder's contents

Genitourinary System

Increases size of kidneys
Encourages renal sodium excretion

Reproductive System

Causes breast changes
    Prepares lobulo-alveolar system for lactation
    Increases glandular tissue
Decreases uterine motility and contractibility
Increases endometrial supply of glycogen, arterial blood, secretory glands,
    amino acids, and water
Develops endometrial glycogen storage cells
Facilitates prolactin secretion in endometrium
Suppresses prolactin secretion in myometrium
Proliferates vaginal epithelium
Secretes thick viscous mucus in cervix

Musculoskeletal System

Relaxes smooth muscle tone of the following:
    Ureters (dilate)
    Bladder (increases capacity)
    Esophagus (decreases tone)
    Stomach (decreases motility; decreases secretion of hydrochloric acid and
        pepsin)
    Intestines (decreases peristalsis; increases gut transit time)
    Trachea (increases volume of air breathed per minute)

Cardiovascular System

Encourages carbon dioxide passage from fetal to maternal circulation

Skin

Increases activity of sebaceous and sweat glands and hair follicles

Metabolic System

Encourages storage of fat
Increases BMR until midpregnancy

Endocrine System

Suppresses action of oxytocin before onset of labor

Immune System

May assist in preventing maternal rejection of fetus (immunologic response)

Pancreas

The fetal demands for fuel for growth deplete the mother's store of glucose. As a result, maternal blood glucose levels are low throughout pregnancy. As the pregnancy progresses, the pancreas is stimulated to increase insulin production, but at the same time the mother's ability to utilize the available insulin decreases; she develops resistance to insulin.

This inability to utilize insulin is a protective measure to ensure that the fetal glucose needs are met before those of the mother. The mother's inability to utilize the available insulin (insulin resistance) sends a signal to the pancreas that is interpreted as a demand for additional insulin production. Insulin demands continue to increase steadily throughout the pregnancy. This physiologic change, coupled with the stress of pregnancy and the antagonistic effect of placental hormones on insulin, can precipitate subclinical diabetes (gestational diabetes) in some clients.

Placenta

The placenta is an organ designed to transmit nutritive substances and oxygen from mother to fetus and carbon dioxide and waste products from fetus to mother. It also secretes hormones that affect virtually every body system during pregnancy. The early chorionic villi of the implanted ovum secrete hCG, which prolongs the life of the corpus luteum. This in turn provides for the continued production of estrogen and progesterone, which are necessary for the maintenance of the endometrium. During pregnancy hCG appears in maternal blood and is excreted in the mother's urine, making urine tests for pregnancy possible.

The placenta takes over the production of estrogen and progesterone from the ovaries. After the first 2 months of pregnancy, the placenta becomes the major source of these two hormones.

The chorionic cells of the placenta produce another hormone, human chorionic somatomammotropin (hCS), also known as human placental lactogen (hPL). This hormone may be found in placental cells as early as the third week after ovulation and in maternal serum by the sixth week of pregnancy. It influences somatic cell growth of the fetus and facilitates preparation of the breasts for lactation.

Musculoskeletal Changes

Postural changes caused by an expanding uterus and hormone-induced pelvic joint relaxation are the primary musculoskeletal alterations related to pregnancy. As abdominal girth increases during pregnancy, the woman's center of gravity shifts. Decreasing abdominal muscle tone, coupled with increased weight, create varying degrees of postural changes, resulting in lordosis (Fig. 7-8). This frequent rearranging and realignment of the lumbosacral curve gives rise to the common complaints of backache and unsure sense of balance. Backache is a particularly common complaint in later months of pregnancy.

The sacroiliac, sacrococcygeal, and pubic joints soften as a result of hormonal influence and have increased mobility. Instability of these joints can also result in pain and walking difficulties. These joints become more mobile to accommodate the passage of the fetus through the pelvis.

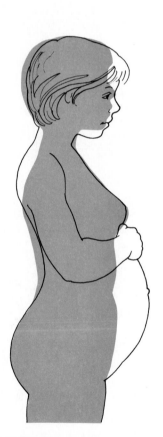

FIGURE 7-8
Postural Changes During Pregnancy. The pregnant woman's head assumes an exaggerated anterior flexion and the shoulders slump anteriorly in an attempt to compensate for the body's gravity shift. The poor lumbrosacral alignment that results from this compensation creates backache and unsure balance.

Cultural Influences on Pregnancy Perception

Recent trends have fostered an increased awareness of the importance and impact of social and cultural factors in both health care and the delivery system. Pregnancy and birth are viewed as very important events in most cultures. The attitudes toward these processes vary considerably between cultures and even within a single society. For example, one societal segment may conceptualize pregnancy and childbirth as a "crisis" situation, whereas another faction of that same society may regard them as a role transition experience. Each of these attitudes has very different implications for the delivery of health care. Health care providers must be aware of the existence of the social and cultural influences that modify expectations in obstetric care. This awareness enables the health care provider to incorporate sociocultural values in client-centered care by doing the following:

1. Identifying and understanding clients' attitudes, behaviors, values, and needs.
2. Planning and implementing effective client-centered, goal-directed nursing care.
3. Modifying plans and care to be consistent with the individual client's needs and values.

The Sick Role, Illness, and Pregnancy

Some societies regard pregnancy as a "normal" state, a passage through which most women will pass. Other societies consider pregnancy as an illness state. Even when pregnancy is viewed as an illness state, the behavioral expectations differ from those for nonpregnant illness. The pregnancy behavior expectations are determined and influenced by the culture's values. They can range from a relatively unstructured to a restrictively structured set of behaviors. When behavioral guidelines are unstructured, the pregnant woman must determine her own parameters. Choosing to assume the "sick" pregnancy role may be one of these parameters.

Societal Trends

Many health care practices in the United States focus on both the pregnant woman and the fetus. Dominant practices include providing prenatal education and care, using ultrasound technology to view the fetus, and providing for delivery to take place in a hospital or birthing center.

Family-Centered Care

The family-centered model for delivering health care has been initiated in response to consumer demands. Consumers want to collaborate actively in their health care planning and decisions. Today's health care consumer has gone from passive to assertive and from being dependent to demanding an active health care role.

Early Discharge

New health care issues and needs have risen from the use of early discharge programs. The health care delivery system has revamped because cost-

⟰ CULTURAL IMPLICATIONS

Values, attitudes, perspectives, and behaviors are influenced and reinforced by the social groups in which one participates. Consequently, health and health care orientation reflect learned ethnic, racial, religious, and social class values.

containment programs mandate early discharge after delivery, meaning the mother's health care skills, information levels, and her infant care skills must be quickly assessed. The health care provider must rapidly plan with the mother and family to implement the needed individualized mother and baby health care maintenance education. The emphasis has shifted from providing care to providing information.

Delayed Childbearing

Cultural changes have resulted in many couples' delaying childbearing until their early to middle thirties. The trend also is to have smaller families. Currently, it is acceptable for the mother to return to work outside the home after a child is born. This trend toward later childbearing and working outside the home has altered traditional practices and values and has created other far-reaching societal impacts.

Effects on Family Members' Roles
Effects on the Couple

Pregnancy and childbirth have an extensive effect on the couple as a unit, starting with how the couple views the pregnancy. Partners with greater mutuality (or "coupleness") in their relationship manage the transition to parenthood better. Pregnancy necessitates shifts in work loads, responsibilities, and authority. Nontraditional roles may need to be assumed. Value systems are affected and altered. Communication takes on new perspectives and parameters. The major task to undertake is reorienting the relationship.

Effect on the Mother

The pregnant woman must accomplish several psychologic tasks. First, she must believe she is pregnant and incorporate the fetus into her body image. The mother's second task is to prepare for the physical separation, or the birth of the infant. Some women are eager to have their baby; however, others do not want to let go of the fetus. A third task is to resolve the identity confusions that accompany role transition and prepare for the smooth functioning of the family unit after birth. She must be ready to assume the caretaking relationship with the baby, i.e., to become a mother. Pregnancy may be the first occasion in the relationship in which the partners realize the extent to which they are interdependent psychologically, socially, and economically.

Effect on the Father

Men undergo far less social preparation than women do for parenthood, and there is little to prepare them for pregnancy per se. Experience with fathers who have actively involved themselves in pregnancy indicates that men, like women, go through various phases during pregnancy. Men experience three phases. The introduction phase comes with the confirmation of the diagnosis of pregnancy and places a father almost immediately into a honeymoon stage. Like his partner, he must assimilate the fact that the baby is his. In the second trimester more thought is given to what it means to be a father, and the plateau stage is entered. The man observes children and pregnant women more intently and becomes more acutely aware of his partner's expanding girth.

As is true for the mother, labor and delivery mark the disengagement-termination phase of the role transition of pregnancy for the father. How they proceed can have a profound effect on the father. Most health providers who have had experience with pregnant couples believe that men who take an active part in the pregnancy are more likely to participate in the birthing with positive psychologic outcomes.

Effect on Sibling(s)

The effect of pregnancy on the children of a family depends a great deal on the age of each child. When and how to tell the children about the expected baby and how to help them prepare for its arrival also depend on the age of each child. Regardless of the age, each of the children needs thorough reassurance that the pregnancy is adding a new member to the family but is not replacing anyone in either parent's affections. Roles of siblings change as they become the older brother or sister of the new baby.

Effect on Grandparents

Recent research has indicated the importance of the grandparent-grandchild relationship. Grandparents act as a potential resource for families, and family systems can be strengthened by the additional support and nurturance of the grandparents. The parent serves as a negotiator in establishing the grandparent-grandchild relationship. Many women report becoming closer to their mothers during pregnancy. The estrangement that began in adolescence disappears as the now-pregnant daughter experiences joys, concern, and anxieties similar to those her mother has felt.

Some grandparents-to-be do not welcome the new role for their daughters or sons. They may see it as a sign of their own aging process or as the victory of the child in obtaining an equal role status with the parent. Most grandparents, however, react more positively to the prospect of a new baby in the family. It reawakens feelings of their own youth, the excitement of giving birth, and their delight in the behavior of the parents-to-be when they were infants. The realization that there is continuity between the past and the present produces satisfaction.

SUGGESTED READINGS

Barranti C: The grandparent/grandchild relationship: Family resources in an era of voluntary bonds. Fam Relat 34:3, July 1985

Fishbein EG: Expectant fathers' stress—due to the mothers' expectations. JOGN 13:325-328, September/October 1984

Greene R, Polivka J: The meaning of grandparent day cards, an analysis of the intergenerational network. Fam Relat 34:2, April 1985

May KA: Active involvement of expectant fathers in pregnancy: Some further considerations. JOGN 7:7-12, March/April 1978

Munroe RL, Munroe RH: Male pregnancy symptoms and cross-sex identity in three societies. J Soc Psychol 89:147-158, February 1973

Parson T: Definitions of health and illness in the light of American values and social structure. In Parson T (ed): Social structure and personality. Glencoe, Ill, The Free Press, 1964, pp 257-291

Phillip CR, Anzalone SJ: Fathering: Participating in Labor and Birth. St. Louis, CV Mosby, 1978

Richardson P: Women's perceptions of change in relationships shared with child during pregnancy. Matern Child Nurs J 12:2, Summer 1983

Segall A: The sick role concept: Understanding illness behavior. J Health Soc Behav 17(20):162-169, 1976

Tenhouten W: The black family: Myth and reality. Psychiatry 33:145-175, 1970

Vogel G: American Indian Medicine. New York, Ballentine Books, 1973

Maternal Nursing Care in the Antepartum Period

IMPORTANT TERMINOLOGY

abortion Termination of pregnancy before fetus has attained stage of viability

antepartum Time between conception and labor; period of pregnancy until onset of labor; prenatal period

gravida Woman who is pregnant

para Refers to past pregnancies that have carried a fetus to viability whether the infant was alive at birth or not

perinatal Pertaining to the time before, during, and after birth; variously defined as time including conception through the 28th day of life or conception through the first year of life

teratogen Nongenetic factor that can cause fetal malformations

viable infant One who weighs at least 500 g and is more than 20 weeks gestation

Optimum **antepartum** care begins with the thorough collection of data about the client's history, physical status, and psychosocial background during the first prenatal visit. Follow-up care at regularly appointed intervals throughout pregnancy allows opportunity to monitor maternal and fetal status, institute treatment and additional diagnostic tests as necessary, and offer ongoing maternal and family support and education.

Client Assessment and History

When a client enters the health care delivery system for antepartum care, the nurse assists in collecting personal history information that may affect the progress and outcome of pregnancy. The history may be obtained by having the client complete a questionnaire, by interviewing the client, or through a combination of both. This initial aspect of assessment provides the nurse with an opportunity to begin building rapport with the client.

Data collected during the first prenatal visit include (1) pregnancy history, (2) current medical history, (3) past medical history, (4) personal characteristics, (5) information about the father of the baby, and (6) family history. Any aspect of the history that changes during the course of the pregnancy should be updated during subsequent visits.

Pregnancy History

Seeking information about the pregnancy before gathering other data conveys interest in the client's primary concern. The current pregnancy history assists the nurse in calculating the expected date of delivery of a fetus that has reached 40 weeks of gestation and alerts the nurse to any complications of pregnancy the client may be experiencing. History of past pregnancies provides a baseline that serves as a predictor of the current pregnancy's outcome.

Current Pregnancy Information

The first day of the last menstrual period (LMP) is recorded and the expected date of confinement (EDC) or expected date of delivery (EDD) is calculated using Nägele's rule (see below). Most women do not deliver on the date calculated but do deliver from 7 days before to 7 days after the EDC.

For additional current pregnancy data that is needed, see Assessment Tool: Client Assessment and History.

Past Obstetric History

Information about the conduct and outcome of past pregnancies is pertinent to guiding the client through the current pregnancy. The course of the current pregnancy may be similar to that of preceding pregnancies.

Some of the information from past pregnancies is summarized and recorded using the terms **gravida** and **para**. For example, Jane Doe is currently pregnant. She had one child born at 39 weeks, twins born at 36 weeks, one spontaneous **abortion** at 10 weeks, and a stillborn fetus at term. Three children are living and well. She is gravida 5 (pregnant five times), para 3 (three deliveries of fetuses that had reached the age of **viability**) and ab 1 (one abortion). Note that the delivery of fetuses from a multiple pregnancy (e.g., twins, triplets) is counted as one pregnancy and one delivery.

Many health care settings use a more detailed approach for recording the client's pregnancy history. In this system the standard gravida is followed by a series of four digits that designate pregnancy outcomes

---

Calculation of EDC Using Nägele's Rule

This rule is based on the average duration of pregnancy, which is 40 weeks. It assumes the menstrual cycle comprises 28 days and that conception occurs on the 14th day. To calculate the EDC, subtract 3 months from the first day of the LMP and add 7 days. Correct for the year if necessary; that is, if the first day of the LMP occurs in January, February, or March through March 25, the EDC will occur in the same year. If the first day of the LMP is after March 25, the EDC will occur during the next calendar year.

$$EDC = \text{First day of LMP} - 3 \text{ months} + 7 \text{ days}$$
$$EDC = \text{June } 10 - 3 \text{ months} = \text{March } 10 + 7 = \text{March } 17 + 1 \text{ year}$$

Client Assessment and History

Current Pregnancy Data

First day of last menstrual period (LMP)
Client's response and adaptation to her pregnancy
Any symptoms experienced since the LMP such as nausea, vomiting, urinary
frequency, and breast changes
Any vaginal spotting or bleeding, with or without cramping, that has
occurred since the LMP

Past Obstetric Data

Year of each previous pregnancy
Outcome of each pregnancy (abortion, preterm, fullterm, living, or stillborn)
Any complications experienced during the antepartum, intrapartum, or
postpartum period
Length of labor
Type of delivery (vaginal or cesarean)
Health status of the neonate
Weight of the neonate

Current Medical History Data

Client's perception of her current health status
Height, weight, and vital signs
Blood type and Rh factor if known
Current use of any licit or illicit substances, including, but not limited to,
alcohol, tobacco, cocaine, heroin, over-the-counter medications, and
prescription drugs
Current acute or chronic disease conditions being treated or monitored by a
primary care practitioner
Any known allergies
Eating patterns (a review of client's food intake for the 3 preceding days
facilitates nutritional assessment)
Exercise routines
Exposure to communicable diseases since the beginning of pregnancy
(especially rubella if not immune)
Illnesses such as colds or influenza since the beginning of pregnancy
Exposure to any teratogenic agent since the beginning of pregnancy

Past Medical History Data

Childhood diseases
Date of immunizations, particularly rubella
Menstrual history, including age at menarche and description of typical cycle
Date of onset and treatment for diseases such as anemia, asthma, blood
dyscrasias, cancer, cardiac disease, diabetes mellitus, endocrinopathy,
hypertension, psychiatric disorders, renal or urinary tract diseases, and
tuberculosis
Date of occurrence and treatment for sexually transmitted diseases
Dates and types of surgery
Dates and reasons for previous hospitalizations
Dates and number of blood transfusions
Injuries, especially to pelvic structure and organs
Contraceptive history and practice
Sexual practices

Personal Characteristics

Age
Racial and ethnic background
Education
Occupation
Support networks, including father of baby, children, other family members,
and close friends

Continued

Client Assessment and History—*continued*

Data About Father of Baby

Age
Height and weight
Racial and ethnic origin
Education
Occupation
Potential health hazards
Current health status
Significant medical history
Any known conditions that are genetically transmitted (self or family)
Use of licit or illicit substances, including, but not limited to, alcohol,
    tobacco, cocaine, heroin, over-the-counter medications, and prescription
    drugs
Blood type and Rh factor
Response to pregnancy

Family History Data

Health status of parents and siblings (if deceased, note cause of death)
Occurrence or history of the following diseases in parents, siblings, and close
    relatives: cancer, cardiopulmonary diseases, complications of pregnancy,
    congenital anomalies, diabetes mellitus, hypertension, psychiatric disorders,
    renal disease, tuberculosis, and vascular disease

and the number of living children. The acronym TPAL, or FPAL, facilitates memorizing the system.

1. *T* or *F* designates the number of infants born at *Term* or *Fullterm*.
2. *P* designates the number of infants delivered *Preterm*.
3. *A* designates the number of pregnancies terminated by either spontaneous or elective *Abortion*.
4. *L* designates the number of *Living* children.

Jane Doe's record would read 52213 (5 pregnancies, 2 term or fullterm deliveries, 2 preterm deliveries, 1 abortion, and 3 living children).

Medical History

The client's current and past medical history provides indicators of her ongoing health status. The caregiver is alert to any deviations in health that might influence the conduct of the pregnancy and its outcome. For example, a woman with insulin-dependent diabetes requires monitoring and guidance to maintain her pregnancy. Also, special concern is directed toward the well-being of her fetus during pregnancy and delivery and toward her neonate after birth.

Current Medical History

The client's height, weight, and vital signs should be measured and recorded during the initial visit, and the weight and blood pressure should be taken and recorded on all subsequent visits. Any significant weight change just before or since the beginning of the pregnancy should be noted. Such weight changes are investigated to determine the cause and potential implications for a high-risk pregnancy.

Current recordings of vital signs and weight become part of the client's ongoing history during the course of her pregnancy and provide a baseline from which to monitor changes that might indicate complications of pregnancy. Additional data to obtain through the client's self-report is found in the assessment tool on pages 149–150. Such information alerts caregivers to potential factors that could affect maternal, fetal, or neonatal well-being. Included among those factors is a detailed drug history to ascertain whether or not the woman is using licit or illicit substances.

Past Medical History

The aforementioned assessment tool delineates the data obtained from the client about her past medical history. This information alerts the caregiver to health factors that may need further investigation or monitoring. For example, special concern is directed toward the guidance and care of a woman who is not immune to rubella because of the severe effects this viral disease has on the developing embryo and fetus.

Personal Characteristics

The assessment tool on pages 149–150 lists pertinent information the caregiver seeks about the client's personal characteristics. As in all areas of the history, rationales for eliciting the information are to alert the nurse and the physician or the certified nurse midwife to potential problems the client might experience during pregnancy. An adolescent female and women more than 35 years of age are at greater risk for experiencing complications of pregnancy. Women in certain occupations may be exposed to **teratogens**, and those of particular ethnic or racial backgrounds may have certain beliefs that influence their behavior and compliance with medically recommended treatment regimens.

Data About Father of Baby

Pertinent information about the father of the baby is found in the assessment tool on pages 149–150. The father's history may reveal factors that will influence the development of the fetus and the outcome of pregnancy. For example, the caregiver is alerted to such things as potential Rh factor and ABO (blood type) incompatability problems in the event that the woman is Rh negative and the man is Rh positive or if her blood type is different from his. The racial or ethnic background of the father may influence the father's participation in the pregnancy and care of the child, and certain genetically transmitted disorders as sickle cell disease are associated with race and ethnicity. As with the woman, it is also important to obtain a detailed drug history on the father. If the father is a substance abuser, he is likely to experience social and health problems that can affect maternal, fetal, and neonatal well-being.

Family History

Pertinent data to obtain about the health history of the family is found in the assessment tool on pages 149–150. This information directs attention toward clients who are at greater risk for experiencing certain health disorders because of a family history of the condition. Also, it may be learned through this information that members of the family have experienced genetically transmitted disorders.

Physical Assessment of the Client

After the client's history is obtained and recorded, a thorough physical examination is performed to establish a baseline for her general state of health and to evaluate the pregnancy. The examination may be conducted by a physician or a nurse practitioner such as a family nurse practitioner or certified nurse midwife.

Before the examination, the woman should empty her bladder because a full bladder is uncomfortable and may interfere with the manipulations performed during the physical assessment. If ordered by the primary care practitioner, a clean-catch specimen may be collected at this time for urinalysis. A full urinalysis, including chemistry and microscopic examination, is usually ordered to help identify clients with unsuspected diabetes mellitus, renal disease, hypertensive disease, and bacteriuria.

During the physical examination particular attention is paid to the client's mouth and throat, thyroid gland and lymph nodes, lungs, heart, breasts, skin, extremities, abdomen, and pelvis. Characteristic changes of pregnancy in each area examined are noted, and signs of infection or systemic disease are identified if present. Table 8-1 lists findings usually associated with pregnancy and abnormal findings that may need treatment or may increase the client's risk for a medically complicated pregnancy.

TABLE 8-1

Components of the Prenatal Physical Examination

Part Examined — Examination Technique	Usual Findings During Pregnancy	Abnormal Findings
Head and Neck		
Palpation, inspection with otoscope or ophthalmoscope, and visual inspection of the mouth	Hyperemia of nasal and buccal mucous membranes, slight diffuse enlargement of thyroid (these changes are associated with pregnancy)	Enlarged lymph nodes, thyroid nodules or irregular enlargement, lesions of eyes or mouth, caries and abscesses of teeth, ear infections
Chest and Heart		
Auscultation with stethoscope, percussion, and visual inspection	Lungs clear, heart in regular rhythm (occasionally a soft, short functional murmur caused by hemodynamic changes of pregnancy)	Rales, wheezes, rhonchi, irregular cardiac rhythm, nonphysiologic murmurs
Breasts		
Palpation and visual inspection	Enlargement of breasts, with increased vascular patterns, darkened areolae with prominent tubercles, colostrum from nipples in later pregnancy; note if nipples are inverted so preparation can be initiated if mother wishes to breast-feed	Masses of nodules, bloody or serosanguineous nipple discharge, nipple lesions, erythema, absence of changes associated with pregnancy
Skin		
Visual inspection	Pigmentation changes (linea nigra, chloasma), enlargement of nevi, appearance of spider angiomas, mottled erythema of hands	Pallor, jaundice, rash, skin lesions
Extremities		
Visual inspection and palpation, percussion with reflex hammer	Mild pretibial and ankle edema in third trimester, slight edema of hands in hot weather	Limitations of motion; varicosities; more than slight pretibial, hand, or ankle edema; edema of face or sacrum; hyperreflexia and clonus

Screening for High-Risk Factors

Physical indicators of a high-risk pregnancy can often be determined during the initial examination (see Assessment Tool: Identification of High-Risk Pregnancy on p. 154). A high-risk pregnancy is one in which maternal deviations in health that are present at conception or occur during the pregnancy compromise the health of the mother or the growth, development, and delivery of the fetus or both.[1,2] The mother and the family need special guidance and assistance throughout the pregnancy in an effort to reduce maternal and **perinatal** morbidity and mortality.

Pelvic Examination

The pelvic examination provides data needed in confirming the pregnancy, determining the length of gestation, and identifying pelvic characteristics and any abnormalities that might produce complications of pregnancy. At the same time specimens are obtained to screen for potential problems that can affect the progress or outcome of the pregnancy. The pelvic examination includes both speculum and bimanual examinations.

The bimanual examination provides information about (1) the consistency of the cervix; (2) the size, shape, and consistency of the uterus; (3)

TABLE 8-1

Components of the Prenatal Physical Examination—continued

Part Examined Examination Technique	Usual Findings During Pregnancy	Abnormal Findings
Abdomen Palpation, visual inspection, auscultation, percussion	Enlarged uterus, palpation of fetal outline in later pregnancy, fetal heart sounds, contractions in last trimester	Uterus too large or too small for dates, absence of fetal heart sounds beyond 10 weeks (using Doppler), transverse lie of fetus, fetal head in fundus, tonic uterine contractions, enlarged liver or spleen
Pelvis Speculum examination, bimanual examination with inspection and palpation, collection of specimens	*Speculum examination:* Bluish discoloration of mucosa of vagina and cervix (Chadwick's sign), congested cervix, ectropion cervix in multigravidas, increased leukorrhea *Bimanual examination:* Soft cervix (Goodell's sign), admits a finger or two (depending on gravida and length of pregnancy); softening of lower uterine segment (Hegar's sign); enlarged uterus; fetal head or parts may be felt in lower uterine segment; gynecoid pelvic configuration *Papanicolaou smear:* Squamous cell metaplasia; negative or normal, adequate or increased estrogen; endocervical cells; hyperplasia that is considered borderline	*Speculum examination:* Yellow, purulent, frothy, cheesy, white or homogeneous gray, foul-smelling discharge; friable, bleeding lesions of cervix; vaginal lesions; bleeding from cervical os; amniotic fluid loss *Bimanual examination:* Cervix dilated and effaced (unless labor has begun); cervical or vaginal masses; excessive amniotic fluid (uterus unusually enlarged); adnexal masses or fullness; rectal masses; hemorrhoids; contractions of the pelvic inlet, midpelvis, or outlet *Papanicolaou smear:* Inflammation; presence of *Trichomonas vaginalis* or fungi; diminished or absent estrogen; atypical or suspicious cells; atypical hyperplasia, dysplasia, neoplasia, or carcinoma

Identification of High-Risk Pregnancy

Sociodemographic Factors

Age
  16 years of age or less
  35 years of age or more
Low socioeconomic status

Factors Arising From Deviations in Health

Obstetric and fetal or neonatal factors
  Parity of 5 or more
  History of spontaneous abortions
  History of ectopic pregnancy
  History of preterm births
  Less than 1 year since previous birth
  History of fetal macrosomia
  History of low birth weight infants
  Contracted pelvis
  Anomalies of the reproductive system
  History of operative deliveries
  History of prolonged true labor
  History of breech deliveries
  History of one or more infants with birth defects
  Rh incompatibility or blood group (ABO) sensitization
  Currently experiencing multiple pregnancy
  Uterine or ovarian tumors
Preexisting medical disorders
  Diabetes mellitus
  Cardiac disease
  Chronic hypertension
  Hemoglobinopathies and other blood dyscrasias
  Hyperthyroidism or hypothyroidism
  Chronic renal disease
  Sexually transmitted diseases
  Malnutrition
  Respiratory disorders such as tuberculosis and emphysema
  Substance abuse, including tobacco
Disorders occurring during pregnancy
  Pregnancy-induced hypertension—preeclampsia and eclampsia
  Gestational diabetes
  Acute infectious diseases
  Sexually transmitted diseases
  Substance abuse, including tobacco
  Hemorrhagic disorders, including placenta previa and abruptio placentae
  Hydatidiform mole
  Pyelonephritis
  Multiple pregnancy

the condition of the fallopian tubes and ovaries; (4) abnormalities of the birth canal such as soft-tissue masses; (5) and the configuration of the bony pelvis.

The fallopian tubes become elongated during pregnancy, and as the uterus rises, their position becomes vertical. Increased vascularity in the ovaries during pregnancy increases their size; the ovary that is larger, however, is the one containing the corpus luteum. Uterine size is useful in determining length of gestation, and pelvic measurements enable a clinical appraisal of potential pelvic contractions that might lead to cephalopelvic disproportion in labor.

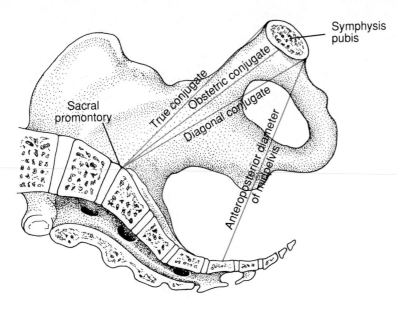

Symphysis pubis

Sacral promontory

True conjugate

Obstetric conjugate

Diagonal conjugate

Anteroposterior diameter of midpelvis

FIGURE 8-1

Anteroposterior Diameters of Pelvic Inlet and Midpelvis. The diagonal conjugate can be measured manually. The obstetric conjugate and the true conjugate are estimated, using the measurement of the diagonal conjugate. The anteroposterior diameter of the midpelvis is the widest portion of the outlet and is of less importance than the transverse diameter of the outlet, which is the narrowest diameter.

The pelvis of every pregnant woman should be measured accurately during the antepartum pelvic examination. The measurements identify conditions that may complicate delivery. Internal and external measurements determine the adequacy of the pelvic inlet and outlet.

Diagonal Conjugate

Internal pelvic measurements reveal the actual diameters of the pelvic inlet (Fig. 8-1). The anteroposterior measurement is of concern since it measures the narrowest portion of the pelvic inlet through which the fetal presenting part must pass at delivery. The most critical anteroposterior diameters cannot be measured directly, so they must be estimated. Calculations are based on the diagonal conjugate, which is the distance between the sacral promontory and the lower margin of the symphysis pubis. With a measurement greater than 11.5 cm, it is justifiable to assume that the anteroposterior diameter of the pelvic inlet is of adequate size for the birth of a term fetus whose weight is appropriate for gestational age. Figures 8-2 and 8-3 demonstrate the technique for measuring the diagonal conjugate.

Obstetric Conjugate

The narrowest portion of the pelvic inlet is the distance from the sacral promontory to the inner surface of the symphysis pubis. This anteroposterior diameter, known as the obstetric conjugate, cannot be measured manually. Instead, the distance is estimated by subtracting 1.5 to 2 cm from the diagonal conjugate.[2] Figure 8-1 demonstrates anteroposterior diameters of the pelvic inlet and the midpelvis.

True Conjugate

The distance between the superior (uppermost) surface of the symphysis pubis and the promontory of the sacrum is the true conjugate, or conjugata vera. This anteroposterior diameter of the pelvic inlet is mentioned since it is often considered the same as the obstetric conjugate, but it is

FIGURE 8-2

Determination of Diagonal Conjugate Diameter. The diagonal conjugate diameter is obtained by measuring the distance from the tip of the middle finger, which is resting on the sacral promontory, to the back of the hand just under the symphysis pubis.

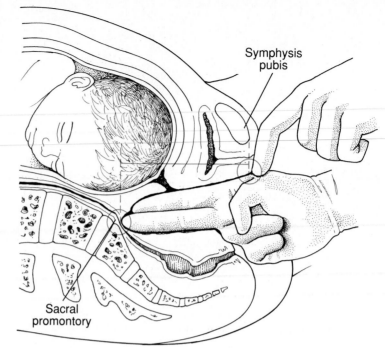

FIGURE 8-3

Measuring Scale. A rigid measuring scale attached to the wall is used to determine the diagonal conjugate diameter by measuring the distance marked on the hand during the manual examination.

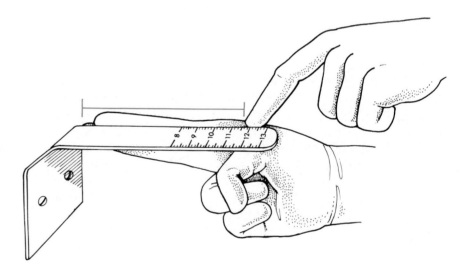

not. Instead, the obstetric conjugate is the narrowest diameter through which the fetal head must pass when descending into the true pelvis. It is for this reason that the obstetric conjugate is estimated (see Fig. 8-1).

Midpelvic Measurements

No precise manual method can estimate the capacity of the midpelvis. Cunningham, MacDonald, and Gant[2] note that midpelvic contraction or narrowing is suggested during the vaginal examination if the ischial spines are prominent, if the pelvic sidewalls converge, if the sacrosciatic notch is narrow, and if the transverse diameter of the outlet is less than 8 cm. Midpelvic contraction is of concern because it can cause transverse arrest of the fetal head during labor.

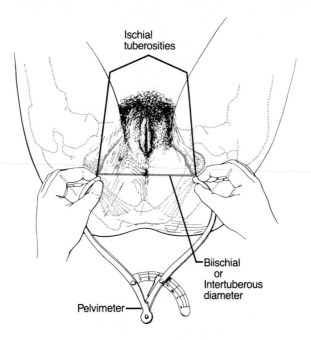

Ischial
tuberosities

Biischial
or
Intertuberous
diameter

Pelvimeter

FIGURE 8-4
Method of Measuring the Biischial, Intertuberous, or Transverse Diameter of the Outlet. Measurement is taken by placing the prongs of a pelvimeter against the innermost and lowermost aspect of the ischial tuberosities on a level with the lower border of the anus. The calibration adjacent to the instrument hinge is read to determine the measurement.

Biischial, Intertuberous, or Transverse Diameter

The most important clinical dimension of the pelvic outlet is the transverse diameter, the distance between the ischial tuberosities. This is the narrowest portion through which the presenting part of the fetus must pass after engagement. The measurement is taken by placing an instrument (usually a Williams' or Thoms' pelvimeter) against the innermost and lowermost aspect of the ischial tuberosities on a level with the lower border of the anus (Fig. 8-4).

The intertuberous diameter may also be estimated by inserting the closed fist against the perineum between the tuberosities. The measured width of the fist can then be used as a reference. A diameter of more than 8 cm is considered adequate for the delivery of a term fetus whose weight is appropriate for gestational age.

Imaging Pelvimetry

Radiologic pelvimetry is the most accurate means of determining pelvic size. The method subjects the maternal ovaries and fetal gonads to a certain amount of radiation. The American College of Radiology and the American College of Obstetricians and Gynecologists have endorsed the concept of limiting the use of x-ray pelvimetry.[2] Thus x-ray pelvimetry is no longer used before labor. Further, its use is considered unnecessary in the management of the labor of a woman who is suspected of having a contracted pelvis unless she is experiencing a breech presentation of the fetus.

Computed tomographic pelvimetry (CT scanning) provides adequate images of the bony pelvis with less radiation exposure than x-ray pelvimetry. Electronic calipers are used to measure the pelvic diameters. Careful positioning of the client is essential to promote accuracy, and minimum maternal movement is necessary to prevent artifacts on the digital radiographs. The nurse's knowledge of this information is important in preparing a client for CT scanning.

Other imaging methods include ultrasonography and magnetic resonance imaging (MRI). Accurate measurements of the maternal pelvis have not been achieved with ultrasound. Although MRI offers the advantages of lack of ionizing radiation, accurate pelvic measurements, soft-tissue analysis, and fetal imaging, use is limited because of cost, time, and equipment availability.

Laboratory Tests

The laboratory tests usually ordered by the primary care provider early in the antepartum period (Table 8-2) include urinalysis and examination of vaginal and cervical secretions and tissues. Blood tests are also ordered. In addition to obtaining a complete blood count, blood specimens are examined to detect conditions of special concern and tested for the Rh

TABLE 8-2

Laboratory Tests During Pregnancy

Test	Purpose
Urine Tests	
Urinalysis	
Sugar	Screens for diabetes; evaluated at each visit
Albumin (microscopic)	Screens for preeclampsia; evaluates for kidney stress or renal problems; done at each visit
Urine culture	Diagnoses urinary tract infection; often done routinely on all pregnant women
Blood Tests	
Blood urea nitrogen (BUN), creatinine, total protein, electrolytes	Evaluates renal function and diagnoses renal disease
Complete blood count (CBC)	
Hematocrit and hemoglobin	Screens for anemia, iron deficiency, folic acid deficiency
White blood cell count	Identifies infectious processes
Differential	Screens for blood disorders and inflammatory conditions
Platelets	Assesses blood clotting mechanism
Hemoglobin electrophoresis	Diagnoses hemoglobinopathies (e.g., sickle cell anemia, thalassemias)
Rh factor and blood type	Alerts care provider to possible incompatibility disease in fetus; identifies blood type in case of hemorrhage
Rh titers	Done when woman is Rh negative and man is Rh positive to assess danger to fetus (rising titer)
Maternal serum α-fetoprotein test (AFP)	Screens for fetal neural tube defects such as anencephaly and myelomeningocele; may also indicate abortion, multiple pregnancy, fetal demise
Rubella antibodies	Determines if woman has developed rubella antibodies
Serologic test for syphilis	Screens for syphilis (if positive, must confirm with fluorescent treponemal antibody absorption [FTA-ABS] test)
Hepatitis viral studies	Screens for hepatitis B antigens and antibodies
Enzyme-linked immunosorbent assay (ELISA)	Screens for human immunodeficiency virus (HIV) in consenting high-risk clients; if positive, must confirm with Western blot test or immunofluorescent antibody assay (IFA)
Other	
Gonorrhea culture of cervical discharge	Diagnoses gonorrhea; often done routinely because gonorrhea is frequently asymptomatic in women
Chlamydia smears of cervical discharge	Diagnoses *Chlamydia trachomatis;* often done routinely because *Chlamydia* infections are frequently asymptomatic
Papanicolaou smear of cervical epithelium	Screens for cervical intraepithelial neoplasia, herpes simplex type 2
Tuberculin skin test	Screens high-risk women for tuberculosis
Electrocardiogram (ECG), chest roentgenogram	Evaluates cardiac and pulmonary function (performed when indicated by acute or chronic diseases)

factor, blood type, Rh titer, if indicated, syphilis, rubella titer, the sickle cell trait (in black women), and hepatitis B antigen. Women considered at high risk for human immunodeficiency virus (HIV) infection may be counseled and tested.

Ultrasonography may be used to determine fetal and placental status. It is a noninvasive diagnostic procedure that is used throughout the antepartum period when indicated to facilitate the management of pregnancy. To date diagnostic sound waves have not been found harmful to maternal or fetal tissues. Sonography can differentiate between some normal and abnormal products of conception as early as the fifth week of gestation.

Assessment of Psychosocial Aspects of Pregnancy

To provide optimum care for clients, nurses must assess the social and cultural context within which the pregnancy occurs; that is, the family and the larger society must be assessed. Pregnancy and childbearing in general have different meanings in various societies and even within any given society.

Assessment of Client's Cultural System

Griffith[3] suggests that childbearing concepts can focus on the following four components of a cultural system:
1. Mores and value systems involving ideas of duty, obligation, and desirability
2. Kinship system prescribing mutual rights, duties, and obligations in relationships resulting from marriage and family ancestry
3. Knowledge and belief system defining conception, labor, and childbearing
4. Ceremonial and ritual systems incorporated into daily lives

Using Griffith's ideas, the nurse may seek information that will facilitate understanding of the client's patterns of belief about childbearing. "Questions involving belief systems surrounding childbearing" may be used by the nurse to facilitate assessment of the client's cultural system (see Assessment Tool: Cultural Considerations on p. 160).

Assessment of the Family

The nurse can function in collaboration with other members of the health team by providing emotional support along with counseling and teaching for the pregnant couple. Thinking of pregnancy as a role transition rather than a crisis helps emphasize the normalcy of the event. Care is structured to support the resources of the couple rather than looking for problems that may not exist. The key to appropriate intervention in this instance is family assessment.

Developmental and situational stress-producing factors that affect the family must be taken into account. Pregnancy, parenthood, and other family life-cycle changes are examples of developmental or normative stressors.[4] Major illness, loss of a job, destruction of property through natural catastrophes, divorce, and separation of families because of war

ASSESSMENT
TOOL

Cultural Considerations

Questions Involving Belief Systems Surrounding Childbearing

Antepartum

Who may have a child?
At what age?
By whom may one have a child?
How many children can one have?
Can one space pregnancies?
What should be the behavior during pregnancy?
Are there restrictions on the father?
Are there any restrictions on sexual activity?
Who may see and touch certain body parts?
How is a fetus formed?
What are the beliefs about conception?

Intrapartum

What causes labor?
How does one behave during labor?
How should one respond to pain?
Should one take medication?
Where should labor take place?

Postpartum

What general behavior is expected?
What behavior is expected of the father and others?
Are there restrictions on food or activity?

Care of the Newborn

When is he or she recognized?
What are the rules for his or her care?
Who cares for the newborn?

Adapted from Griffith S: Childbearing and the concept of culture. JOGN 11(3):181, 1982.

are examples of situational stressors and are termed *extrafamilial stressors*. *Intrafamilial stressors* include problems such as inadequate communication and inadequate or ineffective role relationships. The amount of difficulty the family experiences in adapting to stressful events is related to how well the family members' roles are organized, the extent of their resources, and how flexible they can be in defining positively the discomfort produced by the stressor.

Assessment helps the nurse determine if members of the family are fulfilling expected role behaviors. If they are at this time, the potential problems for the remainder of pregnancy or postpartum period must be determined. If they are not fulfilling roles, the interfamilial and extrafamilial stressors must be determined by the assessment. Assessment Tool: Psychosocial Aspects of Pregnancy on page 161 provides sample questions the nurse may ask when assessing the family.

Nursing Diagnosis

The purpose of the first prenatal visit usually is to confirm the pregnancy. The woman and her family may be excited or upset about her pregnancy. Their reactions and the woman's health status and physiologic response

Assessment of Psychosocial Aspects of Pregnancy

Family Composition

1. Who are the family members (include the extended family)?
   a. What are their ages? What are their relationships to one another?
   b. Where do they live? Do they interact frequently?
   c. Are they "close" emotionally if not physically?
   d. What is the family's relationship to the larger educational community? Is the family involved in community affairs and religious activities? What is its community support structure?

Family Functioning

1. How are the roles allocated and differentiated?
   a. Who does what in the house? Is this mutually satisfactory?
   b. Who makes decisions? How are they made? Is there mutual discussion?
   c. What are the changes that members would like?
   d. How do the parents see their roles being changed with a new infant?
2. How do members usually define situations that happen?
   a. Does the family generally consolidate in times of trouble?
   b. Do they tend to be optimistic, pessimistic, or do attitudes vary with situations?
   c. What are the communication patterns? Who talks to whom? Do problems usually get solved with discussion?
3. What are the family's material and emotional resources?
   a. Is the environment safe and healthful?
      Is housing safe and adequate? Is there appropriate room for the expected infant? If not, what plans are being made to remedy the situation? Is the housing environment structured to prevent accidents? If not, what remedy is planned?
   b. Is the family healthful?
      What is the general health status of the family? Have there been or are there now illnesses? If so, has appropriate medical (or dental) care been sought? Is there a regular source of medical and dental care for the family? Does the woman use maternity services appropriately? If not, why not? How does the family usually pay for health services? Is health insurance or a health maintenance organization (HMO) service available? What are the usual health habits of the family members (exercise, rest, nutrition, smoking, substance abuse)?
   c. Are finances adequate? Who contributes? Will the pregnancy make a difference?
   d. Who turns to whom for emotional support? Who is the woman's main support at this time? Who is the man's main support at this time?
4. Are there interpersonal or intrapersonal difficulties?
   a. Are there long-term problems? What are the attempts to resolve them?
   b. Are there problems specific to this pregnancy?
   c. What alternatives for solution for the existing problems do the parents see?
5. What are the specific plans for the baby and for themselves during pregnancy?
   a. What are their plans for themselves as parents?
   b. What are their plans for the infant?
   c. Are siblings anticipated (if this is the first child)?
   d. What are the plans for siblings?

Focus Assessment

Evaluate family unit for potential stressors impinging on or within the nuclear or extended family (e.g., observed or reported family interactions, illness of family member, socioeconomic status).

Determine cultural expectations associated with pregnancy and birth.

Note factors that may place client in the category of high-risk pregnancy (e.g., age, preexisting or coexisting disorders).

Determine whether or not teratogenic exposure may have occurred.

Calculate gestational age at first visit.

Establish baseline entry status, (e.g., gestational status, nonpregnant weight, vital signs).

Note any significant changes in weight preceding or following onset of pregnancy.

Determine pregnancy-associated physiologic and emotional changes client is experiencing (e.g., nausea and vomiting, urinary frequency, nasal stuffiness, epistaxis, episodic crying, increased sensitivity to stressors).

Identify individual learning needs, motivation, and readiness to learn.

POTENTIAL NURSING DIAGNOSES

Initial Visit

Family Coping: Potential for Growth—related to the developmental tasks of pregnancy (e.g., planning and preparing for changes necessitated by the birth of the infant)

Anxiety—related to fear of or desire for pregnancy

Health Seeking Behaviors—related to desire to achieve a successful pregnancy outcome (e.g., reason for first visit, gestational status, desire to learn and engage in practices that will promote the growth, development, and delivery of a healthy baby)

Altered Nutrition: Less Than Body Requirements—related to nausea and vomiting associated with early pregnancy

Knowledge Deficit—regarding self-care during pregnancy

---

to pregnancy are determined during the client assessment. Analysis of these assessment findings helps the nurse to identify appropriate nursing diagnoses (see Potential Nursing Diagnoses: Initial Visit).

Planning and Intervention

At the initial prenatal visit, counseling and education should be brief and focused on immediate and short-term needs. It is better to postpone further health teaching and counseling until a subsequent visit when the mother is not so overloaded with new stimuli. The lengthy assessment process provides opportunity for the nurse to answer questions that are of immediate concern to the expectant parents. They are given an overview of prenatal care and instructed to write down any questions that arise between visits so that they can be addressed during the next appointment. A suggested nursing care plan for early uncomplicated pregnancy is shown on pages 163-164.

Early Uncomplicated Pregnancy

Goals (Expected Outcomes)	Interventions	Rationale	Evaluation
Anxiety—Related to Adaptation to Pregnancy			
Client or couple will demonstrate behaviors that are indicative of acceptance of the pregnancy and of planning for the pregnancy.	Establish rapport by providing caring, unhurried environment in which couple experiences openness to express their feelings and concerns. Provide opportunity for client or couple to ask questions of concern when they arrive for visit. Answer questions client or couple may have as health history and cultural and family assessment data are obtained.	Helps decrease stress by promoting opportunity to explore feelings and to have questions answered.	Client or couple verbalizes understanding of facts related to diagnosis of pregnancy. Client or couple expresses knowledge of appropriate methods of adaptation to current concerns.
Family Coping: Potential for Growth—Related to Planning and Preparation for Infant			
Client or couple will explore role changes associated with pregnancy. Client or couple will demonstrate behaviors that are indicative of a smooth transition as a growing family.	Provide opportunity to explore methods of resolving extrafamilial stressors. Provide information about community support services if assistance is needed in resolving intrafamilial stressors.	Reduces stressors so client or couple can concentrate on role adaptations related to pregnancy.	Client or couple demonstrates progress in resolving stressors.
	Provide information about community resources that help promote positive adaptation to pregnancy and positive outcomes of pregnancy (e.g., pregnagyms, childbirth education classes, sibling preparation classes, baby care classes). Provide literature for the expectant couple.	Helps to prepare for childbirth experience. Promotes sense of well-being. Encourages active involvement of self and family members. Promotes sense of self-worth.	Client or couple becomes involved in activities (uses resources) that promote role adaptation.
	Provide information from examination findings that suggests confirmation of pregnancy.	Promotes initial bonding as moves through stages of accepting tentative pregnancy as actual pregnancy.	Client or couple verbalizes recognition of pregnancy as real.

Continued

Early Uncomplicated Pregnancy—continued

Goals (Expected Outcomes)	Interventions	Rationale	Evaluation
Knowledge Deficit—Regarding Self-Care During Pregnancy			
Client or couple will demonstrate new knowledge by using health practices that will promote a healthy mother and infant.	Answer questions and clarify misunderstandings and misinformation.	Practices arising from incorrect knowledge may be harmful to woman and developing fetus. Correct information promotes safe practices and a sense of positiveness about self-care.	Client or couple uses self-care practices that promote positive physiologic responses to pregnancy. Client or couple blends cultural beliefs with behaviors that promote a healthy pregnancy and neonate.
	Explain schedule for return visits and assessments and explain care that will be provided during visit.	Promotes confidence in caregivers. Reinforces interest of caregivers in client or couple. Reinforces importance of continuous care throughout pregnancy.	
	Provide anticipatory guidance by giving information that promotes positive adaptations and self-care practices (e.g., exercise, employment, hygienic measures, sexual practices, medication).	Understanding of self-care activities promotes a sense of individual responsibility and interest in achieving expectations.	
	Provide information about teratogens (e.g., environmental substances, licit and illicit drugs, certain infections).	The first trimester of fetal development is essential to positive neonatal outcomes. Couple's awareness of effect of teratogens may promote positive health practices.	
	Encourage client or couple to write down questions that arise between visits so that they can be addressed at next visit.	Demonstrates interest in client or couple and promotes client's active participation in own care.	
Altered Nutrition: Less Than Body Requirements—Related to Nausea and Vomiting Associated With Early Pregnancy			
Client reports reduction in nausea and vomiting and evidences a weight gain of 3 pounds by the end of the first trimester.	Teach to eat foods high in carbohydrates (soda crackers, dry toast) before arising. Teach to eat six small meals per day. Provide information about nutritional needs of mother and fetus.	Decreases gastric acidity, thus reducing nausea and vomiting. Prevents malnutrition and dehydration, which compromise fetal development and physiologic adaptation essential to a healthy pregnancy.	Client is able to retain dry carbohydrate on arising. Client adjusts dietary intake to promote retention of food.

Legal and Ethical Issues

The nurse is required to practice within established legal parameters. Macklin[5] notes that the interests of the client and the client's preference should take priority when planning care. This is often difficult from a legal and ethical perspective. Dilemmas the nurse may encounter when providing care during the antepartum period are described on page 165.

Continuing Client Assessment and Intervention

Regular appointments are scheduled throughout pregnancy. This follow-up care provides the opportunity to continue monitoring maternal and fetal status, institute treatment and additional diagnostic tests as necessary, and offer ongoing maternal and family support and education. The usual schedule of follow-up visits is outlined in the display below. Follow-up visits are scheduled more frequently if complications arise. Routine return visits include the history since the last visit, physical assessment, and

---

Schedule of Return Prenatal Visits

First through sixth month—one visit per month
Seventh and eighth months—one visit every 2 weeks
Ninth month until delivery—one visit per week

Assessments Included in Visits

Each visit

Weight
Blood pressure
Fundal height (McDonald's technique)
Check for edema
Urinalysis for glucose and albumin
Inquiry about symptoms, signs, or problems
Nutrition and appetite
Family and personal problems and adjustment
Prenatal education

10th-12th week and every week thereafter

Fetal heart rate with Doppler ultrasound

20th week and every week thereafter

Fetal heart rate with fetoscope

32-34 weeks

Hematocrit and hemoglobin (more often if anemic)

Middle of ninth month

Pelvic examination (then weekly as indicated)

Others

Rh titers for Rh-negative client with Rh-positive father of baby—if initially negative, twice more during pregnancy; if positive, more often as indicated by titer levels
Urine culture as indicated by symptoms or signs
Other examinations and tests as indicated by symptoms or signs

---

≡ LEGAL AND ETHICAL
≡ CONSIDERATIONS

Antepartum Care

1. An expectant mother in her first trimester of pregnancy has sickle cell anemia. She does not elect to interrupt the pregnancy. Does the woman's decision negate her right to sue for malpractice after she experiences complications associated with pregnancy and sickle cell anemia?
2. A woman reveals that she is a substance abuser. She refuses to enter a treatment program. Does the nurse report the woman to legal authorities for investigation for possession to try to protect her and her fetus?

client education, which is of extreme importance in facilitating a healthy pregnancy and a positive outcome of pregnancy.

Follow-Up Physical Assessment of the Client

Follow-up assessment comprises physiologic data on maternal adaptations to changes of pregnancy, measurements of fetal well-being, identification of signs or symptoms of complications, and determination of client's compliance with medical regimens. The opportunity also is present to identify other health problems within the pregnant family but not directly related to pregnancy such as illness of the father or older children.

General inquiry is made about how the client and family are feeling and any concerns or symptoms. New signs or physical findings such as excess weight gain or glycosuria are explored through a series of questions. The woman is asked about any untoward signs and symptoms, including edema of the fingers or face, bleeding, constipation, and headaches. During these visits the woman is encouraged and given ample opportunity to ask any questions of concern to her.

Weight, blood pressure, and fundal height are measured during each return visit. At approximately the 10th or 12th week the fetal heartbeat can be heard using the Doppler ultrasound device; beginning at this time the fetal heart rate (FHR) is taken and recorded at each visit. The urine is tested during each return visit for sugar and protein (albumin). A graph or flow sheet is used to record all findings.

Legs and feet are examined for edema and development of varicosities. Other aspects of the physical examination are performed if indicated by signs or symptoms.

Vaginal examinations are usually not done on return visits until the client nears term. Frequently, vaginal examinations are begun approximately 2 or 3 weeks before the EDC to assess the status of the cervix, fetal presentation, and the degree of engagement. The hemoglobin and hematocrit values are determined again at 32 to 34 weeks gestation as a precaution against anemia.

Fundal Height

The height of the fundus can be used to approximate the length of gestation by using McDonald's technique. The client must void before the measurement is taken to prevent upward displacement of the uterus by the bladder. A flexible tape measure is used to measure the distance in centimeters from the upper border of the symphysis pubis to the top of the uterine fundus. The tape measure can be curved over the woman's abdomen, or it can be held straight between the fingers with the hand at a right angle to the top of the fundus (Fig. 8-5). When the distance is multiplied by two and divided by seven, the results indicate the duration of pregnancy in lunar months. Gestation of pregnancy in weeks can also be determined (see p. 167). Studies cited by Cunningham, MacDonald, and Gant[2] indicate that McDonald's technique is accurate only for the period between 20 to 34 weeks of gestation.

Fetal Heart Tones

Auscultation of fetal heart tones (FHT) is important because they reflect fetal condition. Before attempting to listen to the FHTs, it is advantageous

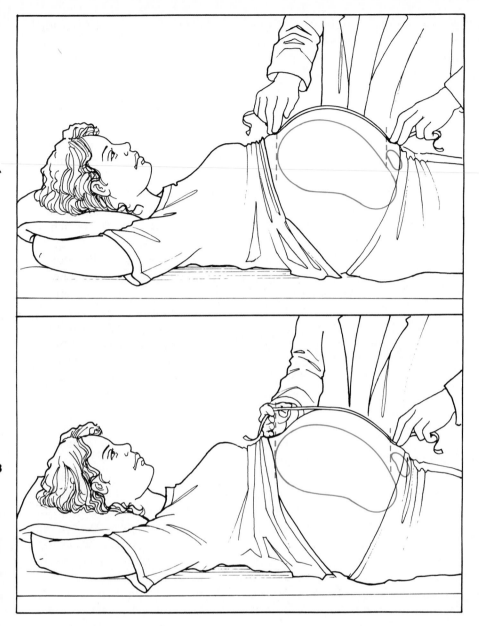

FIGURE 8-5
Measurement of Fundal Height: McDonald's Technique. **A,** Tape measure is curved over the woman's abdomen. **B,** Tape measure is held straight between the fingers with the hand at a right angle to the top of the fundus.

McDonald's Rule for Determining Length of Gestation

Height of fundus (cm) multiplied by 2 and divided by 7 equals gestation in lunar months.

Height of fundus (cm) multiplied by 8 and divided by 7 equals gestation in weeks.

Factors That Influence Fundal Height Measurements

1. Factors such as hydramnios, multiple gestation, a very large fetus, and obesity affect the accuracy of measurement.
2. For women weighing more than 200 pounds, 1 cm is subtracted from the obtained measurement.
3. Technique can vary measurements. The procedure should be standardized when more than one person takes serial measurements.

to determine the fetal position because the FHTs are best heard through the fetus's back. Leopold's maneuvers, as described in Chapter 11, help identify fetal position and presentation.

When assessing the fetal heart, it is important to differentiate between the woman's and the fetus's heart rate. FHRs range from 120 to 140 beats per minute, whereas the maternal rate should be approximately 80 beats per minute. When counting the heart rate, one hand palpates the maternal radial pulse while the FHTs are heard through fetoscope or Doppler device. If the sound heard is not synchronous with the maternal pulse, it is the fetal heartbeat.

Two additional sounds may be heard when listening over the pregnant uterus: the funic souffle and the uterine souffle. The word *souffle* means a blowing murmur or whizzing sound, and *funis* is Latin for umbilical cord. Funic souffle refers to a soft blowing murmur caused by blood rushing through the umbilical cord. Since this blood is propelled by the fetal heart, the rate of funic souffle is synchronous with that of the fetal heart. It is heard only occasionally.

The uterine souffle is produced by blood rushing through the large vessels of the uterus. Since this is maternal blood propelled by the maternal heart, it is synchronous with the maternal heartbeat. Since the uterine souffle can be heard with the fetoscope or Doppler device, it is important to palpate the maternal radial pulse while counting the FHR to ensure the uterine souffle is not mistaken for the fetal heartbeat.

Weight Gain

Obtaining the maternal weight at regular intervals during pregnancy is an important part of antepartum care. Most primary care providers agree that a weight gain of 22 to 27 pounds is desirable for a woman of average prepregnant weight.[2] However, there is increasing evidence among investigators that the weight gain during pregnancy must be individualized for every client, particularly for those who are under and over the average prepregnant weight. If she is underweight before pregnancy, a gain of 30 pounds or more has no deleterious effects on the woman and results in a healthy infant of normal weight. Currently, the emphasis is focused on a balanced nutritional status related to the woman's general physical condition rather than on the amount of weight gained.

Willson et al[1] point out that women should not try to lose or maintain weight during pregnancy because dietary restrictions can interfere with providing nutritional requirements for the developing fetus. Even those women who begin pregnancy significantly overweight must expect to gain additional weight. Overweight women who gain approximately 16 pounds have the lowest incidence of perinatal mortality among overweight women.[6]

The smallest weight gain occurs during the first trimester. Generally a gain of 3 pounds occurs at that time, with a 12-pound gain occurring during each of the last two trimesters. Explaining to the client how pregnancy weight is distributed helps her understand why weight gain is necessary for normal progression of fetal development.

Other Tests

Additional diagnostic tests are ordered as indicated throughout the antepartum period (see Table 8-2). Tuberculin skin testing is advisable for high-risk and symptomatic clients. Renal function tests such as blood urea nitrogen (BUN), creatinine, electrolytes, and total protein excretion are obtained when renal complications are suspected. Some clinics or offices conduct routine urine cultures because of the prevalence of asymptomatic bacteriuria. Urine cultures are indicated for clients with urinary tract infection symptoms or the presence of bacteria or white blood cells on microscopic urinalysis. Additional diagnostic tests may be necessary for high-risk clients, including clients with specific problems such as cardiac disease, pulmonary disorders, and diabetes. The maternal serum a-feto-protein (MSAFP or AFP) test may be offered at the 16th to the 18th week of pregnancy to test for fetal neural tube defects such as myelomeningocele and anencephaly.

Follow-Up Psychosocial Assessment of the Client

The nurse began establishing rapport with the pregnant client and her family during the initial interview. Follow-up appointments provide the opportunity for continuing assessment of client and family needs. Through consistent use of the same tool throughout pregnancy (see Assessment Tool p. 161), can determine if family members are exhibiting behaviors that indicate positive adaptation to the pregnancy and if the family is functioning effectively.

Nursing Diagnosis

Nursing diagnoses direct the focus for continuing care of the client during the antepartum period. Ongoing assessments note any changes in the family's response, in the woman's health status, and in the woman's physiologic and psychologic responses to pregnancy. Integrating knowledge about the normal antepartum processes with the client assessment data facilitates the nurse's selection of appropriate current and potential nursing diagnoses (see Potential Nursing Diagnoses: On-Going Pregnancy on p. 170).

Focus Assessment

Evaluate family unit for potential stressors impinging on or within the nuclear or extended family (e.g., observed or reported family interactions; illness of family member, socioeconomic status).
    Determine cultural expectations associated with pregnancy and birth.
Note the emergence of factors that may place client in the category of high-risk pregnancy (e.g., gestational diabetes, cardiac compromise).
Calculate gestational age at each visit.
Identify current learning needs, motivation, and readiness to learn.
Monitor vital signs, weight, urinalysis, fundal height, and emergence of signs and symptoms commonly occurring at present point in gestation (e.g., quickening).
    Note any significant changes in weight.
As pregnancy progresses, identify the persistence or emergence of new pregnancy-related physiologic and emotional changes client is experiencing (e.g., nausea and vomiting, urinary frequency, backaches, excessive fatigue, constipation, depression, or feelings of insecurity).
Determine client's response to physiologic changes of pregnancy (e.g., weight gain, changing body contours).

Family Coping: Potential for Growth—related to the developmental tasks of pregnancy (e.g., planning and preparing for changes necessitated by the birth of the infant)

Health Seeking Behaviors—related to desire to achieve a successful pregnancy outcome (e.g., reason for first visit, desire to learn and engage in practices that will promote the growth, development, and delivery of a healthy baby)

Knowledge Deficit—regarding the continuing changes during pregnancy and the labor and delivery experience

Body Image Disturbance—related to pregnancy-related changes in appearance

Potential for Infection (Urinary Tract)—related to ureteral dilatation and stasis of urine secondary to compression by the growing uterus and diminished smooth muscle motility caused by the actions of progesterone

Potential for Injury—related to alteration in the woman's center of gravity secondary to the increasing size and weight of the growing uterus

Constipation—related to pressure of the growing uterus on the bowel, iron supplementation, and diminished smooth muscle motility caused by the actions of progesterone

Potential Activity Intolerance—related to normal physiologic changes of pregnancy (e.g., increasing size of gravid uterus, decreased venous return from lower extremities, altered center of gravity)

Planning and Intervention

Nursing interventions during the antepartum period include the following: (1) teaching, (2) support, (3) advice, (4) anticipatory guidance, (5) promotion of self-care preparation, (6) direct physical care, and (7) referral or coordination of services. The scope of nursing care includes helping the client and family to (1) understand and adapt to physiologic and emotional changes of pregnancy; (2) deal with minor discomforts effectively; (3) recognize and, if possible, avoid potentially serious complications; (4) plan for parenthood and integrating the new baby into the family; (5) understand and comply with the medical regimen; and (6) attain optimum health status. Instructions and anticipatory guidance pertinent to the care of clients and their families during the antepartum period are addressed.

Through the psychosocial assessment of clients, emotional and social problems that could interfere with the client's ability to derive full benefit from health services may be identified. For example, a client may have problems such as (1) inadequate funds to provide appropriate nutrition for herself and her family, (2) inadequate funds to obtain necessary supplies for the expected baby, (3) lack of a support system for assistance when returning home with the new baby, and (4) substandard housing. It is the responsibility of the nurse to find out in what ways the client needs help and to make appropriate referrals when indicated (e.g., referrals to the community health nurse, to community service agencies or groups, or to other members of the extended health team, including the medical social worker). Through the use of such referrals lines of communication are kept open between the particular health agency, the community, and the members of the health team. This is one of the nurse's most important functions. Thus comprehensive care for the client is assured.

Evaluation

Throughout the antepartum period the nurse evaluates the client's responses to care and to directions and instructions provided. Further, the nurse evaluates whether or not the client is achieving established goals. Nursing diagnoses may change as the client progresses through the antepartum period, and nursing interventions may be altered according to the client's response.

REFERENCES

1. Willson JR et al: Obstetrics and Gynecology. St. Louis, CV Mosby, 1987
2. Cunningham FG, MacDonald PC, Gant NF: Williams Obstetrics, 18th ed. Norwalk, Conn, Appleton & Lange, 1989
3. Griffith S: Childbearing and the concept of culture. JOGN 11(3):181-184, 1982
4. McCubbin HI, Sussman MB, Patterson JM (eds): Social Stress and the Family: Advances and Developments in Family Stress Theory and Research. New York, Haworth Press, 1983
5. Macklin R: Ethical principles, individual rights, and medical practices. Nat Forum 69(4):25-27, 1989
6. Naeye RL: Weight gain and outcome of pregnancy. Am J Obstet Gynecol 135:3, 1979

SUGGESTED READINGS

Holmes KK et al: Sexually Transmitted Diseases, 2nd ed. New York, McGraw-Hill Information Services, 1990

Johnson FF: Assessment and education to prevent preterm labor. MCN 14(3):157-160, 1989

Merilo KF: Is it better the second time around? MCN 13(3):200-204, 1988

Pagana KD, Pagana TJ: Diagnostic Tests and Nursing Implications, 2nd ed. St. Louis, CV Mosby, 1986

Schneider JW, Griffith DR, Chasnoff IJ: Infants exposed to cocaine in utero: Implications for developmental assessment and intervention. Infants Young Children 3(1):25-34, 1989

Smith JE: The dangers of prenatal cocaine use. MCN 13(3):174-179, 1988

St. Clair PA, Anderson NA: Social network advice during pregnancy: Myths, misinformation, and sound counsel. Birth 16(3): 103-107, 1989

Streissguth AP, LaDue RA: Psychological and behavioral effects in children prenatally exposed to alcohol. Alcohol Health Res World Fall: 6-12, 1985

Tammelleo AD (ed): DC: Amniocentesis unnecessary—child with Down's syndrome liability. Regan Report Med Law 21(3), 1988

Tammelleo AD (ed): MN: Birth defects: Negligent nondisclosure. Regan Report Med Law 23(2), 1988

Tammelleo AD (ed): PA: Blood "tested for AIDS" without consent. Regan Report Med Law 23(2), 1990

Thomson EJ, Cordero JF: The new teratogens: Accutane and other vitamin A analogs. MCN 14(4): 244-248, 1989

Veaalch RM, Fry ST: Case Studies in Nursing Ethics. Philadelphia, JB Lippincott, 1987

Villar J et al: The measuring of blood pressure during pregnancy. Am J Obstet Gynecol 161(4): 1019-1024, 1989

Warren WB et al: Dating the early pregnancy by sequential appearance of early embryonic structures. Am J Obstet Gynecol 161(3):747-753, 1989

Wawrzyniak MN: The painless pelvic. MCN 11(3):178-179, 1986

Nutrition in Pregnancy

IMPORTANT TERMINOLOGY

anemia Condition in which there is a reduction in the number of circulating red blood cells; iron-deficiency anemia results from a greater demand on the stored iron than can be supplied—pregnancy is one cause

amino acids Fundamental structural units of protein

ketosis Accumulation in the body of the ketone bodies: acetone, betahydroxybutyric acid, and acetic acid

lactose intolerance Inability of some people to digest lactose, the sugar in milk; they experience symptoms of gastrointestinal discomfort, i.e., nausea, gas in the abdomen and intestines, abdominal cramping and distention, belching or flatulence, and/or watery stools, after ingestion of lactose from milk or another dairy food

malnutrition Faulty nutrition resulting from poor diet, malassimilation, or overeating

nutrition Process by which living things utilize food for energy, growth and development, and maintenance

nutritional status Condition of health as determined by the nutrients the body receives and utilizes

pica Compulsion for persistent ingestion of unsuitable substances having little or no nutritional value; *geophagia* is the consumption of dirt or clay; *amylophagia* involves the ingestion of a variety of nonfood substances, e.g., ice, burnt matches, hair, stone or gravel, coffee grounds, milk of magnesia, charcoal, and baking soda

recommended dietary allowance (RDA) The levels of intake of essential nutrients that are judged to be adequate to meet the known nutrient needs of practically all healthy persons

vegetarian Person who consumes no animal tissue protein and who may or may not use eggs and dairy products

Nutrition plays a key role in the outcome of pregnancy. A woman's **nutritional status** at conception and the quality of the diet she consumes during the following months help to determine her health and well-being and that of her child. Ensuring optimum nutrition for all childbearing women might not eliminate all the problems of pregnancy, but it is a giant step in the right direction.

If counseling is to be effective and the results lasting, the nurse should strive to elicit wholehearted cooperation from the client. This may be facilitated by involving her in the planning; considering her needs, background, preferences, and attitudes and those of her family; providing information; encouraging and reinforcing appropriate choices and preparation; providing gentle but firm limit setting when indicated; and giving careful, thorough explanation regarding the rationale behind the advice.

If the pregnant woman is helped to understand the importance of good nutrition for herself and her fetus, she may be more motivated than at other times in her life to improve her dietary habits. She should be encouraged to continue her new interest in nutrition after the infant arrives. These improvements can have long-lasting effects on her family. Not only does improved nutrition promote better health for the present family, but it can have a positive effect on future pregnancies of the mother and her children.

Importance of Nutrition During Pregnancy

The importance of maternal nutrition during pregnancy has long been recognized. Evidence was first provided in 1970 in a benchmark study by the National Academy of Sciences. The report, reviewing studies of reproductive experiences, remains the major source of research information on the role of nutrition in human reproduction. Prenatal nutrition is one of the most important environmental factors affecting the health of pregnant women and their babies.[1] As a result of continued research a joint publication was issued by the American College of Obstetricians and Gynecologists and the American Dietetic Association, *Guidelines for Assessment of Maternal Nutrition*. This milestone report acknowledged the first national consensus on the relevant nutritional risk factors during pregnancy. The National Research Council updated the material in its 1981 *Guidelines for Nutrition Services in Perinatal Care*.[2]

Over the years, health care personnel have given a wide variety of dietary advice to the pregnant woman. This has included recommendations ranging from severe restrictions (to limit weight gain) to eating large quantities of food (to promote fetal development). While the effects of nutrition during pregnancy are still being explored, emphasis is currently being placed on the importance of adequate nutrition before, during, and after pregnancy.

Effects of Poor Nutrition

Nutrition plays a key role in the outcome of pregnancy. A woman's nutritional status and the quality of the diet she consumes during pregnancy affect her health and that of her child. Controlled studies on animals have shown a direct relationship between maternal diet and pregnancy outcome. General conclusions to date include (1) maternal **malnutrition** can be one cause of intrauterine growth retardation and low-birth-weight infants; (2) infants who are malnourished throughout gestation because of the mother's restricted diet have reduced head size and a decreased number of brain cells, proportional reductions in the size of other organs, and decreased neuromotor and mental development. Brain development can be further retarded if postnatal malnutrition persists. Continued research is necessary to learn more about fetal growth and development and the consequences of maternal malnutrition.

Although it is difficult to show a direct cause-and-effect relationship between specific nutrients and specific problems in human studies, some correlations have been found. Chronic malnutrition in developing countries and in low-income populations of developed countries has been related to reproductive problems, including difficult labors and deliveries (see display p. 175).[3]

Some historical occurrences have provided study populations that demonstrate the effects of nutritional deprivation under conditions that would not have been approved for scientific experiments. During World War II, a 7-month food embargo of western Holland decreased the population's average daily food ration to fewer than 750 calories. In a retrospective study, women who were pregnant or who conceived during the famine were shown to have a higher incidence of stillbirth and neonatal mortality and decreased infant birth weight.[4] Similar effects on pregnancy were found during the siege of Leningrad in 1941 and 1942. A contrast in the effects of nutritional deprivation on pregnancy outcomes was demonstrated in Great Britain. According to that nation's policy, pregnant and lactating women received top priority for food rations. Such priority is thought to have contributed to an actual decrease in its perinatal mortality during 1940-1945.

Nutritional Needs During Pregnancy

Since adequate maternal nutrition during pregnancy is necessary to attain optimal fetal growth and development, the mother must meet both her nutritional needs and those of the growing fetus (Table 9-1).

TABLE 9-1

Recommended Dietary Allowances for Adult Women (Ages 25 to 50 Years)

	Nonpregnant	Pregnant
Energy (kcal)	2200	+300
Protein (gm)	50	60
Vitamin A (RE)	800	800
Vitamin D (μg)	5	10
Vitamin E (mg)	8	10
Vitamin C (ascorbic acid) (mg)	60	70
Folic acid (μg)	180	+400
Niacin (mg)	15	17
Riboflavin (mg)	1.3	1.6
Thiamin (mg)	1.1	1.5
Vitamin B_6 (mg)	1.6	2.2
Vitamin B_{12} (μg)	2.0	2.2
Calcium (mg)	800	1200
Phosphorus (mg)	800	1200
Iodine (μg)	150	175
Iron (mg)	15	30★
Magnesium (mg)	280	320
Zinc (mg)	12	15

From Food and Nutrition Board, Subcommittee on the Tenth Edition of the Recommended Dietary Allowances, 10 ed. Washington, DC, National Academy Press, 1989.
★30-60 mg of supplemental iron per day is recommended.

*Possible Adverse Effects of Poor Nutrition During the Reproductive Cycle**

Reproductive problems
   Infertility
   Abortion
   Stillbirth
   Neonatal death
Pregnancy problems
   Maternal anemias
   Vitamin deficiencies
   Preeclampsia and eclampsia
   Placental abnormalities
   Gestational diabetes
   Pica-related complications
   Dystocia
   Lactation difficulties
   Slow postpartum maternal recovery
Neonatal problems
   Low-birth-weight infants
   Delayed mental and physical development of infant
   Congenital malformations
   Fetal alcohol syndrome
   Neonatal anemias
   Vitamin deficiencies

*Obviously many other factors influence the occurrence of these problems, but prepregnant status and nutritional status and nutrient intake during pregnancy play a significant role.

Effects of Supplementation

Research on supplementation programs for low-income maternal populations has demonstrated benefits to mothers and their infants. Protein and calorie supplements plus additional food supplies have contributed to a lower incidence of pregnancy-induced hypertension and other diseases of pregnancy, easier deliveries with fewer cesarean sections, lower neonatal morbidity and mortality rates, and infants with greater mean birth weights.[5] Major supplemental studies in Montreal and Guatemala are representative of efforts to assist low-income women and others at risk for reproductive problems.[1]

Recommended Dietary Allowances

The Food and Nutrition Board of the National Research Council sets standards for the daily intake of calories and nutrients by people in the United States.[6] The **recommended dietary allowance (RDA)** is set for 19 of the 40 or so nutrients known to promote growth and maintain health. The allowances are based on available scientific data and are updated periodically.

   The allowances for the adult female are based on the needs of a well-nourished, semisedentary woman between 25 and 50 years of age, who weighs 138 pounds and is 64 inches tall. RDAs are meant to be used as a basic reference and modified according to individual measurements (height and weight) and nutritional needs.

Carbohydrate

The main function of carbohydrate is to produce energy (Table 9-2). Adequate amounts are necessary to spare protein for growth needs. The main sources of carbohydrate in the diet are fruits, vegetables, and grain products. The unrefined carbohydrate sources yield valuable fiber. Sugars and sweets are also sources of carbohydrate but are often called "empty calories" because they do not contribute many nutrients to the diet. The pregnant woman requires approximately 2500 calories per day and 300 additional calories a day during the second and third trimesters.

Fats

Fat is a concentrated source of energy, yielding more than twice as many calories per gram as carbohydrate. Besides providing energy, fat in the diet provides essential fatty acids and supplies and carries the fat-soluble vitamins A, D, E, and K. Fats such as butter, margarine, and salad oil also add to the palatability of food. During pregnancy fats are more completely absorbed for use as energy than in the nonpregnant state.

Protein

The main function of protein is to build and repair all body cells. While most Americans consume more protein than they require, about 10% to 15% of the population have insufficient protein intake. An increased amount is needed during pregnancy for growth and maintenance of maternal and fetal tissues (Table 9-3). Some specific needs for protein are rapid fetal tissue growth, development of the placenta, enlargement of maternal tissues (uterus and breast), increased maternal circulating blood volume, and formation of amniotic fluid.

Proteins are made up of different combinations of the more than 20 **amino acids.** Eight of these are referred to as *essential amino acids*. They cannot be manufactured by the body and must be supplied by the diet. Proteins that contain adequate amounts of all eight essential amino acids are called *complete proteins*. Most animal protein sources fall into this category, but dairy products are the *major* source of complete protein. Only four commonly used foods contain complete protein, namely, milk, cheese, eggs, and meat. Most vegetable protein sources alone are deficient in one or more of the essential amino acids and are "incomplete proteins."

TABLE 9-2

Recommended Calorie Intake

	Age (Years) or Condition	Calories per Day
Females	11–14	2200
	15–18	2200
	19–24	2200
	25–50	2200
	51 +	1900
Pregnant	1st trimester	+0
	2nd trimester	+300
	3rd trimester	+300
Lactating	1st 6 months	+500
	2nd 6 months	+500

TABLE 9-3

Recommended Protein Intake

Nutrient	Amount (Set by National Research Council)		Reasons for Increased Nutrient Need in Pregnancy	Food Sources
	Nonpregnant Adult Need (Age 19 to 24)	Pregnancy Need		
Protein	46 g	76 to 160 g	Rapid fetal tissue growth Amniotic fluid Placenta growth and development Maternal tissue growth: uterus, breasts Increased maternal circulating blood volume, hemoglobin increase, plasma protein increase Maternal storage reserves for labor, delivery, and lactation	Milk Cheese Eggs Meats Grains Legumes Nuts

From Bininger C et al: American Nursing Review for NCLEX-RN. Springhouse, Pa, Springhouse, 1989.

Fruits contain some incomplete proteins but only supplement the other proteins. Two or more incomplete protein sources with different limiting amino acids can be combined in the same meal and are then used by the body as a complete protein (Table 9-4).

The largest spurt of fetal growth and accompanying increased metabolic demands occurs during the last half of pregnancy. Pregnant women during this period requires an additional 60 g of protein a day to meet these increased needs. Milk is a very good source of protein as 8 ounces contain about 8 g of protein. If the caloric intake is less than the required amount, then protein will be used for energy instead of for tissue growth and repair.

Vitamins

Vitamins are organic substances that are essential to life and must be supplied by the diet. The increased vitamin requirements during pregnancy can be met either through food intake or by vitamin supplements (Table 9-5). There are two types of vitamins, fat soluble (Table 9-6) and water soluble (Table 9-7 p. 180). Fat-soluble vitamins A, D, E, and K are stored in the body. Large doses of these, vitamins A and D in particular, can be toxic. Water-soluble vitamins (vitamin C, folic acid, niacin, riboflavin, thiamine, B_6, and B_{12}) are not stored in any significant amount, so deficiencies develop more readily than with fat-soluble vitamins when dietary intake is less than adequate.

TABLE 9-4

Complementary Proteins

Food	Complementary Protein
Grains	Corn tortilla + refried beans + milk
	Corn tortilla + fried egg + milk
	Brown rice + milk custard
	Bagel + cream cheese + milk
	Barley pilaf + ice cream
	Miso soup + fried rice + omelet
	Hominy grits + rice + eggs
	Millet + noodles + milk
	Cracked wheat = dark bread + tomatoes
Legumes	Black-eyed peas + cornbread + corn pudding
	Dried beans + macaroni + cheese + milk
	Soybeans + peanuts + wheat + rice
	Dried peas + mushrooms + yogurt
	Chick-peas + vermicelli + milk
Vegetables	Soya, red, lima beans + rice + ice cream
	Spinach + eggs + ice cream
Nuts and seeds	Sunflower seeds + green peas, beans + peanuts
	Nuts + seaweed + rice cakes

TABLE 9-5

Content of Selected Prenatal Multivitamins★

	Vitamins									Minerals			
	A (IU)	D (IU)	E (IU)	C (mg)	Folate (μg)	Niacin (mg)	Thiamin (mg)	Ribo-flavin (mg)	Pyridox-ine (mg)	Calcium (mg)	Iron (mg)	Mg (mg)	Zinc (mg)
Calinate FA	4000	400	0	50	1000	20	3	3	5	250	60	0.2	0.1
Materna	5000	400	30	100	1000	20	3	3.4	10	250	60	25	25
Mission Prenatal FA	4000	400	0	100	800	10	5	2	10	50	39	—	15
Mission Prenatal HP	4000	400	0	100	1000	10	5	2	25	50	39	—	15
Natafort Film-seal	6000	400	30	120	1000	20	3	2	15	350	65	100	25
Natalins Rx	5000	400	30	90	1000	20	2.6	3	10	200	60	100	15
Pramet FA	4000	400	unknown	100	1000	10	3	2	5	250	60	—	—
Stuartnatal 1 + 1	4000	400	11	120	1000	20	1.5	3	10	200	65	—	25
Zenate Prenatal	5000	400	30	80	1000	20	3	3	10	300	65	100	20

Data adapted from Physicians' Desk Reference 1989.

Minerals

There are 14 or more mineral elements that are essential for adequate nutrition. Some of these are found in fairly large amounts in the body, and others, called *trace elements* or *micronutrients,* are found in minute amounts. Minerals are vital body materials, and some act as regulators and activators of body functions. Their functions play a vital role in both maternal and fetal growth and development (Table 9-8).

TABLE 9-6

Recommended Fat-Soluble Vitamin Intake

Nutrient	Amount (Set by National Research Council)		Reasons for Increased Nutrient Need in Pregnancy	Food Sources
	Nonpregnant Adult Need (Age 19 to 24)	Pregnancy Need		
A	800 mg	800 mg	Cell development, tissue growth (GI, skin epithelium) Fetal tooth bud formation (development of enamel-forming cells in gum tissue) Fetal skeletal formation Glycogen synthesis Light receptive segment production (facilitates adaptive vision)	Egg yolk Butter Cream Fortified margarine Dark green and yellow vegetables Canteloupe Watermelon Apricots Peaches
D	Before age 23, 10 μg; after age 23, 5 μg	10 μg	Absorption of calcium and phosphorus Mineralization of bone tissue Fetal tooth bud formation	Egg yolks Fortified milk Fortified margarine Butter Liver Fatty fish
E	8 mg	10 mg	Tissue growth Cell wall integrity, flexibility Red blood cell integrity in bone marrow	Vegetable fats and oils Leafy greens Cereals, whole grains Meats Eggs Milk
K	65 μg	65 μg	Activation of blood clotting factors	Green leafy vegetables Cabbage Cauliflower Meats (especially liver) Dairy products Fruits

CALCIUM AND PHOSPHORUS. Pregnancy imposes a substantially increased demand for minerals, calcium in particular. Milk contains all the different kinds of mineral elements that are needed for fetal development. The high content of calcium and phosphorus in milk makes it almost indispensable for good growth of bone and teeth. It provides these minerals in the correct proportions and in a digestible form that permits optimum utilization by both mother and fetus. Milk is not only an excellent source of protein but also the most readily digested and easily absorbed of all food proteins. Finally, milk contains some of the most important vitamins, particularly vitamin A, which increases resistance to infection and safeguards the development of the fetus. A quart of milk or its equivalent daily is the recommendation for the expectant mother.

It is interesting to note that most of the additional calcium required during pregnancy is used by the fetus rather than by the mother. The fetus requires much calcium and phosphorus for bone development and draws these vital minerals from the mother's bone stores.

TABLE 9-7

Recommended Water-Soluble Vitamin Intake

| Nutrient | Amount (Set by National Research Council) | | Reasons for Increased Nutrient Need in Pregnancy | Food Sources |
	Nonpregnant Adult Need (Age 19 to 24)	Pregnancy Need		
C (ascorbic acid)	60 mg	65 mg	Tissue formation and integrity Cement substance in connective and vascular tissues Increased iron absorption General metabolism	Citrus fruits Berries Melons Tomatoes Chili peppers Green peppers Green leafy vegetables Broccoli Potatoes
Folic acid	180 µg	400 µg	General metabolism Increased metabolic demand in pregnancy Prevention of megaloblastic anemia in high-risk clients Increased heme production for hemoglobin Production of cell nucleus material	Liver/organ meats Green leafy vegetables Legumes Oranges Bananas Eggs
Niacin	15 mg	17 mg	Coenzyme in energy metabolism, protein metabolism, and cell reactions	Meats, poultry, tuna Peanuts Beans, peas, corn Enriched grains
Riboflavin (B_2)	1.3 mg	1.6 mg	Coenzyme in CHO, fat, and protein metabolism	Milk, yogurt, cottage cheese Liver Whole, enriched grains Dark green leafy vegetables
Thiamine (B_1)	1.1 mg	1.5 mg	Coenzyme in energy metabolism Normal nervous system functioning	Pork, beef, oysters Liver Whole, enriched grains Legumes
B_6 (pyridoxine)	1.5 mg	2.2 mg	Coenzyme in protein metabolism Increased fetal growth requirement Glucose oxidation	Nuts Wheat, corn Liver Meats, poultry Fish, shellfish
B_{12}	2.0 µg	2.2 µg	Various cell reactions Coenzyme in protein metabolism, especially vital cell proteins, such as nucleic acid Red blood cell formation Glucose oxidation	Milk Eggs Meats Liver, kidney Cheese Fish, shellfish

IRON. Adequate intake of iron is particularly important, too. If iron reserves are depleted, the mother's body will reduce red blood cell production rather than use any of the fetal iron reserves. This results in maternal iron deficiency **anemia** that is in turn imposed on the physiologic anemia of pregnancy. For this reason, it is very important for the pregnant woman to take prenatal iron supplements, usually starting in the second trimester.

TABLE 9-8

Recommended Mineral Intake

Nutrient	Amount (Set by National Research Council)		Reasons for Increased Nutrient Need in Pregnancy	Food Sources
	Nonpregnant Adult Need (Age 19 to 24)	Pregnancy Need		
Calcium	1200 mg	1200 mg	Fetal skeletal formation Fetal tooth bud formation Increased maternal calcium metabolism Nerve impulse transmission Necessary component in blood clotting	Milk, ice cream Cheese Whole grains Leafy vegetables Canned salmon Oysters Sardines Dried beans Eggs
Phosphorus	1200 mg	1200 mg	Fetal skeletal formation Fetal tooth bud formation Increased maternal phosphorus metabolism	Milk Cheese Lean meats Whole grains Legumes Nuts
Iron	15 mg	30 mg (or 30 mg supplement)	Increased maternal circulating blood volume, increased hemoglobin (carries O_2 to brain) Fetal liver iron storage (primarily in third trimester) High iron cost of pregnancy	Oysters Liver Red meats Egg yolks Whole or enriched grains Dark green leafy vegetables Nuts Legumes Dried beans, fruits
Iodine	150 μg	175 μg	Increased basal metabolic rate through increased thyroxine production	Iodized salt Seafood
Magnesium	280 mg	320 mg	Coenzyme in energy and protein metabolism Enzyme activator Tissue growth, cell metabolism Muscle action	Bananas Nuts Soybeans, dried beans Cocoa Seafood Whole grains Dried beans and peanuts
Zinc	12 mg	15 mg	DNA, RNA synthesis CNS development Protein synthesis Hydrochloric acid production	Meat Liver Eggs Milk Seafood Whole grains Cereals Nuts Seeds Cocoa
Sodium	500 mg	500 mg	Fluid volume electrolyte balance Adequate renal, placental blood flow	Salt Foods of animal origin

SODIUM. Sodium is present in foods of animal origin and in some vegetables, but the major dietary source is salt. There is increasing recognition of the importance of adequate sodium intake during pregnancy.

In the past, like calorie restriction, salt restriction was thought to be an important factor in the prevention of pregnancy-induced hypertension (formerly called toxemia). Clinical and laboratory data now indicate that the sodium requirement is increased during pregnancy. Restriction, therefore, can be harmful when indiscriminately imposed. The use of diuretics for reduction of edema that was previously thought to be associated with sodium retention caused by excessive salt in the diet has also been discontinued. Flowers[7] has noted that there is a mechanism present in pregnancy that increases sodium reabsorption and retention when there is a reduction in sodium intake. An adequate renal and placental blood flow demands an adequate circulating blood volume. A stringent reduction in sodium intake causes a reduction in circulating blood volume, which is intolerable during pregnancy and causes damage to both mother and fetus. Many physicians now advise clients early in pregnancy to simply salt their food to taste. However, this does not mean that salt intake needs to be increased because the usual diet of most women in the United States easily meets the sodium requirements for pregnancy.[8]

Water and Other Fluids

Water is often omitted when nutrients are listed, but it is, in fact, a very essential nutrient. It is an important solvent that is necessary for digestion, nutrient transport to cells, and removal of body wastes. It is also a lubricant and helps regulate body temperature. A pregnant woman should drink 7 to 8 glasses of water a day.

Pregnant Adolescent Nutritional Needs

Nutritional needs for the pregnant adolescent vary according to age, weight, and activity. Needs are determined by adding nutrient requirements for the nonpregnant girl to the additional amount needed in each category for pregnancy requirements (see display below). Nutritional needs for the young adolescent (12 to 14 years old) will be higher than

---

Calculating Calorie Requirements for Pregnant Adolescents★

1. Allow calories for maximum daily growth needs: 123 calories
2. Add RDA† of calories for pregnancy: 300 calories
3. Add average RDA† of calories for age and growth percentile for nonpregnant female: <u>2100 calories</u>
     2523 total daily calories
4. *Underweight.* Add 500 additional calories per day, 16% of which should be protein (20 g):   3023 total daily calories
5. *Overweight.* Use lower range of "normal" suggested values or 38 calories/kg or 17 calories/lb pregnancy weight.

From Frank D et al: J. Calif Perinatal Assoc 3(1):21, 1981.
★These calculations are based on the maximum calorie allowance for growth. The best indication of whether a pregnant female is getting sufficient calories is to monitor her growth with a prenatal growth grid. If inadequate or excess weight gain occurs, consultation with a nutritionist is recommended.
†Recommended daily dietary allowance.

those of the woman whose growth has been completed. Although the RDAs are based on chronologic age, they are probably the best available figures to use if the pregnant female is still growing. However, if mature (15 years and older), the pregnant adolescent's nutritional needs would approach those reported for pregnant adults.[9]

Additional amounts of vitamins, minerals, and calories are needed to meet growth needs of the pregnant adolescent and her infant and to correct deficiencies due to inadequate intake of nutrients before, during, and after pregnancy. Iron supplements are needed to provide for the growing muscle mass and blood volume increase in the pregnant teen.[10] These supplements also can provide the iron needed even though iron intake is poor.

An additional 0.4 g calcium are needed to meet adolescent pregnancy requirements. A total supplement of 1.6 g may be needed if milk and milk products or significant calcium sources are omitted from the diet for any reason.

Folic acid is another vital nutrient in adolescent pregnancy. The RDA of 400 g is increased in pregnancy for females of all ages. A supplement is suggested as most diets cannot supply the additional sources needed.[6]

Zinc and other trace elements are often lacking in the teenage diet. Multivitamins and mineral supplements can supply these important requirements.

Adolescent Dietary Habits

Adolescent dietary habits are well established. Due to irregular eating habits, resistance to adult advice, and a life-style coupled with peer food practices and media influences, the pregnant adolescent usually has an inadequate diet that increases risk for premature and low-birth-weight babies.[11] Inadequate calcium and iron intake add to these risk factors, creating anemias in both mother and infant. Adequate nutrition may also be of low priority to the pregnant adolescent, who may be much more concerned with meeting her social and emotional needs, for example, acceptance by peers and physical appearance. This may be more evident early in unplanned pregnancy.

Food Choices

The teenager's food choices may be influenced by those of her peers and often include many "fast foods" and high sugar snacks. If the pregnant teen lives at home with parents or other caregivers, she may have little or no control over what foods are available, thus limiting food choices at home. Poor food choices contribute to an inadequate intake of fresh fruits and vegetables, meats, and other sources of iron, calcium, potassium, and vitamins A and C.[6] Limited milk and milk products further reduce adequate intake of vitamins D and B, protein, and calcium.

Adolescent Weight Gain

Weight-conscious teenagers may resist continuous weight gain, especially if they gain a lot in early pregnancy. They need extra help in understanding the dangers of dieting during pregnancy. The underweight pregnant adolescent needs an additional 500 calories and protein daily. Adjustments are also needed for the overweight pregnant teen.

TABLE 9-9

Components of Weight Gain During Pregnancy

	lb
Fetal components	
Fetus	7½
Placenta	1½
Amniotic fluid	2¼
Maternal components	
Uterus and breasts	3½
Blood	4½
Extracellular fluid	3½
Other tissue (fat)	1¾

Maternal Weight Gain During Pregnancy
Weight Gain Components and Patterns

For some time, maternal weight gain was considered adequate if it consisted only of the amount necessary for the products of conception and that anything more would just be stored as "unwanted fat." Although the exact components of weight gain and the proportions of each are not known, and probably vary from one pregnancy to another, the distribution of an average weight gain is shown in Table 9-9. These figures are rough estimates only, and if actual weights could be measured, they might differ. The fat component is sometimes quoted as being closer to 2 kg, and in some analyses, part of the maternal gain is credited to lean muscle mass.

It is apparent from Figure 9-1 that most of the gain during the second trimester is related to maternal tissues, while the fetus gains the most during the third trimester. The pattern of total weight gain is also illustrated in this figure. This pattern is believed to be much more important than the actual amount of weight gained. The usual pattern consists of a 1 kg to 2 kg (2 lb to 4 lb) weight gain during the first trimester, followed by an average gain of 0.4 kg (0.9 lb) per week during the last two trimesters.[12]

FIGURE 9-1

Pregnancy Weight Gain. Pattern and components of cumulative gain in weight during pregnancy, assuming total gain of 11 kg.

Pitkin RM: Nutritional support in obstetrics and gynecology. Clin Obstet Gynecol 19(3):491, September 1976.

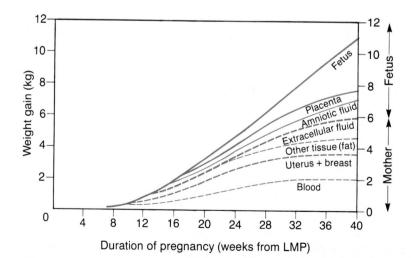

Insufficient Weight Gain

Weight gain is an important risk factor during pregnancy. Today emphasis focuses on insufficient weight gain during pregnancy, as this condition is shown to be correlated with low-birth-weight infants and may indicate poor maternal and fetal nutrition. Insufficient weight gain is considered to be an increase of 1 kg (2.2 lb) or less per month during the second or third trimester.[13] Others suggest failure to gain 10 lb by the 20th week of pregnancy identifies the woman at risk.[8]

Excessive Weight Gain

The RDA for a pregnant woman is 300 kcal/day above the woman's usual RDA. Individual needs could vary according to many factors, including client size and activity. Vermeersch suggests calculating individual needs by allowing approximately 40 kcal/kg of pregnant body weight or about 18 kcal/lb.[14]

Obesity is defined as weight 20% above the standard for height. The obese maternity client is at risk for developing hypertension, gestational diabetes, and thrombophlebitis. Obesity may also indicate less than optimum nutritional habits. The obese woman, like the adolescent, may attempt to diet during pregnancy, which can have adverse effects for her infant. Severe caloric restrictions that result in weight loss causes maternal ketonemia, a catabolic state in which fat stores are used for energy. The fetus tolerates this weight loss poorly. There is evidence that ketonemia causes a lowering of the infant's IQ.[8]

Excessive weight gain is described as a gain of 3 kg or more per month.[13] Some studies have shown that pregnancy outcome continues to improve as maternal weight gain increases, but others indicate that problems can develop past a certain optimum gain. Still others challenge the assumption that weight gain reflects a nutritionally balanced diet.[15] Those favoring unrestricted weight gain cite concern that any limitation will possibly limit needed nutrients.

Many studies have shown the relationship between maternal weight gain and birth weight. It is these findings, coupled with concern over the relatively high United States perinatal mortality rate, that have led to the recommendation of more liberal weight gain for the mother during pregnancy. The weight gain recommended varies from one source to another. Some suggest that unlimited weight gain might be best to ensure an adequate intake of nutrients. Others advocate a minimum gain of 24 lb to 25 lb, with a range of 24 lb to 30 lb. Aaronson and Macnee[15] have raised questions about the value of caloric intake as a reflection of adequate nutrition.

Women who gain weight rapidly during the first two trimesters may reach what they consider to be maximum gain by the seventh month. They then attempt to decrease what they eat to avoid gaining any more weight. This deprives them of adequate nutrients at the time when fetal brain cells are growing the fastest and when the fetus is depositing a protective layer of fat.[13] These women need encouragement to continue eating adequately.

Clients need reassurance that gaining over 20 lb is beneficial for both themselves and the baby. They must be helped to understand the rationale for adequate weight gain throughout the pregnancy and to consider the weight gain as temporary.

Making calories count is not the same as saying that pregnant women should count their calories. They should understand the importance of eating only nutritionally dense foods that contribute necessary nutrients to the diet. "Empty calories," mainly foods such as doughnuts, candy bars, and sugar-containing sodas, should be avoided. The obese woman also benefits from dietary instruction, not only during pregnancy but also in planning a weight reduction program after pregnancy. "Eat to appetite" is a good slogan to promote adequate weight gain during pregnancy, but it is only valid when the woman does not have an eating disorder and is taught which foods to eat to obtain the most nutrients.

Ethnic Dietary Preferences
Cultural Influence

Food and eating are culturally and socially defined. The religious, racial, and ethnic background of the client and her family is an important consideration. Certain foods may be highly desired and others excluded entirely from the diet. Methods of food preparation also greatly vary. Many families are fond of their regional or national diet and often prefer it to the American regimen.

Ethnic or Language Differences

Ethnic or language differences may contribute to nutritional problems in the pregnant woman. She may not be able to find the foods she is used to cooking, and substitutions may not furnish the same nutrients. Also, if English is not spoken, she may misunderstand or misinterpret dietary instructions, recipes, or information on food container labels.

Assessing the client's ethnic background can be helpful in understanding her dietary habits and potential risk factors. The nurse must *always* remember that great food preference variations exist within an ethnic group. Dietary assumptions should not be made about a client based solely on surname, primary language spoken, or identifiable ethnic group.

Dietary Alternative
Vegetarianism

Vegetarianism has become the dietary choice of an increasing number of people in recent years. Some abstain from eating meat for religious reasons, while others choose vegetarianism as a means to more efficiently use the world's resources or to economize on their food bills.

Types of Vegetarian Diets

Various types of **vegetarian** diets differ in the extent to which they exclude animal sources of protein. Semivegetarians include meat and other animal proteins occasionally. Lactoovovegetarians exclude meat but include eggs and dairy products. Some who only occasionally eat fish, poultry, and liver consider themselves lactoovovegetarians. Lactovegetarians exclude all animal protein sources except dairy products, i.e., meat, poultry, fish,

TABLE 9-10

Food Guide for Lactoovovegetarian and Vegan Diets

Food (Serving Size)		Minimum Number of Daily Servings	
		Lactoovovegetarians	Vegan
I	Whole grains (1 cup) or breads (1 slice)	6	7 (9)★
II	Legumes (1 cup)	2	3
	Nuts and seeds (3 T)	1	1
III	Milk (1 cup) or milk products (1 slice)	4	4†
	Eggs	1-2	—
IV	Fruits (1/2 cup juice) or vegetables (1/2 cup cooked/raw)	5	5 (7)★
V	Oils (T)	2	2

From Dimperio D: Florida's Guide to Maternal Nutrition, Tallahasee, State of Florida, Department of Health and Rehabilitation Services, 1986.

★The higher amount in parenthesis is suggested when soy milk is not used.

†Soy milk, fortified with calcium and B_{12}.

seafood, and eggs. A small minority of vegetarians in the United States are "pure" vegetarians, or vegans, who exclude all animal sources of protein. Besides the obvious need to make sure the pregnant vegetarian obtains enough high-quality protein, it is also important for the nurse to be aware that some vegetarians, especially the vegans, may have diets lacking other nutrients. Their caloric intake may be low, leading to low prepregnancy weight and low pregnancy weight gain. Elimination of dairy products from the diet can result in calcium or B_{12} deficiencies. Vegetarians will need assistance in finding sources of information and in planning menus (Table 9-10).

Other Dietary Problems

Lactose Intolerance

Food intolerances must also be considered when assessing nutrition risk factors during pregnancy. Intolerance, especially to milk sugar lactose, should be noted. This is a particular problem during pregnancy because it is difficult to meet the pregnant woman's need for calcium, protein, and certain vitamins and minerals without using milk and milk products.

Many adults have difficulty digesting milk because they have an insufficient amount of the enzyme lactase in the small intestine. Lactase breaks down lactose (milk sugar) into glucose and galactose. If the available lactase is not sufficient to hydrolyze the amount of lactose ingested, fermentation occurs in the large intestine and causes abdominal cramps, diarrhea, bloating, and flatulence.

High-Risk Groups

High-risk groups for lactose intolerance include those whose traditional cultural food habits do not include much milk in the adult diet. These include Eskimos, aborigines of Australia, natives of New Guinea, Chinese, Thais, Filipinos, and most African blacks.[16] On the other hand, not every pregnant woman who says "I don't like milk" or "Milk doesn't agree with me" is lactose intolerant.

Dietary Plan for Lactose Intolerance

If the client does not like milk or is intolerant of it, the nurse should develop a plan to make milk more palatable or include adequate substitutes. The instant nonfat and whole dry milk may be used in a quantity that provides an adequate intake. Approximately 5 tablespoons of dried skim milk equals 1 pint of fluid milk. Acidophilus milk is available in supermarkets for those who cannot tolerate regular milk.

In counseling lactose-intolerant clients, special attention should be directed to meeting calcium, protein, vitamin, and mineral requirements. Some dairy products are lower in lactose than others and can be used in place of milk (Table 9-11). Unless alternatives are planned to assist the client to meet nutrient requirements, the client may continue to suffer major side effects from milk sugar lactose that are counterproductive. Lactase enzyme replacement therapy may be helpful. The nurse should reinforce compliance with this therapy if it is used by the client in treating lactose intolerance.[17]

Preexisting Medical Problems

Other preexisting medical problems, including anemia, cardiac disease, diabetes, hypertension, and infections, may affect the ingestion, absorption, or utilization of nutrients. These clients will need nutritional guidance to meet their pregnancy needs and to incorporate any diet therapy for the particular condition.

Psychologic Conditions

Mental illness such as depression and eating disorders such as anorexia nervosa or bulimia may lead to a reduced caloric and nutrient intake. The result may be poor maternal weight gain with the possibility of low-birth-weight infants and increased perinatal mortality. Clients with low self-esteem, especially some pregnant teens, may be too shy or feel powerless to demand adequate food intake. This is expecially true in a multi-member household.

Dietary Faddism

Dietary faddism refers to diets that are very restrictive or food habits that concentrate on certain foods or food groups to the exclusion of others. Such food regimens can result in dehydration, loss of lean tissue mass, kidney damage, and severe fatigue due to chronic **ketosis;** in some cases, coma and death have resulted from severe brain malfunction. As these diets are extremely unbalanced, they are nutritionally unsound and dangerous for even a nonpregnant woman, especially if followed for a prolonged period. They should be avoided by the pregnant woman.

Pica

Pica has existed for a long time and is not limited to any race, culture, geographic area, or status. It is a common practice among pregnant

TABLE 9-11

Lactose Content of Selected Milk and Milk Products

Product	% Lactose (g/100 g)	Unit	Lactose (g/U)
Whole milk[1,3,4]	4.5-4.7	1 cup (244 g)	11.0-11.5
Low-fat milk, 2% fat[4]	3.7-5.3	1 cup (244 g)	9.0-13.0
Skim milk[1,3,4]	4.6-5.7	1 cup (245 g)	11.2-14.0
Chocolate milk[1,4]	4.0-4.8	1 cup (250 g)	10.0-12.0
Sweet acidophilus[4]	3.7-4.1	1 cup (244 g)	9.0-10.0
Buttermilk, cultured[1,4]	3.7-4.5	1 cup (245 g)	9.0-11.0
Condensed, whole, sweetened[1,3,4]	10.2-14.3	1 fl oz (38.2 g)	3.9-5.5
Evaporated, whole[1,3]	9.5-11.3	1 fl oz (31.5 g)	3.0-3.6
Dried, whole[1,3,4]	37.5-39.4	¼ cup (32 g)	12.0-12.6
Nonfat dry milk, instant[1,4]	50.5-51.0	1 ⅓ cup (91 g)★	46.0-46.4
Whipped cream topping[4]	13.3	1 T (3 g)	0.4
Medium cream, 25% fat[1]	3.6	1 T (15 g)	0.5
Light cream[1,4]	4.0	1 T (15 g)	0.6
Half and half[1]	4.1	1 T (15 g)	0.6
Sour cream[1]	3.2	1 T (12 g)	0.4
Yogurt			
Plain[2] (8 g protein per 8 oz)	4.7	8 oz (227 g)	10.6
Plain lowfat[2] (12 g protein per 8 oz)	7.0	8 oz (227 g)	16.0
Plain skim[2]	7.7	8 oz (227 g)	17.4
Flavored[2]		See footnote 2.	
Cheese			
Blue[4]	2.5	1 oz (28 g)	0.7
Camembert[4]	0.4	1 oz (28 g)	0.1
Cheddar[1,4]	1.4-2.1	1 oz (28 g)	0.4-0.6
Colby[4]	2.5	1 oz (28 g)	0.7
Cottage, creamed[1,4]	2.1-2.9	1 cup (210 g)	4.4-6.0
Cottage, lowfat (2%)[1,4]	3.1-3.5	1 cup (226 g)	7.0-8.0
Cottage, dry curd[1]	0.7	1 cup (145 g)	1.0
Cream[1,4]	2.0-2.9	1 oz (28 g)	0.6-0.8
Gouda[4]	2.1	1 oz (28 g)	0.6
Limberger[4]	0.4	1 oz (28 g)	0.1
Parmesan, grated[4]	2.9	1 oz (28 g)	0.8
Cheese, pasteurized, processed			
American[1,4]	1.7	1 oz (28 g)	0.5
Pimento[1,4]	1.8-6.1	1 oz (28 g)	0.5-1.7
Swiss[1,4]	1.4-2.1	1 oz (28 g)	0.4-0.6
Butter			
Salted[1,4]	0.8-1.0	1 pat (5 g)	0.04-0.05
Unsalted[1]	0.8-1.0	1 pat (5 g)	0.04-0.05
Whipped[1]	0.8	1 pat (3.8 g)	0.03
Ice cream			
Vanilla, regular[1,4]	6.8-7.1	1 cup (133 g)	9.0-9.4
French, soft[4]	5.2	1 cup (173 g)	9.0
Ice milk, vanilla[1,4]	7.4-7.6	1 cup (131 g)	9.7-10.0
Sherbet, orange[1,4]	2.0-2.1	1 cup (193 g)	3.9-4.0

★Reconstitutes to 1 qt.
[1] Average Composition of Sealtest Foods Products. Kraftco Corporation, 1971.
[2] Lactose content of yogurt. National Dairy Council, 1983 (included in Paradigms 9-10 83).
[3] Paul AA, Southgate DAT: McCance and Widdowson's The Composition of Foods. London, Elsevier/North-Holland Biomedical Press, 1978.
[4] Walsh JD: Bowel carbohydrate malabsorption. In Bayless TM (ed): Current Therapy in Gastroenterology and Liver Disease 1984-1985. Philadelphia, BC Decker, Inc., 1984.

women. *Pica* is defined as the craving for and ingestion of nonnutritive substances such as clay, dirt (*geophagia*), laundry starch, raw flour, ice, coffee grounds, or baking soda (*amylophagia*). In some cases there are regional preferences for certain pica substances. Anemia is frequently linked to pica. Some studies suggest that pica is related to iron deficiency anemia as either a cause or an effect. Other studies suggest the ingested substances could lead to anemia by displacing iron-containing foods, but others have demonstrated that iron therapy can stop the cravings.[18] When large quantities of the pica substance are ingested, there is usually some displacement of nutritious foods to the detriment of the woman's nutritional status. Theory attempts to explain pica have been explored in psychologic, cultural, sensory, nutritional, microbiologic, and physiologic arenas (Table 9-12).

Herbal Remedies

Use of herbal remedies and teas must be noted, as their risks and adverse effects on the pregnant woman and infant have been reported (Table 9-13).[5]

Excessive Substance Use

Excessive use of alcohol, drugs, or tobacco must be assessed, as they can interfere with appetite and utilization of some nutrients. Their use can sometimes result in congenital anomalies, low birth weight, and, in the case of alcohol and drugs, withdrawal symptoms in the infant after delivery.

TABLE 9-12

Areas Impacted and Possible Cause of Pica

Area	Possible Cause
Psychologic	Attention-seeking mechanism
Cultural	Habit passed from mother to daughter
Sensory	Relief from hunger and nausea
Nutritional needs	Instinctive searching for needed nutrient
Microbiologic	Clay absorbs gastric juices and quells intestinal spasms
Physiologic	Possible alleviation of pregnancy-increased salivation

TABLE 9-13

Herbs: Their Use and Potential Risks

Herb	Use	Risk
Chamomile	Relaxant	Allergic reaction (up to anaphylactic shock)
Ginseng	Health food remedy	Painful, swollen breasts
Mandrake	Sold falsely as ginseng	Contains scopolamine
Pennyroyal oil	Abortifacient	Toxicity, teratogenesis, increased risk of medical abortion
Sassafras	Tonic for a variety of unsubstantiated uses	Possible carcinogenesis, hepatotoxin, potentiator of drugs
Snakeroot	Sold falsely as ginseng	Contains reserpine
Tonka beans, melilot, sweet woodruff (tea)	Seasonal tonic	Hemorrhage
Devil's claw root	Abortifacient	Sodium and water retention, hypokalemia, hypertension, cardiac failure/arrest
Ginger root tea	Morning sickness remedy	Unknown

From Dimperio D: Florida's Guide to Maternal Nutrition. Tallahasee, State of Florida, Department of Health and Rehabilitation Services, 1986.

Socioeconomic Status

Low income limits the amount of money available for food and may be the reason for an adequate nutrient intake. Low maternal nutrient stores may also be a problem owing to chronic malnutrition. There is an increased likelihood of low-birth-weight infants and other reproductive problems in low socioeconomic groups.

Assessment

Assessing Dietary Intake

Since optimum nutrition is necessary to produce a healthy infant, nutritional assessment should be done at the beginning of prenatal care. Nutritional evaluation is continued throughout the pregnancy. Individual nutritional habits are influenced by social, cultural, religious, and psychologic factors. The nurse must consider these factors when helping the pregnant woman choose a nutritionally sound diet during pregnancy.

The Adult Diet Assessment Form[19] (see p. 192) is a useful tool in assessing the client's food habits. The nutrition questionnaire should be completed by the client on her first prenatal visit. If the client completes the assessment, the nurse validates the client's answers to ensure accuracy. The nurse uses this information as the basis for discussing current dietary habits. A diet history can be used to determine actual eating patterns and intake for past 24 hours. This dietary recall (Fig. 9-2) includes the time, the type, and the amount of food or beverage eaten. Terms like *breakfast, lunch,* or *snacks* should be avoided, as the client may not associate foods eaten with these terms.[19] For example, a woman who considers snacks as chips or cookies may not report having a sandwich or glass of milk as a snack. Such confusion may prevent obtaining an accurate history. This dietary recall data can be used to determine if the intake meets nutritional requirements for the mother and her fetus.

Another method of obtaining the information is to have the client keep a diary of everything she eats or drinks for 2 or 3 days. She should be advised to do the following: (1) avoid holidays or days with atypical diet patterns, (2) record everything as soon after eating as possible, (3) note amounts of each food as accurately as possible, and (4) describe sauces and condiments, such as cheese sauce or soy sauce. Some women have difficulty remembering to write down their food intake, but if the diary is incomplete, it can still provide useful information.

Assessing Nutritional Status

Three types of data—anthropometric evaluation, laboratory tests, and general physical assessment—can assist in assessing a client's nutritional status.

Anthropometric Evaluation

Height and weight are the most common anthropometric evaluation measurements used. Comparing height and weight can identify an underweight person. Recording weight at intervals throughout the pregnancy provides data that can be compared with the recommended pattern.

ADULT DIET ASSESSMENT FORM--PART 1

Name_____

ID#_____

CLIENT NUTRITION QUESTIONNAIRE

Birthdate_____

Comments

Please answer these questions by putting a circle around either "Yes" or "No."

1. Have you ever talked to anyone about what you have been   Yes No
   eating before today? If "Yes", when_____
   What were you told?_____

2. Have you ever had any problems with your weight? If "Yes",   Yes No
   what were they?_____

3. Have you ever been on a special diet? (low salt, diabetic,   Yes No
   weight reduction, low-fat, etc.)
   If "Yes," what kind of diet?_____

4. In the past two weeks, have you had: Heartburn   Yes No
                                              Constipation   Yes No
                                              Diarrhea   Yes No
                                              Nausea   Yes No
                                              Vomiting   Yes No
                                              Weight Loss   Yes No
                                              Weight Gain   Yes No

5. Are you taking any of the following: Vitamins/Minerals Yes No
                                              Laxatives   Yes No
                                              Antacids   Yes No
                                              Diet Pills   Yes No
                                              Birth Control Pills Yes No

6. How many times a week do you generally eat out or away
   from home? _____   Where do you generally go
   for these meals? _____

7. Do you buy and prepare most of your own food?   Yes No
   If "Yes," how many people do you cook for? _____
   If "No," who does most of the cooking for you?_____

8. Have there been any changes in your appetite in the past   Yes No
   few months? If "Yes," explain_____

9. Do you have a working: Refrigerator   Yes No
                                              Stove   Yes No

10. Do you receive: Food Stamps   Yes No
                                              AFDC   Yes No
                                              Medicaid/Medicare Yes No
                                              Meals on Wheels   Yes No
                                              WIC   Yes No

11. Do you have any trouble chewing your food?   Yes No

12. How much exercise do you get every day? (please circle)
    a little   moderate   a lot
    (desk work, watching T.V., (walking,   (running, farm work,
    cooking)   light house work)   heavy house work)

PREGNANT WOMEN ONLY	POSTPARTUM WOMEN ONLY
1. When is your baby due? _____	1. When was your baby born? _____
2. If you have been pregnant before, how many pounds did you gain during your last pregnancy? _____ lbs.	2. How many pounds did you gain during your pregnancy? _____ lbs.
3. Do you plan to breastfeed or bottlefeed? Breastfeed___ Bottlefeed___ Both___	3. Are you breastfeeding? Yes____ No____

HRS—H Form 3086E, Oct 87 (Obsoletes previous editions which may not be used)
(Stock Number: 5744-00E-3086-3)

DIET RECORD

Food Frequency

Circle any of the following foods or drinks you have eaten in the last two days.

Milk	Bread	Oranges	Broccoli	Coffee
Cheese	Rolls	Grapefruits	Carrots	Tea
Ice Cream	Cereals	Orange Juice	Greens	Coke/Soda
Yogurt	Grits	Grapefruit Juice	Spinach	Diet Soda
	Rice	Other fruit or juice	Sweet Potatoes	Koolaid
Meat	Spaghetti	What kind?	Tomatoes	Water
Fish	Noodles		Pumpkin	Beer
Eggs	Cornstarch	_____	Other vegetables	Wine
Dried Peas	Clay/Plaster		What kind?	Liquor
Dried Beans				Tobacco
Peanut Butter			_____	Street Drugs

24-Hour Recall

Please write down everything you had to eat or drink (including water) in the last 24 hours:

Time	Food or Beverage	Amount

Is this the way you usually eat?   Yes____   No____

Reviewed by:_____
              Name, Title

Date_____

FIGURE 9-2

Diet Record. The diet record enables the nurse to evaluate the pregnant woman's nutritional needs, which allows the nurse to suggest different foods to ensure the woman's nutritional requirements are met.

From Dimperio D: Florida's Guide to Maternal Nutrition. Tallahassee, State of Florida, Department of Health and Rehabilitation Services, 1986.

TABLE 9-14

Guide to Hematologic Laboratory Tests

Test	Nonpregnant Normal Values	Deficiency
Ferritin (μg/L)	40–160	≤12
Serum Iron (μg/dl)	65–165	<42
Transferrin (TIBC) (μg/dl)	300–360	>400
% Saturation	25–40	<15–20
Mean corpuscular volume (MCV) (fl)	82–92	<80 (iron) >96 (folate)
Mean corpuscular hemoglobin concentration (MCHC) (%)	32–36	<32
Mean corpuscular hemoglobin (MCH) (pg)	27–31	<27
Protoporphyrin (μg/dl RBC)	30	>100

From Dimperio D: Florida's Guide to Maternal Nutrition. Tallahasee, State of Florida, Department of Health and Rehabilitation Services, 1986.

The weight gain grid (Fig. 9-3) shows the recommended pattern for weight gain. It can be used to plot the pattern of each individual's weight gain and to detect any deviation. For example, a sudden, sharp increase in weight after the 20th week may indicate excessive fluid retention and the onset of preeclampsia. Inadequate weight gain or weight loss can also be noted.

Evaluation of Laboratory Tests

Laboratory tests are used to determine the presence and level of various nutrients (Table 9-14). These tests can identify or confirm specific nutrient-related problems. Special attention is given to hemoglobin and hematocrit results as these two measurements reflect nutritional status. Hematologic laboratory tests also are important diagnostic tools for identifying iron and folate deficiencies.

Physical Assessment

The nurse regularly reviews the pregnant client's objective physical assessment data. While these data can provide useful nutritional assessment information, they must be used in conjunction with laboratory tests and dietary history to obtain useful clues that would indicate need for further investigation.

Assessing Nutritional Risk Factors

Certain factors place women at risk for nutritional problems related to pregnancy and require special attention to nutritional needs. These factors can be grouped into categories (Table 9-15).

Nursing Diagnosis

Nursing diagnoses derived from nutritional assessment data are concerned with altered nutrition and relate to factors of increased risk for the expectant mother or fetus (see Potential Nursing Diagnoses p. 197).

WEIGHT GAIN GRID
(Prenatals Only)

Height (without   shoes)_____

Standard Weight_____

Prepregnancy Weight_____

E.D.C._____

Height w/o Shoes (Inches)	Standard Weight (Pounds)	90% of Std. Weight (Pounds)
4' 9"	102	92
4'10"	105	95
4'11"	108	97
5' 0"	111	100
5' 1"	114	103
5' 2"	118	106
5' 3"	121	109
5' 4"	126	113
5' 5"	130	117
5' 6"	136	121
5' 7"	138	124
5' 8"	142	128
5' 9"	146	131
5'10"	150	135

Modified from 1959 Metropolitan Life Insurance Co.

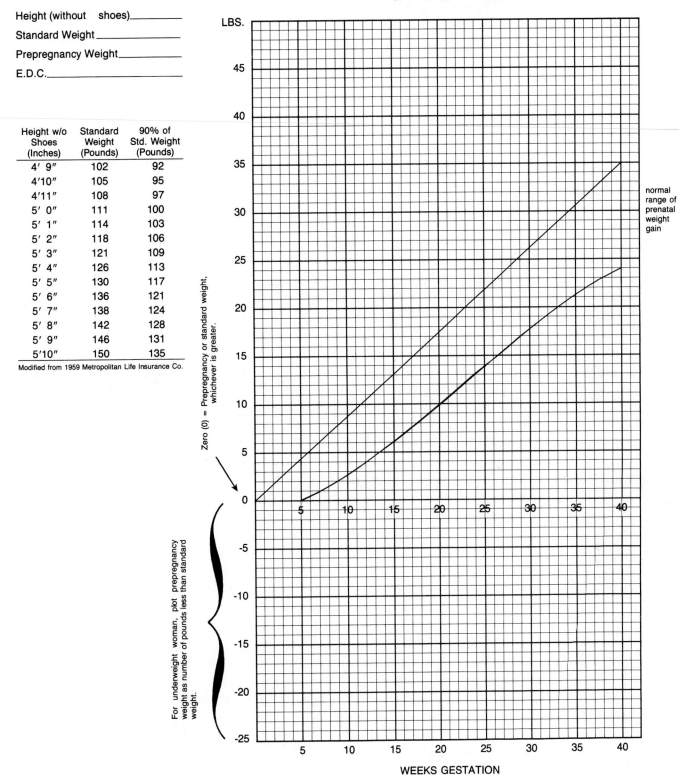

FIGURE 9–3

Weight Gain Grid. The weight gain grid plots the weight gained by the pregnant woman. It allows the nurse to evaluate the pregnant woman's normal weight gain and to alert her to control her eating habits to prevent complications that can occur when too much weight is gained.

From Dimperio D: *Florida's Guide to Maternal Nutrition.* Tallahassee, State of Florida, Department of Health and Rehabilitation Services, 1986.

TABLE 9-15

Nutritional Risk Factors

Category	Factor	Significance
Age	Adolescence	Increased nutritional needs; possible poor food habits; noncompliance
	Older gravidas	Possible increased incidence of other risk factors
Obstetric history	High parity or frequent conceptions	Depletion of maternal nutrient stores
	Previous obstetric complications	Possible nutritional relationship may recur
Medical history	Preexisting medical problems	May affect ingestion, utilization, or absorption of nutrients
Complications of current pregnancy	Development of complications such as anemia, preeclampsia, or gestational diabetes	Development of nutritional deficiencies due to increased nutritional needs
Maternal weight	Low prepregnancy weight	Increased incidence of pregnancy and neonatal complications
	Insufficient weight gain	Indication of poor maternal and fetal nutrition; increased number of low-birth-weight infants
	Obesity	Possible poor nutritional habits; increased incidence of pregnancy complications
	Excessive weight gain	If sudden, may indicate preeclampsia; lack of agreement on other possible risks
Dysfunctional dietary patterns	Dietary faddism	Diets often inadequate to meet fetal or maternal nutritional needs
	Pica	Displacement of nutritious foods, often related to iron deficiency anemia
	Excessive use of alcohol, drugs, or tobacco	Interference with appetite and with utilization of some nutrients
Socioeconomic status	Low income	Limited ability to buy sufficient food; possible chronic malnutrition
Cultural or ethnic group	Ethnic or language differences	Interference with ability to find usual foods; misinterpretation of dietary instructions
	Herbal remedies	Allergies, abortifacient effect
Psychologic conditions	Depression, anorexia nervosa	Possible reduced caloric and nutrient intake

Planning and Implementation
Nutritional and Dietary Counseling

Using the collected assessment data the nurse can plan and implement care for the pregnant client. Nutritional counseling should be initiated during the first prenatal visit. The nurse should consult with the dietician or the nutritionist and the physician in developing a dietary plan that provides adequate client nutrition. In some clinical settings, the nurse is the primary provider of nutrition information. If more than one counselor is involved in the planning, it is important that each member of the team be consistent in the nutritional information and advice presented (see display p. 197).

Ongoing Counseling

Dietary counseling should be an ongoing aspect of prenatal care. There should be discussion of nutrition at each follow-up visit, with reinforcement or additional suggestions provided as needed. Include the client's

Potential for Injury (Fetal)—related to inadequate intrauterine nutrition required for normal growth and development secondary to maternal nutritional deficits

Potential for Injury (Maternal)—related to complicated pregnancy secondary to nutritional deficits

Altered Nutrition: Less Than Body Requirements for Pregnancy—related to inadequate dietary intake, lactose intolerance

Altered Nutrition: More Than Body Requirements for Pregnancy—related to excessive caloric intake

Knowledge Deficit—regarding nutritional needs during pregnancy

Focus Assessment

Calculate number of weeks since last menstrual period.
Establish baseline entry weight.
  Determine average (nonpregnant) weight during past year.
  Measure height and current weight. Compare client's height and reported nonpregnant weight with established standards for height and age.
  Note reports of recent weight gain or loss, complaints of nausea and vomiting, food intolerances.
Appraise clinical signs of nutritional status (e.g., hair, skin, skinfold thickness).
Review client's usual dietary practices and daily intake for nutritional and caloric adequacy.
  Review client's report of food intake during previous 24 hours. If necessary for further information, request client keep a 3-day food intake record just prior to next visit; include one weekend day.
  Identify foods client prefers or dislikes, food allergies, current dietary intolerances.
  Note cultural or ethnic influences on diet, special dietary practices.
  Identify nutritive value of ethnic foods if needed.
Rule out body responses to nutritional deficiencies.
  Explore unusual cravings, e.g., laundry starch, clay. (Ice ingestion may indicate anemia.)
Monitor weight pattern throughout pregnancy.
  Weigh at each prenatal visit. Compare current weight with weight at previous visit.
  Review laboratory findings: complete blood count, hemoglobin and hematocrit values.

Nutritional and Dietary Guidelines

1. Include client's family, when appropriate, in nutritional planning.
2. Incorporate client's food choices and preferences in the nutritional plan.
3. Assist client to increase her knowledge of needed nutrients.
4. Encourage and reinforce correct choices and willingness to make adaptations.
5. Provide firm guidance when indicated.
6. Document dietary counseling sessions, including printed materials and client's understanding of information.

family when possible in the dietary planning and counseling sessions. Let the client make food choices whenever possible. Assist her in increasing her knowledge about nutrition and nutrients, encourage and reinforce correct choices or willing adaptations, and provide firm guidance.

Listening to the client, allowing her to express feelings, beliefs and needs without fear of reprimand are essential nursing skills in successful counseling. This approach is especially crucial when working with the pregnant adolescent.

The nurse must have a tolerant and nonjudgmental attitude and should respect the client's right to reject dietary information. This attitude may be difficult for the nurse to achieve, since health care providers traditionally expect their advice to be followed. However, more may be gained in the long run by accepting the "client's right to choose." A client is more likely to seek care from those she feels respect her views, even when these views differ from those of the provider. Providing this conducive atmosphere cannot be overemphasized.

Periodic Dietary Review

Periodic use of diet recall or a food diary can be helpful in assessing the extent to which the suggestions are being followed. The nurse must be alert for signs of rapid and excessive weight gain or loss. Preexisting medical conditions (thyroid dysfunction, anemia, chronic medical or surgical disorders of the GI tract, etc.) or the onset of medical disorders must be considered. The client may also gorge herself or, on the other hand, starve herself or take a diuretic prior to the prenatal visit. If this is evident from diet recall or client interview, the nurse must explore these behaviors in a matter-of-fact way with firm guidance. Frequent follow-up to prevent complications from noncompliance is necessary.

Many clients' diets are adequate. They may only need reinforcement of present dietary habits and encouragement to continue good nutrition. For those women whose dietary intake is not adequate or whose history indicates one or more risk factors, consistent counseling and other nursing interventions aimed at optimum nutritional intake is vitally important.

Counseling Clients With Special Needs

VEGETARIANS. Vegetarians will need help in finding dietary information sources and in planning menus. The nurse counsels the client who wishes to maintain her vegetarian dietary pattern to follow guidelines presented in Table 9-10 so that all food groups are included. Using soy milk fortified with calcium and B_{12} will facilitate adequate nutrient intake. Vitamin B_{12} supplements should be recommended if a vegan diet has been followed for more than 5 years.[5]

LACTOSE-INTOLERANT CLIENTS. When counseling lactose-intolerant clients, special attention is directed to meeting calcium, protein, vitamin, and mineral requirements. Some dairy products are lower in lactose than others and can be used in place of milk (see Table 9-11). Alternatives to calcium-containing food items must be planned so the client meets nutrient requirements. It is counterproductive for the client to suffer major side effects from milk sugar lactose intolerance. Custards, quiches, and milk in other cooked forms such as yogurt, cottage cheese, and canned macaroni and cheese are sometimes better tolerated by these clients.[20] Lactase-treated milk (Lactaid and Lactrace) is also available commercially.[20] If lactase enzyme replacement therapy is prescribed to treat lactose intolerance, the nurse reinforces compliance.[21]

Counseling Adolescents

In counseling the pregnant adolescent, the nurse focuses on immediate problems of nutritionally related discomforts. This establishes rapport and belief in the nurse's abilities to provide immediate intervention. The teenage client is generally more interested in her bodily changes and labor and delivery than in nutrition.[5]

The nutrition counseling plan should be simple, based on the client's readiness for more detailed information, and behavior oriented. It is not realistic to expect the pregnant teen to forego all symbolically important foods, such as potato chips and sodas. A realistic "exchange" can be devised by the nurse in encouraging the client to drink two glasses of milk for each soda she drinks. This example of a realistic counseling strategy helps build a trusting nurse–client relationship, which can become a prime motivator early in the pregnancy. As the pregnancy progresses, especially when fetal movement is felt, the teenage client is more likely to become motivated to comply with diet counseling if she understands how nutrition affects the health of her developing infant.

Group interaction and participation in nutrition classes taught by the nurse can provide peer reinforcement and support to each client. Adolescent clients working together to plan meals during these sessions provides a positive and supportive group approach to nutrition counseling.

Encouraging family or significant others to participate in dietary counseling should be approached cautiously with the pregnant teen. Invite the family members to attend during later sessions in the pregnancy. Working with the client first encourages an open exchange for the shy teen or the client who has a poor self-concept. She needs time and freedom to gain confidence in her own abilities to learn about her pregnancy and begin to take an active role in her own care. The nurse should be alert to the particular needs of the individual pregnant adolescent and to plan counseling sessions appropriately to meet her needs.

Available Resources

The nurse should be aware of available resources for nutritional counseling, education, and support. When client consultation with a nutritionist is needed and one is not available on the clinic or hospital staff, it may be possible to locate one in the area through the local community health department or a home economist's office. Printed materials and visual aids may be obtained from city, county, and state health departments. The March of Dimes Birth Defects Foundation also provides many teaching aids and printed materials about nutrition during pregnancy. Other valuable sources for dietary information are listed on page 200.

WIC Program

A source for obtaining supplemental food and nutritional counseling and education is the Special Supplementary Food Program for Women, Infants and Children, better known as WIC. Funds for the program come from the United States Department of Agriculture and are administered at the state and local levels by state health departments.[12]

Agency Sources for Nutrition Publications

The following associations are only a few of the resources that the nurse and the physician have to assist their clients in planning for adequate nutrition.

Adolescent Pregnancy Program
Public Health Service
Department of Health and Human Services
200 Independent Avenue S.W., Room 725H
Washington, D.C. 20201

American Home Economics Association
2010 Massachusetts Avenue N.W.
Washington, D.C. 20036

Adolescent Pregnancy Program
Public Health Service
Department of Health and Human Services
200 Independent Avenue S.W., Room 725H,
Washington, D.C. 20201

American Medical Association
535 North Dearborn Street
Chicago, Illinois 60610

American Public Health Association
1015 15th Street N.W.
Washington, D.C. 20005

Bureau of Foods
Division of Nutrition
Federal Building 8
200C Street, S.W.
Washington, D.C. 20204

Food and Drug Administration
5600 Fisher Lane, Room 15B-32
Rockville, Maryland 20857

The Food and Nutrition Board
2101 Constitution Avenue
Washington, D.C. 20418

Food and Nutrition Information and Educational Materials Center
National Agricultural Building, Room 304
Beltsville, Maryland 20705

National Dairy Council
6300 North Dairy Road
Rosemont, Illinois 60018

The United States Government Printing Office
Superintendent of Documents
Washington, D.C. 20402

This program was initiated in 1974 to provide specific foods for pregnant, lactating, and postpartum women, infants, and children up to 5 years of age who are determined to be at risk nutritionally and who otherwise would be unable to afford an adequate diet. Food vouchers or supplemental foods are distributed at designated health clinics. The WIC program seeks to do more than just provide food for needy families. Nutrition education is mandated to be an integral part of the program.

Sample Narrative Charting

16 wks' gestation. Wt: 105. Gained 1 lb past 4 wks (see weight gain grid); Hb: 10; Hct: 32. Easily fatigued; no energy; looks tired, pale. Discussed 24-hr diet record, chronic fatigue, food budget and transportation problems, noncompliance with pamphlet "Food for You." Stressed need for additional calories, iron, increased protein for her and fetus. 3200 calorie diet, sample meal given and discussed; Rx for Natafort Filmseal with instructions; verbalized understanding of dosage, side effects, nursing considerations. Verbalized understanding of diet and vitamins but needs assistance for buying both. Referred to nutritionist to plan meals, WIC for eligibility (pamphlet given). Instructed to make appt. this week; verbalized compliance. To submit 3-day diet diary for review; recheck wt., counseling in follow-up visit × 2 wks. Requested report from nutritionist prior to next visit. Repeat Hb, Hct × 4 weeks. Will refer to Dr. Jones for work-up pending results.

Documentation

The nurse records all interventions on the client's clinical record. A sample narrative charting is shown above.

Evaluation

Outcomes related to nutrition in pregnancy are linked directly to assessment of client's needs and problems, diagnoses, client goals, and effectiveness of nursing interventions. Documentation of client progress and nursing care effectiveness should be ongoing and complete, both from a legal-ethical viewpoint and from a practical perspective in that client goals must be measured against progress noted on the nursing care plan.

NURSING
CARE
PLAN

Insufficient Weight Gain

Goals (Expected Outcomes)	Interventions	Rationale	Evaluation
Altered Nutrition: Less Than Body Requirements—Related to Inadequate Dietary Intake			
Client will maintain adequate prenatal nutritional status and meet energy demands of pregnancy effectively.	Explain physiologic demands of pregnancy and need for increased caloric intake.	Increased maternal metabolic rate and fetal growth require large amounts of energy. Calories provide energy for maternal body processes, thermal balance, physical activity, and for building and maintaining maternal and fetal/placental tissue. Nutrients are vital to growth and maintenance of healthy tissue and for effective function of body processes.	Client exhibits expected pattern of weight gain throughout the pregnancy: First trimester: 1 to 4 pounds Second trimester: 10 to 12 pounds. Third trimester: 10 to 12 pounds. No complaints of fatigue or lack of energy to perform normal activities.

Continued

NURSING
CARE
PLAN

Insufficient Weight Gain—continued

Goals (Expected Outcomes)	Interventions	Rationale	Evaluation
Knowledge Deficit—Regarding Nutritional Needs in Pregnancy			
Client will explain benefits of high caloric and nutrient intake during pregnancy, identify foods high in protein, vitamins, and iron and list foods high in "empty" calories.	Discuss dietary requirements during pregnancy. Emphasize relationship to maternal and fetal health.	Poor maternal nutrition is associated with a higher incidence of: complicated pregnancy (e.g., spontaneous abortion, intrauterine fetal growth retardation, stillbirth), reduced fetal brain cell development, and developmental lags in infancy. Increases client's understanding of the importance of eating a well-balanced, high protein, high caloric diet during pregnancy. Facilitates compliance with dietary management.	Client requests pamphlets to take home and denies cultural taboos or influence on food choices or eating habits.
	Refer to nutritionist for meal planning, menus; WIC for eligibility for food buying assistance. Distribute and discuss "Food for You" and "What is WIC" pamphlets. Assist in identifying acceptable substitutes for foods disliked or not tolerated well, e.g., milk and milk products.	Increases potential for compliance with dietary management.	Client reports appointments with WIC; using food checks to purchase food and vitamins. Client presents own menus developed with assistance of nutritionist. Daily dietary record verifies compliance with recommendations; reveals 3200 calories, 16% protein (76 g). Client reports taking prenatal supplements (vitamins, iron, folic acid) as directed for individual management and denies pica. Hemoglobin and hematocrit remain within acceptable limits. Hemoglobin: 10 g or more Hematocrit: >35%

REFERENCES

1. Delgado H et al: Nutrition and length of gestation. Nutri Res 2:117, 1982
2. Worthington-Roberts BS, Rees JM: Nutritional needs of the pregnant adolescent. In Worthington-Roberts BS, Vermeersch J, Williams SR (eds): Nutrition in Pregnancy and Lactation, 3rd ed. St. Louis, Times Mirror/Mosby, 1985
3. Burtis G, Davis J, Martin S: Applied Nutrition and Diet Therapy. St. Louis, WB Saunders, 1988
4. Rosso P, Cramoy C: Nutrition and pregnancy. In Winick M (ed): Nutrition—Pre- and Postnatal Development. New York, Plenum Press, 1979
5. Dimperio D: Florida's Guide to Maternal Nutrition. Tallahassee, State of Florida, Department of Health and Rehabilitation Services, 1986
6. Food and Nutrition Board Subcommittee: Recommended Dietary Allowances, 10th ed. Washington, DC, National Academy Press, 1989
7. Flowers CE: Editorial: Nutrition in pregnancy. J Reprod Med 7:264-274, November 1971
8. Jacobsen HN: Diet therapy and the improvement of pregnancy outcomes. Birth 10 (1):29-31, Spring 1983
9. Frank D et al: Calif Perinatal Assoc 3(1):21, 1981
10. McCormick MC, Shapiro S, Starfield B: High risk young mothers: Infant mortality and morbidity in four areas in the US, 1973-1978. Am J Pub Health 73 (12):18, 1983
11. Williams SR: Essentials of Nutrition and Diet Therapy, 4th ed. St. Louis, Times Mirror/Mosby, 1986
12. Ritchey SJ, Taper LJ: Maternal and Child Nutrition. New York, Harper & Row, 1983
13. Pitkin RM: Assessment of nutritional status of mother, fetus, and newborn. Am J Clin Nutr 34(4):658, 1981
14. Vermeersch J: Physiological basis of nutritional needs. In Worthington B (ed): Nutrition in Pregnancy and Lactation, 3rd ed. St. Louis, CV Mosby, 1985
15. Aaronson L, Macnee C: The relationship between weight gain and nutrition in pregnancy. Nurs Res 38:223-227, July/August 1989
16. Luke B: Lactose intolerance during pregnancy: Significance and solutions. MCN 2 (2):92-96, March/April 1977
17. Stevens K, Pavlides C: Individualized prenatal nursing care of pregnant adolescents makes a difference, JOGN November/December 1989, pp 521-522
18. Key TC, Horger EO, Miller JM: Geophagia as a cause of maternal death. Obstet Gynecol 60(4): 525-526, 1982
19. Doenges M, Kenty J, Moorhouse M: Maternal/Newborn Care Plans. Philadelphia, FA Davis, 1988
20. Holland B, Unwin ID, Buss DH: Milk Products and Eggs: Fourth Supplement to McCance and Widdowson's The Composition of Foods. Rosemont, Ill, The Royal Society of Chemistry and Ministry of Agriculture, Fisheries and Food, National Dairy Council, 1989
21. Solomons NW: An update on lactose intolerance. Nutri News, 49 (1):1-3, 1986

SUGGESTED READINGS

Ademowore AS, Courey NG, Kime JS: Relationships of maternal weight gain to newborn birthweight. Obstet Gynecol 39:460, 1972

Bininger C et al: American Nursing Review for NCLEX-RN. Springhouse, Pa, Springhouse, 1989

Nutrition During Pregnancy and Lactation, Maternal and Child Health Unit, California Department of Health, 1975

Higgins A: Montreal diet dispensary study. In Nutritional Supplementation and the Outcome of Pregnancy: 93-110. Washington, DC, National Academy of Sciences, 1973

Knor E: Decision Making in Obstetrical Nursing. Philadelphia, BC Decker, 1987

Physician's Desk Reference. Oradell, NJ, Medical Economics, 1989

Stritfield PP: Congenital malformation: Teratogenic foods and additives. Birth Family J 5:1, Spring 1978

US Department of Agriculture: Food and Nutrient Intakes of Individuals in One Day in the United States. Nationwide Food Consumption Survey 1977-1978. Preliminary Report No. 2. Washington, DC, US Government Printing Office, 1980

Williams, S: Handbook of Maternal and Infant Nutrition. Berkeley, Calif, SRW Productions, 1982

Williams SR: Nutrition and Diet Therapy, 5th ed. St. Louis, Times Mirror/Mosby, 1985

Worthington-Roberts BS, Williams SR: Nutrition in Pregnancy and Lactation, 4th ed. St. Louis, Times Mirror/Mosby, 1989

Prenatal Education

IMPORTANT TERMINOLOGY

active relaxation Ability to relax voluntary muscles of the body either consciously or on suggestion

coach Person who shares the birth experience and offers support, encouragement, and understanding

comfort measure Any measure that eases discomfort in labor

conditioned response Response acquired through repeated training and practice

focal point Object in direct line of vision; used to increase concentration and focus attention on something other than the contraction

hyperventilation Imbalance of carbon dioxide and oxygen that results from breathing too fast or too deep

prenatal classes Classes focusing on first and second trimester of pregnancy

psychoprophylaxis Lamaze approach to prepared childbirth; physical and psychologic preparation

Prenatal education is an essential component of family-centered maternity care. It prepares the pregnant woman and her support person(s) for the physical and emotional experiences of childbearing. The goal of this educational process is to smooth the transition from pregnancy to birth and parenthood. Expectant parents and families of all socioeconomic levels and cultures are entitled to quality childbirth preparation. The childbirth educator must be prepared to meet the needs of individual clients as well as groups. Childbirth preparation programs include accurate information that meets the needs of the clients and assists them to do the following:

- Make informed decisions about health care
- Adjust to the changes of pregnancy and be aware of risks and warning signs
- Follow the guidelines given to maintain a healthy pregnancy
- Develop a positive attitude and cope with the stresses of childbearing
- Develop confidence in meeting the demands of early parenthood to promote a positive parent-child relationship

The process of childbirth is dynamic and is much like the nursing process. The needs of individual clients are assessed and the course content designed to meet those needs. Objectives are established. The content is presented using various teaching strategies as indicated by the needs assessment. The learning process is then evaluated by reassessment to ensure that course objectives were met.

Role of the Childbirth Educator

The childbirth educator is responsible for providing expectant parents with accurate, current information that enables them to maintain a healthy pregnancy and promotes a positive pregnancy outcome.

To achieve effective childbirth education, the childbirth educator must function as an active member of the health care team. Health care team

TABLE 10-1

Settings for Childbirth Education Classes

	Community	Health Care Provider	Private Setting
Sponsorship	Childbirth education associations Fitness centers High schools American Red Cross Clinics Employers Churches Public health departments Teen centers College/University	Hospitals Health maintenance organizations (HMO) Independent practice associations (IPA) Preferred provider organizations (PPO) Health departments Nursing centers	Self Partnership Incorporation
Financial arrangements	Fee for service (Hourly) salary No fee (community service) Contract arrangements	Salary Contracting (fee for service) Reimbursement Percentage	Direct fee for service Third party reimbursement
Location	Hospital School Church Community center Home	Health care facility Classroom Auditorium Medical library	Home Private offices Community center
Key considerations	Flexibility in sponsorship, location, and financing of classes Opportunity for community service Support group through Childbirth Education Association Central registrar to reduce administrative time Limited opportunity to educate and orient about hospital services Limited contact with health care providers	Familiarizes parents with health care environment Enhances communication with childbirth educator and childbirth team members Programs may be restricted to health care facility's philosophy Potential role conflict—employee vs. parent advocate Health care facilities' rules/policies may cause barriers to communication	Must be self-supporting programs Program reflects personal philosophy Role of parent advocate does not jeopardize employee status Responsible for publicity

From NAACOG: Competencies and Program Guidelines for Nurse Providers of Childbirth Education. Chicago, The Association, 1987.

members share their knowledge and skills to provide accurate and consistent quality information in the educational process.

Program Development

Developing an educational program is similar to preparing a teaching plan for an inpatient client. The steps are similar to those used in the nursing process.

The first step is to determine consumer needs and identify other maternity client education programs currently offered in the community. Each group of clients has different needs. Although the material presented during each course is somewhat standardized, it should be presented in a manner that meets the needs of those attending the course. Consideration must be given to the cultural differences, ages, socioeconomic status, educational levels, and personal values of the clients. Other considerations include location of the program and availability of client transportation (Table 10-1).

Once the needs have been assessed, they are prioritized, and a teaching plan is developed that includes measurable objectives. Objectives provide direction for development of the teaching materials and are a means of evaluating client learning.

Next teaching strategies are developed, and they must reflect the principles of adult learning to maintain client interest in the material and to facilitate learning (Table 10-2).

TABLE 10-2

Teaching Strategies

Strategy	Strengths	Limitations
Lecture	Transmission of facts	One-way communication
Discussion	Problem solving and transmission of attitudes; may enhance esteem	Time-consuming
Demonstration/return demonstration	Group member involvement Learning skills Teaching psychomotor skills	Extensive equipment may become expensive
Films, slides, tapes, records, audio and video tapes*	Examples	Hardware and software may become prohibitively expensive
Role playing	Problem solving and attitude building	Outcome not predictable; facilitator must be experienced in group techniques
Tours	Myths dispelled	Not always convenient; cannot always predict experience
Handouts†	Reinforcement of content	Can be expensive
Lending library	Class supplementation (may be required)	Books often are not available; often not returned

From NAACOG: Competencies and Program Guidelines for Nurse Providers of Childbirth Education. Chicago, The Association, 1987.

*Material must be previewed before presentation/showing to parents, is not a substitute for teaching, and requires introduction and discussion to achieve closure.

†May be assembled in booklet form and distributed to class members.

Evaluation is the next step and is an ongoing process that is part of each class. The childbirth educator continually reassesses the clients' needs and determines if those needs are being met. Program evaluation is obtained through learner feedback, class evaluation forms, birth evaluation forms, and feedback from other health care team members.

Teacher and Facilitator

The primary role of the childbirth educator is as an interactive client educator. For effective teaching to occur adult learning principles must be understood (see display below). In accepting the teaching responsibility, the childbirth educator also becomes a facilitator of the learning process.

Client Advocate

The childbirth educator is a client advocate. To be effective in this role, he or she must understand and accept the clients' different cultural and socioeconomic backgrounds and respect their rights and beliefs. Through client advocacy the childbirth educator assists the client in obtaining the information needed to make an informed decision and to obtain the best possible health care.

Certification and Continuing Education

Childbirth educators usually are nurses. However, the childbirth educator does not have to be a nurse nor must he or she be certified. Many non-certified maternal-child nurses provide childbirth education. However,

Adult Learning Characteristics

1. Learners and teachers bring with them a variety of experiences, skills, attitudes, and beliefs that have personal meaning to them.
2. Each member of the class has different abilities, even though the members are there for the same purpose.
3. Learning and teaching styles are a manifestation of self-concept. Teaching methods should allow for the differences in style.
4. Learning may be defined as a change in behavior; the childbirth education program should plan for meeting that change.
5. Learning requires the learner to take an active role.
6. Learners learn what they desire to learn and what they accept.
7. The learning process is enhanced by the learner's taking responsibility for his or her own learning.
8. The physical and social environment facilitates learning.
9. Learning occurs on successively deeper levels, from the known to the unknown.
10. Learning is facilitated by the opportunity to apply learning in as realistic a situation as feasible.
11. Learners are motivated when they understand the purpose of learning.
12. Learners are motivated by successful experiences.
13. Learners are motivated by teacher acceptance.
14. Learners are motivated when they can relate new learning to previous learning.
15. Learners are motivated when they find usefulness of the learning in their own personal terms.

From Sasmor J: Childbirth Education: A Nursing Perspective. New York, John Wiley & Sons, 1979.

both the noncertified childbirth educator and the obstetric nurse must be aware of content taught in the certification program so there can be follow-through of information and continuity of care.

Childbirth education certification programs are available to both nurses and people with expertise in other fields such as physical therapy or education. After successful completion of the certification program, the individual is verified as having the knowledge and professional expertise required to provide childbirth preparation programs. Certification recognizes that the individual has an understanding of the physiologic components of pregnancy, a knowledge of the principles of adult learning, comprehensive understanding of childbirth preparation, and good communication and counseling skills. These specialized competencies are built on existing professional skills and knowledge.

To provide accurate and current educational information, the childbirth educator participates in continuing education programs to maintain and expand skills and knowledge. These programs address issues such as technologic advances in maternity care, changes in the health care system, medical, legal and ethical health care considerations for the childbearing family, and updating of educational skills.

Scope and Availability of Maternity Education Programs

A variety of educational programs about pregnancy, childbirth, and infant care are available. Programs range from those focusing on preconception care to those addressing infant care and early child development (Table 10-3). Pregnant women and their support persons demand information and are eager to learn.

Health care providers are becoming increasingly aware of the importance of preparation for parenthood and are encouraging their clients to attend classes. Resources are available to provide all pregnant women with the needed preparation for pregnancy and childbirth regardless of financial constraints. The childbirth education program must include information about available resources.

Prenatal Program

Prenatal classes cover the physical and psychosocial needs during the first and second trimester of pregnancy. The goal of these classes is to encourage a healthy regimen during this phase of pregnancy. This program educates the client about normal physical and psychologic changes, fetal growth and development, developmental tasks of pregnancy, and proper care to ensure a healthy pregnancy.

Program Content

The mother is taught about the normal pregnancy-induced changes that take place in her body during the first and second trimester. Education can help her accept those changes and be alert for any abnormalities that must be reported to her health care provider. Common discomforts such as nausea and vomiting, frequency of urination, breast tenderness, and fatigue are discussed, and relief measures are suggested. If the mother understands the cause of the discomforts, they may become more easily

TABLE 10-3

Prenatal Teaching Guide (1st Through 32nd Weeks)

1st-12th Weeks	12th-24th Weeks	24th-32nd Weeks
Woman more concerned with herself, physical changes with pregnancy, and her feelings about the pregnancy.	Woman has usually resolved the issue of the pregnancy and becomes more aware of the fetus as a person.	Woman becomes more interested in baby's needs as a corollary to her own needs now and after birth.
Changes that are normal for pregnancy	Growth of fetus	Fetal growth and status
Breast fullness	Movement	Presentation and position
Urinary frequency	Fetal heart tones (FHT)	Well being—FHT
Nausea and vomiting	Personal hygiene	Personal hygiene
Fatigue	Comfortable clothing	Comfortable clothing
Expected date of confinement—calculate and explain	Breast care and supportive bra	Body mechanics and posture
Compare with uterine size	Recreation, travel	Positions of comfort
Expectation for care	Vaginal discharge	Physical and emotional changes
Initial visit	Employment or school plans	Sexual needs/changes; intercourse
Subsequent visits	Method of feeding baby	Alleviation of
Clinic appointments	Breast or bottle	Backache
Need for iron and vitamins	Give literature re methods	Braxton Hicks contractions
Resources available	Avoidance or alleviation of	Dyspnea
Education	Backache	Round ligament pain
Dental evaluation	Constipation	Leg ache or edema
Medical service	Hemorrhoids	Confirm infant feeding plans
Social service	Leg ache, varicosities, edema, cramping	Prepare for breast or bottle feeding
Emergency room	Round ligament pain	Nipple preparation
Danger signs	Nutritional guidance	Massage and expression of breast
Drugs, self-medication	Weight gain	Preparation for baby
Spotting, bleeding	Balanced diet	Supplies
Cramping, pain	Special nutritional needs	Household assistance
		Danger signs
		Preeclampsia
		Headache, excessive swelling, blurred vision
		Tubal ligation (papers prepared ahead)

From Roberts J: Priorities in prenatal education. JOGN 5:17-20, May/June 1976.

tolerated. Psychologic changes such as ambivalence about the pregnancy, changing self-image, mood swings, and sexual adjustments are discussed.

The support person is encouraged to attend classes with the mother. His or her attendance may help the support person gain a greater understanding of what the mother is feeling and also identify and understand what he or she is feeling. When the client and her support person share their feelings, a communication line is created that facilitates the educational process (Fig. 10-1).

Nutritional needs are discussed, and clients are taught how good nutrition facilitates a positive pregnancy outcome. Caloric and nutritional intake needed to maintain fetal and maternal well-being and recommended weight gain increments are discussed. Clients with specific nutritional needs are referred to a dietician. The nurse must be aware of individual dietary needs so they can be discussed with other members of the health care team.

Discussion includes risks to avoid during pregnancy, including use of drugs (other than those prescribed by the health care provider who is aware of the pregnancy), smoking, and use of alcohol. Recommendations about the safety of caffeine and use of artificial sweeteners vary among health care providers. Therefore the childbirth educator must know the

32nd–36th Weeks	36th Week to Term

Woman anticipates approaching labor and caring for baby after birth.

Fetal growth and status
Personal hygiene
  Positions of comfort
  Rest and activity
  Vaginal discharge
Alleviation of discomfort
  Backache
  Round ligament pain
  Constipation or hemorrhoids
  Leg ache or edema
  Dyspnea
Recognition of "false labor"—Braxton Hicks contractions
  How to cope and "practice" with these
Nature of "true labor"—signs. Difference between "bloody show" and bleeding
What happens during labor
  Labor contractions and progress
  What she will experience
Relaxation techniques
Breathing techniques
  Abdominal
  Accelerated pattern
  Panting and pushing
Involvement of husband or significant other
Provision for needs of other children
  Anticipation of baby
  Care for children at home while mother is in hospital

Woman should feel "ready" for labor and for the assumption of caretaking responsibilities for baby, even though she may feel anxious about both of these as well.

Review signs of labor (or teach)
Review or continue instruction re relaxation and breathing techniques
Finalize home preparations
Anticipation of hospitalization
  Admission (emergency room and labor admitting room)
  Examination, IV, shave, possible enema
  Care in labor
  Medication and anesthesia available
  Postpartum care
  Supplies needed: bra, personal items, money
  May have two visitors
  Tour of maternity unit
Confirm plans to get to hospital; care of other children; when to go and where
Consider family planning needs
Emergency arrangements
  Precipitate delivery
  Premature rupture of bag of waters with or without contractions
  Care away from home
  Vaginal bleeding

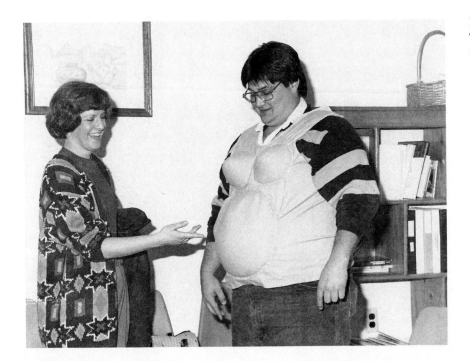

FIGURE 10-1

The Empathy Belly. The empathy belly allows the coach to feel how much weight a woman gains during pregnancy and helps him or her understand the effects this weight has on a woman's physical and psychologic well-being.

recommendations of each to avoid presenting conflicting information. Other risks the client is instructed to avoid include immunizations, exposure to communicable diseases, radiation exposure, and sexually transmitted diseases.

A discussion about prenatal screening tests such as amniocentesis, α-fetoprotein screening, and ultrasonography can decrease client anxiety about them. In-depth discussion of particular tests is done on an individual basis with those clients scheduled for the tests. Clients slated to undergo genetic testing such as amniocentesis may need counseling in addition to education. The childbirth educator must be prepared to provide support and identify resources for the client.

Personal hygiene and **comfort measures** that address the physical changes of pregnancy are recommended. Exercises for the relief of discomforts such as backache, leg cramps, and ankle edema are demonstrated. The client is also instructed about using good body mechanics and getting appropriate exercise because these measures can prevent or decrease many of the minor discomforts of pregnancy (see Client Self-Care Education: Proper Body Mechanics). Some programs include a physical therapist who teaches this class.

Throughout the course the client and support person are provided with ample opportunity to ask questions and express concerns. Many have issues and concerns that can be resolved by the group members' sharing ideas and information and discussing feelings.

The prenatal course provides an opportunity for the childbirth educator to assess the clients' needs for other childbearing programs, which can be communicated to the childbirth educator who will be teaching classes about later pregnancy. This communication provides continuity of care.

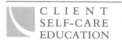 **CLIENT SELF-CARE EDUCATION**

Proper Body Mechanics

1. **Standing:** Do not let your head hang forward. Think tall; pull yourself up from the crown of your head. Keep your pelvis tilted back by tightening your abdominal muscles and tucking your buttocks under.

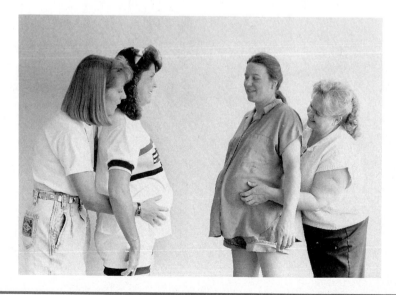

Adapted from Noble E: *Essential Exercises for the Childbearing Year.* Boston, Houghton-Mifflin, 1982.

Proper Body Mechanics—continued

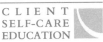

CLIENT
SELF-CARE
EDUCATION

2. **Sitting:** While sitting in a chair, be sure the entire length of your thigh is supported. Your knees should be kept even with your hips. Your feet should be supported on the floor or a stool, and your legs will be more comfortable when spread slightly apart. Periodically your feet should be elevated and some ankle rotation exercises done to aid in circulation. Tailor sitting, or sitting cross-legged on the floor, is an excellent position to use because it strengthens the pelvic muscles and stretches the thigh muscles.

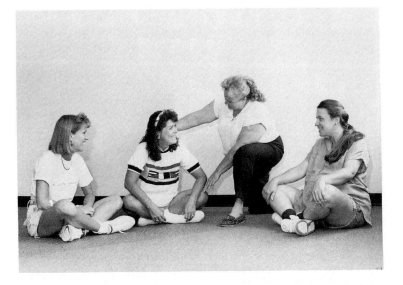

3. **Lying:** Lying flat on your back should be avoided as much as possible. The weight of the growing baby and uterus compresses your major blood vessels, which can result in lowered blood pressure. If you must lie on your back, be sure your head is elevated on a pillow, the small of your back is well supported, and your feet are elevated whenever possible. Sidelying is the most comfortable lying position in pregnancy and labor. Compression of the major vessels is avoided. Your upper leg and foot should rest on a pillow placed between the legs. Your back can be supported by a pillow folded lengthwise and tucked under the back and buttocks.

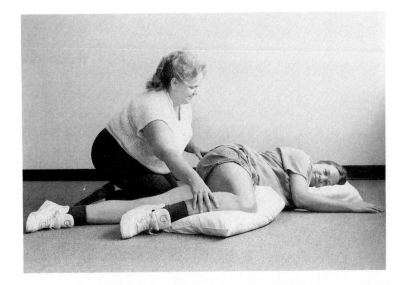

Continued

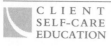
CLIENT
SELF-CARE
EDUCATION

Proper Body Mechanics—continued

4. **Lying down and getting up:** Sit with your legs off to one side; slowly lower your body onto the bed, using your arms, then roll to your back. When getting up, roll to your side, push off with your arms until you are in a sitting position, and place your legs over the edge of the bed.

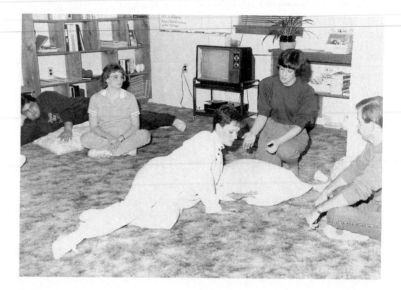

5. **Lifting:** Never use your back for lifting; this has potential for back injury even when you are not pregnant. Legs are for lifting. When picking up objects at the floor level, squat, keep your back straight, and come up from your knees, allowing your legs to do the lifting.

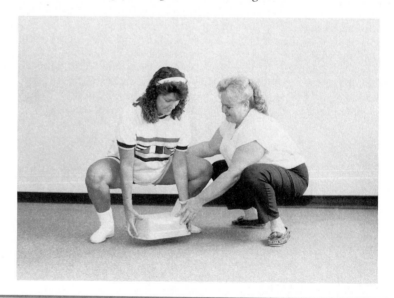

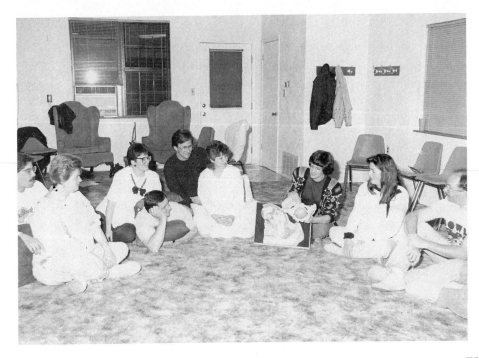

FIGURE 10-2
Childbirth Preparation Classes. One of the roles of the childbirth educator is to explain the physical mechanisms of the labor process.

Childbirth Preparation Classes

Childbirth preparation classes can be thought of as a continuation of the prenatal classes. They offer similar information but concern the third trimester of pregnancy and emphasize preparation for labor and delivery (Fig. 10-2). The goal of a childbirth preparation program is to prepare the childbearing family for the physical and emotional experience of childbirth. As a team, the prepared couple assumes an active role as they gain knowledge, confidence, and a positive attitude.

Program Content

There are several methods of childbirth preparation, with most having roots in the original work of Dr. Grantly Dick-Read. Dick-Read theorized a cycle in which the fear and anticipation of pain in childbirth create tension. This tension causes a resistance in the musculature, resulting in pain; pain increases the fear, therefore creating a vicious, continuous cycle until delivery (Fig. 10-3). Dick-Read perceived the interactive process of mind and body as a whole and went on to identify conditions that could influence labor. His approach to childbirth preparation focused on (1) adequate education during the antenatal period to ensure a physically and mentally healthy mother; (2) replacing the fear with confidence and understanding of the labor process; and (3) preparing for the childbirth experience using exercise, relaxation, and breathing techniques. The goal was to eliminate the fear-tension-pain cycle.

Fear is diminished when the mother understands the childbirth process. She learns about the anatomy and physiology of labor and the procedures that will be performed. This knowledge reduces her anxiety and uncertainty (see Client Self-Care Education: Events Taking Place During Labor and Delivery Process). Exercises are taught that increase the flexibility,

Text continued on page 219.

FIGURE 10-3

The Continuum of Responses in Prepared and Unprepared Women. A significant difference can be seen in the responses of the prepared and unprepared woman. Self-help tools are part of the childbirth preparation that enables the woman to break up the cycle to promote a more comfortable labor.

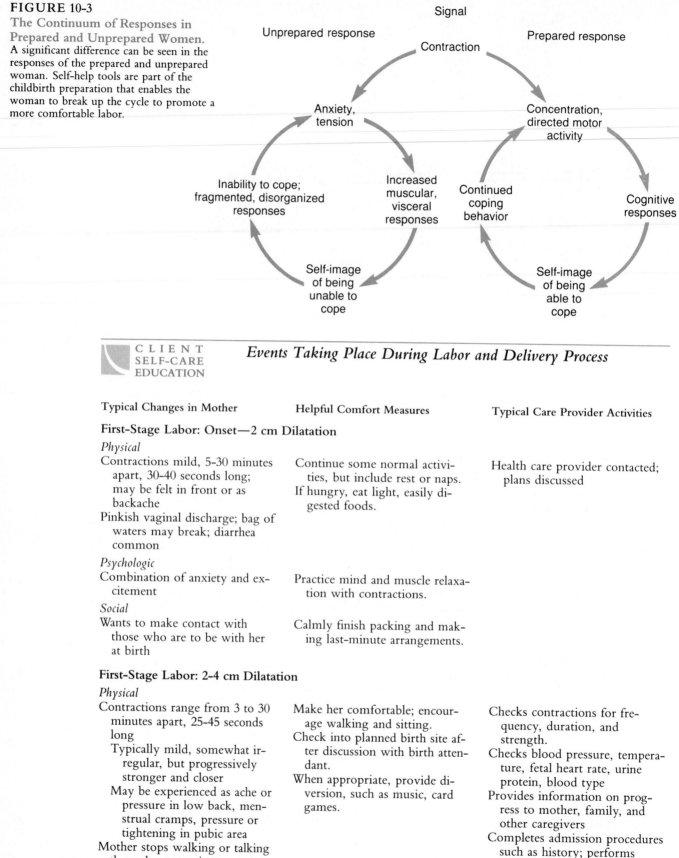

CLIENT SELF-CARE EDUCATION

Events Taking Place During Labor and Delivery Process

Typical Changes in Mother	Helpful Comfort Measures	Typical Care Provider Activities
First-Stage Labor: Onset—2 cm Dilatation		
Physical		
Contractions mild, 5-30 minutes apart, 30-40 seconds long; may be felt in front or as backache	Continue some normal activities, but include rest or naps. If hungry, eat light, easily digested foods.	Health care provider contacted; plans discussed
Pinkish vaginal discharge; bag of waters may break; diarrhea common		
Psychologic		
Combination of anxiety and excitement	Practice mind and muscle relaxation with contractions.	
Social		
Wants to make contact with those who are to be with her at birth	Calmly finish packing and making last-minute arrangements.	
First-Stage Labor: 2-4 cm Dilatation		
Physical		
Contractions range from 3 to 30 minutes apart, 25-45 seconds long	Make her comfortable; encourage walking and sitting.	Checks contractions for frequency, duration, and strength.
Typically mild, somewhat irregular, but progressively stronger and closer	Check into planned birth site after discussion with birth attendant.	Checks blood pressure, temperature, fetal heart rate, urine protein, blood type
May be experienced as ache or pressure in low back, menstrual cramps, pressure or tightening in pubic area	When appropriate, provide diversion, such as music, card games.	Provides information on progress to mother, family, and other caregivers
Mother stops walking or talking through contractions at approximately 4 cm dilation		Completes admission procedures such as history; performs enema and/or shave when indicated

Events Taking Place During Labor and Delivery Process— continued

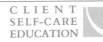

CLIENT
SELF-CARE
EDUCATION

Typical Changes in Mother	Helpful Comfort Measures	Typical Care Provider Activities
Psychologic Typically comfortable, smiling, excited, ready for labor experience May show anxiety through tears or talkativeness; may gasp for breath, make fists and rocking motion	Observe response to contractions; check relaxation and breathing. Encourage mother not to start breathing techniques too soon; emphasize relaxation. Listen closely; praise efforts.	Becomes acquainted with mother and family and tells them what to expect Encourages mother's participation in decisions about her care
Social Typically sociable, interested in what is going on, asking questions, reporting symptoms, enjoying diversion May or may not want family member present during admission procedures	Accept behavior. Provide privacy if desired by mother for vaginal examinations or other procedures. Provide entertainment and company as desired by mother.	Observes support of family/ friends and encourages them to provide help and company

First-Stage Labor: 5-7 cm Dilatation

Physical Contractions range from 2-5 minutes apart, 40-60 seconds duration; stronger intensity, longer peaks, and becoming more uncomfortable and annoying May experience dry mouth, nausea or vomiting, diaphoresis (perspiration), diarrhea May appear flushed or pale; if unprepared, may breathe deeply, rapidly, or unevenly and may hyperventilate (experienced as dizziness or tingling of lips or fingers)	Support mother's desires through assistance with relaxation and breathing patterns; remind her of focal point; add effleurage (fingertip massage). Anticipate physical needs; encourage hourly urination; offer lip balm, ice chips, position changes, cool damp cloth to forehead as desired, or hot towels to areas of discomfort. Rub back or apply counterpressure to lower back as desired by mother. Try pelvic rocking; encourage position changes.	Continues assessment of infant heart rate, blood pressure, dilation, and contractions Straightens sheets and changes pads to increase comfort Provides medication requested as an adjunct to support, rather than a substitute for it; considers mother-baby safety as well as mother's desires
Psychologic If she tires, may become more restless, less relaxed, and uncertain of her ability to cope May moan or cry	Keep mother informed between contractions; use simple, short phrases.	Encourages family support; teaches and supplements labor support as appropriate
Social Typically more serious; less talkative, attentive, and able to understand Desires companionship Easily upset by restriction, assessment procedures, or even attempts to support her	Someone should stay with mother. Family members should eat and take rests to prepare themselves for the birth; ask for nurse or other family member to substitute during breaks.	Assists family members in meeting their own needs for breaks, foods, comfort

Continued

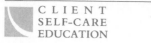

CLIENT
SELF-CARE
EDUCATION

Events Taking Place During Labor and Delivery Process—*continued*

Typical Changes in Mother	Helpful Comfort Measures	Typical Care Provider Activities
First-Stage Labor: 8-10 cm Dilatation		
Physical		
Contractions range from 1-3 minutes apart, 50-90 seconds long, peaking almost immediately, frequently with double peaks and urge to push	Provide cool sponging of face or warm blankets as needed.	Continues assessment of infant heart rate, blood pressure, dilation, station, position
Typically perspires; increased vaginal discharge	Provide firm low back pressure or back rub as desired.	Avoids new medications since the worst is nearly over for the mother and it is not desirable to give medications close to infant's birth; strong coaching should get mother through this difficult but brief part
May have severe low backache, hiccoughing, belching, nausea or vomiting, shaking of upper thighs, pulling sensation in pelvis, cramps in legs, buttocks	Instruct to pace breathing if nauseated, possibly breathing into a paper sack.	
Bag of waters may break	Encourage appropriate breathing to prevent pushing if the urge to push occurs too early.	
Drowsy between contractions		
Psychologic		
Typically less responsive; indecisive, restless, and irritable; loses perspective	Work with her in a calm, organized manner. Stay with her.	
If awakened during a contraction, she may be unable to cope effectively with that contraction	Provide strong coaching with establishment of eye-to-eye contact when instructing.	
Often feels unable to go on	Anticipate contraction with palpation or clock and wake mother, helping her begin breathing and other coping strategies. Let her sleep between contractions if can arouse before contractions.	
Natural amnesia; may not remember much of this part		
Social		
Totally focused on self	Provide perspective, encouragement. This is the most difficult part, but often lasts only 12-20 contractions.	
Desires constant companionship		
Second-Stage Labor: Birth		
Physical		
Contractions less frequent, every 2-5 minutes, 45-90 seconds long	Assist in pushing with contractions by getting her into an advantageous position such as an upright position where gravity can help.	Encourages coaching from family, instructs them, helps them accept her behavior; gives her support and provides companionship
Rectal bulging, flattening of perineum, bloody show	Help her avoid excessive breath holding during pushing by having her let a small amount of air escape from her mouth while pushing with abdominal muscles and relaxing pelvic muscles.	Allows mother to try pushing a few times before urging a decision on anesthesia
Becomes awake, alert, gets "second wind," usually has strong urge to push with contraction unless regional block such as epidural given	Encourage her to take a new breath every 5 to 6 seconds while maintaining abdominal pressure. This avoids drops in infant heartbeat, which can occur with prolonged breath holding.	Especially if second stage progress is slow, encourages mother to experiment with positions such as squatting if appropriate
Pushing with contractions felt as a great relief; also accompanied by sensations of stretching, burning, and "splitting" until baby moves down and creates a natural anesthesia		Continues to check infant heart rate and blood pressure, especially if mother has had an epidural or saddle
Could find pushing painful if mother fails to relax pelvic floor or if infant's head is still rotating		

Events Taking Place During Labor and Delivery Process—continued

CLIENT
SELF-CARE
EDUCATION

Typical Changes in Mother	Helpful Comfort Measures	Typical Care Provider Activities
Psychologic May panic, especially if unprepared; first attempts at pushing often uncoordinated	Keep someone at mother's head during birth to avoid all eyes on her bottom.	Explains birth procedures as they occur Provides mirror for birth if desired
Social Likely to be totally involved during contractions but eager for interaction between contractions; desirous of family presence especially if there are complications	Encourage, stay with mother.	Avoids situations where mother is asked to blow instead of push because she must wait for staff
Third Stage and Recovery *Physical* Contractions temporarily cease with infant birth, then resume Detachment of placenta accompanied by upward rise of uterus in abdomen Recovery period accompanied by vaginal bleeding, shaking, chills, bladder filling; uterus should stay firm but may relax, increasing bleeding	If infant will breastfeed, mother should offer breast during first hours. Healthy infants are typically awake and alert.	For infant, provides care, observes, footprints For mother, continues to monitor her blood pressure and bleeding; assists in urinating; covers with warm blankets; teaches to massage own uterus; evaluates need for medication
Psychologic Asks questions about labor and delivery events, recalls events vividly, may feel apologetic for labor behavior Seeks reassurance that infant is normal May be very alert or may want to sleep	Reassure regarding acceptance of labor behavior with no apology needed. Praise regarding labor accomplishment.	Explains details of birth experience as desired Explains recovery routines Plans to visit the next day to allow mother to review labor and birth events
Social Typically alert, happy, tired, expressing feelings through talking, laughing, and/or crying Seeks contact with infant Expresses feelings with family	Share experiences and feelings Spend time with infant; begin process of becoming a family	Delays administration of medication to infant's eyes until after family has been together Encourages mother-father-infant interaction through touching, cuddling, breast-feeding

Adapted from Humenick S: Your labor guide. Lamaze Parents Magazine, 1989, pp 72-77.

strength, and endurance of the specific muscles used in childbirth. Breathing techniques and relaxation exercises are designed to focus the mother's attention on something other than the contractions. Relaxing allows her uterus to do the work of labor, and she uses her muscles effectively. Relaxation reduces tension and decreases pain, and the client experiences a more comfortable labor without the need for excessive amounts of medication.

RELAXATION TECHNIQUES. The ability to relax is one of the most important skills the client will develop during the childbirth preparation program. This skill requires much practice and development of body awareness (see display on p. 221). The first step toward achieving a state of relaxation is to become aware of tension. Then the client can learn how to relax and reduce the tension. In teaching relaxation the childbirth educator begins with an exercise that allows the client to focus on perceiving the difference between tension and relaxation. Once the client has an understanding of how being relaxed feels, other techniques that can reduce the tension are taught (Table 10-4).

TABLE 10-4

Relaxation Techniques

Name and Type	Description	Feedback
Progressive relaxation (modifies muscular responses)	Consists of systematically tensing and releasing muscles; developed by Edmond Jacobson, modified by J. Wolpe into a 6-week approach with home practice.	Primary feedback initially described as the awareness of participant who focuses on the sensation of tensing and relaxing each muscle. Either a coach or electromyograph can provide feedback.
Neuromuscular dissociation (modifies muscular responses)	Follows progressive relaxation by asking the participant to tense some muscles and relax others simultaneously; introduced in this country by Elisabeth Bing.	Feedback by having the coach check relaxation and tension was introduced by Karmel and Bing—not mentioned in books by either Fernand Lamaze or Irwin Chabon.
Autogenic training (mental control modifiying muscular and autonomic systems responses)	Training through suggestions including "my right arm is heavy" or "my left arm is warm"; includes slowing the heart and respiration and cooling the forehead; developed by J. Schultz and W. Luther.	Feedback initially described as the awareness of the participant with no outside feedback; has been used with biofeedback equipment, thermometers.
Meditation (modifies vascular and neurotransmitter responses)	Defined by Herbert Benson as dwelling on an object (repeating a sound or gazing at an object) while emptying all thoughts and distractions in a quiet atmosphere in a comfortable position; used in transcendental meditation and yoga.	Concentration on a focal point and on breathing patterns would be forms of meditation by Benson's definition. Participant can monitor self but also receives coach's feedback on both activities.
Visual imagery	Includes techniques such as visualizing oneself on a warm beach or as a bag of cement or going down a staircase; often precedes introduction of other kinds of relaxation; may also be used to visualize and potentially affect specific body parts as in cancer therapy; may be used in desensitization in which one relaxes while visualizing a potentially threatening situation; used in labor rehearsals.	
Touching/massaging	Touch has always been a way for one person to calm another. There is evidence of actual transfer of energy taking place in some forms of touching. In childbirth preparation touching is associated with muscular relaxation (Sheila Kissinger).	Feedback from coach includes informing when muscle tension is felt, necessitating advanced coaching. Coaches may need first to discern relaxation by moving a limb.
Biofeedback	Electromyograph measures neuromuscular tension. Thermometer measures skin temperature at extremities. Galvanic skin reflex records conductivity changes because of the action of sweat glands at the surface of the skin. Electroencephalograph distinguishes alpha, beta, and theta waves in the brain.	Feedback from all of these machines is in one or more of these forms: visualization of a meter, listening to a sound, or watching a set of flashing lights.

From Humenick S: Teaching relaxation. Childbirth Educator, Summer 1984.

Suggestions for Promoting Relaxation

Before beginning a relaxation exercise:
1. Provide a calm, relaxed environment with quiet music.
2. Make sure you will not be interrupted during the exercise.
3. Empty your bladder.
4. Assume a comfortable position with all limbs supported with pillows.

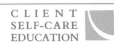

POTENTIAL
NURSING DIAGNOSES

Couples Participating in Training for Relaxation for Pregnancy or Labor and Birth or Life Stress

Knowledge Deficit—regarding relaxation skills

Noncompliance—related to partner's lack of knowledge regarding the importance of relaxation skills to coping with stress, e.g., during labor

The client benefits from use of relaxation techniques are: (1) decreased perception of pain, (2) reduction in fatigue, (3) possible decrease in the length of labor, and (4) interruption of the fear-tension-pain cycle. The **coach,** or support person, learns to identify signs of tension and assists the woman in obtaining a state of relaxation (see Client Self-Care Education: The Role of the Coach in Relaxation). Relaxation skills should be emphasized as life skills, not just as a technique for childbirth (see display on p. 222 and Nursing Care Plan on p. 223).

The Role of the Coach in Relaxation

CLIENT
SELF-CARE
EDUCATION

Action

1. Make a visual check of your partner's position.

2. During the exercises check your partner periodically for relaxation by picking up her arm.

3. If you note any tension, relax it away by using a light massage on the tense part and verbally reminding her to relax.

Rationale

1. Signs of tension include frowning, rigid neck and shoulders, and clenched fists.

2. If she has achieved a state of relaxation, the upper arm, lower arm, and wrist should move separately and feel heavy in your hands. She should not move or lift her arm for you.

3. Verbal communication reminds the mother that she is tense. The touch communication identifies area of tension.

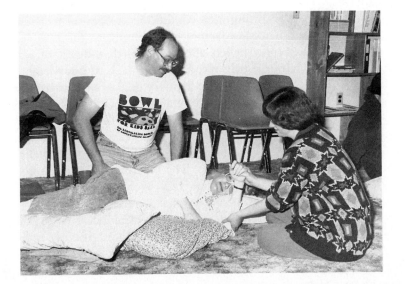

Focus Assessment

Identify readiness to learn.
    Identify couple's expectations of the training program.
    Determine couple's current knowledge regarding self-care techniques for stress management.
Explore their usual methods of coping with stressful situations.
Observe the couple's patterns of interaction and decision making, i.e., interactions with each other, nurse-instructor, and other couples.
    Note evidence of dominance or mutual support.
Identify areas where individualized teaching and support is needed.
    Note type of questions asked, response to teaching methods, and participation in learning activities.

Lamaze or Psychoprophylactic Method

The Lamaze method of childbirth preparation, **psychoprophylaxis,** is the most widely used method in the United States. The psychoprophylactic method was first used in Russia by Drs. Nicolaiev and Velvovsky. It is based on Pavlov's theory of conditioned reflexes and the role of reflexes in the response to pain. Dr. Ferdinand Lamaze, a French obstetrician, studied the technique in Russia and introduced it in France. The Lamaze method was introduced in the United States in the late 1950s after an American woman, Majorie Karmel, wrote a book about her Lamaze birth experience. Along with Marjorie Karmel, Elizabeth Bing was instrumental in the success of the Lamaze method in the United States and in the formation of The American Society for Psychoprophylaxis in Obstetrics, Inc. (ASPO).

Theory Basis

Dr. Lamaze perceived pain during labor as a **conditioned response** that can be suppressed by forming new conditioned responses to counteract and eliminate the pain. Other factors contributing to the pain of labor include culturally accepted beliefs about childbirth and fear of pain and complications, which primarily results from a lack of knowledge about the childbirth process. Therefore the primary goal of the Lamaze method is to eliminate the fear first by educating about the childbirth process, the mechanism of labor, and the neurologic pathway of pain. With this understanding, much of the apprehension and fear can be replaced with new conditioned reflexes such as use of breathing techniques initiated during a contraction (see display on p. 224). The breathing techniques not only function as a diversional activity that inhibits the pain stimulus but also provide adequate oxygenation and encourage relaxation.

A positive attitude is reflected in all the components of psychoprophylaxis, which reinforces positive coping behavior. Another important component is the coach, or support person, who is a key contributor to positive coping behaviors. The support person must understand the childbirth process to be effective.

NURSING
CARE
PLAN

Couples Participating in Training for Relaxation for Pregnancy/Labor and Birth/Life Stress

Goals (Expected Outcomes)	Interventions	Rationale	Evaluation
Knowledge Deficit—Regarding Relaxation Skills			
Client will demonstrate relaxation techniques and state their benefits in everyday life and for reducing labor pain.	After determining what woman and partner know, explain other benefits of relaxation. Include benefits for right now, labor and birth, and later life. Give other examples in everyday life that may be familiar, e.g., "tension headache" (tension causes increased pain).	Client can easily relate relaxation techniques to everyday occurrences.	Client verbalizes understanding, may contribute some benefits and has no further questions.
Noncompliance—Related to Partner's Lack of Knowledge About Importance of Relaxation Skills			
The partner will be able to participate in and understand the need for relaxation exercises.	Include partner in teaching when possible. Discuss health benefit for partner also. Have partner participate by doing relaxation with woman as you teach. Teach partner how to assess woman's level of relaxation and how to give positive nonjudgmental feedback to her.	Partner, as part of the team, is instrumental in having the client achieve a state of relaxation.	Partner assists with woman's learning, practice, and evaluation; gives appropriate feedback during practice.
	Explain it will take time and daily practice (15-20 min) to be effective in labor/stress.	Partner may mutually benefit from relaxation techniques.	Couple practices, evidenced by verbal reports and by woman's increasing ability to relax as observed by nurse during practice sessions: Relaxed jaw; Slow, regular breathing; Smoothed facial muscles; Legs rolled out and feet at 45 degree angle to each other. Couple acts as team during observed practice session.
	Motivate by making sure couple understands benefits and physiologic consequences resulting from unnecessary tension. Help couple plan specific home practice schedule with self-reward system to help motivate.		

Program Content

Although emphasis is placed on breathing and relaxation techniques, additional information is provided during Lamaze classes (see display on p. 224), including aspects of the third trimester such as physical changes, discomforts and relief measures, anatomy and physiology related to childbirth, exercises for pregnancy and delivery, and fetal growth and devel-

Psychoprophylactic Self-Help "Tools" for Prepared Childbirth

Body conditioning exercises: to prepare specific muscles used during childbirth

Active relaxation: to be able to relax the voluntary muscles of the body either consciously or on suggestion

Focal point: to increase concentration and narrow attention to something other than the contraction

Breathing techniques: to provide a concentrated effort toward breathing, thus diverting attention away from the contraction and reducing the intensity of discomfort while providing a good supply of oxygen to mother and baby

Comfort measures: to ease discomfort in labor by using comfort-promoting activities

Coach: to provide support, encouragement, understanding, and assistance in using the other tools

Medication: to promote relaxation and comfort so that the other tools may be used more effectively (Dr. Lamaze refers to the psychoprophylactic method as an analgesic maneuver and believes use of medication is not necessary when the method is applied properly)

Example of General Goals for a Childbirth Preparation Program

The childbearing couple will attend a 6-week series of classes in Lamaze Prepared Childbirth in which they will learn basic anatomy and physiology of pregnancy, body conditioning exercises, relaxation techniques, and breathing techniques, as well as other tools to use as comfort measures during the childbirth experience. The preparation they receive will allow them to approach labor informed and knowledgeable about what to expect, thus decreasing fear and tension. Explanations of possible complications and unknown factors will be given so that the couple may be fully prepared. The classes will promote childbirth as a positive experience and will encourage communication and support among the couples.

opment. The labor process is discussed in detail from the physiologic and psychologic changes that occur to options for childbirth. Alternative childbirth methods, including cesarean delivery, use of instruments such as forceps and vacuum extraction, and induction of labor, are discussed. This information provides the client with adequate knowledge and reduces the anxiety she may experience should one of these situations occur. The final class in the program covers the topics of early parenting, infant feeding, postpartum adjustments and coping skills, and contraception.

Client Goals

The client's success in childbirth preparation is not based on a perfect performance in labor and delivery or on her ability to live up to the expectations of others. It is based on the client's individual goals for the childbirth experience and her ability to use the knowledge and skills gained through the childbirth preparation program. The childbirth educator must remain flexible in his or her teaching method to assist the client in setting realistic goals by meeting individual client needs.

Lamaze Breathing Techniques

Four breathing techniques are taught in Lamaze classes: slow paced breathing, modified paced breathing, pattern paced breathing, and breathing while pushing.

The breathing techniques used depend on the phase and stage of labor (see Client Self-Care Education: Breathing Techniques).

Breathing Techniques

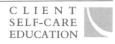

1. Slow-paced breathing

Inhale   Exhale   Inhale   Exhale   Inhale   Exhale   Inhale   Exhale   Inhale

This is relaxed breathing at a slower rate than usual. You may use your nose or mouth to inhale or exhale, whichever is more comfortable. Slow paced breathing provides good oxygenation and is conducive to relaxation.

Practice guide

Always begin and end your practice contractions with a cleansing breath. As you practice slow paced breathing, find a focal point; as you breathe, count "in 2, 3, 4—out 2, 3, 4," to keep your pace slow.

Practice "having" contractions of varying lengths, beginning with a simulated 30- or 45-second contraction and increasing the length as you progress to the other breathing techniques.

After you have mastered slow paced breathing, you may move on to modified paced breathing.

2. Modified paced breathing

Inhale   He   He   He   He   He   He   He   He   He   He   He

This is breathing at a slightly faster rate than usual. The breaths are shallow, and hyperventilation is possible if you breathe too rapidly. Begin slowly with the contraction and increase the pace with the intensity of the contraction.

Practice guide

a. Breathe in a manner that is most comfortable for you so you can concentrate on the diversional activity of the breathing rather than on feeling as though it is an effort to breathe.

Breathe at a pace no faster than two times your normal respiratory rate taking shallow breaths. Be aware of signs of hyperventilation (dizziness, light-headedness, and tingling around the mouth and in the hands) and the corrective measures (cupping hands over nose and mouth and rebreathing the exhaled air, or breathing into a paper bag).

During the practice session your coach should be observing you for signs of tension (frowning, rigid neck and shoulders, clenched fists). He or she should make sure you are aware of tension and help you relax.

Continued

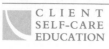

CLIENT
SELF-CARE
EDUCATION

Breathing Techniques—continued

3. Pattern paced breathing

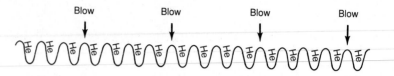

a. This is performed at the same rate as modified paced breathing, but a soft blow is added at regular intervals to create a rhythmic pattern. This technique requires much concentration and is valuable in the more active stages of labor.

Practice guide

The coach gives verbal cues that create the breathing pattern. For example, he or she selects a number between one and four, which is the number of breaths the woman will take, followed by a short blow. The coach then selects another number.

The numbers, or pattern, should be varied so the mother's concentration focuses on the breathing rather than on the contraction.

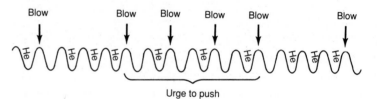

b. This alternate pattern, using one breath and one blow, can counteract the desire to push.

Practice guide

To practice for a premature urge to push, the coach gives a cue that the urge to push is felt. The woman then uses a panting type breathing to control the urge.

4. Pushing

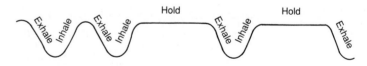

This technique assists in delivering the baby.

Practice guide

Begin the contraction with two cleansing breaths. Take a third breath and hold it for a count of six while exerting downward force with your abdominal muscles. When you need more air, take a quick breath and repeat the process until the contraction is over. End the contraction with a cleansing breath. Be sure the muscles used in Kegel exercises are relaxed as you are pushing.

SLOW PACED BREATHING. In the early phase of labor when the contractions are slightly uncomfortable, the slow paced breathing technique is conducive to relaxation while providing distraction from the contractions. Slow paced breathing is relaxed breathing at a rate one-half the client's normal resting respiratory rate. It does not matter whether the client breathes through the nose or mouth. The key point is that she breathes comfortably and slowly.

MODIFIED PACED BREATHING. Once the contractions become stronger, the client finds it more difficult to concentrate on her breathing. She moves to a faster paced breathing technique called modified paced breathing. With modified paced breathing the breaths are more shallow, and the rate is one and one-half to two times faster than the normal resting respiratory rate.

Hyperventilation is possible with the faster paced breathing techniques if the client blows off too much CO_2, resulting in an imbalance of CO_2 and O_2 in the maternal system caused by her breathing too fast or too deep. It is important to instruct the client about signs and symptoms of hyperventilation and demonstrate ways to correct the CO_2-O_2 imbalance. The symptoms of hyperventilation include dizziness, light-headedness, and tingling around the mouth and in the hands. To correct the CO_2 imbalance the client cups her hands over her nose and mouth and re-breathes the exhaled air. Another technique to correct the imbalance is to breathe into a paper bag.

PATTERN PACED BREATHING. Pattern paced breathing techniques are used when the client needs much distraction to keep her mind off the contraction. Pattern breathing is performed at the same rate as modified paced breathing, but a soft blow is added at regular intervals to create a rhythmic pattern. This technique is very helpful in the transitional phase of labor particularly when the client feels a premature urge to push. If needed, this pattern can be altered, using one breath and one blow to counteract the urge to push.

BREATHING WHILE PUSHING. During the second stage of labor there are several breathing techniques that can be used to assist in delivery of the baby. The Valsalva maneuver, or breath holding, is done by taking two deep cleansing breaths at the beginning of the contraction. Then a third breath is taken and held while a downward force is exerted by the abdominal muscles and the perineum is relaxed. The coach counts to six; then the mother takes a quick breath, and the entire process is repeated until the contraction is over. The contraction is ended with a deep cleansing breath.

When a gentle pushing technique is desired, for example, during delivery of the shoulders, a deep breath is taken but is slowly exhaled while pushing.

If at any time during the pushing stage it becomes necessary to stop pushing, the client is instructed to use a panting type breathing in which she alternates using one breath and one blow.

The client is encouraged to practice the relaxation and breathing techniques by using them to manage stressful or uncomfortable situations during the day. A specific amount of time should be set aside each day for the mother and her support person or coach to practice the skills (see Client Self-Care Education: Suggestions for Practicing Breathing Techniques). Through repeated practice the skills learned in class become the new conditioned responses that are needed for a positive childbirth experience.

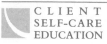

Suggestions for Practicing Breathing Techniques

When practicing the breathing techniques, always remember the following:

1. The breathing techniques do not work alone; relaxation is the key component to success.
2. Always begin with slow paced breathing because it provides a physiologic calming effect and decreases the impact of stressors. After that the breathing techniques do not have to be used in any prescribed order. Use the breathing techniques that best promote control during labor.
3. Coaches also need to practice all the breathing techniques with their partner to assist the mother with getting the pattern. Time should be set aside for the coach and mother to practice together.
4. Breathing should be practiced in a calm, relaxing environment with quiet music. Use music that you enjoy. You will develop an awareness of the music and an association with relaxation that can be beneficial in labor.
5. Develop an awareness of breathing.
   a. When practicing the relaxation exercises, pay attention to your rate and depth of breathing.
   b. Use a cleansing breath by breathing in slowly and deeply through the nose and out slowly through the mouth to promote relaxation.
   c. Notice how different positions affect your breathing and use this information during labor.

Other Childbirth Methods

There are other approaches to childbirth preparation, with some more popular in certain geographic areas than others. Although the methods vary in their approach and techniques, many are based on the fear-tension-pain cycle.

Bradley Method

The Bradley method uses many techniques similar to psychoprophylaxis but stresses working with the body to have a natural labor. This method focuses on husband-coached childbirth and uses techniques of deep breathing, relaxation, and physical conditioning. Use of medication in labor is strongly opposed. Bradley instructors are educated through the Academy of Husband-Coached Childbirth and must have a high rate of medication-free deliveries to maintain their certification.

Psychosexual Method

The Psychosexual method was developed by Sheila Kitzinger and is based on the belief that childbirth is part of the spectrum of sexuality in a woman's life. Kitzinger associates pregnancy with the entire psychosexual dimension of the woman and her relationship with her family. This method is also based on Dick-Read's work. Emphasis is placed on understanding the physiologic processes and working in harmony with the body. Imagery is one of the major techniques used to promote relaxation. Also used is touch relaxation with the support person using tactile stimulation to decrease tension. Another area of emphasis is relaxation of the perineum by voluntary release of the perineal muscles.

Childbirth Refresher Classes

Some childbirth educators and institutions offer childbirth refresher classes. These classes are intended to meet the needs of the client who has had a previous pregnancy. If the last pregnancy was some time ago or was shared with another partner, it is beneficial for the client to attend a full series of childbirth preparation classes. The client must be comfortable with the techniques used during the childbirth process.

Program Content

A refresher class reviews anatomy and physiology, the labor and delivery process, breathing techniques, and relaxation skills the client learned in the first program. A brief discussion of cesarean birth, induction procedures, and variations in the labor and delivery process are included in case the client experiences one of these variations. In meeting the needs of this client it is important to know how the previous childbirth experience was perceived and what the mother needs from the refresher course. Since there are differences both in childbirth preparation methods and teaching styles, it may be necessary to have the client demonstrate the previously learned skills. Updates or corrections in information are discussed along with explanations and reasons for the changes.

It is often more difficult for the couple taking childbirth refresher classes to find time to practice breathing and relaxation techniques because of the demands of their child or children. The childbirth educator offers suggestions for making time to practice and encourages them to focus on the skills they believe were weakest during their previous childbirth experience.

Cesarean Birth Classes

Cesarean classes are offered for those clients who have either had a previous cesarean delivery or anticipate a cesarean delivery. The goal of the cesarean class is similar to the goal of any childbirth preparation program, i.e., to prepare the client physically and psychologically for childbirth.

Program Content

A positive approach refers to cesarean delivery as a birth, not as an operation. Many clients who have experienced cesarean birth feel dissatisfied with their birth experience either because they were not prepared for this type of delivery or because they were prepared for a vaginal delivery and were disappointed when a cesarean birth was required. By opening the class with a discussion of previous experiences and feelings, the client is given the opportunity to identify and talk about both negative and positive feelings. Negative feelings can be resolved and avoided with this birth if the childbirth educator addresses them and teaches ways to promote positive outcomes. This type of introduction allows the childbirth educator to determine the client's needs.

The content of the cesarean birth class should include information that prepares the client mentally, physically, and psychologically for the birth. Discussing indications for cesarean birth promotes greater understanding. When discussing the indications for cesarean birth, the subject of vaginal birth after a cesarean (VBAC) is introduced for those clients having their first cesarean birth. VBAC may be an alternative for selected clients, and if interested, they can discuss it with their health care provider.

Physical fitness preparation is essential for the client having a cesarean birth. Body conditioning prepares her for the stress of a surgical birth and promotes faster recovery. Exercises that improve physical fitness, muscle tone, and circulation are taught. The exercises are the same as those taught to mothers who expect to deliver vaginally.

Relaxation is as important in cesarean childbirth preparation as it is in preparation for a vaginal birth. Many times there is more stress and tension associated with a cesarean birth because of the nervous anticipation of surgery and fear of pain and complications. Relaxation techniques are beneficial in coping with this stressful period.

A discussion of the hospital admission procedure, including laboratory tests, x-ray procedures, amniocentesis to determine fetal lung maturity, and preparation for surgery, prepares the client and decreases fear. This discussion also includes use of analgesic medications and anesthesia for cesarean birth. If clients have particular concerns about anesthesia, they can be referred to their health care provider.

The process is described from admission, to the operating room, to recovery. This detailed discussion promotes realistic client expectations. A film showing a cesarean birth can relieve many of the concerns and help resolve any misconceptions the client may have.

The coach is included in the cesarean birth preparation classes, and his or her role is discussed. Each individual hospital policy concerning the coach attending the cesarean birth must be known by the childbirth educator so this information can be relayed to the client.

The postpartum period for the cesarean client varies in length of recovery time and the amount of discomfort. Immediate postpartum care is discussed, and the client is informed about the medications that are available to relieve discomfort. Self-help comfort measures are also discussed. A demonstration of various positions that can be used for infant feeding promotes client comfort and assists her to have a successful breast-feeding experience.

Infant Care and Postpartum Classes

The postpartum period can be a stressful and challenging period in a parent's life. The mother is undergoing many postpartum physical changes and at the same time is confronted with the psychologic demands of parenthood. The father is also adjusting to his parenting role and changes in his family responsibilities. These adjustments may occur smoothly, or the family may need outside education and counseling to cope with the changes. Maternal–child nurses can provide the information new parents need to adjust in the postpartum period and to provide the care required by their new baby.

Program Content

Many childbirth educators and organizations offer postpartum and infant care classes. The content of postpartum classes varies according to the needs of the clients. Most classes include discussions about care of the newborn, family adjustment to a new family member, breast care, care of the perineum, postpartum emotions and depression, involution, contraception, sexuality, and postpartum exercises.

Some childbirth educators incorporate a postpartum and parenting class into their program as a class reunion that the clients attend with their new infants. This reunion can provide an opportunity for the parents to share ideas, concerns, and experiences.

Special Interest Programs

Special interest programs are designed to meet the additional educational needs of clients. These programs include classes in sibling preparation, grandparenting, and breast-feeding, as well as classes for pregnant adolescents. Many of these programs are offered through hospitals, public health departments, organizations such as the YMCA, support groups, and childbirth educators in private practice. These programs have a dual purpose: they provide current information for the participants, and they are a source of group support.

Sibling Preparation Program

Sibling preparation classes are available for families with other children. The goal of this program is to prepare the child or children for the introduction of another family member. The class usually includes a tour of the postpartum and nursery areas. Seeing where the mother and new baby will be can help the child feel more comfortable about mother's going to the hospital. Activities directed at preparing the child for a new baby in the house are designed in a way that promotes a positive feeling for the new family addition.

If the siblings will be present at the birth, an additional class to prepare them and their caretaker for what will occur may be held.

Grandparent Program

Grandparent classes are a part of the concept of family-oriented maternity care. This program is offered to grandparents who want to learn more about grandparenting skills. The family is the major focus in obstetric care today. Years ago when the grandparents were having their children, the focus was much different. Grandparents often have many questions about currently available birthing options because so few options were available to them during their childbirth experiences. Grandparent classes can familiarize grandparents with the changes that have occurred in maternity care so they can better understand the type of care their children and grandchildren will be receiving. If grandparents will be present for the birth in a labor, delivery, and recovery room, they will need special preparation. Many hospitals permit grandparent visitation so the grandparents can visit the new baby and hold and care for the infant. These practices help the grandparents make a smooth transition into their new role and facilitate communication with the new parents.

Programs for Pregnant Adolescents

The number of adolescent pregnancies continues to increase. To meet the needs of this growing group, it is essential to provide special educational opportunities for them. Many hospitals offer classes for pregnant teenagers, and public health departments include educational programs as a requirement for those clients participating in the Women, Infants, and Children (WIC) program. The pregnant adolescent greatly needs information related to nutrition and prenatal care to ensure a healthy pregnancy. Support groups are also available for single mothers.

The childbirth preparation program must make the pregnant adolescent feel welcome and comfortable so she can benefit from the experience. If a separate program exclusively for pregnant adolescents is not available, measures must be taken to prevent the client from feeling isolated when attending the prenatal classes. The coach is not referred to as "husband" or "father" because many times the pregnant adolescent has someone other than the baby's father as her coach. If she feels she is a part of the group and is encouraged and praised frequently, she may be more inclined to seek additional information if needed. Many times she is not receiving support at home or from her peers, and a nonjudgmental and caring attitude can boost her self-esteem.

In addition to educational needs, this group has needs related to financial problems, lack of education, and possibly lack of family and social support. Unfortunately, the pregnant adolescent does not always seek educational programs and support groups. An understanding childbirth educator with a positive attitude plays a very important role in educating and assisting the pregnant adolescent. This educator must continually revise the teaching plan to meet the individual and sometimes complex needs of the client. In many cases the nurse also provides counseling. When identified counseling needs are beyond the educator's scope, the client is referred to a counselor who deals effectively with teenagers.

Breast-Feeding Classes

Most childbirth preparation programs offer information on breast-feeding. Expectant parents must receive adequate information about feeding choices to make a decision about whether to breast-feed or bottle-feed. The pros and cons of each method are discussed in class, and booklets and handouts with additional information are distributed. If breast-feeding is to be successful, both the mother and support person must be comfortable with the decision. Adequate time is made available for answering questions. The childbirth educator is often able to identify special needs and concerns of the client and assist in meeting those needs to promote a successful breast-feeding experience.

Breast-feeding classes provide information about the care of the breasts, proper positioning of the infant for feeding, techniques of nursing, proper diet, and treatment and prevention of problems associated with breast-feeding. Included in the class forum is time for mothers to share their ideas and concerns. Mothers who have previously breast-fed are encouraged to attend because they can be very supportive to a mother nursing for the first time. The needs of special clients such as mothers whose infants are in the neonatal intensive care unit or who have been transferred to another hospital or mothers of twins can be addressed in a special breast-feeding program or individually if they are uncomfortable attending the regular classes.

SUGGESTED READINGS

Bing E: Six Practical Lessons for an Easier Childbirth. Bantam Books, 1967

Brinkley G, Goldberg L, Kukar J: Your Child's First Journey. Wayne, NJ, Avery Publishing, 1982

Donovan B: The Cesarean Birth Experience. Beacon Press, 1977

Durham L, Collins M: The effect of music as a conditioning aid in prepared childbirth education. JOGN 15(3):268-270, 1986

Green M, Naab M: Lamaze Is for Chickens, a Guide to Prepared Childbirth. Avery Publishing, 1985

Hassid P: Textbook for Childbirth Educators. Philadelphia, JB Lippincott, 1984

Humenick S: Your labor guide. Lamaze Parents Magazine. 1989, pp 72-77

Kitzinger S: The Complete Book of Pregnancy and Childbirth. New York, Alfred A Knopf, 1980

Lawrence RA: Breastfeeding: A Guide for the Medical Profession, 2nd ed. St. Louis, CV Mosby, 1985

Lindell SG: Education for childbirth: A time for change. JOGN 17(2):108-112, 1988

Maloni JA, McIndoe JE, Rubenstein G: Expectant grandparents class. JOGN 16(1):26-29, 1987

NAACOG: Competencies and Program Guidelines for Nurse Providers of Childbirth Education. Chicago, The Association, 1987

Noble E: Essential Exercises for the Childbearing Year. Boston, Houghton-Mifflin, 1982

Poole CJ: Fatigue during the first trimester of pregnancy. JOGN 15(5):375-379, 1986.

Riordan J: A Practical Guide to Breast Feeding. St. Louis, CV Mosby, 1983

Sasmor J: Childbirth Education: A Nursing Perspective. New York, John Wiley & Sons, 1979

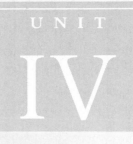

The Family in the Intrapartum Period

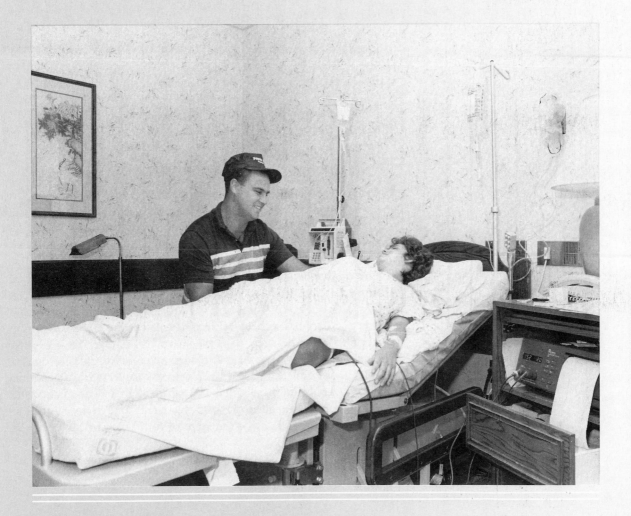

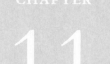
Obstetric Analgesia and Anesthesia

IMPORTANT TERMINOLOGY

analgesia Stage I of anesthesia; loss of memory of and sensitivity to pain; consciousness and protective reflexes (swallowing) not affected

anesthesia Encompasses all techniques used to create loss of sensation, e.g., general anesthesia, analgesia, regional and local anesthesia

pudendal block Infiltration of anesthetic into perineum near pudendal nerve to anesthetize perineum during late first stage and second stage of labor, delivery, and episiotomy repair

regional anesthesia Injection of local anesthetic agent to provide pain relief to a region by directly affecting nerve impulse transmission (also known as conduction anesthesia)

spinal block Injection of local anesthetic agent directly into spinal fluid of spinal canal at L2 to L5 to provide anesthesia for vaginal delivery or at level of T6 for cesarean delivery

Pain is whatever the experiencing person says it is, existing whenever he or she says it does. The client may express her pain in a number of ways that are different from what the nurse might expect. The client may show less pain or seem to have more pain than would be expected for that time in labor.

The quality of labor discomfort (pain) is difficult to describe. Any painful sensation can have various qualities, including burning, prickling, aching, sharpness, or "shooting." Pain can be deep or superficial. Labor contractions are felt as deep aching. Words commonly chosen by women in labor to describe their pain are sharp, cramping, aching, throbbing, stabbing, hot, shooting, heavy, tiring, exhausting, intense, and tight.

Clients describe the pain during delivery as pressure, stretching, splitting, or burning of the vaginal and perineal area. The client usually has an overwhelming urge to push at this time, and many say the pushing relieves the pain and causes a degree of numbness in the perineum.

Evaluating Pain

As the nurse begins caring for the client in labor, valuable insight can be gained by reviewing when labor began since prolonged labor intensifies pain because of fatigue and discouragement. During the first stage of normal labor, pain or discomfort results from the involuntary contraction of the uterine muscle. As labor progresses, the intensity of each contraction increases, resulting in a greater potential for pain or discomfort.

As the woman describes her contractions, her attitude toward labor in general is revealed and can be assessed. The degree of fear or anxiety experienced is of special importance since these feelings profoundly affect pain. They decrease pain tolerance and increase the perceived intensity of the pain. Anxiety or fear also increases muscle tension and can increase painful stimuli during labor by interfering with contractions and can decrease oxygenation to the fetus.

Pain During Transition

Uterine contractions are most intense and occur most frequently during transition. The woman experiences the most pain and has the most difficulty coping with her discomfort during transition when the pain is more intense than that felt during delivery.

To obtain more detailed and useful information about the intensity of contractions, the nurse can ask the client to rate the contraction on a scale of 1 to 10, with 1 being mild and 10 very intense (very strong). It is also helpful to encourage her to describe other characteristics of the contraction such as where the sensation begins and where it is felt most intensely. This information often suggests the need for specific pain relief measures. For example, if the contraction begins in the lower back and is felt most intensely there, rubbing that area and applying counter pressure may provide considerable comfort.

If the client reaches a point where she can no longer cope or relax between contractions, the nurse should offer to get an order for an analgesic agent. Both the client and her support person should be praised for how well they are managing labor.

Back Labor Pain

In addition to uterine contractions, approximately 24% of women in labor also have to cope with the pain or discomfort of back labor, which occurs when the fetus is in an occiput-posterior position. With each contraction the occiput of the fetus presses on the woman's sacrum, causing extreme pain as the intensity of contractions increases. Back labor is more painful for the woman than labor in which there is an anterior-occipital position.

Nonpharmacologic Methods of Analgesia

Sometimes fetal and maternal needs are in conflict during labor. The woman's needs may include relief of pain, but the fetal needs or problems may prohibit medication administration. Nonpharmacologic methods have been developed to help control rather than eliminate the pain (see display on p. 238). The laboring woman who can control her pain

---

Nursing Guidelines for Pain Relief Measures

Use a variety of pain relief measures.

Use pain relief measures *before* pain becomes severe. (It is easier to prevent severe pain and panic than to alleviate them once they occur.)

Include those pain relief measures that the client believes will be effective.

Take into account the client's ability to be active or passive in the application of the pain relief measure.

Regarding the potency of the pain relief measure needed, rely on the client's experience of the severity of pain rather than the known physical stimuli.

If a pain relief measure is ineffective the first time it is used during a contraction, encourage the client to try it at least one or two more times before abandoning it.

---

requires less medication. The nurse (and physician) who is sensitive, empathetic, and nonjudgmental can do far more to alleviate anxiety and pain than can the injection of pharmacologic substances. However, if the woman is becoming more tense and uncomfortable, the nurse should notify the primary care provider so the use of pain medication can be considered.

Positioning

During first stage labor the woman is encouraged to assume any position of comfort (Fig. 11-1), although she may not lie supine since to do so interrupts uteroplacental blood flow. Moving and walking enhance contractions and often increase comfort. Getting onto her hands and knees may ease the pain when the fetus is in the occiput-posterior position. Lying on the side avoids compression of the inferior vena cava and aorta so cardiac output and uterine blood flow are optimum. Sitting or semi-upright positions aid fetal descent and cause stronger expulsive efforts.

Changing position approximately every 30 minutes may promote comfort and encourage rotation and descent of the fetus. It is important the mother have freedom of movement during labor. Figures 11-2 through 11-6 indicate positions that can prevent or alleviate dystocia in labor.

Relaxation

Many authorities regard the ability to release tension under stress as the most important skill taught in childbirth education classes. It is the core of all other childbirth skills, including breathing and expulsion techniques. The woman and her labor partner should practice relaxation exercises during the last weeks of pregnancy.

Tensing during labor is a natural response to the contracting uterus. Tension causes exhaustion and oxygen depletion, which lower the pain threshold and prolong labor. Research has documented that increased relaxation significantly decreases labor. The skill of relaxation is not only helpful for birth but is a lifelong skill that can be called on during the daily stresses of life.

Distraction

Distraction is an effective method of pain relief. Common sense suggests that pain is more tolerable if the client becomes less aware of it. The nurse

Text continued on page 242.

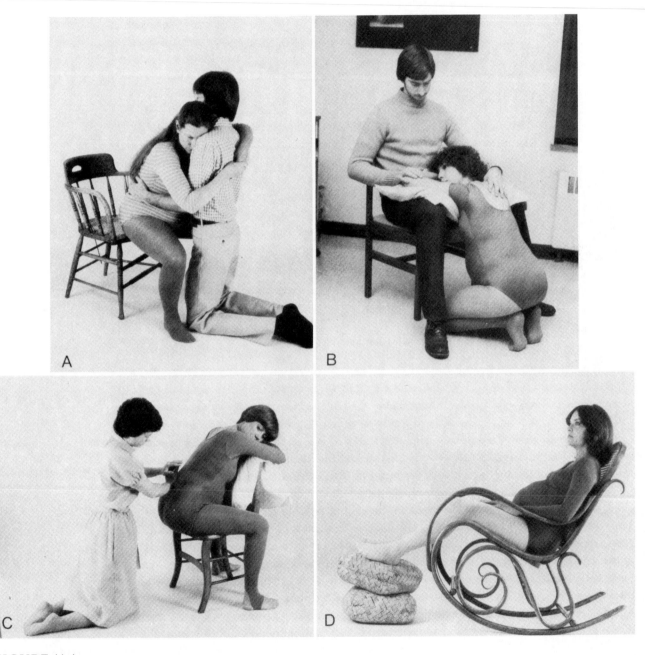

FIGURE 11-1

Positions for Labor. **A,** Sitting forward with her partner supporting her may offer
flexibility for a woman during labor. **B,** While squatting during labor, a woman can
support her balance by leaning against her partner. **C,** Firm pressure on the sacral area
of the woman's lower back often relieves back pain that accompanies some labor. **D,**
Many women find rocking during labor both relaxing and comfortable.   *Continued*

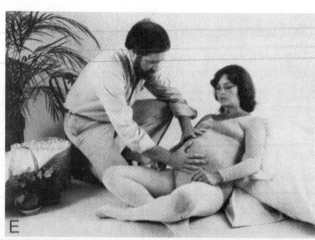

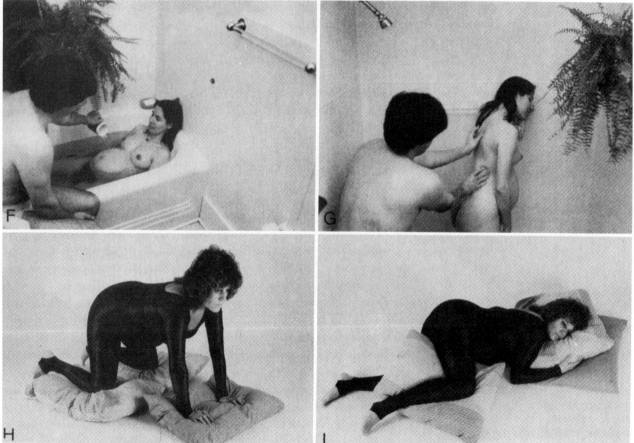

FIGURE 11-1 cont'd

E, Effleurage (light rhythmic stroking) may be soothing during labor and can be performed by the woman or her support person. **F,** Many women find that relaxing in a tub of warm water relieves discomfort in early labor. **G,** Laboring in a shower during early labor may be comforting. Warm water streaming down the woman's back may relieve back pain. **H,** Assuming a hands-knees position and rocking her pelvis may help a woman to relieve back pain during labor. **I,** During labor a position of comfort may be sidelying with pillows supporting the woman's shoulders and legs.

From Phillips CR: Family-Centered Maternity Care. St. Louis, CV Mosby, 1987.

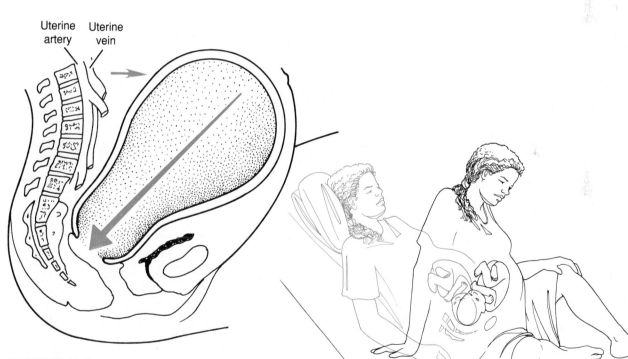

FIGURE 11-2
Maternal Positioning to Prevent or Alleviate Dystocia in Labor. When she is supine or standing, the plane of the woman's pelvic brim is not perpendicular to the spinal axis. When the spine is flexed and the lower abdominal muscles tightened, the pelvis is tilted, thus reducing the lumbar (sacral) curve. Note the s curve is simplified to a c curve, aligning the fetus with the birth canal and resulting in a more efficient labor pattern, descent, flexion, and internal rotation.

Uterine artery   Uterine vein

FIGURE 11-3
With the woman in an upright position, the uterus falls forward, away from her spine and pelvic vessels. When the uterus is supported by the anterior abdominal wall, most of the weight is directed toward the pelvic inlet. Gravity adds 10 to 35 mm Hg to the pressure exerted on the presenting part, and contractions are stronger, more efficient, and less painful in an upright position.

FIGURE 11-4
Multiple positions present a variety of angles between the fetal head and the pelvic inlet, providing more chances to help the deflexed, asynclitic, transverse, or posterior head to find the "right fit."

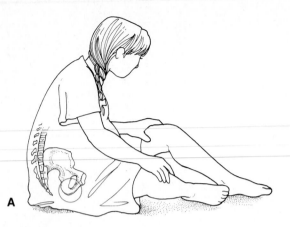

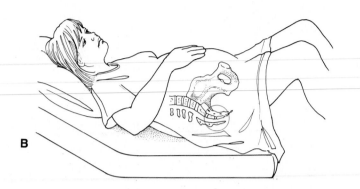

FIGURE 11-5
A, Upright positions (standing, squatting, sitting forward) result in maternal weight on the ischial tuberosities and cause movement of the sacrum, which may enhance rotation and descent. **B,** When a woman is in a modified lithotomy position, her weight is borne largely by the sacrum and coccyx, restricting posterior movement of the sacrum.

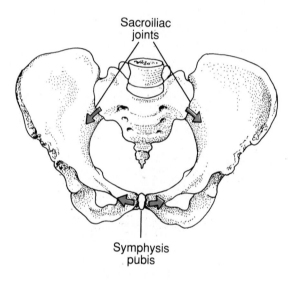

FIGURE 11-6
The joint-softening effect of relaxin allows the pelvis to hinge open at the pubic and sacroiliac joints. Pressure (through sitting) on the ischial tuberosities increases the size of the woman's pelvic outlet by 0.7 to 1.5 cm.

assists in finding a method for distraction that works for the client (see display on p. 243).

Breathing Patterns

Childbirth education programs teach various breathing techniques. One such technique is abdominal breathing. The client is taught to take long, slow, deep abdominal breaths. Another variation teaches the woman to raise her abdominal wall and use chest breathing during the contraction and then slowly to lower the abdominal wall at the end of the contraction. This permits the uterus to rise as it contracts.

As contractions become more painful, relaxation and abdominal breathing are combined. This requires vigilant coaching by the support person and often the nurse as well. As labor progresses, more and more concentration is needed to achieve relaxation.

Another method of breathing is taught in the Lamaze or psychoprophylactic education. These breathing patterns use several levels of inter-

Distraction Techniques

Concentrating on a focal point (staring at an object during a contraction)
Tapping out the rhythm of a song
Performing rhythmic head movements
Using a rhythmic breathing pattern while concentrating on relaxation
Concentrating on imagery (thinking the infant down and out)
Changing positions and massaging the abdomen (effleurage)
Using breathing techniques

costal breathing (using only the chest muscles) combined with active concentration on relaxing the muscles not involved in labor.

Slow, deep chest breathing is another breathing technique used in early labor. When this breathing pattern is no longer effective (usually at approximately 4 cm dilatation), the woman does slow, even pant breathing. As labor progresses, she may use faster breathing at the beginning and end of each contraction. During transition the breathing pattern changes to a rapid, light part-blow. Breath is blown out forcefully at intervals, and shallow panting is done during contractions.

Concentration on breathing and relaxation is most effective when there are minimum distractions. If focused breathing does not maintain relaxation and tenseness is increasing, the nurse should work with the client to concentrate on relaxation. However, if these attempts fail, it is essential that the breathing patterns be discontinued. Relaxation should be the focus of attention. When the woman becomes tense, she tends to hold her breath or hyperventilate. Both cause decreased maternal and fetal oxygenation. Administration of an analgesic may be necessary to increase relaxation so adequate oxygenation of woman and fetus is maintained.

Natural Childbirth

Both health professionals and the lay public have come to realize that heavy sedation and narcotic use during labor can have pronounced and prolonged depressing effects on the neonate. Prepared or natural childbirth has become popular because women wish to experience the birth process fully and be able to relate to their newborn immediately after birth. Approaches to natural childbirth include the Lamaze and Bradley techniques. The keys to a successful natural childbirth experience are motivation and preparation. There are times, however, when a woman who undertakes natural childbirth requires pharmacologic **analgesia** or even **anesthesia** before she delivers.

Hypnosis

Hypnosis has been used sporadically for pain relief in obstetric patients. It is touted as a method that assists clients through labor and delivery with minimum or no medication. In actual practice hypnosis has limited application.

Although the use of formal hypnosis may be limited, informal hypnosis involving prepared childbirth practices of breathing and relaxation, suggestion, encouragement, and reassurance is a valuable tool that can be safely used by those responsible for client care.

Acupuncture

The use of acupuncture for analgesia during labor and vaginal delivery has had little success. Classic Chinese medicine has never advocated its use for this purpose. Acupuncture has been used successfully for cesarean delivery in some women, but, like hypnosis, it is not effective for vaginal delivery.

Transcutaneous Electric Nerve Stimulation

Transcutaneous electric nerve stimulation (TENS) can provide analgesia through electric stimulation of the afferent nervous system. Skin electrodes made of a conductive adhesive are applied symmetrically on either side of the T10 to L1 level of the spine. Smaller electrode pads are applied to the sacral area. An electric current of a low level of stimulation is conducted continuously during labor. During contractions the stimulation is increased, with the degree of stimulation needed varying from client to client. The best analgesia is provided when the current is increased to the point that muscle activity is stimulated in the area of stimulation. TENS is especially helpful for back labor. TENS provides noninvasive analgesia without risk to mother and fetus and can be administered by the labor and delivery nurses or by the primary health care provider. Its effect can also be reversed almost immediately.

A rare complication of TENS is signal artifact, electric interference with the fetal heart tracing. If it occurs, the TENS machine can be turned off to interpret the fetal heart rate (FHR) tracing.

Support During Labor

The presence of a nurse, coach, or significant other helps support the woman's efforts during labor. From the beginning of labor the woman needs to have someone with her at increasingly frequent intervals and to know that someone is available at all times. Toward the end of labor she needs someone with her constantly.

At times the nurse's greatest contribution is to assist the support person so he or she in turn can support the client. Some believe the significant other should not be the official support person but that the couple needs a support person who can provide support for both. It is important that the nurse be increasingly present as labor progresses, even though the coach is present, to provide support for the coach. Most coaches need help with the application of the comfort techniques and may not remember them all. Coaches also get frightened at the intensity of labor and need to feel that the nurse is readily available to them. Sometimes a nurse hesitates to interrupt couples during labor if they seem to be doing well. Nevertheless, the nurse must check frequently on the couple in order to be there when needed.

Providing Information

Feeling powerless provokes anxiety. Understanding what is happening during labor seems to increase the woman's sense of control over the event. Knowledge can increase feelings of control and reduce anxiety, which in turn can motivate the woman to tolerate the pain.

Information about the progress of labor such as degree of cervical dilatation and descent of the fetus is important for the woman to know. It serves as a reminder that labor does end, and the end is getting closer. Especially toward the end of labor when discomfort increases, the knowledge that the ordeal is almost over enables the woman to tolerate pain that she would otherwise find unbearable.

Effective Use of Touch

Many of the physical care activities that nurses perform consist, in part at least, in "laying on of hands." Touch can be valuable in establishing and maintaining rapport and an effective relationship with both of the prospective parents. Even the intrusive procedures that are so often painful or distasteful, if done with gentleness and skill, show the client that her dignity and integrity are respected.

Psychosocial Support During Contractions

Particularly during the late active phase there is a need for human contact—someone to hold onto—during the severe contractions. The client responds less well to other physical contact such as stroking or sponging. She may even say, "Leave me alone," meaning "Don't disturb me" (see below). However, it may be helpful for her to have someone's hand to hold, and she should be allowed to do this if she indicates the need. During this time both she and the coach must constantly be reinforced with praise for using the techniques that enable her to cooperate with the natural forces of labor.

Pharmacologic Analgesia

The goal of using analgesics during labor is to provide maximum pain relief with minimum risk to the woman and fetus (Table 11-1). Analgesic agents include narcotics, sedatives, and tranquilizers.

Narcotics

Narcotics are the keystone of systemic pain relief medications. The major difference among the various narcotics is in the duration of their action. Knowledge of the duration of action facilitates rational selection of the appropriate narcotic. In general, all narcotics, when administered in analgesic doses, produce some degree of respiratory depression in both mother and newborn.

Ways of Responding to Pain

Moaning and groaning
Crying out
Becoming very "turned-in" and withdrawn
Displaying anger and hostility
Feeling a need to inflict pain on another

TABLE 11-1

Common Medications Used for Analgesia During Labor

Drug	Category	Dosage and Route	Actions	Comments
Meperidine hydrochloride (Demerol)	Narcotic: a nonopiate, addicting analgesic	IM: 50-100 mg, repeated 3-4 hr prn IV: 25 mg, repeated 1-2 hr prn	Peaks IM: Onset 10 min Peaks 60 min Duration 2-3 hr IV: Onset 5 min Duration 1-2 hr	Maternal effects: analgesia, sedation, nausea, vomiting Fetal effects: loss of variability of fetal heart tone; can cause respiratory depression at birth; can cause decreased muscle tone at birth
Butorphanol tartrate (Stadol)	Nonnarcotic analgesic	IM: 2 mg repeated 3-4 hr prn IV: 1 mg repeated 3-4 hr prn	Peaks IM: Onset 10 min Peaks 30-60 min Duration 1-4 hr IV: More rapid onset and peak Duration 3-4 hr	Maternal effects: sedation, vertigo, nausea, sweating, lethargy, headache, flushing Fetal effects: loss of variability of fetal heart rate; can cause respiratory depression at birth; can cause decreased muscle tone at birth
Hydroxyzine hydrochloride (Atarax, Vistaril)	Antianxiety agent (minor tranquilizer), antihistamine, antiemetic	IM: 25-50 mg, repeated 4-6 hr prn IM or IV injection	Sedative, antiemetic	Can reduce amount of narcotic needed Never given by SC, intraarterial
Promethazine hydrochloride (Phenergan)	Antihistaminic, antiemetic	Sedation early labor: 12.5-50 mg Sedation active labor: 25-50 mg with 25-75 mg of meperidine; may be repeated Nausea and vomiting: 12.5-25 mg, repeated 4-6 hr prn	Antihistaminic effects occur within 20 min after IM injection Duration of action 4-6 hr	

Narcotics such as meperidine administered in reasonable doses during labor have some mild neurobehavioral depressant effects on the newborn (see Drug Guide: Meperidine Hydrochloride). However, these effects are of short duration and usually dissipate by the second day of life. Both the analgesic and the depressant properties of all the narcotics can be rapidly antagonized in the mother and newborn by administering naloxone (Narcan), a specific narcotic antagonist (see Drug Guide: Naloxone Hydrochloride).

Butorphanol (Stadol) is a new synthetic agonist-antagonist narcotic analgesic drug that is used when no narcotic drug (morphine or meperidine) is present in the body (see Drug Guide: Butorphanol Tartrate on p. 248). It is given in doses of 1 or 2 mg intramuscularly or 1 mg IV every 3 to 4 hours during labor and is effective for pain relief and safe for the neonate. Butorphanol may not be used if a narcotic agent has already been administered because its antagonist effect reverses the analgesic effects.

⊖ DRUG
⊖ GUIDE

Meperidine hydrochloride (Demerol): A narcotic analgesic that interferes with pain impulses at the subcortical level of the brain; used during labor for analgesic effect.

Obstetric Action: Enhances analgesia by altering the physiologic response to pain; suppresses anxiety and apprehension of labor.

Labor and Delivery Administration: Average dose is 50-100 mg intramuscularly (IM) every 3-4 hr or 25-50 mg by slow intravenous (IV) push every 3-4 hr.

Maternal Contraindications: Hypersensitivity to meperidine, asthma, central nervous system or respiratory depression, nonreassuring fetal heart rate patterns.

Potential Side Effects and Complications: Respiratory depression, nausea and vomiting, dry mouth, drowsiness, dizziness, flushing, transient hypotension, bradycardia, palpitation.

Nursing Implications:
1. Assess client's history, initial data base for history of hypersensitivity.
2. If given IV, administer meperidine slowly just as contraction subsides to minimize effect of rapid absorption on fetus.
3. If given IM, administer deeply into muscle (given IM if there is no IV line).
4. Instruct client to remain in bed with bed rails up; have signal cord within her reach.
5. Observe client for maternal side effects such as dizziness or nausea.
6. Evaluate effectiveness of drug in relieving pain of labor.
7. Assess client's bladder for distention (at least every 2 hr) and encourage her to void.
8. Assess fetal monitor strip for reactivity and variability.
9. Assess newborn respiratory status and muscle tone at delivery.

⊖ DRUG
⊖ GUIDE

Naloxone hydrochloride (Narcan): A narcotic antagonist that reverses respiratory depression induced by a variety of narcotics.

Obstetric Action: Used in clients who have received epidural (intraspinal) morphine to decrease or relieve completely its side effects.

Postpartum (After Epidural Morphine) Administration: Average dose is 0.1-0.2 mg IV repeated as necessary if respiratory depression is noted.

Maternal Contraindications: Known client hypersensitivity to the drug; use cautiously if client is suspected of being physically dependent on opioids.

Potential Side Effects and Complications: Hypotension, hypertension, ventricular tachycardia, fibrillation, and pulmonary edema have been reported most often in clients with preexisting cardiovascular disorders or who have received other drugs that may have similar adverse cardiovascular effects. Abrupt reversal of narcotic depression may result in nausea, vomiting, sweating, tachycardia, increased blood pressure, and tremulousness. In postoperative clients, larger than usual doses of naloxone may result in significant reversal of analgesia and in excitement. Seizures have been reported infrequently.

Nursing Implications:
1. A vial of naloxone (1 ml, 0.4 mg) must be readily available at the nurse's station for immediate administration if respiratory depression occurs.
2. An airway, oxygen suction, and emergency life support drugs should be available.
3. Nurses caring for these clients should be currently certified in community cardiopulmonary resuscitation (CPR) or basic life support (BLS).
4. Since naloxone may be present in breast milk, the client should not breast-feed until the epidural analgesia has ended.
5. Naloxone should not be mixed with any other drug unless its effects on the chemical and physical stability of the solution have been established.

Sedatives (Hypnotics)

Sedative-hypnotic drugs are used for clients who need pharmacologic intervention to reduce anxiety and fear. These drugs produce drowsiness, tranquility, and a feeling of well-being. They should be used in conjunction with continuous supportive attendance. The drugs do not produce amnesia, nor do they raise the pain threshold; thus they are poor

⊖ DRUG
⊖ GUIDE

Butorphanol tartrate (Stadol): A synthetic nonnarcotic analgesic for relief of moderate to severe pain.

Obstetric Action: Effective for pain relief in labor, although the exact mechanism of the drug is unknown. It is thought to act on the subcortical portion of the central nervous system.

Labor and Delivery Administration: Average dose is 2 mg IM every 3-4 hr or 1 mg IV every 3-4 hr.

Maternal Contraindications: History of hypersensitivity; should be used with caution in woman delivering a premature baby.

Potential Side Effects and Complications: The most frequent reactions are nausea, clamminess, and sweating. Less frequent reactions are headaches, vertigo, a floating feeling, dizziness, lethargy, confusion, and light-headedness.

Nursing Implications:
1. Assess client's history and initial data base for hypersensitivity to butorphanol.
2. If analgesic is given IV, administer it slowly just as a contraction is subsiding to minimize effect of rapid absorption on fetus.
3. If giving intramuscularly, administer deeply into muscle (given IM if there is no IV line).
4. Instruct client to remain in bed with side rails up; have signal cord within reach.
5. Observe for maternal side effects (decreased respirations, increased blood pressure, nausea, increased perspiration).
6. Evaluate effectiveness of pain relief.
7. Assess client's bladder at least every 2 hr for distention and encourage her to void.
8. Assess fetal monitor strip for reactivity and variability.
9. Assess newborn respiratory status and muscle tone at delivery.

analgesics. If used during the latent phase of the first stage, labor may be slowed. Barbiturates produce no analgesia and may even cause excitement and disorientation if given for severe pain. Barbiturates rapidly cross the placenta and can cause depressing effects on the fetus. Barbiturates may be used in very early labor when delivery is not anticipated for 12 to 24 hours.

Tranquilizers

Tranquilizers are used to relieve anxiety, reduce narcotic requirements, and control emesis. These drugs also cross the placenta rapidly but do not cause neonatal depression when given in recommended doses. They do cause a decrease in beat-to-beat variability of the FHR.

Psychologic Benefits of Pain Relief

The adequate relief of pain also results in psychologic benefits (Table 11-2). The client who experiences tolerable discomforts during labor is able to cooperate with examinations and work with her contractions. Consequently, she facilitates efforts by the health team members to obtain information, and she avoids prolongation of labor. After childbirth she is less fatigued.

Assessment

One of the most important responsibilities of the nurse in labor and delivery is the careful observation and monitoring of maternal

TABLE 11-2

Benefits of Pain Control in Labor and Delivery

Emotional Advantages	Physiologic Advantages
Positive experience with a significant step toward parenthood	Woman can cooperate with examinations
Feeling of actual participation in birth of own child	Woman can work with contractions
Fostering growth of relationship between parent and child	Woman is less fatigued after labor and delivery
Fostering growth of relationship between parents	Successful use of nonpharmacologic pain relief reduces risk to infant
	Complications such as pain-related decrease in oxygen can be avoided in the fetus already at risk

Adapted from Northrup C, Kelly M: Legal Issues in Nursing. St. Louis, CV Mosby, 1987; and The Organization of Obstetric, Gynecologic and Neonatal Nurses: Nursing Responsibilities in Implementing Intrapartum Fetal Heart Rate Monitoring. NAACOG, 1988.

≡ LEGAL AND ETHICAL
≡ CONSIDERATIONS

Liability for negligence in the labor and delivery period generally centers around the failure to attend to the client or to monitor the progress of the fetus during labor. The American College of Obstetricians/Gynecologists (ACOG) recommends that auscultation of the fetal heart be done at 15 to 30 minute intervals during the active phase of first stage of labor and at 5 to 15 minute intervals during second stage of labor for high-risk and low-risk clients respectively.

Evaluation of the FHR information when continous electronic monitoring is done may take place at the intervals suggested for auscultation or more frequently depending on the individual client-care situation. Written documentation is also in accordance with institutional policy and procedure. The length, duration, and intensity of uterine contractions should be palpated or monitored. These periodic monitorings must be recorded. The court views an item that was not documented as one that was not done.

and fetal status (see Legal and Ethical Considerations). This is true also when analgesic medications are being used or there is a potential for their use.

A rule of thumb for determining a client's need for analgesia is her inability to relax between contractions. When the client requests medication for pain, the nurse assesses her progress in labor and the contraction pattern (frequency, duration, intensity, and regularity of contractions), as well as the resting tone of the uterus and her vital signs. The FHR is assessed to determine fetal well-being. This information is charted. If the physician has not previously written an order for pain medication, the nurse reports the assessment findings to him or her so that an order for analgesia can be obtained (see display on p. 250).

Nursing Diagnosis

Nursing diagnoses concerned with coping and comfort may be relevant to most clients at some point during labor (see Potential Nursing Diagnoses: Analgesia and Anesthesia on p. 250).

Focus Assessment

Determine client's current level of knowledge about the use of analgesia and anesthesia during labor and delivery.

Identify individual client's nonverbal indicators of pain.

Monitor client's behavioral response to uterine contractions.

Determine client's need or desire for analgesia.

Monitor client's physiologic and psychologic response to analgesia, e.g., vital signs, nonverbal indicators of pain, level of consciousness.

Monitor fetal response to analgesia, i.e., heart rate.

Monitor time elapsed between administration of analgesia and signs of impending delivery.

POTENTIAL NURSING DIAGNOSES

Analgesia and Anesthesia

Potential for Injury (Fetal)—related to intrauterine stress secondary to effects of analgesic and decreased plantental perfusion

Pain—related to uterine contractions during labor and delivery and to inadequate analgesia

Ineffective Individual Coping—related to lack of knowledge about the process of labor and delivery, anxiety, fear, inability to control own response to painful stimuli, or fear of losing control

Fatigue—related to high energy expenditure required during labor

Knowledge Deficit—regarding use of analgesia and anesthesia during labor and delivery

Impaired Gas Exchange—related to effects of anesthesia

Potential for Injury (Maternal)—related to postural hypotension

Sensory Alteration—related to cutaneous hyperesthesia (pruritus) secondary to side effect of epidural anesthesia

Urinary Retention—related to inability to perceive bladder distention secondary to epidural anesthesia

---

Planning and Intervention

The woman and her coach need frequent reports of how the labor is progressing and the steps being taken by health care personnel to assist during the labor and to alleviate pain. Before administering the medication prescribed to promote analgesia, the nurse informs the client that the medication will make her more comfortable and help her with the labor. This information can potentiate the effectiveness of the drug.

Before the medication is given, the client should empty her bladder. Also, fetal heart tones (FHTs), contraction pattern, and the woman's vital signs are taken and recorded before medication administration. Once analgesic therapy has been instituted, the client is instructed to remain in bed and use the call lights when she needs assistance.

The environment must be conducive to rest. Most institutions require side rails be up when the client is medicated, even when someone is in attendance. The necessity for use of side rails is explained to both the client and her partner to avoid undue fears or misinterpretations. The support person in particular should understand the importance of keeping the rails up after attending to the woman's needs.

Comfort measures (see p. 251 and Fig. 11-7) lessen the client's anxiety, fear, and tension. The prepared client can be supported also by the nurse or coach who "talks her through" the contraction. Often this technique decreases or eliminates the need for medication. If an analgesic is administered, this action should be recorded on the fetal monitor strip, in the nurses notes, or on the delivery record.

Nursing Support and Comfort Measures

Position client with pillows and blankets behind her back and between and under her legs to promote relaxation, reduce tension, and eliminate pressure points.

Encourage use of relaxation techniques.

Encourage use of breathing techniques.

Encourage use of effleurage (Fig. 11-7).

Organize procedures to provide for rest.

Control who is present during labor and delivery.

Assure privacy and prevent exposure.

Explain the process and progress of labor.

Keep client clean and dry.

Provide mouth care.

Offer washcloth for wiping face.

Give back rub.

Apply heat or cold to client's lower back.

Suggest client empty her bladder.

Give medication for pain or anxiety.

Provide support during vaginal examinations.

Use physical touch.

Apply heat to lower abdomen.

Control environment to decrease noise.

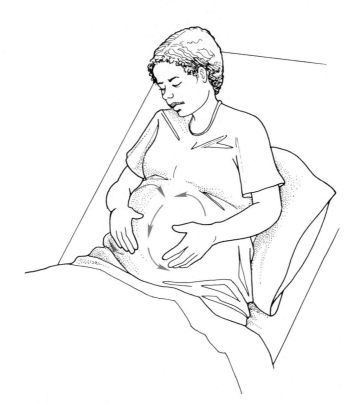

FIGURE 11-7

Effleurage Pattern. Effleurage is another childbirth education (Lamaze and other psychoprophylactic methods of childbearing) tool that may provide psychologic and physiologic relief of pain—psychologic because it involves concentration and physiologic because it increases circulation to the lower abdomen, which aids in decreasing pain.

Evaluation and Reassessment

The nurse assesses the client 20 to 30 minutes after medication administration to determine its efficacy. The findings are documented.

The contraction pattern is assessed for any change in it, and the FHR is assessed to determine well-being of the fetus. All drugs have some effect on the fetal heart, particularly on variability, so the effect on variability should be noted on the chart. Documentation is required after each evaluation and reassessment. *Text continued on page 255.*

NURSING
CARE
PLAN

Pain Management During Labor

Goals (Expected Outcomes)	Interventions	Rationale	Evaluation
Potential for Injury (Fetal)—Related to Decreased Placental Perfusion Secondary to Effects of Analgesia or Anesthesia			
Client will maintain adequate placental perfusion as evidenced by the continued absence of signs of fetal distress. Fetal status is unaffected by analgesia.	Encourage maternal use of upright or left or right lateral position during labor.	Enhances placental perfusion; minimizes potential for supine hypotensive syndrome.	Maternal blood pressure remains within normal limits.
	Support effective self-management of labor pain, e.g., effective breathing patterns.	Reduces potential need for analgesia.	FHR consistently remains at 120 to 160.
	Institute immediate actions to counteract effects of maternal hypotension.	Minimizes interruption of blood flow to placenta and fetus.	FHR has absence of late decelerations.
	Turn client on left side or manually displace or support fetus to the maternal left.	Increases placental perfusion.	Compromised fetus responds promptly to interventions; FHR returns to normal range.
	Administer oxygen by face mask at 6 to 8 L/min.	Increases level of oxygen in circulating blood available for maternal and fetal use.	Amniotic fluid is clear with no evidence of meconium caused by hypoxia.
	Notify primary health care provider immediately if actions are unsuccessful.	Enables diagnosis and effective treatment.	At birth infant's Apgar score is 8 to 10 at 1 and 5 min.
Pain—Related to Uterine Contractions and the Process of Labor			
Client will experience effective management of her labor discomfort or pain.	Work through support person.	Reinforces couple's pre-established working relationship.	Couple works effectively together.
	Assist with frequent change of position.	Maintaining one position increases tension and discomfort. Moving allows client a sense of control over some aspect of the experience; promotes comfort; provides distraction.	Client verbalizes that position changes and comfort measures reduce tension and increase comfort.
	Encourage use of upright and left-lateral positions.	Supine position may result in compression of inferior vena cava, causing supine hypotensive syndrome. Left-lateral position enhances placental perfusion.	
	Encourage use of breathing techniques practiced in childbirth education classes. If coach is absent or ineffective, assist with breathing pattern as necessary.	Reinforces previous learning; facilitates and supports application of coping patterns. Assists woman in maintaining control of her behavioral response to pain; enhances and supports coping.	Client verbalizes relief of pain or uses breathing patterns correctly. Client is visibly relaxed throughout and after contractions. Client is coping effectively with labor. FHR indicates good placental perfusion.

NURSING
CARE
PLAN

Pain Management During Labor—continued

Goals (Expected Outcomes)	Interventions	Rationale	Evaluation
Pain—Related to Uterine Contractions and the Process of Labor—continued			
	Alert client that contraction is beginning.	Warning signal allows woman to begin use of appropriate breathing/relaxation techniques.	
	Let client know the progress of the contraction, i.e., identify the increment, acme, decrement.	Facilitates short-term coping (one contraction at a time).	
	Provide positive reinforcement by complimenting her contraction management.	Supports continuing positive self-image; motivates efforts to maintain control over pain responses.	
	Provide comfort measures; dry bed, back rubs; perineal care; ice chips, mouth care with lemon and glycerine swabs, wiping face with cool washcloth.	Minimizes annoyance of additional discomforts; allows woman to focus on coping with contractions.	
	Keep client or couple informed of labor's progress.	Provides psychologic boost, i.e., enhances belief that labor will soon end.	
	Encourage and assist with relaxation with and between contractions.	Relaxation maximizes uteroplacental perfusion, conserves woman's energy, increases coping abilities, and enhances her comfort.	
	Provide client teaching: For clients who have had no previous preparation for childbirth, discuss and demonstrate abdominal and chest breathing; institute other above-described interventions.	Encourages client to focus on breathing rather than on pain. Assists in coping with contraction discomfort or pain; allows woman to control her response to pain.	Client begins using abdominal or chest breathing effectively. Client is visibly more relaxed during contractions. Client relaxes after contraction ends. Client verbalizes increased comfort.
	If woman does not relax between contractions, offer analgesic for pain; answer questions; let client or couple know the decision is theirs. Inform primary health care provider of woman's need or request for aid in coping with her contractions and regaining control over her response to pain.	Anxiety and tension increase discomfort and lessen coping ability; lack of relaxation can impede labor progress.	

Continued

NURSING
CARE
PLAN

Pain Management During Labor—*continued*

Goals (Expected Outcomes)	Interventions	Rationale	Evaluation
Pain—Related to Uterine Contractions and the Process of Labor—*continued*			
	Note and record maternal pulse, respirations, and blood pressure and FHR before administering medication. Administer analgesic as ordered. Note and record maternal and fetal response to analgesic.	Identifies present status and provides baseline for future comparisons.	Client verbalizes relief of discomfort; visibly regains control over response to labor pain. Maternal vital signs and FHR remain within normal limits.
	Ensure immediate availability of narcotic-antagonist medications and resuscitative equipment.	Enables prompt treatment of potential complications caused by narcosis.	
Ineffective Individual Coping—Related to Lack of Knowledge About Process of Labor, Anxiety, Fear, Fatigue, Inability to Control Own Response to Painful Stimuli, Fear of Losing Control			
Client exhibits successful self-management of the psychologic stress of labor. Client fulfills her expectations for a safe and satisfying childbearing experience.	Encourage client to deal with contractions one at a time and relax as they end.	Anticipating the next contraction causes tension and discomfort during the rest period; anxiety and tension reduce tolerance to pain.	Client is coping effectively with labor.
	Explain sensations that can be expected with progressing labor and procedures.	Reduces anxiety and fear of the unknown.	
	Assist with relaxation and distraction.	Supports coping abilities; relaxation enhances uteroplacental blood flow.	Client is visibly relaxed throughout and after contractions. Client is coping effectively with labor.
	Encourage active participation of support person.	Reduces distress and increases cooperation and comfort; supports established relationship.	The couple works effectively together.
	Reinforce effective use of breathing techniques. Provide encouragement and praise.	Supports coping abilities and positive self-image. Communicates understanding of couple's stress and needs and the desire to help.	Client uses breathing patterns correctly. Client or couple actively participates in second stage of labor.
	Maintain therapeutic use of self, e.g., tone of voice, touch, nearness.	Maintains rapport and facilitates effective nursing support of the client or couple.	
	Institute other measures as described under Pain as needed.	Facilitates effective pain management; assists successful coping and satisfactory outcome.	Client expresses satisfaction with labor and delivery management.

Pain Management During Labor—continued

Goals (Expected Outcomes)	Interventions	Rationale	Evaluation
Fatigue—Related to Energy Expenditure Required During Labor, Loss of Sleep, Lack of Food			
Client will experience minimum fatigue during labor.	Provide a quiet, restful environment; minimize noise and light as possible.	Encourages relaxation.	Client is using breathing techniques effectively.
	Encourage active participation of support person.	Enhances client's sense of security; supports effective collaboration and coping.	Client is responsive to nursing measures, client verbalizes increased comfort and ability to relax.
	Reinforce effective breathing techniques.	Assists in coping with contractions.	Client dozes between contractions.
	Encourage relaxation with and after contractions.	Conserves energy.	
	Provide comfort measures (e.g., dry bed, back rub, ice chips).	Encourages relaxation.	
	Offer analgesic if client unable to relax and losing control (see Pain).	Reduces perception of pain, assists relaxation, enables return of control.	
Knowledge Deficit—Regarding Use of Analgesia for Labor and Delivery			
Client will make an informed decision about use of analgesia during her labor.	Explain the actions and anticipated effects of the drug(s).	Identifies the advantages and disadvantages of the specific drug(s).	Client verbalizes understanding of anticipated effects of specific drug on labor and the maternal and fetal status.
	Encourage client or couple to ask questions.	Allows verbalization and exploration of concerns.	
	Explain that the effects will be monitored closely.	Provides reassurance of prompt management of untoward effects.	Client expresses satisfaction with management of pain, labor, and delivery.
	Support (and implement) their decision.	Assures their control over pain management during labor and delivery.	Client or couple self-determines acceptance or refusal of analgesia.

Obstetric Anesthesia

In the past 3 decades there have been great improvements in obstetric anesthesia. The client today has several choices for pain relief. Many clients wish to be alert and to participate actively in the labor and delivery process (see displays on p. 256). Thus client choice is a factor in choosing a method of anesthetic pain management; clients want to choose what they believe best suits their health care needs.

Regional Anesthesia for Labor and Delivery

Regional anesthesia administered during labor and vaginal and cesarean delivery is widely used. It is effective and, when properly administered,

Selection of Anesthetic or Analgesic

The ideal analgesic or anesthetic for labor and delivery would satisfy the following conditions:

It provides satisfactory alleviation of pain for the individual parturient.

It does not interfere significantly with the normal mechanics or progress of labor and delivery.

It is not associated with undue risk to the client.

It is associated with minimum fetal and newborn depression.

It provides safe and satisfactory conditions for the delivery.

It allows early interaction between the mother and her newborn, preferably in the delivery room.

However, no single technique of pain relief fulfills all of the above objectives for every woman.

Pregnancy's Physiologic Implications for Anesthetic Techniques

Pregnancy is associated with an increased sensitivity to most anesthetics, analgesics, and tranquilizers, which makes overdose more likely.

Upper airway edema, normally present in late pregnancy, increases the possibility for airway obstruction.

Changes in pulmonary function and an increased oxygen requirement predispose the parturient to the rapid development of hypoxia, particularly in the second stage of labor or during induction of anesthesia. A 40% increase in pulmonary minute ventilation at term, which may increase further to 300% in the second stage of labor, makes induction of anesthesia with inhalation drugs rapid.

Gastrointestinal tract changes brought about by pregnancy and labor affect many drugs used in labor. Increased nausea and vomiting, prolonged gastric emptying time, and the fact that the maternity client may have recently eaten subject her to an increased risk of pulmonary aspiration of gastric contents with its devastating morbidity and mortality.

Changes in the cardiovascular system, particularly those associated with aortic and vena caval compression by the gravid uterus, predispose the obstetric client to sudden hypotension and cardiovascular collapse and her fetus to hypoxia and acidosis at the time of general or major conduction anesthesia.

Forms of Regional Anesthesia

Subarachnoid block
  Spinal
  Saddle
Peridural (epidural) block
  Lumbar epidural
  Caudal epidural
Paracervical block
Pudendal block
Local infiltration

safe (Table 11-3). Regional anesthesia allows the client to be awake and to participate actively in the birth of her infant. It also decreases the potential for drug-induced systems depression in the fetus and aspiration pneumonia in the client (because she is awake). There are several forms of regional anesthesia (see above). Figure 11-8 illustrates the pain pathways that are active during labor and delivery.

TABLE 11-3

Effects of Selected Regional Analgesic or Anesthetic Methods and Agents

Types of Regional Analgesia/Anesthesia	Therapeutic Effect	Maternal Side Effects	Fetal or Newborn Side Effects	Miscellaneous Information
Subarachnoid block: spinal and saddle	High degree of pain relief for delivery	Maternal hypotension Occasional postspinal headache Urinary retention post partum	None unless maternal hypotension occurs	No pain relief during first stage of labor Excellent pain relief for delivery
Peridural (epidural) block: lumbar and caudal	High degree of pain relief for first and second stage labor and delivery	Frequent mild hypotension; loss of bearing-down reflex in second stage	None unless severe sustained maternal hypotension occurs	May slow labor Epidural blocks pain at each stage of labor Incorrect placement of caudal needle could result in puncture of maternal rectum or fetal head

Paracervical block	Temporary block of pain during labor	Transient depression of contractions
		Rare maternal side effects
			Fairly high incidence of bradycardia of 25%–85%
			Contraindications:
			  Premature fetus
			  Fetal compromise
			  Placental insufficiency
			  Vaginal infection
				Provides analgesia during labor but no perineal anesthesia; does not interfere with pushing

Pudendal block	Nerve block for second stage of labor	Loss of bearing-down reflex	Rarely any	Does not relieve contraction pain; anesthetizes perineum

Subarachnoid Block

Spinal Block Anesthesia

Spinal block anesthesia is technically easy to administer (Fig. 11-9). It is one of the most useful blocks for obstetrics because the amount of anesthetic agent is less than that required for any other obstetric block (approximately one-fifth less anesthetic agent than if using the epidural route). Because of this low dose, maternal and fetal anesthetic toxicity is not a problem. Essentially every obstetric procedure not requiring depression of uterine activity can be done using spinal block anesthesia.

As a prerequisite for spinal anesthesia, the woman is well hydrated with intravenous fluids as a precaution to minimize the degree of hypotension if it does occur. Hypotension is a potential side effect that can result from vasodilation caused by blocking of sympathetic nervous system (Table 11-4 on p. 260).

Spinal block anesthesia is administered just before delivery. The woman is positioned on her side or in a sitting position and is assisted in flexing her back (curling forward around her fetus). The needle-insertion area is prepared and draped, and a spinal needle is inserted into the subarachnoid space. The anesthetic is injected through the needle immediately after a contraction. If the drug were administered before or during a contraction, the contraction could force the anesthetic agent higher in the subarachnoid

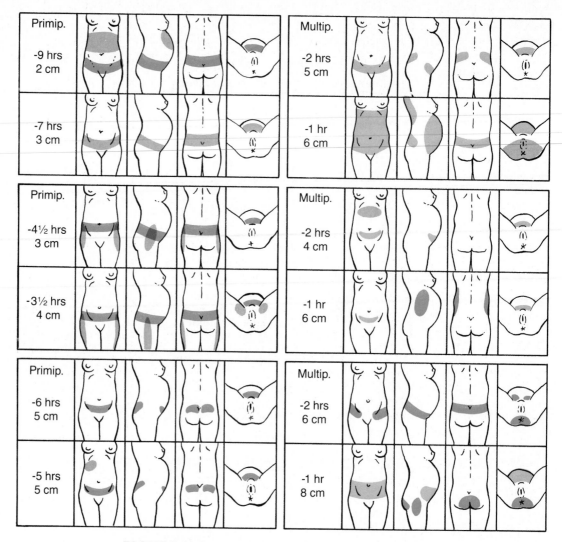

FIGURE 11-8

Distribution and Intensity of Pain During Labor. Shaded areas show the distribution of pain in six women at various points during labor before delivery. *Stipple* = mild pain; *crosshatch* = moderate pain; *black* = severe pain.

Adapted from Melzack R et al: Severity of labour pain: Influence of physical as well as psychological variables. Can Med Assoc J 130:579-584, 1984.

space, possibly resulting in a higher anesthetic level, which could be dangerous.

Onset of spinal anesthesia is very rapid, usually complete within 5 minutes. After anesthesia administration the woman's blood pressure is monitored every 1 to 2 minutes for the first 10 minutes and then every 5 to 10 minutes for the next hour to ensure hypotension is not occurring.

Saddle Block Anesthesia

Late in labor a subarachnoid block injected at the S1 to S5 level provides perineal anesthesia and allows forceps delivery and repair of episiotomy. This is called a true saddle block. A modified saddle block (anesthesia affecting T10 to S5) completely eliminates both uterine and perineal pain. Saddle block anesthesia can also be used during cesarean section when increased to the level of T4.

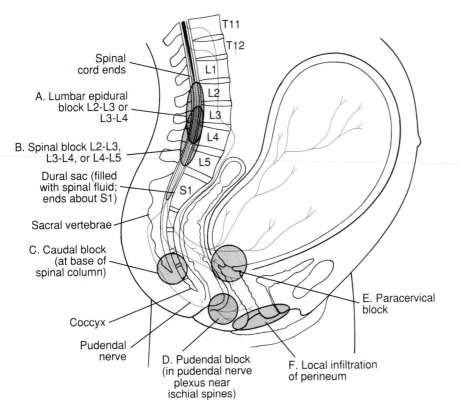

FIGURE 11-9

Sites for Anesthetic Administration During Labor and Delivery. *A*, Site for lumbar epidural block. Lumbar epidural block is usually continuous and provides analgesia and anesthesia from active labor through delivery. Client may be sitting or in a lateral position for insertion. The catheter remains in place so additional doses of medication can be administered. *B*, Site for spinal block, often called a saddle block. This block is administered just before delivery. A local anesthetic drug is injected directly into the spinal fluid in the spinal canal (subarachnoid space) with client in a sitting or lateral-recumbent position. *C*, Site for caudal block. Local anesthetic is injected into the caudal canal. A catheter may be inserted to give additional doses of the anesthetic. This block is given when active labor is established and results in loss of sensation to the cervix, lower vagina, and perineum. *D*, Site for pudendal block. This block is administered vaginally by the obstetrician. Anesthetic is given transvaginally and bilaterally into the pudendal nerve to provide anesthesia for episiotomy, delivery, and episiotomy repair. *E*, Site of paracervical block. To insert the spinal needle for this block, the client is placed in the lithotomy position. The needle with the guide is inserted into the lateral fornix of the vagina and then 3 to 4 mm further into the vaginal wall. Anesthetic is injected at 4 o'clock and 8 o'clock. This block provides brief pain relief but provides no perineal or vaginal anesthesia. Therefore some additional anesthesia is required for delivery. *F*, Local infiltration site. The client is placed in a lithotomy position just before delivery, and anesthetic is injected into the site of the anticipated episiotomy.

Peridural (Epidural) Block

Lumbar Epidural Anesthesia (Analgesic)

Lumbar epidural block can provide adequate analgesia for all obstetric procedures not requiring depression of uterine activity. Its use provides a pain-free labor in an alert and cooperative woman who requires no additional medications for pain. However, this anesthesia route requires a larger dose of anesthetic agents than does the spinal block route. Also, an epidural block does not require the woman to remain in a flat position after delivery as is required with a saddle block. Lumbar epidural anesthesia has largely replaced caudal epidural anesthesia.

TABLE 11-4

Deviations from Expected Patterns During Spinal Block Anesthesia

Deviation	Causes	Intervention
Total subarachnoid block	Injection of anesthetic into subarachnoid space before or during a contraction	Correct hypotension with intravenous (IV) fluids, and displace uterus from inferior vena cava and aorta (place wedge under client's right hip). Support oxygenation with bag and mask ventilation using oxygen under positive pressure. Intubate with a cuffed endotracheal tube.
Maternal hypotension	Vasodilation secondary to sympathetic block	Hydrate with 1 L of isotonic IV fluids to increase circulatory volume to decrease incidence of hypotension. Place wedge under client's right hip to displace uterus.
Loss of urge to push and increased incidence of persistent occiput-posterior position	Complete perineal analgesia; muscle tone required for occiput to rotate to anterior position is not available	Decrease concentration of anesthetic agent to produce sensory but not motor block.
Postspinal headache	Leakage of cerebrospinal fluid through spinal needle insertion hole	Use small-gauge needles (25 gauge or less) for administration of spinal anesthetic. Provide adequate hydration with IV fluid before and after spinal anesthetic. Apply tight abdominal binder when client in upright position after delivery. Administer analgesics. Ensure bed rest in prone, flat position after delivery for prescribed number of hours. Apply epidural blood patches to seal hole in dura. Inject client's own noncoagulated blood into epidural space to create a seal for dura hole (the seal stops the leak within a few minutes approximately 90% of the time).

Before a lumbar epidural block can be administered, labor must be well established and must have progressed to the active phase. This means that contractions must be regular (approximately 3 to 3½ minutes apart, lasting 60 to 75 seconds), the fundus firm (50 to 60 mm Hg), and cervical dilatation 5 to 6 cm in most clients.

Other prerequisites for epidural anesthesia are an intravenous line in place and prehydration of the woman as ordered usually with 500 to 1000 ml of an isotonic solution). Hydration increases circulating volume and minimizes the potential for hypotension in the woman and hypoxia in the fetus.

For catheter insertion the client lies on her side and curls forward around her fetus or is in a sitting position. A needle is inserted through one of the intervertebral spaces in the lumbar region (L2-3, L3-4, or L4-5) into the epidural space (Fig. 11-10). With the needle's lumen as the guide, a small polyethylene catheter is threaded through and beyond the needle tip. The needle is then withdrawn, leaving the catheter in place. The catheter is taped to the woman's back with the distal end pinned to her gown so it is accessible for subsequent injections of the anesthetic agent(s).

After the catheter is in place, a test dose of anesthetic is given to rule out accidental subarachnoid or intravenous placement. Once placement is confirmed, 4 to 10 ml of local anesthetic is administered. As nerve roots leave the spinal cord, they pass through the epidural space and are bathed in the local anesthetic agent that has been injected into the epidural space, creating anesthesia.

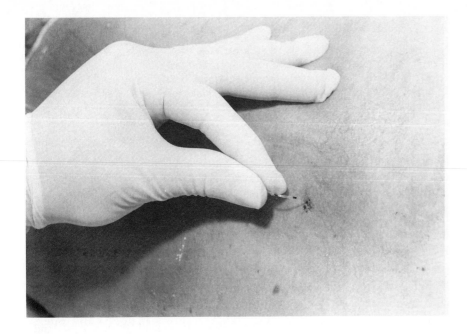

FIGURE 11-10

Lumbar Epidural Catheter Placement. After needle is placed into the epidural space, the plunger of the syringe is aspirated to ensure proper placement (if blood or spinal fluid are aspirated, epidural placement cannot be confirmed). An epidural catheter is then inserted, and a test dose of anesthetic agent is administered to rule out subarachnoid placement or intravenous placement. Analgesia is then established by injecting 4 to 10 ml of local anesthetic.

After the epidural catheter is in place, the client is positioned to avoid uterine compression of the aorta and vena cava. Placing a wedge under the client's right hip minimizes this complication. Sometimes she is placed on one side for epidural catheter insertion and anesthetic administration and then is turned to the opposite side. Table 11-5 outlines deviations from the expected patterns during epidural anesthesia.

A technique being used with greater frequency is a continuous infusion of a dilute local anesthetic, e.g., infusing 10 to 12 ml/hr of 0.25% to 0.5% bupivacaine. This low-dose anesthetic administration technique maintains a continuous sensory block with a minimum motor block.

TABLE 11-5

Deviations From Expected Patterns During Epidural Anesthesia

Deviation	Cause	Interventions
Greater amount of drug required for epidural route	Large area into which drug is administered	Use drugs that metabolize more quickly (procaine and chloroprocaine).
Maternal hypotension	Vasodilation	Eliminate uterine compression of aorta and vena cava (place wedge under client's right hip); prehydrate (blood volume expansion) with isotonic intravenous fluids; administer oxygen; position client as needed.
Loss of urge to push	Complete perineal anesthesia eliminates urge to push	Use low concentration of drug (i.e., 0.25% bupivacaine or 1% lidocaine); decrease rate of continuous epidural infusion; wait until urge returns.
Permanent neurologic damage	Needle's slipping into subarachnoid space	Monitor carefully to confirm medication is administered in epidural space.

Focus Assessment

Closely monitor vital signs and fetal heart rate.

Identify client's response to contractions (diminished pain, mobility).

Examine epidural catheter for placement, kinks, breaks, evidence of leakage.

Observe for signs of side effects of epidural anesthesia (e.g., respiratory embarrassment, hypotension, allergic reactions, nausea, loss of urge to bear down during second stage).

Monitor bladder status.

It is important that the anesthetic dose is adequate to relieve pain when the fetus begins its descent (usually late in the first stage of labor during transition). However, too much anesthetic can retard fetal descent. Progress of labor and the anesthetic dose must be assessed and managed carefully (see above).

When delivery is imminent, the client is assisted to a sitting position, and 10 to 20 ml of lidocaine (or chloroprocaine) are injected into the lumbar epidural space to produce rapid onset of analgesia and muscle relaxation. Table 11-6 describes characteristics of local anesthetics commonly used in obstetrics.

TABLE 11-6

Regional Analgesic and Anesthetic Agents

Local Anesthesic and Trade Name	Characteristics	Route	Comments
Chloroprocaine (Nesacaine)	Very low toxicity, most rapidly metabolized anesthetic, with little accumulation and rapid onset but poor spread; short duration of action	Caudal, epidural, spinal, pudendal	Ideal drug for epidural; rapid onset, rapid rate of hydrolysis; low fetal or maternal toxicity
Tetracaine (Pontocaine)	Poor spread, very slow onset	Spinal (subarachnoid block)	Only made for spinal block (too toxic for epidural or caudal)
Lidocaine (Xylocaine)	Most versatile local anesthetic, moderate toxicity, rapid onset, moderate duration, excellent spread	Caudal, epidural, spinal, pudendal, and paracervical block	With epidural use, possible suppression of some reflexes in newborn; recent studies question this conclusion
Mepivacaine (Carbocaine)	Rapid onset, moderate duration, moderate toxicity but very slow metabolism, marked accumulation with repeated dosage	Caudal, epidural, spinal, paracervical block, pudendal	Epidural use associated with minimum decrease in temporary neonatal muscle tone
Bupivacaine (Marcaine, Sensorcaine)	Slow onset, long duration, marked cardiac toxicity; low concentrations give excellent sensory and little motor block, ideal for obstetrics	Caudal, epidural, paracervical block, pudendal	Inadvertent intravascular injection associated with cardiovascular collapse
Etidocaine (Duranest)	Rapid onset, long duration, marked cardiac toxicity; produces profound motor block and often poor sensory block, making it a poor drug for obstetrics	Caudal, epidural, paracervical block, pudendal	Inadvertent intravascular injection associated with cardiovascular collapse

Caudal Epidural Anesthesia

A caudal block may also be administered after labor is well established and in the active phase. The woman is positioned on her side or prone with wedges under her thighs. The sacrum is prepared and draped, and a needle inserted in the caudal canal (Fig. 11-11). A catheter is threaded through the needle and a test dose of anesthetic given to ensure the dura has not been punctured. The catheter is taped securely in place. Fifteen to 20 ml of anesthetic agent are given initially, and additional doses of approximately 15 ml are given as needed thereafter to maintain analgesia during labor and for delivery.

The catheter is removed during the first 1 to 2 hours after delivery. Caudal anesthesia is used less often than epidural block because it is more difficult to administer and is more painful to the client during needle placement. Caudal anesthesia does have one advantage over epidural block in that when given just before delivery, its onset of perineal anesthesia and muscle relaxation is more rapid.

FIGURE 11-11

Caudal Anesthesia. Woman assumes modified knee-chest or lateral Sims' position to permit access to sacral hiatus. Once needle and catheter are in place, she may assume any position in bed.

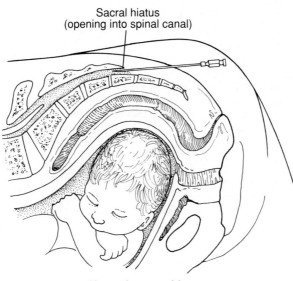

Sacral hiatus
(opening into spinal canal)

Knee-chest position

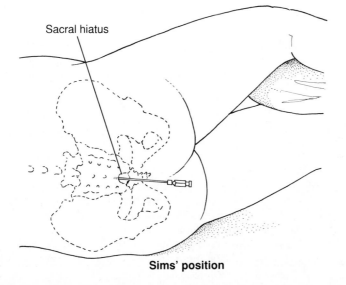

Sacral hiatus

Sims' position

Epidural Anesthesia

Goals (Expected Outcomes)	Interventions	Rationale	Evaluation
Impaired Gas Exchange—Related to Effects of Anesthesia			
Client will exhibit normal respiratory function.	If respiratory depression occurs, notify anesthesiologist immediately.	Enables expert management of client status.	Client's vital signs are stable (respirations >10 per min; systolic blood pressure [BP] >100 mm Hg).
	Institute actions to support respiration. Establish an airway to ventilate (bag and mask) with O_2 until endotracheal intubation is accomplished to ventilate and prevent aspiration.	Establishes airway and maintains respiration status with positive pressure ventilation.	Gas exchange is maintained.
	Increase IV fluids.	Increases venous return to heart.	Client exhibits no signs of respiratory depression.
	Place in Trendelenberg position to displace uterus to the left.	Maintains uteroplacental perfusion.	Fetal heart rate baseline maintained at 120 to 160. Fetus is reactive. No deceleration present.
Potential for Injury (Maternal)—Related to Postural Hypotension			
Client will experience no fall in blood pressure with position change.	Assist client with position changes.	Reduces risk of postural hypotension; protects client from falling.	Client's BP remains stable; she has no complaint of dizziness or light-headedness. Client changes positions without incident.
Potential for Injury (Fetal)—Related to Maternal Hypotension			
Client will exhibit normal fetal heart rate (FHR) on monitor tracing.	Turn client on left side and administer oxygen, at 6-10 L/min.	Increases placental perfusion; raises blood oxygen level.	Fetus exhibits no late decelerations on monitor. FHR remains stable at 120-140 bpm.
Pain—Related to Uterine Contractions and Ineffective Anesthesia			
Client will verbalize her freedom from pain.	Notify anesthesiologist if pain relief is inadequate.	Enables expert evaluation; ensures effective anesthesia.	Client states she is comfortable and free of pain.
Urinary Retention—Related to Inability to Perceive Need or Urge to Void			
Client will experience no bladder distention.	Encourage voiding as need is indicated by palpating bladder.	Client is unaware of bladder distention. A full bladder can impede the oncoming fetal head.	Client voids spontaneously on request and empties bladder. Client voids spontaneously and empties bladder within 8 hours of removal of epidural catheter.
Knowledge Deficit—Regarding Effects of Epidural Anesthesia			
Client will verbalize understanding of anticipated effects.	Reinforce explanation of anesthesiologist.	Allays concern about the procedure or the ability to maximize comfort during labor. Ensures reporting of signs and symptoms.	Client cooperates during placement of epidural catheter. Client reports her state of comfort and any adverse reactions.

Paracervical Block Anesthesia

Paracervical block is another method of providing anesthesia during labor. Local anesthetic is injected submucosally into the fornix of the vagina lateral to the cervix (Fig. 11-12). Paracervical block affects sensory nerve fibers in the uterus, cervix, and vagina and provides adequate analgesia for the first stage of labor. This technique does not anesthetize the perineal sensory nerve fibers, so it is not effective for episiotomy or delivery.

One disadvantage of paracervical block is the increased potential for fetal bradycardia after the block. Bradycardia can be caused by (1) fetal absorption of some of the anesthetic, which slows the FHR; (2) vasoconstriction of the uterine vessels by the local anesthetic, causing a significant decrease in the utero-placental-fetal blood flow; or (3) uterine hypertonus secondary to either use of the local anesthetic or trauma after the injection (Fig. 11-13).

Because of the potential for fetal bradycardia, many physicians believe this technique should not be used if there is evidence of uteroplacental insufficiency or if the fetus has a nonreassuring FHR pattern. If the paracervical block is used, the drug dosage must be small and the FHR and maternal blood pressure monitored continuously for approximately 5 minutes after administration. If fetal bradycardia does not occur, the opposite lateral side is infiltrated with anesthetic. After the opposite fornix is infiltrated, the FHR and maternal blood pressure are again closely monitored. Pain relief lasts 40 to 90 minutes. The block may be repeated at intervals until the cervix has reached approximately 8 cm dilatation.

Pudendal Block

For vaginal delivery bilateral pudendal nerve block (Fig. 11-14) is perhaps the safest and one of the most useful of all the regional anesthetic blocks. Although **pudendal block** provides no relief from uterine pain and no analgesia for cervical or uterine manipulations, it does alleviate most of the vaginal and perineal pain associated with delivery and produces adequate analgesia for episiotomy and repair and for most uncomplicated outlet forceps deliveries. Since pudendal block does not completely anesthetize the perineum, it does not eliminate the bearing-down reflex of the second stage of labor. Its administration is not painful, and when local anesthetic toxicity is avoided, it has no ill effects on the mother or her newborn. Pudendal block does not cause maternal hypotension and is the only regional anesthesia that does not affect autonomic innervation of the uterus.

Local Perineal Infiltration Anesthesia

Local infiltration was used widely in the past because of the apparent lack of depression in the newborn. Unfortunately, local infiltration seldom produces complete and satisfactory maternal anesthesia, and frequently the mother required supplemental general anesthesia after delivery. Other problems with local infiltration include the time required to produce analgesia and the large amount of local anesthetic drug required. With the refinements in major conduction anesthesia and general anesthesia, using local infiltration is seldom justified unless no skilled anesthetist is available.

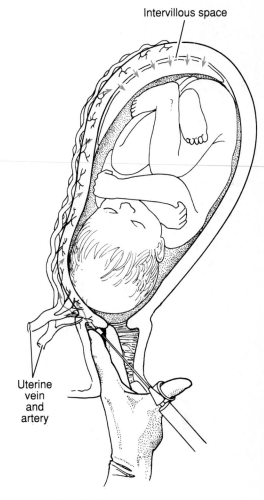

Intervillous space

Uterine vein and artery

FIGURE 11-12

Paracervical Block. Paracervical block is an effective and relatively simple method of relieving pain during labor. Five to 10 ml of a low-concentration anesthetic agent are injected into the vaginal fornix at 3 o'clock and 9 o'clock or at 4 o'clock and 8 o'clock to provide rapid but brief pain relief from labor contractions. It does not, however, provide perineal or vaginal pain relief for delivery. After the drug is injected, the client is turned to a sidelying position.

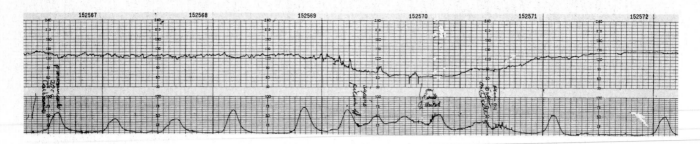

FIGURE 11-13

Course of Fetal Bradycardia Induced by Paracervical Block. Tracing reflects the client's placement in the supine position and administration of paracervical block during active labor. After approximately 11 minutes an episode of fetal bradycardia is noted, as is an increase in uterine tone. Treatment is initiated; the client is turned to her side and oxygen is given, resulting in return of normal uterine tone and normal fetal heart rate.

From Parev JT: Handbook of Fetal Heart Monitoring. Philadelphia, WB Saunders, 1983.

FIGURE 11-14

Pudendal Block. Pudendal nerves are located lateral to tips of ischial spine. A bilateral block requires only 10 ml to 20 ml of a dilute local anesthetic solution such as 1% lidocaine or 1% to 2% chloroprocaine hydrochloride and is usually administered by the obstetrician or midwife who is delivering the baby.

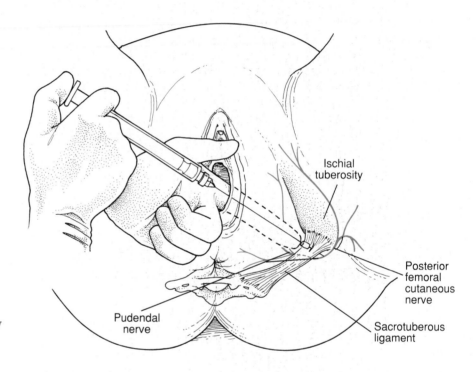

Ischial tuberosity

Posterior femoral cutaneous nerve

Sacrotuberous ligament

Pudendal nerve

Local infiltration of the perineum provides anesthesia for episiotomy and repair at the time of delivery. The anesthetic agent is injected into the subcutaneous tissue of the perineum just before delivery. Local anesthetic agents have no effect on FHR or maternal vital signs. This type of anesthesia is used by the primary care provider if the client chooses to have natural childbirth or in areas where there is very limited anesthesia coverage.

A summary of intrapartum nursing interventions during regional anesthesia is presented in Table 11-7.

Intravenous Anesthetic Drugs

Intravenous sedation is usually used in special circumstances (e.g., emergency forceps delivery for fetal distress) when a quick, short, unanticipated procedure is necessary. The client does not have an excessive depth

TABLE 11-7

Summary of Intrapartum Nursing Interventions During Regional Anesthesia

Parameter	Frequency
Blood pressure, pulse, respirations	Check every 5 min for 20 min after anesthesia is initiated and after each additional dose of anesthesia until client is stabilized.
Position	Avoid supine position. Position client on right or left side, alternating sides every 30-60 min.
Fetal heart rate	Monitor continuously per electronic fetal monitor or every 10-15 min if auscultating it.
Contractions	Monitor frequency, duration, quality (intensity), shape, and resting tone continuously with electronic fetal monitor or every 30 min if palpating with hand.
Temperature	Take every 4 hr unless elevated, then every 2 hr.
Bladder	Have client try to void at least every 2 hr. Palpate for bladder distention every 2 hr. Obtain order for catheterization if client unable to void and bladder is very distended.
Intake and output	Measure and record each shift.
Reporting	Keep primary care provider and anesthesia person aware of labor progress and position of fetus. During transition phase of first stage and second stage, client must be aware of contractions to ensue pushing is effective and progress in labor is occurring.

Adapted from Knuppel RA, Drukker JE: High Risk Pregnancy: A Team Approach. Philadelphia, WB Saunders, 1986.

of sedation and can respond to a verbal command. This state can be induced by several drugs such as barbiturates, narcotics, or diazepam. One drug, ketamine, is an intravenous induction agent that produces analgesia, amnesia, and a sleeplike state. Ketamine increases both maternal blood pressure and pulse and can be helpful if hypotension is a concern; however, its use is contraindicated if the client is hypertensive. Ketamine is safe for the woman and fetus in low doses; however, if it is used with other drugs such as narcotics maternal aspiration may be a risk. Higher doses of ketamine are associated with loss of reflexes, increased uterine tone, and neonatal depression.

Thiopental sodium is a very short-acting barbiturate that depresses the central nervous system and produces loss of consciousness within 30 seconds of administration. Since is has a rapid action and very little potential for nausea and vomiting, it is useful for sedation and induction of general anesthesia.

General Anesthesia

General anesthesia is rarely used for vaginal delivery unless an emergency exists (e.g., difficult breach delivery, shoulder dystocia, or internal version of a second twin). It poses too great a risk for the woman since pregnant clients are already predisposed to vomiting and aspiration as a result of delayed gastric emptying and increased gastric acid secretions during the third trimester.

Because general anesthesia obliterates protective laryngeal reflexes, the client must be quickly intubated to prevent aspiration. Intubation stimulates the oropharynx and trachea, causing increased cardiac output, heart rate, and blood pressure. These elevations could be disastrous for clients with severe pregnancy-induced hypertension or heart disease.

Agents used for general anesthesia do cross the placental barrier but usually do not cause depression in the infant if the interval between induction and delivery is rapid. Agents used for general anesthesia are halothane and methoxyflurane (Penthrane). Halothane is used when uterine relaxation is necessary. It also improves fetal oxygenation by decreasing uterine tonus. Methoxyflurane provides light anesthesia but also creates a slight to moderate fall in maternal arterial pressure, which can produce a decrease in uterine blood flow. This agent also can cause uterine relaxation in the postpartum period, resulting in increasing uterine bleeding.

Anesthesia for Cesarean Birth

Cesarean delivery is usually performed using (major conduction) regional anesthesia, subarachnoid block (spinal), or epidural block, particularly when trained anesthesiologists are available. Figure 11-15 shows levels of anesthesia for both vaginal and cesarean deliveries.

Regional anesthesia requires maternal hydration with 500 to 1000 ml of an isotonic intravenous solution before the block is administered. It takes several minutes to insert the spinal needle. After the needle is in place, anesthesia is produced in less than 5 minutes. If the cesarean section is an emergency, the time delay may be prohibitive. In an emergency situation general anesthesia is used because it can be induced in less time.

ADVANTAGES. One advantage of the regional anesthesia method is the anesthetic agent does not cross the placenta and depress the fetus, thus eliminating the necessity for a quick delivery. Regional anesthesia allows the woman to be awake during the cesarean delivery, to be comfortable, and to see and relate early to her infant. If hypotension and local anesthetic toxicity are avoided, the risk of pulmonary aspiration is minimum.

FIGURE 11-15

Levels of Regional Conduction Anesthesia for Obstetrics: Spinal (Subarachnoid) Block and Lumbar Epidural. **A,** Anesthesia for cesarean section must extend from xiphoid process of sternum (near the level of T8) to provide analgesia of entire abdominal cavity. **B,** Anesthesia for vaginal delivery extends from umbilicus or symphysis pubis to provide analgesia for delivery and repair of episiotomy.

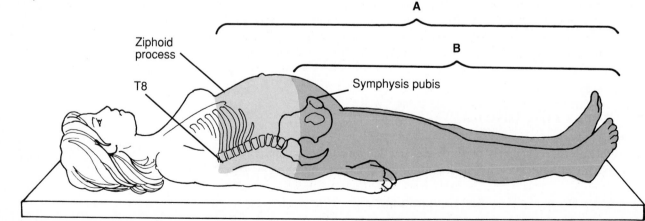

DISADVANTAGES. The disadvantages of conduction anesthesia for cesarean birth are that (1) it provides inadequate analgesia if the block level is below T10, (2) it involves the risk of maternal hypotension, and (3) the time required for its onset may delay urgent surgical intervention.

CONTRAINDICATIONS. Maternal fear and refusal to have regional analgesia are absolute contraindications. Maternal hypovolemia or shock from any cause is a contraindication because these conditions can be exacerbated by the sympathetic block, causing decreased uteroplacental blood flow. Sepsis or localized infection at or near the site of injection is an absolute contraindication because of the danger of causing an epidural abscess or inflammation (arachnoiditis). Abnormal maternal blood coagulation contraindicates the use of conduction analgesia because of the increased risk for bleeding (e.g., formation of an epidural hematoma).

Postpartum Epidural Morphine

Women receiving epidural blocks for their cesarean delivery (or a more complicated operative vaginal delivery) may benefit from epidural morphine administered after delivery (see Drug Guide: Epidural Morphine Sulfate on p. 270). Since the epidural catheter is still in place after delivery, the client is given the option of receiving 5 mg of epidural morphine sulfate. If she chooses to receive it, the morphine is injected through the catheter into the epidural space before removal of the catheter. Onset of anesthesia occurs 30 to 60 minutes after administration, and there is no motor and sympathetic block or associated hypotension. Clients experience little or no discomfort or pain during recovery and for up to 24 hours. Epidural morphine can be used with any client who has an epidural catheter in place except when there is an allergy to morphine.

Women receiving epidural narcotics require frequent observation to ensure adequate respirations. Other side effects of epidural narcotics include nausea and vomiting, itching, urinary retention, and rarely, somnolence. As is true of respiratory depression, these side effects are rapidly antagonized by naloxone.

Assessment

The nurse is responsible for assessing and monitoring maternal and fetal states during labor, particularly when the client requires analgesia or anesthesia. The nurse must be able to recognize the signs and symptoms of complications early and know what action to take until the anesthesiologist or anesthetist is available. Maternal and fetal physiologic responses to labor, analgesia, and anesthesia are assessed. Electronic FHR monitoring and contractions are evaluated.

The most frequent side effects associated with anesthesia are maternal hypotension, which may be heralded by nausea, and fetal bradycardia. Occasionally, the client will have signs and symptoms of an allergic or toxic reaction to local anesthestic agents, including light-headedness, dizziness, slurred speech, metallic taste, numbness of tongue and mouth, muscle twitching, loss of consciousness, and generalized convulsions.

Epidural morphine sulfate: An exogenous opiate that weakens signals to the brain by binding opiate receptors at many sites in the central nervous system, the brain (cortex), brain stem (thalamus), and spinal cord (dorsal horn), altering both the perception and emotional response to pain through an unknown mechanism.

Obstetric Action: Intense analgesic effect from direct action on the opiate receptors of the spinal cord rather than from systematic absorption. Onset is slower, but duration of analgesia is longer.

Dosage: 5-7.5 mg—provides analgesia for approximately 24 hours.

Maternal contraindications: Allergy to morphine.

Potential Side Effects and Complications:
Pruritus
Itching may be mild or severe; generally begins within 3 hours and lasts up to 10 hours. Naloxone (0.1 to 0.2 mg IV bolus or infusion of 0.4 to 0.6 mg/hr) will relieve symptoms; if client can tolerate itching, she can avoid taking naloxone, which counteracts the pain relief benefit.
Nausea or vomiting
Can occur 4 to 7 hours after morphine injection. Naloxone alleviates the symptoms without affecting the analgesic effect of the epidural morphine. Diphenhydramine (Benadryl) or trimethobenzamide (Tigan) can be given.
Urinary retention
Onset is early and lasts 14 to 16 hours; not usually a problem since client has Foley catheter in place.
Respiratory depression
Rare, with rate <12%. Can occur during first 1 to 2 hours or as late as 8 to 16 hours after instillation; less likely to occur if mother is in semi-Fowler's position.
Newborn effects
Since the morphine is injected into the catheter after the infant is born, there are no adverse effects.

Nursing Implications:
1. Assess for client's sensitivity to narcotics on admission.
2. Have a vial of naloxone (Narcan) (1 ml, 0.4 mg) readily available for immediate administration in case of respiratory depression.
3. Answer questions about analgesia and anticipate questions when possible.
4. Assess respiratory function hourly for 24 hours, as well as client's level of consciousness or sedation and color of mucous membranes; may use apnea monitor for 24 hours to determine if there is a decrease in respirations.
5. Assess pain relief and notify anesthesiologist if not adequate.
6. Observe for allergic reactions such as itching, edema, or respiratory difficulties.
7. Observe for nausea or vomiting.
8. Administer comfort measures such as lotions, cool or warm packs, cool or light clothing, or diversional activities.
9. Administer medications such as diphenhydramine or naloxone as ordered to alleviate side effects.
10. Monitor output if Foley catheter in place; ensure it is patent and draining (assist client with bedpan or to bathroom when Foley catheter is discontinued and motor and sensory function have returned).
11. Instruct the client to rest (since tendency is to be active much sooner after cesarean delivery).

⊡ POTENTIAL
NURSING DIAGNOSES

Regional or General Anesthesia

Ineffective Breathing Pattern—related to regional anesthetic level's depressing respirations

Urinary Retention—related to loss of sensation

Ineffective Airway Clearance—related to regional or general anesthesia

Anxiety—related to ability to cope with childbirth

Ineffective Individual Coping—related to labor pain

Knowledge Deficit—regarding use of analgesia or anesthesia for labor and delivery

Nursing Diagnosis

Several nursing diagnoses may be appropriate for a client receiving general anesthesia. They are concerned with her breathing pattern, urinary retention, airway maintenance, anxiety, coping, and knowledge deficit.

Planning and Intervention

The nurse assists in preparing the family for the analgesia or anesthesia method they have requested. This includes providing orientation to the

TABLE 11-8

Client Care Summary for Anesthesia★

	Intrapartum	Recovery and Postpartum
Regional Anesthesia		
Blood pressure (BP), pulse (P), respirations (R)	Every 5 min × 20 min initially and after each reinjection (every 5 min should be continued longer if client is not stabilized in 20 min; after stabilization, every 15 min	Every 15 min × 4 Every 30 min × 2, then on discharge to PP (recovery period is usually about 2 hr)
Temperature (T)	Every 4 hr	On admission, then every 4 hr, then on discharge to PP
Position	Alternate sidelying (right and left) initially; once anesthetic effective, left lateral preferred but can rotate	—
Fetal monitoring (FM)	Continuous FM during anesthesia, preferably with internal monitor; without monitor, every 10-15 min	—
Contractions: frequency, duration, quality, resting tone	Continuous FM during anesthesia every 30 min if no monitor	—
Input and output (I and O)	Every shift (if client has no other complications); by anesthesia standards	—
General Anesthesia (for cesarean section)		
BP, P, R		Every 15 min × 4; if stable, every 30 min × 2; if stable every 1 hr until stable; then every 4 hr
T		On admission to recovery room, then every 4 hr, then on discharge to PP
I and O		Every shift in recovery room and until IV discontinued and voiding established

Adapted from Knuppel RA, Drukker JE: High Risk Pregnancy: A Team Approach. Philadelphia, WB Saunders, 1986.

★Nurse-client ratio = 1:1 until stabilization; 1:2 after stabilization.

selected procedure, answering questions, assisting the client with positioning for the anesthesia procedure, and encouraging and praising the client for doing well during the procedure. During labor the nurse evaluates the woman's bladder for urinary retention caused by decreased bladder sensation. Contractions are evaluated to determine progress of labor. Maternal comfort level and return of sensation are evaluated. If adverse maternal or fetal responses occur, the nurse initiates emergency measures. Table 11-8 provides a client care summary for anesthesia.

Evaluation and Reassessment

The nurse assesses the analgesic or anesthetic effects, both physical and psychologic, on the woman. The mother will require reassurance if she believes she handled labor poorly or it did not meet her expectations. If the mother is very chatty, she may need to review her labor and delivery experience. Clients who have difficulty coping with the pain of labor must be reassured that responses to pain are individual and are not related to her ability to mother. Evaluation also includes the interaction of all family members present.

SUGGESTED READINGS

Gibbs CP: Anesthesia in pregnancy. In Knuppel RA, Drukkin JE (eds): High Risk Pregnancy: A Team Approach. Philadelphia, WB Saunders, 1986

Hanson-Smith B: Nursing care planning guide for childbearing families. Baltimore, Williams & Wilkins, 1989

Henrikson ML, Wild LR: A nursing process approach to epidural analgesia. JOGN (September/October):316–319, 1988

Lefevre M: Obstetric anesthesia. Am Fam Physician 27(6):146–154, June 1983

Lipkin GB: Drug therapy in maternal care. In Spencer RT et al: Clinical pharmacology and nursing management, 2nd ed. Philadelphia, JB Lippincott, 1986

Malinowski JS, Pedigo CG, Phillips CR: Nursing Care During the Labor Process. Philadelphia, FA Davis, 1989

Maresh M, Choong KH, Beard RW: Delayed pushing with lumbar epidural. Analgesia in labour. Br J Obstet Gynaecol 90:623–627, July 1983

Neeson JD: Clinical Manual of Maternity Nursing. Philadelphia, JB Lippincott, 1987

Reisner LS: Obstetric analgesia and anesthesia: Current concepts part I. The first stage of labor. Perinatal Neonatal (May):27–30, 85, 1983

Reisner LS: Obstetric analgesia and anesthesia: Current concepts part II. The second stage of labor. Perinatal Neonatal (June):39–44, 1983

Shnider SM, Levinson G: Anesthesia for Obstetrics, 2nd ed. Baltimore, Williams & Wilkins, 1987 (a fine overall text on subject of obstetric analgesia and anesthesia)

Slavazza KL et al: Anesthesia, analgesia for vaginal childbirth: Differences in maternal perceptions. JOGN (July/August):321–329, 1985

First Stage of Labor

IMPORTANT TERMINOLOGY

bloody show Pinkish mucous vaginal discharge that results from mixing mucus with blood from ruptured capillaries

cervical effacement Thinning of the cervix

cervical dilatation Opening of the cervix during labor for delivery of the fetus

fetal attitude Relationship of fetal parts to the rest of the fetus; normally flexed

fetal lie Relationship of long axis of the fetus to long axis of the mother; normally a longitudinal lie

fetal position Relationship between presenting parts of the fetus and the maternal pelvis

fontanels Unossified spaces consisting of bands of connective tissue between the cranial bones of the skull; anterior is diamond-shaped; posterior is triangular

lightening Settling of the presenting part into the true pelvis

linea terminalis Imaginary line separating the false and true pelves

presentation or presenting part Part of the baby entering the pelvis first

rupture of membranes Breaking of the amniotic sac

sutures Membranous interspaces that separate bones of the fetal head

This chapter presents the anatomic and physiologic landmarks that indicate labor is beginning. It discusses the change in the mother's pelvic structures that allow the fetus to descend and the delivery problems associated with the position of the fetus. Three phases of the first stage are discussed, as well as the premonitory signs of labor. The nurse's role is one of support person for the mother and coach and to maintain the well-being of the mother and fetus during this initial stage.

Factors That Influence Labor

For labor to progress and birth to occur:
1. The **pelvic parameters and measurements** must be normal in size and shape to facilitate the descent, rotation, and expulsion of the infant.
2. The **fetus** must be of appropriate size and shape to pass through the varying dimensions of the pelvis.
3. **Uterine contractions** must be consistent in frequency, duration, and intensity.
4. Various **psychologic factors** help the mother cope and have self-confidence during the birthing experience.
5. **Maternal positioning** influences the pattern of uterine contractions and effectiveness.

Factors That Influence Labor

The process of labor is dependent on five factors: pelvic structure; fetal size, position, and presentation; contractions; client psyche; and position of the client during labor and delivery (see above).

Pelvic Structures

Pelvic Types

There are four general classifications of pelvic shapes: gynecoid, android, anthropoid, and platypelloid (Fig. 12-1). Factors that can alter the size and shape of the pelvis are race, general body build, nutrition, developmental defects, and disease or injury of the spine, pelvis or lower extremities. The shape of the pelvis affects how the fetus will be able to pass through the birth canal and, consequently, the progress of labor.

The shapes of male and female pelves are very different (Fig. 12-2). The most conspicuous difference is in the angle of the pubic arch, which is much wider in women. The female pelvis is shallow and rounded,

FIGURE 12-1

Caldwell-Maloy Classification of Pelvic Types. *Top,* The typical shape of the inlet for each type is shown. A line has been drawn through the widest transverse diameter, dividing the inlet into an anterior and posterior segment. The longitudinal line illustrates the anteroposterior diameter of the inlet. *Bottom,* The typical interspinous diameter of each type is depicted. This diameter is the narrowest point through which the fetus must pass. **A,** Gynecoid: feminine type; inlet rounded or blunt, heart shaped. **B,** Android: male type; funnel or cone shaped. **C,** Platypelloid: flat; inlet oval in shape transversely. **D,** Anthropoid: inlet oval in shape from front to back.

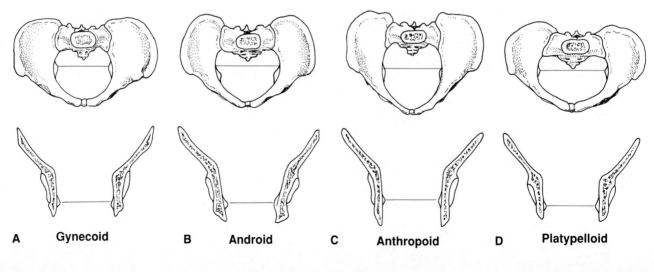

| A | Gynecoid | B | Android | C | Anthropoid | D | Platypelloid |

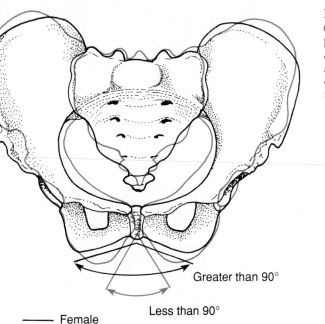

Greater than 90°

Less than 90°

—— Female

Male

FIGURE 12-2
Comparison of the Male and Female
Pelvis. A, The male pelvis is narrow and
compact; the pelvic arch is less than a right
angle. **B,** The female pelvis is broad and
capacious; the pubic arch is greater than a
right angle.

lighter in structure, and smoother in texture. The male pelvis is longer, conical, compact, and rough in texture. Male and female pelves are identical in type until puberty. Changes in pelvic inclination and shape reflect bipedal locomation due to incomplete ossification of pelvic bones during childhood. If a client has had longstanding ovarian or adrenal dysfunction, she may have a pelvis with android features.

Pelvic Parameters and Measurements

The entire childbirth process centers on the safe passage of the fully developed fetus through the pelvis. Slight irregularities in the structure of the pelvis may delay the progress of labor and any marked deformity may render delivery through natural passages impossible.

Early in the pregnancy, often during the first or second visit, the client will have a pelvic examination to assess adequacy of the pelvis. The exam assesses size and shape of the pelvic inlet, midpelvis, and the pelvic outlet. It is helpful to know in advance whether there are abnormalities in the size or shape of the pelvis.

The pelvis is divided into two portions, the false pelvis and the true pelvis (Fig. 12-3). The false pelvis, or upper part, is located above the **linea terminalis** and supports the weight of the enlarged pregnant uterus. The true pelvis, or lower part, forms the bony canal through which the fetus must pass during labor. For descriptive purposes the true pelvis is divided into three parts: an inlet, or brim; a midpelvis, or cavity; and an outlet.

PELVIC INLET. Continuous from the sacral promontory and extending along the ilium on each side in circular fashion is a ridge called the linea

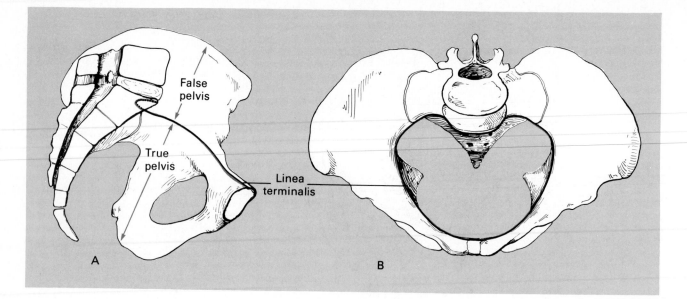

FIGURE 12-3
Views of the True and False Pelvis.
A, Side view of true and false pelvis. **B,**
Front view showing linea terminalis (pelvic
brow). The false pelvis provides skeletal
stability. The size and shape of the false
pelvis have no obstetric significance. The
size and shape of the true pelvis are
important obstetrically as the pelvis must
allow fetal passage during labor and
delivery. If the true pelvis is inadequate, a
cesarean delivery must be performed.

terminalis, or brim. This is the inlet, the entryway, through which the fetal head must pass to enter the true pelvis. The pelvic inlet is heart-shaped, and the promontory of the sacrum forms a slight projection into the inlet from behind.

The inlet is widest from side to side and narrowest from back to front (i.e., from the sacral promontory to the symphysis). The fetal head enters the inlet of the average pelvis with its longest diameter (anteroposterior) in the transverse diameter of the pelvis (Fig. 12-4). The greatest diameter of the head accommodates itself to the greatest diameter of the inlet.

The internal diameter of the inlet is the most important measurement of the pelvis. The majority of pelvic structure abnormalities affect the anteroposterior diameter of the inlet. Three measurements are needed to assess the adequacy of the pelvic inlet: the diagonal, the obstetric, and the true conjugates. See Chapter 8 for further information about pelvic measurements.

Diagonal conjugate. The chief internal pelvic inlet measurement is the diagonal conjugate, or the distance between the sacral promontory and the lower margin of the symphysis pubis. This measurement in and of itself is not important, but its importance lies in its use as the basis for calculating the true conjugate. If the measurement is greater than 11.5 cm, the pelvic inlet is judged to be adequate.

Obstetric conjugate. The second pelvic inlet measurement influencing labor and delivery is the obstetric conjugate. This measurement is the distance from the sacral promontory to the inner surface of the symphysis pubis, a few millimeters below its upper margin. The obstetric conjugate is the smallest anteroposterior diameter through which the fetal head must pass in its descent into the true pelvis. An obstetric conjugate measurement of 10 cm or more is adequate.

True conjugate. The true conjugate is the distance between the posterior aspect of the symphysis pubis and the promontory of the sacrum. Because

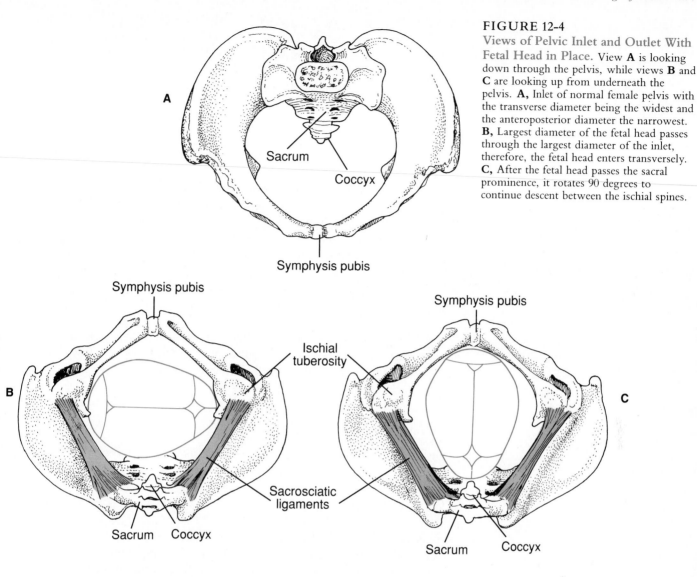

FIGURE 12-4
Views of Pelvic Inlet and Outlet With
Fetal Head in Place. View **A** is looking
down through the pelvis, while views **B** and
C are looking up from underneath the
pelvis. **A,** Inlet of normal female pelvis with
the transverse diameter being the widest and
the anteroposterior diameter the narrowest.
B, Largest diameter of the fetal head passes
through the largest diameter of the inlet,
therefore, the fetal head enters transversely.
C, After the fetal head passes the sacral
prominence, it rotates 90 degrees to
continue descent between the ischial spines.

this measurement cannot be easily obtained physically, it must be estimated based on the diagonal conjugate measurement. This is the smallest
diameter of the pelvic inlet through which the fetal head must pass.

MIDPELVIS (PELVIC CAVITY). The boundaries of the midpelvis are the
ischial spines laterally, the lower margin of the symphysis anteriorly, and
the sacrum (S3 to S4) posteriorly. The transverse diameter of the midpelvis
is the narrowest in the pelvis and is the distance between the ischial spines.
The diameter is greater if the spines are very blunted as opposed to
prominent and sharp.

During delivery the head must descend until it almost reaches the level
of the ischial spines and then curve forward. The inclination of the midpelvis determines the direction the fetus takes as it progresses through
the pelvis in the process of delivery.

PELVIC OUTLET. When viewed from below, the pelvic outlet is the area
confined by the symphysis pubis in the front, the ischial tuberosities on

the sides, and the tip of the coccyx in back. The size of the pelvic outlet is determined by measuring the transverse diameter between the inner surfaces of the ischial tuberosities (the biischial diameter or intertuberous diameter). This is the smallest diameter through which the infant must pass as it descends through the pelvic outlet.

Pelvic Soft Tissues

The maternal pelvic soft tissues also influence the progress of labor. The levator ani muscles are the main soft tissue components of the pelvic floor. They play a role in the descent and expulsion of the fetus because the birth canal (uterus, cervix, and vagina) pass through these tissues. Also the condition of the uterus and vagina can affect the progress of labor. Excessive rigidity or scarring of these tissues decreases the flexibility and increases the resistance to the descent of the fetus.

Fetal Size

The fetal head is usually the presenting part. If the head can pass through the birth canal, there is usually no difficulty in delivering the rest of the body, although occasionally broad shoulders can present a problem.

Fetal Position

Assessment of **fetal position** can be done in several ways: abdominal palpation, vaginal examination, and auscultation.

Abdominal Palpation

It is extremely helpful to palpate the abdomen to assess fetal position before listening to the fetal heart tones (FHT). The region of the abdomen in which the fetal heart is heard varies according to the presentation and the extent to which the presenting part has descended. Use the four Leopold maneuvers to determine fetal position before listening for FHTs (Fig. 12-5).

Have the client empty her bladder before beginning the procedure. This contributes to her comfort and aids in gaining more accurate information in the latter part of the procedure. The client lies flat on her back, with knees flexed to relax the abdominal muscles. The examiner lays both hands gently and, at first, flat on the abdomen so the abdominal muscles are not stimulated to contract.

The first three maneuvers are conducted at the side of the bed facing the client. During the last maneuver, the examiner stands to the side facing the client's feet.

Vaginal Examination

A skilled examiner can identify landmarks (**fontanels** and **sutures**) on the fetal head and determine fetal position. Important information about the position of the fetus and the degree of flexion of its head can be obtained by palpating the fontanels through the dilated cervical os.

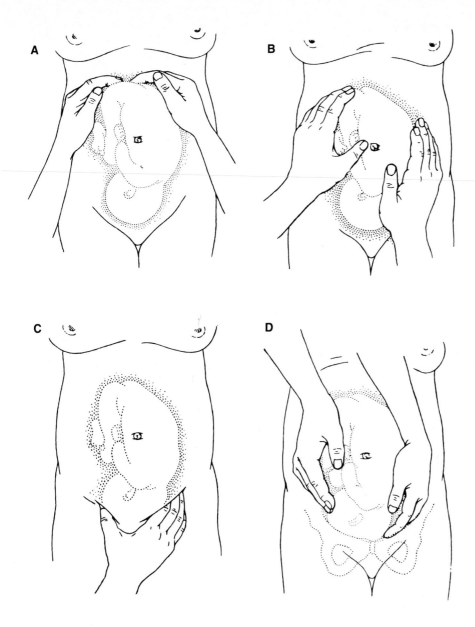

FIGURE 12-5

Leopold Maneuvers. **A,** First maneuver helps determine fetal presentation, or the part of the fetus presenting at the inlet of the pelvis; usually presentations are head or breech. The examiner faces the client's head and uses the tips of the fingers to palpate the fundus of the uterus. The fetal head feels smooth, globular, and firm and is mobile and ballotts. However, breech presentation feels irregular, rounded, and soft and is less mobile. **B,** Second maneuver helps to determine fetal position, or identifies the relationship of the fetal back and small parts to the front, back, or sides of the maternal pelvis. The examiner continues to face the client's head and places hands on either side of the uterus. While one hand stabilizes one side of the uterus, the other hand palpates the opposite side of the uterus to determine fetal back or small parts. Then the other side of the uterus is stabilized and palpated to locate the fetal back. The back is a long, smooth, hard plane. The small parts feel irregular and knobby and may be moving. **C,** Third maneuver helps to determine presenting part. While continuing to face the client's head, the examiner uses the thumb and fingers of one hand to grasp the client's lower abdomen just about the symphysis pubis and notes the contour, size, and consistency of the presenting part. The head feels firm and globular and is mobile if unengaged and immobile if engaged. A breech presentation feels smaller, softer, and irregular. **D,** Fourth maneuver helps to determine fetal attitude, or the greatest prominence of the fetal head over the brim of the pelvis. The examiner faces the client's feet and, using the tips of the first three fingers of each hand, presses deep in the direction of the pelvic inlet. The fingers of one hand will encounter a bony cephalic prominence. If the cephalic prominence is located on the opposite side from the back, it is the infant's brow, and the head is flexed. If the cephalic prominence is located on the same side as the back, it is the occiput, and the head is extended.

Auscultation

The location of the fetal heart sounds as heard through the fetal stethoscope yields some information about fetal position but is not dependable.

In cephalic presentations, the fetal heart sounds are heard loudest midway between the umbilicus and the anterior superior spine of the ilium (Fig. 12-6). In general, left occipitoanterior (L.O.A.) and left occipitoposterior (L.O.P.) positions, the fetal heart sounds are heard loudest in the left lower quandrant. The same applies to the right lower quandrant for right occipitoanterior (R.O.A.) and right occipitoposterior (R.O.P.) positions. In posterior positions of the occiput (L.O.P. and R.O.P.), the sounds are heard loudest well down in the flank toward the anterior superior spine. In breech presentation, the fetal heart sounds usually are heard loudest at the level of the umbilicus or above.

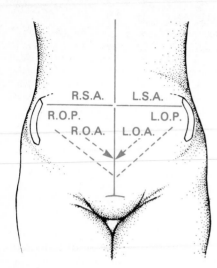

FIGURE 12-6
Fetal Heart Tones and Fetal Position.
Location of fetal heart sounds on the
abdominal wall indicates possible
corresponding fetal position and the effects
of the internal rotation of the fetus.

Fetal Lie

The **lie** of the fetus refers to the relationship of the long axis of the fetus to the long axis of the mother. Figure 12-7 illustrates longitudinal and transverse lie. When the long axis of the fetus forms an acute angle in relation to the mother, it becomes an oblique lie. An oblique lie is usually converted during the course of early labor to either a longitudinal or a transverse lie. The common causes of the transverse lie are abnormal relaxation of the abdominal wall due to grand multiparity, pelvic contraction, and placenta previa.

Fetal Attitude

The **attitude** of the fetus describes the relationship of the fetal parts to one another. The most striking characteristic of the fetal attitude is flexion. The spinal column is bowed forward, the head is flexed with the chin against the sternum, and the arms are flexed and folded against the chest. The lower extremities also are flexed, the thighs are on the abdomen, and the calves are against the posterior aspects of the thighs. In this state of flexion, the fetus assumes a roughly ovoid shape, occupies the smallest possible space, and conforms to the shape of the uterus. In this attitude, fetus is about half as long as it would be if it were completely stretched out.

Fetal Presentation

The term ***presentation***, or ***presenting part***, is used to indicate that portion of the infant's body that lies nearest the internal os. It is the portion that is felt by the examining fingers (Fig. 12-8). Presentation can be cephalic (vertex or face), breech, or shoulder.

Cephalic Presentation

Head, or cephalic, presentations are the most common. They are seen in about 97% of all births at term. Cephalic presentations are divided into

FIGURE 12-7
Fetal Lie. Fetal lie refers to the relationship
of the long axis of the fetus to the long axis
of the mother. **A,** Longitudinal lie; **B,**
transverse lie; **C,** oblique lie.

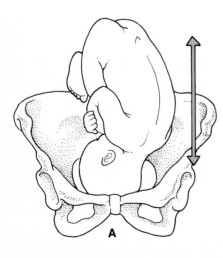

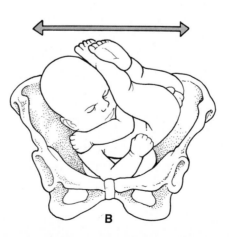

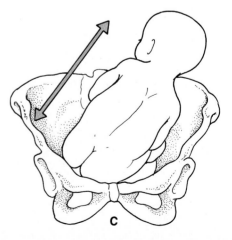

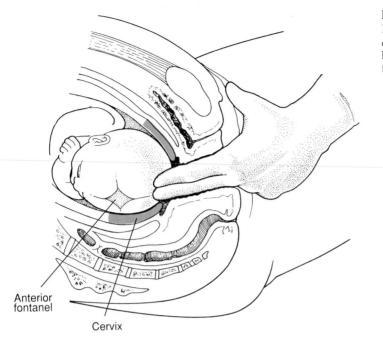

Anterior
fontanel

Cervix

FIGURE 12-8
Determination of Fetal Position. The
examiner's fingers identify the fetal cephalic
landmarks to determine the position of the
fetal head.

groups (Fig. 12-9) according to the relation of the infant's head to its
body. Most common is the vertex presentation in which the head is
sharply flexed with the chin touching the thorax. Thus the vertex is the
presenting part.

Breech Presentation

Breech presentation is the next most common presentation. The fetal
buttocks are the presenting part. It occurs in about 3% of births. In breech
presentations the thighs may be flexed and the legs extended over the
anterior surface of the body (frank breech presentation), or the thighs
may be flexed on the abdomen and the legs on the thighs (complete breech
presentation), or one or both feet may be the lowest part (foot or footling
presentation) (Fig. 12-10).

Shoulder Presentation

When the fetus lies crosswise in the uterus, it is in a transverse lie, and
the shoulder is the presenting part. Shoulder presentations are relatively
uncommon, and with very rare exceptions, the spontaneous birth of a
fully developed child is impossible in a "persistent transverse lie."

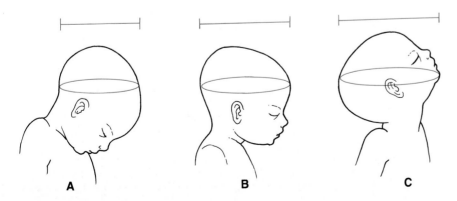

A   **B**   **C**

FIGURE 12-9
Cephalic Presentations. **A,** Complete
head flexion allows the smallest diameter of
the head to enter the pelvis. **B,** Moderate
extension causes the larger diameter of the
head to enter the pelvis. **C,** Marked
extension forces the largest diameter of the
head against the pelvic brim, but the head is
too large to enter the pelvis.

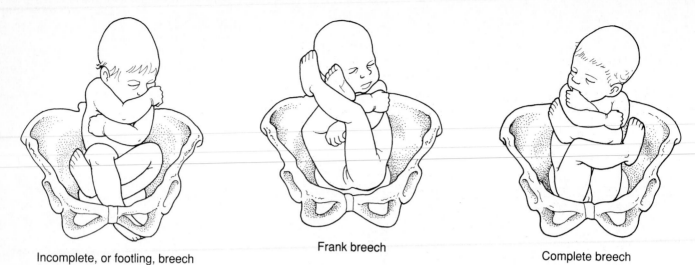

Incomplete, or footling, breech

Frank breech

Complete breech

FIGURE 12-10

Breech Presentation. Breech presentation is more common when the infant is premature or there is multiple gestation. The reasons for breech presentation are not always apparent, although associated factors include great parity, twinning, hydramnios, hydrocephalus, placenta previa, and implantation of the placenta in the cornual fundal regions of the uterus. Frank breech is the most favorable position for vaginal delivery because the buttocks fit into the pelvis more evenly, helping to prevent cord prolapse and acting as a better cervical dilator than other breech presentations. However, the current trend is to deliver breech presentations by cesarean section.

Fetal Position

In addition to identifying the presenting part of the baby, it is important to know the exact position of the presenting part in relation to the maternal pelvis.

Presentation is determined by identifying the relationship of the fetal landmarks to the part of the mother's pelvis (see Fig. 12-8). Thus in a vertex presentation, the back of the head (occiput) may point to the front or back of the pelvis. The occiput rarely points directly forward or backward in the median line until the second stage of labor, but usually it is directed to one side or the other—transverse. The occipital anterior positions are considered the most favorable for both mother and baby. Of these the left occipitoanterior (L.O.A) position is the most common.

Abbreviations for Fetal Presentations

Certain reference points on the presenting surface of the baby have been arbitrarily chosen as points of direction in determining the exact relation to the presenting part of the quadrants of the pelvis. In vertex presentations, the occiput is the guiding point; in face presentations, the chin (mentum); in breech presentations, the sacrum; and in shoulder presentations, the scapula (acromion process).

Vertex Presentation

Left occipitoanterior: L.O.A.
Left occipitotransverse: L.O.T.
Left occipitoposterior: L.O.P.
Right occipitoanterior: R.O.A.
Right occipitotransverse: R.O.T.
Right occipitosposterior: R.O.P.

Breech Presentation

Left sacroanterior: L.S.A.
Left sacrotransverse: L.S.T.
Left sacroposterior: L.S.P.
Right sacroanterior: R.S.A.
Right sacrotransverse: R.S.T.
Right sacroposterior: R.S.P.

Face Presentation

Left mentoanterior: L.M.A.
Left mentotransverse: L.M.T.
Left mentoposterior: L.M.P.
Right mentoanterior: R.M.A.
Right mentotransverse: R.M.T.
Right mentoposterior: R.M.P.

Shoulder Presentation

Left acromiodorse-anterior: L.A.D.A.
Left acromiodorso-posterior: L.A.D.P.
Right acromiodorso-anterior: R.A.D.A.
Right acromiodorso-posterior: R.A.D.P.

The various positions are usually expressed by abbreviations made up of the first letter of each word that describes the position (see display on p. 282). The same system of terminology is used for the face, breech, and shoulder presentations. The display below summarizes information about positions and presentations.

Summary of Fetal Positions and Presentations

A. Attitude of fetus—customary position that baby assumes in utero
   1. Relationship of one part of the fetus to another
      a. Spine, arms, legs, and head usually flexed
      b. Fetus assumes ovoid shape, i.e., conforming to uterus shape
B. Lie
   1. Relationship of long axis of fetus to the long axis of mother can be
      a. Longitudinal
      b. Transverse
      c. Oblique
C. Presentation
   1. Presenting part is that part of fetus which engages at inlet and can be felt through the cervix by the examining fingers
      a. Head (cephalic) presentation occurs in 97% of cases
      b. Breech occurs in about 3% of cases
D. Position
   1. Determined by some arbitrarily predetermined position of fetus to right or left side and front or back of mother's pelvis
      a. Position may affect the length and difficulty of the labor process
      b. Pelvis is divided into four regions to assist in describing the position of the presenting part of the fetus; the regions are
         (1) Left anterior
         (2) Left posterior
         (3) Right anterior
         (4) Right posterior
         (5) Transverse, right or left (note: neither anterior nor posterior)
   2. Longitudinal lie—long axis of fetus parallel to long axis of mother
      a. Cephalic positions
         (1) Vertex (head sharply flexed so that vertex presents)
            (a) Occiput is the point to determine this position, i.e., R.O.A. right occiput anterior, means that the occiput faces the right front of the mother's pelvis
         (2) Face (neck extended, face presents)
            (a) Chin (mentum) is point for position, i.e., LMA left mentum anterior, means that chin faces left front of mother's pelvis
         (3) Brow (siniciput) (neck partially extended and brow presents and is point for position)
            (a) Rare and difficult to deliver
            (b) Frequently converts spontaneously or by version to vertex or face
      b. Breech positions—sacrum used as point of position
         (1) Frank breech (buttocks presenting part, thighs flexed and legs extended)
         (2) Full breech (buttocks present, thighs flexed on abdomen and legs flexed on thighs)
         (3) Footling breech (one or both feet present)
         (4) R.S.P., right sacroposterior, sacrum faces right posterior portion of mother's pelvis
   3. Transverse lie—long axis of fetus horizontal (perpendicular) to long axis of mother
      a. Shoulder presentation—scapula (or acromium process) is the point used for determining position in a tranverse lie
         (1) Very rare and must be delivered by cesarean section

Uterine Contractions

Contraction Characteristics

A contraction is the intermittent shortening of a muscle. Contractions propel the fetus through the birth canal. Contractions during labor are involuntary and their action is independent of both the mother's will and extrauterine nervous system control.

Each contraction has three phases, a period during which the intensity of the contraction increases (increment), a period during which the contraction is at its height (acme), and a period of diminishing intensity (decrement). The increment phase is longer than the other two combined.

The contractions of the uterus during labor are intermittent with periods of relaxation between. The interval between contractions gradually decreases from about 10 minutes early in labor to about 2 to 3 minutes in the second stage of labor. These periods of relaxation provide rest for the uterine muscles and for the mother. These rest periods are also essential to fetal welfare because unremitting contractions decrease placental blood flow, which in turn decreases oxygen supply to the fetus and results in fetal distress.

Contraction Physiology

During labor the uterus differentiates into two identifiable sections, the upper segment and the lower segment (Fig. 12-11). The upper segment is the active contractile portion of the uterus. Its function is to expel the fetus. The intensity of the contraction is greatest at the fundus and decreases from the fundus downward. With each contraction the muscle fibers of the upper segment become shorter and the upper segment becomes thicker.

CERVICAL DILATATION. As labor progresses, a passive lower segment is developed. The muscle fibers of the lower section stretch with each con-

FIGURE 12-11

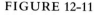

Uterine Segmental Activity.
Differentiation of two identifiable uterine segments into the upper active segment and the lower, passive segment occurs during labor to aid delivery. At the time of vaginal delivery, the active upper segment of the uterus retracts about the fetus as the fetus descends through the birth canal. The passive lower segment has considerable less myometrial tone.

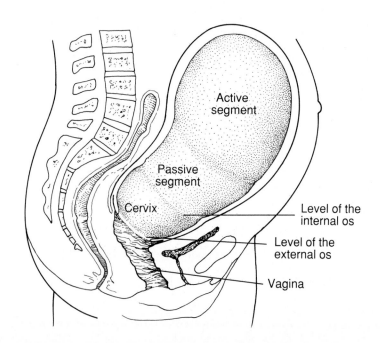

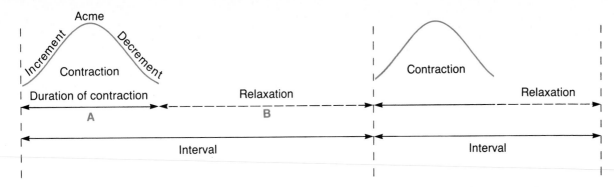

FIGURE 12-12

Timing of Contractions. Five factors are involved in the timing of contractions. Frequency—interval of time between the beginning of one contraction and the beginning of the next contraction. Duration—time measured from the beginning to the end of one contraction. Intensity—strength of the contraction assessed by palpation (or internal uterine pressure if internal uterine catheter is in place); Tonus—degree of relaxation between contractions. It is imperative that the uterus be completely relaxed between contractions. Shape of graph curve—should be bell shaped. Each contraction exhibits a wavelike pattern, beginning with a slower increment, gradually reaching the acme and then diminishing rather rapidly.

traction, and the area becomes thinner. This results in dilatation and thinning of the cervix. Dilatation is further enhanced by the amniotic sac burrowing into the cervix in pouchlike fashion and exerting further dilating action with each contraction.

Cervical dilatation is measured during the pelvic examination. The diameter of the cervical opening is estimated and expressed in centimeters. Dilatation of the cervix in the first stage of labor is solely the result of involuntary uterine contractions.

Timing of Contractions

Frequency, duration, and intensity of the contractions are closely monitored by palpation or recorded when an electronic fetal monitor is used. Use fingers to palpate rather than the palm of the hand when timing contractions because fingers are more sensitive. The fingers must have adequate contact with the abdomen because insufficient contact results in inaccurate assessment of contraction intensity and resting tone (Fig. 12-12).

The time is noted when the contraction begins. It starts with the gradual tensing and rising forward of the fundus and continues through its three phases (increment, acme, and decrement) until the uterus relaxes again.

The mother is unreliable to indicate when a contraction begins as she is often unaware of the contraction for 5 to 10 seconds after it starts. Sometimes she is unaware until the contraction reaches its acme. It is important to observe the frequency and duration of the contractions to be assured that the uterine muscle does relax between contractions. Table 12-1 describes characteristics of uterine contractions for latent, active, and transition phases of the first stage of labor. The display below lists contraction warning signs.

Client Psyche

Some studies have suggested the possibility of an interrelationship between difficulty during labor and delivery and sociocultural or psycho-

---

Deviations From Expected Patterns: Contraction Warning Signs

1. Hypertonus: relaxation between contractions not adequate; if IUP in place, resting tone is greater than 20 mm Hg
2. Relaxation phase between contractions less than 60 seconds
3. Contractions greater than 90 seconds in duration
4. Contractions exceeding 90 mm Hg in intensity

TABLE 12-1

Characteristics of Uterine Contractions in First Stage of Labor

	Latent Phase of Labor	Active Phase of Labor	Transition Phase of Labor
Frequency	5 min	3-3½ min	2-2½ min
Duration	30-50 sec	60-75 sec	60-90 sec
Intensity			
Internal monitor	25-40 mm Hg intrauterine pressure	40-60 mm Hg intrauterine pressure	60-75 mm Hg intrauterine pressure
External monitor: palpation of contraction at peak by nurse	Fundus dents at peak	Fundus firm at peak difficult to indent	Fundus very firm or hard at peak
Uterine tonus			
Internal monitor	Average 8-12 mm Hg	Same	Same
	No greater than 15-20 mm Hg	Same	Same
External monitor: palpation by nurse between contractions	Relaxed	Same	Same
Shape of contractions	Bell-shaped	Bell-shaped	Bell-shaped

logic factors. Some data suggests there is a relationship between anxiety and uterine dysfunction. If a woman perceives pregnancy as an illness, there may be the likelihood of a longer labor. Therefore, it is very important to assist mothers psychologically during their labor. This can be done by supporting and encouraging both the mother and her coach and by providing information to reduce anxiety.

Position of the Client

The position of the client during labor is very important. The first consideration for positioning is that the mother must not lie on her back. When in the supine position, there is an increased risk of both inferior vena caval and aortic compression (Fig. 12-13). Vena caval compression can cause hypotension in the mother because of decreased venous return and decreased cardiac stroke volume. Aortic compression causes no symptoms to the mother but may produce decreased uteroplacental perfusion, which results in decelerations or bradycardia in the fetus.

It is important to maintain the mother's position on her side or slightly upright. It is also important to alternate positions about every 30 minutes. Other benefits of a more upright or lateral position are

1. Contractions are more intense.
2. Maternal comfort increases.
3. Rate of descent of fetal presenting part may be increased.
4. The fetal diameters correspond better with the wider pelvic diameters.
5. Length of labor may be reduced.
6. Chance of compression of inferior vena cava and aorta decreases.

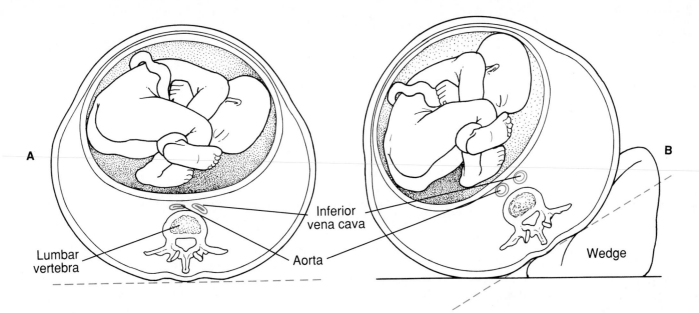

FIGURE 12-13
Relief of Aortic and Vena Caval
Compression. **A,** When the client lies on
her back (supine position), the uterus and its
contents compress the aorta and vena cava,
which decreases venous blood flow
returning to the mother's heart. Cardiac
output is decreased, and oxygenation to the
uteroplacental fetal compartment is
compromised, particularly during a
contraction. **B,** Uterine displacement with
wedge under right hip to relieve aortocaval
compression. Note: If the mother must be
placed on her back, a wedge should be
placed beneath her right hip.
From Ostheimer GW: Regional Anesthesia
Techniques in Obstetrics. New York, Breon
Laboratories, 1980.

Overview of Labor

Labor is the work of the uterus to expel the uterine contents (fetus, fluids, placenta, and membranes). The process of labor is divided into four distinct stages: first, second, third, and fourth.

The *first stage* of labor, or the dilating stage, begins with the first true contractions and ends with the complete dilatation of the cervix. **Cervical dilatation** is the enlargement of the cervical os from an opening that is a few millimeters in diameter to one large enough (approximately 10 cm) to permit the passage of the fetus. When the cervix can no longer be felt, dilatation is complete.

First stage labor is further divided into the latent, active, and transitional phases (Tables 12-2 and 12-3).

The *second stage* of labor, or the stage of expulsion, begins with the complete dilatation of the cervix and ends with the delivery of the baby.

The *third stage* of labor, or the placental stage, begins with the delivery of the baby, continues through expulsion of the placenta, and ends 1 to 2 hours after delivery or when the mother is stable.

The *fourth stage* of labor, or the recovery stage, begins with the delivery of the placenta and ends when the mother's physical status has stabilized and she can be transferred to the postpartum nursing unit.

TABLE 12-2

*Phases and Work of First State of
Labor*

Phases	Work
Latent (dilation, 0-4 cm)	Regular contraction pattern and effacement
Active (4-7 cm)	Dilatation
Transition (7 cm to complete dilatation)	Descent

	First Stage	Second Stage	Third Stage
Primigravida	8-12 hr	30 min-2 hr	10 min
Multipara	6-8 hr	5-30 min	10 min

First Stage of Labor

Latent Phase

The work of the latent phase of first stage labor is **cervical effacement**. Effacement is the shortening of the cervical canal from a structure that is 1 or 2 cm in length to one in which there is no canal (Fig. 12-14). The former canal becomes a circular orifice with paper-thin edges.

FIGURE 12-14

Stages of Cervical Effacement and Dilatation. Cervical effacement and dilatation comprise several stages. The edges of the internal os are drawn several centimeters upward so the former endocervical canal becomes part of the lower uterine segment.

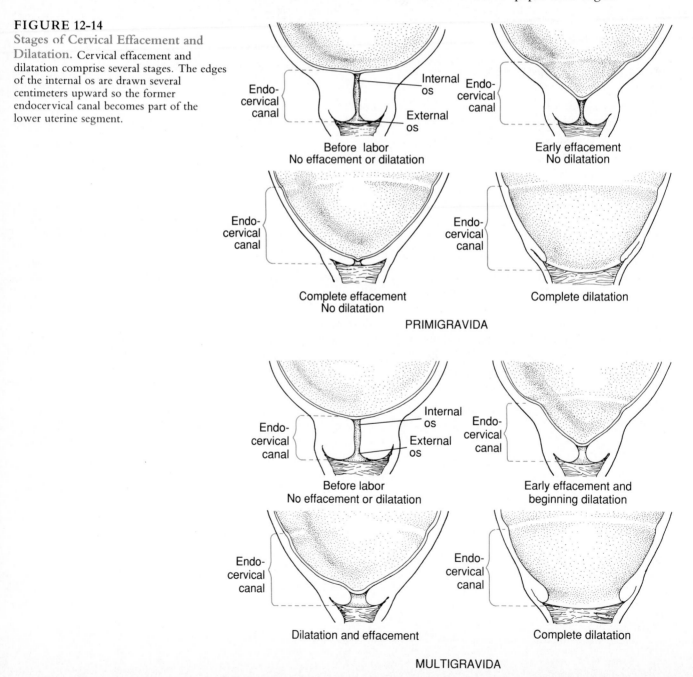

PRIMIGRAVIDA

MULTIGRAVIDA

At the beginning of the first stage the contractions are short, mild, and approximately 5 minutes apart and may not cause the client any particular discomfort. She may walk and is generally quite comfortable between contractions. Early in the first stage the discomfort is usually located in the small of the back, but as time goes on, it sweeps around, girdlelike, to the anterior part of the lower abdomen. Over time, contractions occur more frequently and are more regular in duration and intensity.

The latent phase is often the longest segment of labor. In the primigravida the latent phase ends with complete effacement and cervical dilatation of approximately 4 cm. In the multipara effacement is rarely complete so that dilatation proceeds with the cervical canal's having rather thick edges.

Active Phase

The work of the active phase of first stage labor is dilatation of the cervix. The active phase begins when contractions become regular and dilatation progresses from 4 cm to 7 cm. Contractions are more frequent (2 to 5 minutes apart), last longer (45 to 60 seconds), and are more intense (moderately hard by palpation or 50 to 60 mm Hg by intrauterine pressure monitoring).

Primigravida dilatation should progress approximately 1.2 cm/hour and multiparas approximately 1.5 cm/hour. When labor has progressed to the active phase, the woman usually prefers to remain in bed. Ambulation is no longer comfortable. During this phase the client becomes intensely involved in her labor and the sensations within her body. She tends to withdraw from the surrounding environment.

Transition Phase

The work of the transition phase is beginning fetal descent. As cervical dilatation progresses from 7 to 10 cm, the contractions reach peak intensity. The transition phase is often the most difficult and painful period of labor for the woman.

During this phase there is usually a marked increase in the amount of **bloody show** as a result of the rupture of capillary vessels in the cervix. Contractions occur 2 to 2½ minutes apart, last 60 to 90 seconds, and are hard if palpated or measure 60 to 75 mm Hg if using intrauterine pressure monitoring.

Once fetal descent begins, it should be progressive at approximately 1 cm/hour for primigravidas and 2 cm/hour for multiparas. If descent is not progressing at the expected rate, the fetus could be malpositioned. Fetal descent continues into the second stage of labor.

See the display on page 290 for clues that identify the phases of first-stage labor.

Causes of Onset of Labor

Various theories have been proposed to explain the onset of labor. Apparently several mechanisms are involved in initiating and maintaining labor. The display on page 290 describes the leading theories.

Clues to Identifying Phases of First-Stage Labor

Latent Phase

Talkative, outgoing
Excited and happy (smiling)
Unsure if contractions are true or false labor
Some fear and anxiety
Relief that labor may have begun
Anticipation of what lies ahead

Active Phase

May grimace
Introspective
Becoming more serious
Restless
Apprehensive
Less relaxed, more tense
May doze between contractions
Becomes more dependent; desires and needs coach

Transition Phase

Difficulty in controlling behavior
Fatigued
Discouraged
Talks only in phrases or words
May be nauseated; may vomit
Legs may shake
May be irritable

Theories to Explain Onset of Labor

Progesterone Deprivation Theory: Before to onset of labor, maternal
  estrogen/progesterone ratio shifts. Progesterone levels decrease, and
  estrogen levels increase.
Oxytocin Theory: Oxytocin is not the role initiator of labor; however, the
  closer to term, the greater is the sensitivity of the uterus to oxytocin.
  Oxytocin's effect may be significant in combination with other substances.
Fetal Endocrine Control Theory: Suggested mechanism of action is that fetal
  steroids stimulate the release of precursors to prostaglandins, which then
  produce uterine contractions.
Prostaglandin Theory: Prostaglandins rise sharply in early labor. They induce
  uterine contractions at any time during pregnancy. Prostaglandin inhibitors
  suppress uterine activity. Therefore the release of prostaglandins forms the
  major, final pathway in the stimulation of labor.

Premonitory Signs of Labor

During the last few weeks of pregnancy a number of physical changes
occur indicating that the time of labor is approaching. These changes
include **lightening**, bloody show, and **rupture of membranes**.

Lightening

Lightening is the settling of the fetal head into the pelvis. This may occur
at any time during the last 4 weeks of pregnancy, but occasionally it does

not occur until labor begins. Lightening usually occurs 2 to 3 weeks before the onset of labor in primigravidas. In multigravidas lightening frequently occurs just before labor's onset or after labor begins. It can occur suddenly. The expectant mother may arise one morning relieved of abdominal tightness and diaphragmatic pressure that were present the day before. Although there is relief in the upper abdomen, pressure in the lower abdomen may be increased. This increased lower abdominal pressure causes frequency of urination because of additional pressure exerted by the fetus on the bladder. There may also be leg pain caused by fetal pressure on the sciatic nerve.

Show

Cervical dilatation dislodges the mucus plug. After the cervical mucus plug is expelled, the pressure of the descending fetus causes capillaries in the cervix to rupture. The blood-tinged mucus, bloody show, must be differentiated from frank bleeding.

Rupture of the Membranes

The membranes sometimes rupture before labor starts. Labor usually begins within 24 hours after membranes rupture. Rupture of membranes can also occur during early or advanced labor. Whenever the membranes rupture, it is important for the client to notify the physician promptly because membrane rupture increases risk for cord prolapse and intraamniotic infection.

Close attention and care are needed to minimize the risk of infection and to assess for cord compression.

True Labor vs. False Labor

The terms *contractions* and *labor* are not synonymous. Braxton Hicks uterine contractions do not result in cervical dilatation, whereas labor contractions do.

Braxton Hicks contractions occur throughout most of pregnancy, but as term approaches and the uterus is more distended, they may occur more frequently, are more intense, and cause discomfort to the mother. The mother may even believe the Braxton Hicks contractions are beginning labor. She may be admitted to the hospital and be assessed for a period of time. If cervical dilatation occurs, there is true labor. If dilatation does not occur, she is experiencing false labor and will be discharged (see Client Self-Care Education: Onset of Labor) (Table 12-4).

When to Go to Hospital or Birthing Center

Patients should notify the primary care provider when contractions become regular. A primigravida is instructed to wait at home until contractions occur every 5 minutes, are regular, and last for 60 seconds or occur every 5 minutes for 2 hours. Multigravidas are instructed to notify their primary care provider when contractions are 5 to 10 minutes apart and regular. Other situations requiring immediate primary care provider notification are breaking of the bag of water and any vaginal bleeding.

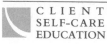

CLIENT
SELF-CARE
EDUCATION

Onset of Labor

Intervention	Rationale
1. Time contractions. When contractions are occurring but are uncomfortable, continue activities but time frequency and duration.	1. Determines if contractions are becoming more frequent, are lasting longer, and are more regular
2. Notify primary care provider when contraction pattern is regular. a. *Primigravida:* regular contraction pattern of every 5 min for 2 hr b. *Multigravida:* regular contraction pattern of every 5–10 min	2. Guides timing of hospital admission
3. Notify primary health care provider of the following: a. Rupture of bag of water b. Vaginal bleeding c. Decreased fetal movement (report time it takes to perceive 10 fetal movements)	3. Alert physician of increased risk or signs of labor

Note: If there is any delay in getting in touch with the primary health care provider, the client should go directly to the hospital.

Intervention	Rationale
4. Perform self-care during early labor. a. Rest, relax. b. Take a warm bath; do some walking. c. Occupy time with distractions that are pleasant. d. Limit intake to clear fluids such as water, juices, tea, popsicles. e. Empty bladder frequently. f. Time contractions. g. Practice relaxation; save breathing techniques for time of greater discomfort.	4. Conserves energy for the later work of labor

---

TABLE 12-4

Differential Factors in True and False Labor

Factor	True Labor	False Labor
Contractions		
Intervals	Regular	Irregular
Location	Starts in back and sweeps around to front of abdomen	Chiefly in abdomen
Intensity	Increases; increase also in duration; intensifies with walking	Remains the same or is variable; any change in position and activity gives relief; does not intensify with walking
Frequency	Increases	No increase
Bloody show	Usually present; pink-tinged mucus	Usually not present
Cervix	Effaces and then dilates	No change
Sedation	May not interrupt contraction pattern	May stop contractions

Preparing to Go to the Hospital

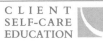

Action

1. Learn signs of impending labor.
   a. Lightening
   b. Increased Braxton Hicks contractions
   c. Weight loss of 2-3 pounds 3-4 days before onset of labor
   d. Increased vaginal mucous discharge
2. Pack suitcase, simplify housekeeping duties, plan for meals during absence, review last-minute details for child care during absence.
3. Balance activity and rest.
4. Review preparations for coming to hospital.
   a. Transportation
   b. Travel route to hospital
   c. Travel time
   d. Parking
   e. Admission entrance
   f. Admission procedure

Rationale

1. The more understanding the client and her support person have, the better prepared they are for the onset of labor.

2. Actions decrease worry and stress once labor begins. Efficient implementation may be needed if client is hurried because of active labor or an emergency.
3. Avoids overexhaustion.
4. Familiarity decreases stress.

When contractions first begin, they may be 15 to 20 minutes apart and last only 20 to 30 seconds. Over time, contractions should become more frequent, last longer, and be more intense. During early labor it is important for the client to keep busy or be distracted in order to stay relaxed and permit time to pass.

Childbirth education classes and the primary care provider's instructions assist the couple to have a better understanding of labor and to know when it is appropriate to go to the hospital (see Client Self-Care Education: Preparing to Go to the Hospital).

Entering the Labor and Delivery Unit
Client's First Impressions

The kind of greeting the client receives as she enters the labor and delivery unit is extremely important and sets the tone for future interaction with the health team.

The mother and support person need to feel welcome and expected. Many hospitals are allowing not only the coach to accompany the mother but also other support persons the mother chooses to have with her during labor and delivery.

The mother and the coach need to know what is expected of them and what they in turn can expect of the staff. The mother is then helped, if necessary, to change into the hospital gown and is made comfortable in a chair or, if she wishes, in bed.

Client Orientation

The client and coach are oriented to the general environment. The nurse assesses what they already know to determine what needs to be included in this introductory orientation.

In general, the client and support person need to know what procedures and activities will be performed and the reasons for them. In addition, they should know the mother's activity limitations and any food and fluid restrictions. Information about what the client and the coach can expect regarding the progress of labor should also be included (i.e., what will be happening physically, how the mother will be feeling, how she and her partner can participate in the labor experience).

Establishment of Nurse-Client Relationship

For a woman in labor, admission to the maternity unit may be her first acquaintance with hospitals as a patient. Her immediate feelings may be strangeness, loneliness, and homesickness, particularly if the coach is not permitted to stay with her in the labor room. Regardless of the amount of preparation for this event, whether she is happy or unhappy, whether she wants this infant or not, every mother enters labor with a certain amount of tension and anxiety.

It is important for the nurse to develop a rapport with the couple as soon as possible after admission. This relationship comprises relating thoughts and feelings that express empathy, compassion, interest, and respect for each as a unique individual.

Assessment

≡ LEGAL AND ETHICAL
≡ CONSIDERATIONS

A \$268,036 jury verdict was obtained for the wrongful death of a fetus before delivery. The mother came to the hospital as a high-risk client with ruptured membranes. Five and one-half hours passed before the hospital staff checked the fetal heart tones and discovered they were absent. The nurses were charged with negligence in failing to continuously monitor a high-risk client.

The admitting process includes a review of the prenatal record, if available, with data including the client's blood group and Rh factor, antibody detection, serology, and any diagnostic or therapeutic procedures done prenatally.

A nursing history and physical assessment assist the nurse in evaluating the client's risk status. The physician is notified of any identified risk factors because they can alter the type of labor and delivery experience the client desires (see Assessment Tool: Admission History and Nursing Assessment).

After the admission data base has been completed, the primary care provider is notified of the client's admission. The nurse gives a summary of the admission assessment findings (see display on p. 296).

General Physical Condition

The client should be asked the reason for her admission to the hospital. The nurse should not assume it is labor. Other reasons include leaking of amniotic fluid, bleeding, or decrease in fetal movement. Use open-ended questions to elicit basic information. However, more direct questioning may be necessary for further clarification.

Admission History and Nursing Assessment

1. Date and time of admission
2. Primary care provider (obstetrician, family practice physician, or certified nurse midwife)
3. Infant's physician or pediatrician
4. Estimated date of confinement (delivery)—note if determined by dates or by ultrasound
5. Gravida, para, abortions
6. Allergies
7. Maternal medical-surgical history (i.e., heart disease, diabetes, high blood pressure, any other problems)
8. Medications or drugs taken during pregnancy
9. Any problems with previous pregnancies
10. Any problems with this pregnancy
11. When labor began, when contractions became 5 min apart and regular (primigravida) as 5 to 10 min and regular (multipara)
12. Contractions on admission: frequency, duration, frequency, relaxation
13. Vaginal discharge
    a. Membranes intact or ruptured? Date, time, amount, appearance, color, and odor if ruptured
    b. Bloody show or frank bleeding? Type, amount, color (include when it began)
14. Last oral intake: what and when
15. Vital signs: temperature, pulse, respirations, blood pressure
16. Fetal heart rate: rate, location, regularity
17. Vaginal examination findings: dilatation, effacement, presentation, and station
18. Labor plans discussed with primary care provider

Sample Narrative Charting: ADMISSION NOTE—Primigravida admitted to Labor, Delivery, Recovery Room (LDR) No. 5 in labor. Changed clothes and into bed. Oriented to surroundings. Contractions 3-3½ minutes apart, lasting 60 seconds, and good quality. States "contractions hurt." Husband present and coaching through contractions. Working well together. BP 110/60 (between contractions on left side). TPR 98.6-84-18. Vaginal exam done. External fetal monitor applied, hooked into central station. Oriented to monitor. Signal cord within reach. Dr. Edmiston notified of admission and assessment.

Estimated Date of Confinement

This date can be obtained from the prenatal record. Term is achieved beginning on day 1 of 38 weeks of gestation and extending through day 7 of 41 weeks, a time span of 4 weeks. The date of the client's last menstrual period allows the nurse to calculate the estimated date of confinement (EDC) by using Nägele's rule or a gestation wheel, which provides the number of weeks and partial weeks of gestation.

Fetal Heart Rate

It cannot be overstressed that the nurse is caring for at least two clients, the mother and her fetus(es); therefore nursing assessment includes each one (see Assessment Tool: Initial Fetal Assessment).

Fetal heart rate (FHR) should be assessed very early in the admission process. The normal FHR of the term fetus is 120 to 160 beats/minute. FHR is assessed using electronic fetal monitoring, auscultation with a

Information Reported to Physician After Client's Admission

- Name of client
- Gravida, para, abortion
- Estimated date of confinement
- Vital signs
- Fetal heart rate (FHR)
  - Baseline FHR
  - Accelerations or decelerations
- Vaginal examination information
  - Dilatation and effacement of cervix
  - Presenting part
  - Station
  - Bloody show or bleeding
- Amniotic membrane status
  - Intact or rupture
  - If ruptured, amount, color, thickness or thinness of fluid, odor (if present)
- Contraction pattern
  - Duration
  - Frequency
  - Intensity
  - Resting tonus
- Type of analgesic or anesthetic client desires
- Any unusual or abnormal assessment

ASSESSMENT
TOOL

Initial Fetal Assessment

1. Is the fetus mature? What is the due date?
2. Are the client's membranes ruptured? If so, what is the color of the amniotic fluid (clear, meconium stained)? Consistency of fluid (thick, thin)? Odor? Any bloody show or bleeding?
3. Does the mother look as though she is carrying a term fetus? Measure fundal height and correlate with gestational age.
4. Is the fetus active? Has the mother noticed any changes or decrease in fetal movement?
5. Auscultate the fetal heart for baseline rate and rhythm, or apply the electronic fetal monitor and run a strip of tracing to assess baseline FHR, reactivity, and any periodic changes.

fetoscope, or Doppler. When auscultating the FHR, the nurse counts the rate for 1 full minute. The heart rate must be checked before, during, and after a contraction so that any slowing or irregularities can be detected. FHR assessment is particularly important in assessing fetal reaction to the contraction. See Table 12-5 for parameters of baseline FHR.

With an electronic FHR monitor applied (see Nursing Procedure: Application of External Fetal Monitor), the nurse obtains the baseline FHR. The FHR during contractions (periodic FHR) is monitored to identify any associated accelerations or decelerations. Variability (the interplay between the sympathetic and parasympathetic nervous system) is also assessed.

If the client has ruptured membranes and the cervix is dilated at least 2 cm, an internal fetal monitor can be applied. This procedure is done

TABLE 12-5

Fetal Heart Rate★

Finding	Rate (bpm)
Normal baseline range at term	120–160
Mild tachycardia	160–180
Marked tachycardia	>180
Mild bradycardia	100–119
Marked bradycardia	<100

★Baseline FHR is the rate between contractions (or when the client is not in labor).
FHR = fetal heart rate; bpm = beats per minute; > = greater than; < = less than.

Application of External Fetal Monitor

NURSING
PROCEDURE

Intervention

1. Explain procedure to mother (and coach).
2. Lay out transducer (to monitor the contraction pattern) and tocodynamometer (toco).
3. Place both monitor belts beneath mother's back.
4. Plug transducer and toco into monitor and press button for power.
5. Place toco on mother's abdomen at level of her umbilicus. Secure toco according to manufacturer's guidelines so that contractions can be recorded. Note: Toco only records frequency, duration and shape of contractions.
6. Apply ultrasonic gel to underneath side of transducer.
7. Place transducer on area of abdomen identified as appropriate for receiving best fetal heart signal.
8. Increase volume and listen for FHR. If signal not optimum, readjust transducer placement (wait 3-4 sec between moves of transducer).

9. When placement of monitor is complete, document the following:
   a. Application of external monitor
   b. Date and time of application
   c. Average baseline FHR
   d. Monitor connected to central bank (some hospitals have displays at nurses' station (or other locations) that receive the most recent 7-8 min of fetal heart and contraction tracings from each client's room)

Rationale

1. Helps to dispel anxiety and fear
2. Orients couple to monitor and its attachments.

3. For securing transducer and toco after placement in appropriate area on abdomen
4. All equipment now ready to function

5. If toco placed above umbilicus, monitors mother's respiratory rate instead of FHR.

6. Aids in transmission of sound waves

7. Initial transducer placement; some adjustment may be needed

8. Locates best site for receiving fetal heart signal; 3-4 sec pause between adjusting permits monitor to develop its memory of information received
9. Documentation necessary for every procedure

---

by labor and delivery nurses or the primary care provider. Additional information on FHR monitoring is presented in Chapter 13.

Amniotic Fluid Status

On admission the mother will be asked if her bag of waters is intact or ruptured (see display on p. 298). Ruptured membranes are often difficult

Significance of Ruptured Membranes

1. If the presenting part is not fixed in the pelvis, the possibility of cord prolapse and cord compression is maximized.
2. Labor is likely to occur soon if the pregnancy is at or near term.
3. If the fetus remains in the uterus 24 hours or more after the membranes rupture, the probability of intrauterine infection and neonatal sepsis is increased.

to diagnose unless there is a gush of fluid from the vagina. The nitrazine test determines whether or not the membranes have ruptured. The nitrazine paper used for the test is impregnated with a dye that reacts with the vaginal material. Its color is compared to a standard color chart. Bloody show can give a false reading. If there is gross amniotic fluid, the nitrazine paper will turn dark blue. If the nitrazine test does not confirm ruptured membranes, a fern test may be done.

The sterile speculum examination and collection of fluid for the fern test may be done by the nurse or the primary health care provider. A long-stick cotton swab is inserted as deeply into the cervix as possible for moistening with the amniotic fluid or secretions present. The swab is withdrawn and smeared on a glass slide. The dried slide is examined under a microscope. If membranes are ruptured, the dried fluid or secretions will have a fern pattern. The presence of ferning indicates a positive test result. If there is no ferning, the results are negative. If membranes are ruptured and there are no contractions, labor may be stimulated by starting an oxytocin infusion. Often the physician will wait for some time to see if labor begins spontaneously.

Initial Vaginal Examination

Early in the admission process the primary care provider or staff nurse performs a vaginal examination to determine cervical dilatation and effacement and fetal presentation and position. The client is positioned on her back with a wedge placed under her right hip to prevent compression of the vena cava and aorta. A vaginal examination should not be performed if bleeding is noted. One major reason for bleeding is placenta previa. A vaginal examination could initiate a major hemorrhage. If the client is bleeding, the primary health care provider should be notified and the vaginal examination deferred until the reason for the bleeding is determined.

Ongoing Assessment
Fetal Heart Rate Monitoring

Results of repeated auscultation of the FHR or continuous or intermittent monitoring of it must be recorded. FHR is documented every hour during early labor and every half hour once regular contractions are established.

The FHR can be assessed by auscultation or with electronic FHR monitoring. An external monitor can be applied to the mother's abdomen, or if membranes are ruptured, an internal monitor can be applied. More extensive information about fetal heart monitoring is in Chapter 13.

≡ LEGAL AND ETHICAL
≡ CONSIDERATIONS

Nurses working in the postpartum and labor and delivery room areas are advised to obtain a client's consent before conducting any physical examination. Clients have a legal right to be free from unconsented touchings, and this right is protected by the tort of battery.

In addition, the FHR is checked *immediately* after the rupture of membranes, whether rupture occurred spontaneously or was instigated artificially by the primary care provider. This check is important because the rush of amniotic fluid that follows the rupture could cause the cord to prolapse. Any indication of fetal distress from pressure on the umbilical cord can be detected by a decrease in FHR. The nurse is alert for decelerations in the FHR and determines if the pattern warrants notification of the physician.

Characteristics of Contractions

Contractions are assessed for frequency, duration, intensity, tonus, and shape. An external or internal fetal monitor may be used, or contractions can be palpated manually by the nurse. Uterine contractions gradually increase in frequency, duration, and intensity as labor continues.

Uterine contractions can be assessed by abdominal palpation when intrauterine pressure reaches approximately 20 mm Hg. The laboring mother perceives discomfort from a contraction at an intrauterine pressure of approximately 25 mm Hg. The resting tone should remain below 15 to 20 mm Hg (intrauterine measurement) for adequate uteroplacental perfusion.

Further information about contraction monitoring is in Chapter 13.

Vital Signs

Normally, the client's temperature, pulse, and respirations (TPR) should not be elevated on admission with the exception of a transient pulse increase caused by excitement. Temperature is monitored and documented every 4 hours as long as the membranes are intact and temperature is normal. If temperature is >99.6° F or if membranes are ruptured, temperature is assessed every 2 hours.

Elevated temperature or pulse can indicate dehydration. If temperature or pulse is elevated, the mother's fluid intake is assessed. If the temperature is >99.6° F (37.2° C) orally, infection is suspected. The pulse will also be elevated if infection is present.

Blood pressure is monitored and recorded every hour during the first stage of labor. It is taken when a contraction ends and well before the next one begins. Since anxiety can increase blood pressure, the blood pressure should be taken when the client is relaxed. Client position also affects blood pressure. She should be upright or lying on her side (preferably the left side). Whenever the blood pressure is elevated, it must be rechecked with the mother lying on her side.

Blood pressure that is 30 mm Hg systolic or 15 mm Hg diastolic higher than the baseline amount recorded prenatally must be reported to the primary health care provider.

Pulse during normal labor ranges in the 70s or 80s and rarely exceeds 100 beats/minute. Pulse should be assessed between contractions.

Respirations can also increase slightly during labor. The primary health care provider is notified if the pulse rate is >100 beats/minute or the respiratory rate is >20/minutes.

After the assessment is completed, the primary care provider is notified of the admission and is given a summary of the assessment findings. The assessment findings are documented in the client's chart (Table 12-6).

TABLE 12-6

Nursing Care Documentation Guide
for First Stage of Labor

Nursing Care	Frequency/Description
Blood pressure, pulse, respirations	On admission; then every hour
Temperature	On admission; then every 4 hr until membranes rupture or if labor prolonged
Fetal heart rate	Auscultation: every 30 min (listen through two or three contractions)
	External fetal monitor: intermittent or continuous
	Internal fetal monitor: continuous
Contractions: frequency, duration intensity, resting tone	Palpation: every hour. Fetal monitor: continuous (if using external monitor, palpation still necessary)
Vaginal discharge	Bloody show, amniotic fluid; describe and estimate amount, color, and odor
Position changes	Left or right, lateral or upright Note: Avoid supine position.
Nursing support	Ice chips, warm blankets, mouth care, dry linens, back rubs
Bladder assessment; complaints of pain	Voiding encouraged every 2-3 hr; then assess every hour
Coping mechanisms: support person present, visitors	Every hour

Nursing Diagnosis

Potential nursing diagnoses appropriate for the first stage of labor address comfort, fear, tissue perfusion, knowledge deficiency, and coping.

Since the birth of an infant is viewed as a major event in life, the nursing diagnoses not only address the mother's and fetus' needs but also needs of other family members such as the father, grandparents, aunts, uncles, and friends. Diagnoses dealing with fear, knowledge deficit, and ineffective family coping can be applicable to other family members.

Focus Assessment

Monitor maternal position, vital signs, level of consciousness closely.
Monitor fetal heart rate.
Determine individual client and family information needs.
Identify client's nonverbal signs of pain.
Compare client response to uterine contractions with fetal monitor recording of contraction frequency, duration, strength, and interval.
Identify nonverbal signs of distress in significant other.
Identify patterns of coping with pain.

POTENTIAL
NURSING DIAGNOSES

First Stage of Labor

Altered Tissue Perfusion—related to impaired maternal venous return (secondary to uterine compression of the vena cava while the woman is in the supine position), i.e., supine hypotensive syndrome

Potential for Injury (Fetal)—related to decreased placental perfusion (secondary to maternal supine hypotensive syndrome)

Knowledge Deficit—regarding hospital procedures and the process of labor

Fear—related to hospital surroundings, procedures, and labor/delivery

Pain—related to uterine contractions and mechanical dilatation of the cervix

Ineffective Individual Coping—related to hospitalization and pain of active labor

Initial Planning and Intervention
Vulvar and Perineal Preparation

A complete vulvar shave was once a routine admission procedure. Currently, shaving of vulvar hair is infrequently done. A small area around the vagina or between the vagina and rectum may be shaved in anticipation of performance of an episiotomy. If shaving is done, a pad is placed under the client's buttocks. The client is instructed to turn on her side to permit adequate exposure of the perineal area. The area to be prepared is soaped from front to back and the brief shave performed. A scissor clip may be done instead of a shave.

Enema

Until recently, an enema was another routine admission procedure. However, experience and research indicate that the enema is not as necessary as once believed. Although some hospitals may still require an enema, in many that decision is made by the nurse and the client. It is wise for the nurse to assess the client's need for an enema as the nursing history is being completed. If the client has had a bowel movement in the last 1 or 2 days, she may not need an enema. If she is constipated, an enema can be helpful. The type of enema given usually uses tap water or a disposable prepared solution. Soapsuds enemas should not be used because they have been associated with acute colitis, bowel perforation, gangrene, and even anaphylaxis.

Ongoing Planning and Intervention

Because contact with the client during the labor and delivery process is short term, the nurse is challenged with the problem of providing high-quality care in a short space of time. The nurse must effectively use whatever time is available to provide an atmosphere of receptivity to the client's needs. The ability to identify client needs rapidly is paramount.

Once essential nursing care is implemented, the nursing care focuses on therapeutic communication and technical understanding. Providing "supportive care" includes both emotional support and physical care. Providing for the mother's well-being and comfort assists her in maintaining her emotional equilibrium.

As labor progresses, the mother's mood becomes more serious, and she is more attuned to her body processes as she works to cope with the discomfort and pain. Both the mother and support person need reassurance and reinforcement that they are doing well. The nurse remains with the client, providing care in an organized, calm manner. Instructions must be short and direct. The nurse encourages the support person to assist the mother and makes ice chips and a cool washcloth for the mother's forehead available. The support person may provide counterpressure on the sacrum during contractions for easing low back pain. The nurse keeps the mother's perineum clean and dry and maintains a quiet environment. She also updates both of them on the progress of the labor.

Evaluation

All assessment and interventions are directed at ensuring appropriate progress during the first stage of labor, physical and emotional care for the mother, and reassurance and support for mother and support person, as well as ensuring optimum uteroplacental and umbilical blood flow so that the fetus is well oxygenated (see Nursing Care Plan: First Stage of Labor).

NURSING
CARE
PLAN

First Stage of Labor

Goals (Expected Outcomes)	Interventions	Rationale	Evaluation
Ineffective Individual or Family Coping—Related to Hospitalization or Client's Being in Pain			
Client and her support person benefit from having worked together as a team throughout the first stage of labor.	Encourage support person's participation in care.	Promotes effective coping by binding client and support person closer.	Support person assists client in coping with labor.
	Work through support person for change of position or change in breathing.	Helps support person feel needed and good about involvement.	Support person states he or she feels part of the labor process.
	Provide explanations to client and support person.	Assists support person in helping the client.	Client states she benefits from support person's presence and support.
	Identify and reinforce adaptive coping behavior.	Makes support person aware of importance of job and that job is being well done (essential part of the team).	Support person feels that he or she is doing a good job.
	Provide support to support person (refreshments and breaks).	Promotes support person's ability to cope since he or she also needs refreshments and breaks but often feels guilty about leaving unless suggestion comes from nurse.	Support person expresses gratitude that breaks are suggested.
Fear—Related to Hospital Procedures and Surroundings and Labor (and Impending Delivery)			
Client reports increased comfort with hospital procedures and process of labor and delivery.	Provide calm, quiet environment.	Assists client to be calm.	Client is relaxed, showing no anxiety and fear.
	Anticipate unasked questions and give explanation for everything to be done.	Eliminates fear of unknown.	Client appears more confident about progress.
	Give positive feedback for progress.	Increases her confidence in herself, reducing anxiety.	Client states she is grateful for praise.
	Reinforce that client and baby are both doing well if realistic (i.e., all vital signs of both are normal).	Accentuates the positive, gives mother more confidence that she and her infant are doing OK. Promotes positive feelings.	Client verbalizes she is more confident and less fearful.

NURSING
CARE
PLAN

First Stage of Labor—continued

Goals (Expected Outcomes)	Interventions	Rationale	Evaluation
Alteration in Tissue Perfusion—Related to Supine Position Causing Compression of Inferior Vena Cava and Aorta and Decreased Placental Perfusion to Fetus			
Client and fetus progress through first stage of labor with no problems.	Maintain position of client in lateral or upright position.	Prevents compression of inferior vena cava and aorta by uterus and fetus.	Client remains normotensive and voices no complaints of nausea or dizziness.
	Place wedge under client's right hip for vaginal examinations, induction of epidural anesthesia, and any other procedures requiring a supine position.	Offsets uterus and fetus from the inferior vena cava and aorta.	Fetus maintains normal baseline rate (absence of tachycardia, bradycardia or late decelerations).
	Place wedge under client's right hip if supine position necessary.	Keeps uterus and fetus off aorta and vena cava.	Blood pressure and FHR remain stable.
Acute Pain—Related to Progress of Labor			
Client demonstrates an understanding of how to help and participate, to maximize her comfort, and to help determine if and when analgesia will be used.	Change position every one-half hour (side lying and upright).	Promotes comfort and maintains contraction pattern.	Client appears relaxed between contractions and has stable contraction pattern.
	Permit ambulation until membranes rupture and presenting part engaged.	Promotes comfort and facilitates contractions and progress in labor.	Client has regular stable contraction pattern and states pain is tolerable.
	Encourage relaxation and distraction.	Passes time, decreases discomfort, facilitates progress of labor.	Client is relaxed and participates in making decisions about position changes and use of analgesia.
	Promote effective breathing techniques as long as they are helpful.	Aids coping with contractions.	Couple works together well with breathing and relaxation.
	Encourage use of visual imagery.	Provides distraction.	Client verbalizes coping success with contractions.
	Provide warm shower or bath if physician agrees (if bag of water intact).	Promotes relaxation and progress.	Client states she is relaxed and feels good about coping skills.
	Assist with comfort measures: giving back rub, performing effleurage, wiping face, keeping bed straightened and dry, maintaining comfortable room temperature, giving perineum care as needed.	Aids in promoting comfort.	Client states all comfort measures are helpful and facilitate effective coping.
	Promote privacy and quiet environment.	Promotes comfort.	Client appears relaxed and verbalizes that environment is restful.
	Assist with regulation of visitors.	May need assistance in regulating who stays and who leaves.	Client verbalizes positive responses to limiting visitors.

Continued

NURSING
CARE
PLAN

First Stage of Labor—continued

Goals (Expected Outcomes)	Interventions	Rationale	Evaluation
Acute Pain—Related to Progress of Labor—continued			
	Provide clear fluids or ice chips.	Provides oral hygiene and hydration.	Client states mouth does not feel dry at present.
	Administer intravenous fluids as ordered; observe for bladder distention.	Provides hydration.	Client is able to void approximately every 2 hr.
	Encourage voiding every 1–3 hr.	Full bladder may impede descent of fetus.	Client's bladder is empty, and fetus is descending.
	Provide encouragement to mother and her support person.	Both need reassurance they are doing well.	Client and support person verbalize pleasure at a job well done.
	Administer analgesic as ordered when mother unable to relax between contractions.	Assists with pain management and relaxation to facilitate fetal oxygenation.	Client is coping well and is more relaxed after receiving analgesic. FHR pattern is normal.
Knowledge Deficit—Regarding Process of Labor and Hospital Procedures and Routine			
Childbirth plans are fulfilled and satisfied.	Explain what sensations to expect in each phase of first stage of labor, e.g., contraction pattern will increase.	Assists understanding of each phase of labor and why contractions are more frequent, last longer, and are more intense.	Client verbalizes and demonstrates understanding of labor, hospital procedures, and routine.
	Explain procedures to be done, what to expect, and reason for each.	Prepares for what is to be done and why it is done.	Client verbalizes understanding of procedures; states it is easier when she knows what to expect.
	Encourage questions; clarify and explain as needed.	Provides optimum atmosphere for providing information.	Client asks questions to clarify understanding.
	Explain need to call for nurse if bag of water ruptures.	Assures client knows why calling for nurse is important.	Client calls for nurse when membranes rupture.
	Explain need for ambulation (if indicated), position changes, emptying of bladder, relaxation.	Increases knowledge and positive working with the labor.	Client initiates changes in position and is cooperative.
	Reinforce good work that both are doing.	Causes them to try even harder.	Both respond to praise and work harder to do well.

NURSING
CARE
PLAN

Admission of Client in Labor

Goals (Expected Outcomes)	Interventions	Rationale	Evaluation
Acute Pain—Related to Uterine Contractions and Cervical Dilatation			
Client will experience effective management of pain during labor and delivery.	Assess client's response to pain; give encouragement to couple. Assist with pain-relief techniques.	Determines effectiveness of coping and ensures couple is given help to experience what they desire from this childbearing experience.	Client reports satisfaction with the pain control experienced during labor.
	Encourage and support client's participation in choice of technique to cope with pain.	Both client and coach need to feel they are in control and doing a good job.	Client verbalizes satisfaction with labor experience and support of nurse.
	Encourage relationships by providing quiet, restful environment, keeping client clean and dry, and monitoring breathing techniques.	Helps in coping with labor pain.	Client appears relaxed during contractions.
	During contractions assist coach to give sacral pressure for backache.	Counter pressure to sacrum often decreases severity of backache.	Client reports that severity of backache decreases with sacral massage.
	Encourage client to ambulate if permitted.	Decreases pain perception.	Client reports contractions are less painful while ambulating.
	Offer ice chips, lip balm.	Prevents dry mouth and cracked lips; may help decrease thirst.	Client reports that ice chips decrease thirst.
	Support client in choice of analgesia or anesthesia.	Client makes informed choice to meet her pain needs.	Client expresses choice of analgesia or anesthesia.
Altered Placental Perfusion to Fetus—Related to Mother's Supine Position			
Client will maintain sidelying or upright position.	Teach importance of never lying in supine position.	Minimizes potential for supine hypotension; maximizes venous return of blood to heart and maximizes cardiac output.	Client avoids supine position, displays no signs of hypotension; FHR baseline is stable.

Continued

NURSING
CARE
PLAN

Admission of Client in Labor—*continued*

Goals (Expected Outcomes)	Interventions	Rationale	Evaluation
Ineffective Individual Coping—Related to Lack of Support Systems			
Client will cope effectively with contractions.	Encourage presence of support person(s). Nurse will assist with support if no support person is available.	Studies have shown that mothers and fetuses do better if support person is present.	Client maintained appropriate breathing patterns; relaxes between contractions.
	Assist support person in coaching breathing techniques.		
	Make sure support person gets breaks.		
	Praise support person.		
	Talk to mother and support person as a team, giving encouragement and praise.		
	Instruct support person.		
	Wipe mother's face with cool wash cloth.		
	Offer ice chips.		
	Tell mother when contraction begins and when it is ending.		
	Rub mother's back.		
	Instruct support person about how to determine if mother is relaxing.		
Knowledge Deficit—Regarding Process of Labor and Body Changes			
Client will gain understanding of what is happening to her and what to expect.	Establish relationship with client and support person.	Provides reassurance, care and effective communication.	Client and support person are familiar with the new environment and "settle in."
	Learn how clients want to be addressed (e.g., first name).	Increases psychological comfort.	Client states how she wants to be addressed.
	Provide orientation to the unit and labor process.	Decreases tension or anxiety related to the "unknown".	Client understands equipment, procedures, expectations.
	Convey attitude that the couple is expected and welcomed.	Provides warm, comfortable, and therapeutic atmosphere.	Client states she is comfortable with the environment and the nurse.
	Individualize teaching plan to cover expectations and restrictions of the environment; review or teach relaxation methods and answer questions.	Personalizes the labor experience.	Client and support person(s) state they feel rapport with the nurse(s).
	Explain the fetal monitor and how it works.	Provides confidence and eliminates fear of technology.	Client states she feels reassured by hearing the infant's heart beat.

SUGGESTED READINGS

Bean CA: Methods of Childbirth. New York, Dolphin Books, 1982

Bing E: Six Practical Lessons for Easier Childbirth. New York, Grosset & Dunlap, 1982

Bowes WA Jr: Clinical aspects of normal and abnormal labor. In Creasy RK, Resnik R (eds): Maternal-Fetal Medicine: Principles and Practice. Philadelphia, WB Saunders, 1989

Cunningham FG, MacDonald PC, Gant NF: Williams' Obstetrics. Norwalk, Conn, Appleton & Lange, 1989

Fenwick K, Simkin P: Maternal positioning to prevent or alleviate dystocia in labor. Clin Obstet Gynecol 30:1, March 1987

Gulanick M, Klopp A, Galanes S: Nursing Care Plans: Nursing Diagnosis and Intervention. St. Louis, CV Mosby, 1986

Hanson-Smith B: Nursing Care Planning Guides for Childbearing Families. Baltimore, Williams & Wilkins, 1989

Howe CL: Physiologic and psychosocial assessment in labor. Nurs Clin North Am 17(1)49-56, March 1982

Kilpatric SJ, Laros RK: Characteristics of normal labor. Obstet Gynecol 74:1, July 1989

Kintz DL: Nursing support in labor. JOGN, March/April 1987, pp 126-130

Lupe PJ, Gross TL: Maternal upright posture and mobility in labor. Obstet Gynecol 67(5):727-730, May 1986

Malinowski JS, Pedigo CG, Phillips CR: Nursing Care During the Labor Process. Philadelphia, FA Davis, 1989

Nesson JD: Clinical Manual of Maternity Nursing. Philadelphia, JB Lippincott, 1987

Russell KP: The course and conduct of normal labor and delivery. In Pernall ML, Benson RC (eds): Current Obstetric and Gynecologic Disorders. New York, Appleton & Lange, 1987

Varney H: Nurse-Midwifery: Boston, Blackwell Scientific, 1987

Zlatnik FJ: Normal labor and delivery and its conduct. In Scot JR et al (eds): Danforth's Obstetrics and Gynecology. Philadelphia, JB Lippincott, 1990

CHAPTER 13

Second Stage of Labor

IMPORTANT TERMINOLOGY

analgesia Loss of perception of pain

anesthesia Loss of ability to perceive touch, pain, and other sensations

baseline fetal heart rate Average fetal heart rate during 10 minutes of fetal monitoring

baseline variability Changes in the fetal heart rate (away from the baseline), resulting from interplay between sympathetic and parasympathetic nervous systems

crowning Appearance of vertex (head) at external vaginal opening

deceleration Slowing of fetal heart rate in the baseline or during a contraction (periodic)

fetal bradycardia Baseline fetal heart rate <110 beats/minute during a 10-minute period of continuous monitoring

fetal tachycardia Baseline fetal heart rate >160 beats/minute during 10-minute period of continuous monitoring

hypoxia Deficient amount of oxygen

The second stage of labor begins with complete dilatation of the cervix and ends with delivery of the baby. A vaginal examination is done to confirm the cervix is completely dilated. However, the experienced nurse often suspects dilatation is complete by observing changes in the client's behavior (e.g., involuntary pushing with contractions). The usual duration of second stage labor is approximately 1 hour for the primigravida and ½ hour for the multipara.

Maternal Response to Second Stage Labor
Cardiovascular System

A contraction can obstruct or decrease the blood flow to the uterus. As a contraction increases in frequency and intensity, blood supply to the uterus and the intervillous space decreases correspondingly. During a contraction the blood previously routed to the uterus and the intervillous space remains in the general circulation and causes an increase in peripheral vascular resistance. Increased peripheral vascular resistance in turn increases maternal systolic blood pressure and pulse rate.

Cardiac output increases 30% to 50% during the second stage of labor. During the period of increased intensity and peak (increment and acme) of contractions, cardiac output increases further but decreases as the contraction subsides (decrement) in intensity. Cardiac output peaks at approximately 80% immediately after delivery and then decreases.

Blood Pressure

Since increased cardiac output causes systolic blood pressure to rise during contractions, blood pressure must be assessed midway between contractions. The mother's blood pressure is affected by her position. If she is in the supine position for pushing, there is potential for compression of the inferior vena cava and aorta. Vena caval compression can precipitate hypotension, and aortic compression (aortocanal hypotension) can cause a 50% decrease in pulse pressure in the lower half of her body. These blood pressure problems can be avoided if the mother uses the upright position or side-lying positions for second stage labor.

Fluid and Electrolyte Balance

During second stage labor the mother is working (laboring) to push the fetus down and out of the birth canal. Response to this hard work is an increase in muscle activity and a rise in the respiratory rate. The end result of increased muscle activity is perspiration, which can deplete the fluid volume. Increased respiratory rate is accompanied by further evaporative water loss caused by the need to warm the inspired air to body temperature. Oral intake is limited to occasional ice chips because of the potential for vomiting and aspiration. Therefore intravenous fluids are given to ensure adequate hydration.

Gastrointestinal System

Gastric motility and absorption are reduced and gastric emptying time is prolonged as a result of hormonal influences during pregnancy.

Respiratory System

During the second stage of labor O_2 consumption increases 100%. Breath-holding during labor decreases maternal and fetal oxygenation; rapid breathing (hyperventilation) causes retention of CO_2. When closed-glottal (complete closure of glottis, allowing no air to escape) pushing is used, the mother is instructed to push for 10 seconds, grab a quick breath, and push again for 10 seconds so there are three 10-second pushes with each contraction. This method of pushing during second stage labor can prevent maternal and fetal acidosis.

Hematopoetic System

Leukocytosis may occur during labor and is attributed to the vigorous muscle activity and stress of labor. It is not unusual for a laboring mother to have a leukocyte level of 25,000/mm.

Renal System

As the presenting part of the fetus descends (as the result of second stage contractions and maternal pushing), it increases pressure on soft tissues, which can decrease blood and lymph drainage from the bladder and lead to edema of the surrounding soft tissues. This condition can result in the mother's inability to void, particularly after delivery.

A full bladder during the second stage of labor can slow descent of the fetus. Performing bladder assessment and emptying by catheter if necessary are important to aid progress of labor and minimize soft-tissue trauma.

Pain

Pain studies have demonstrated the anticipation of pain can increase the anxiety level. Increased anxiety causes the client to react sooner to less pain, and small amounts of pain are perceived as much greater. Furthermore, other sensations such as pressure and stretching may be misinterpreted as pain. This increased perception causes the client to complain that vaginal examinations or touching the abdomen "hurts."

The nurse can help break the cycle of pain anticipation or prevent it from becoming established by intervening at the anticipation-anxiety junction. This is accomplished by reminding the client that a contraction is over and the pain is gone and that since another contraction is not expected for several minutes, there is time to relax and rest. This technique may decrease pain anticipation.

Pain during the first stage of labor is caused by dilatation of the cervix, hypoxia of uterine muscle cells during contractions, stretching of the lower uterine segment, and pressure on adjacent structures. It is felt in the lower abdominal wall and the low lumbar and upper sacral regions.

Factors that affect maternal response to pain include her culture, fatigue, previous pain experience, and anxiety.

⟰ CULTURAL
IMPLICATIONS

In some cultures it is natural to communicate pain; in others, pain is stoically accepted.

Fetal Response to Labor
Biomechanical Effects

As labor progresses and fetal descent occurs, contractions create pressure on the fetal head and may cause partial compression of the umbilical cord. The increasing pressure on the head causes transient **hypoxia,** which stimulates the fetal vagus nerve. It in turn stimulates the parasympathetic nervous system and briefly slows the fetal heart rate (FHR).

Partial cord compression decreases blood flow to the fetus, stimulating the fetal sympathetic nervous system. The response is an increase in FHR.

Both nervous system responses are physiologic and reflect the expected fetal responses.

Hemodynamic Effects

Blood flow to the fetus is temporarily decreased during a uterine contraction. During labor the most important placental functions are the transfer of O_2 and glucose to the fetus and of CO_2 from the fetus to maternal circulation. If the fetus receives insufficient O_2 during labor and accumulates an increased amount of CO_2, metabolic acidosis results (decreased PO_2, increased CO_2, decreased pH).

Fetal Position Change

Certain fetal position changes are necessary for the smallest diameter of the fetal head to pass through the birth canal. The display below and on pages 312 and 313 outlines the mechanisms of labor. Figure 13-1 indicates stations that measure fetal descent through the pelvis.

Mechanisms of Labor in Vertex Presentation

Certain movements are necessary for the smallest diameter of the fetal head to pass through the birth canal.

Engagement: Point at which largest transverse diameter of the head has passed through the pelvic inlet.

Descent: Gradual progressive fetal movement throughout labor; progress is measured by station of fetal head (relationship of vertex to ischial spines).

Flexion: Position with chin flexed and head tipped forward presents smallest head diameter to birth canal, allowing further descent.

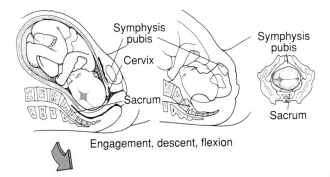

Engagement, descent, flexion

Internal Rotation: Head is turned to side on the diagonal so it can pass under the symphysis pubis (longest diameter of fetal head is aligned with largest diameter of pelvis).

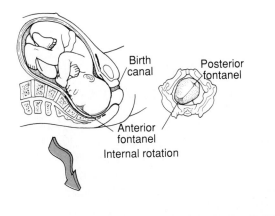

Internal rotation

Continued

Mechanisms of Labor in Vertex Presentation—continued

Extension: Head is pushed forward through vulva (outlet) because it offers
    least resistance.

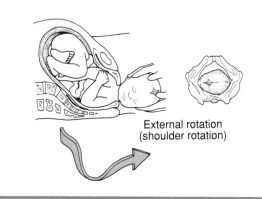

Restitution: Immediately after head is born, it rotates back to original position
    (left occipitotransverse and right occipitotransverse).

FIGURE 13-1

Stations of Fetal Head. Station 0 is the
level of the ischial spines. Above the ischial
spines the measurement is −1 cm to −4
cm. Below the ischial spines the
measurement is +1 cm to +4 cm.

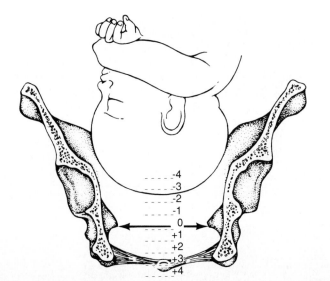

Mechanisms of Labor in Vertex Presentation—continued

External Rotation: Shoulders change from transverse to anterior-posterior position for delivery.

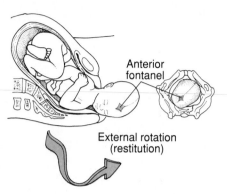

Anterior fontanel

External rotation (restitution)

Expulsion: Delivery of rest of baby.

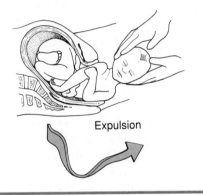

Expulsion

Assessment

Specific signs and symptoms, both behavioral and physical, herald the onset of the second stage of labor (see below). If these signs are overlooked, a precipitous delivery could occur without benefit of appropriate medical attention.

The second stage of labor is shorter and more intense than the first stage. The nurse must be alert for rapidly changing conditions and keenly observe labor progress as delivery time approaches. Both the mother and the fetus must be watched for signs of complications because the potential

Signs and Symptoms Indicating Onset of Second Stage of Labor

- Involuntary bearing down caused by the Ferguson reflex when the presenting part is near or on the perineal floor.
- Sudden increase in bloody show caused by exposure of cervical capillaries as a result of increasing cervical dilatation (and effacement).
- Rupture of membranes, which may occur at any time but occurs frequently at the beginning of the second stage.
- Urge to defecate, caused by pressure of the presenting part against the rectum.
- Bulging of perineum and dilatation of anal orifice.
- Increased apprehension and irritability or relief and elation at being able to push to shorten time of delivery.

for complications increases during this time. Signs of complications include the following:

- Bleeding
- Hypertonus (loss of uterine resting tone)
- Precipitous delivery
- Fetal distress

When the cervix is completely dilated, the nurse assesses the client's urge to push during a contraction. If there is no urge to push, the presenting part is at 0 station or above (see Fig. 13-1). When the presenting part is in this position, there is no pressure or triggering of the Ferguson reflex; thus, there is no urge to push and often no descent of the fetal presenting part.

Previously physicians believed the second stage of labor should be rushed by forced pushing so that delivery would occur within 2 hours. Presently, fetal assessment has improved with the use of electronic FHR monitoring, and the natural duration of second stage labor is no longer associated with an increased mortality and morbidity.

Uterine Activity and Fetal Heart Monitoring

Noninvasive (external) and invasive (internal) methods are available for monitoring uterine activity and FHR. FHR can be monitored using an ultrasound transducer, and contractions can be either manually palpated or electronically recorded using a tocotransducer (Table 13-1). These are noninvasive means of monitoring. Invasive methods use a fetal scalp electrode to monitor FHR and a pressure-sensing catheter inserted between the fetal head and uterine wall to monitor contraction activity.

During labor FHR is assessed continuously when electronic monitoring is used. Electronic monitoring can detect nonreassuring FHR patterns early so interventions can be initiated. If a fetoscope is used, FHR is assessed every 15 minutes during second stage labor for low-risk clients, and the FHR is observed for significant changes. Subtle changes cannot be detected with fetoscope.

Uterine contractions are assessed for frequency, duration, intensity, resting tonus, and resting phase (Fig. 13-2).

TABLE 13-1

Characteristics of Uterine Contractions During Second Stage

Frequency	Duration	Intensity	Uterine Tonus	Shape of Contractions
3-3½ min	60-75 sec	Internal monitor: 40-60 mm Hg intrauterine pressure	Internal monitor: average 8-12 mm Hg; >15-20 mm Hg is hypertonus	Bell shaped
		External monitor: palpation of contraction at peak by nurse—fundus firm; client pushing with contractions	External monitor: fundus palpation by nurse between contractions to ensure it is relaxed	

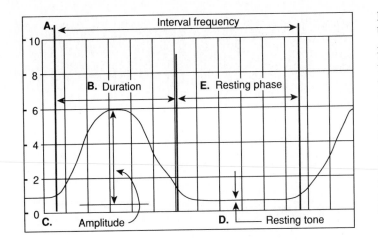

FIGURE 13-2

Uterine Activity Monitoring.
A, Frequency of contractions: from the beginning of one contraction to the beginning of the next. *B,* Duration: from the start to the end of a contraction. *C,* Amplitude: strength, (intensity), of a contraction measured by palpating with the hand or in mm Hg with intrauterine pressure monitoring. *D,* Resting tone should be complete between contractions. (Average resting tone is 8 to 12 mm Hg of intrauterine pressure.) *E,* Resting phase: time between contractions when uterine muscle relaxed resulting in maximum uteroplacental blood flow.

Manual Contraction Palpation

If a uterine monitor is not being used, contractions can be palpated with the hand. The nurse keeps her fingers lightly on the fundus. Using the fingers is recommended because they are more sensitive than the palm. However, for some nurses using the whole hand (palm and fingers) is helpful. Finger contact with the abdomen must be adequate because insufficient contact results in inaccurate timing of contractions.

External Monitoring (Noninvasive)

Both the FHR and uterine contraction activity can be externally monitored. An ultrasound transducer (Fig. 13-3) to monitor FHR is secured on the mother's abdomen after Leopold's maneuvers indicate which site is most conducive for receiving FHR signals. Sound waves are bounced off the fetal heart, and when properly positioned, the transducer receives signals indicating movements of the fetal heart chambers. These signals

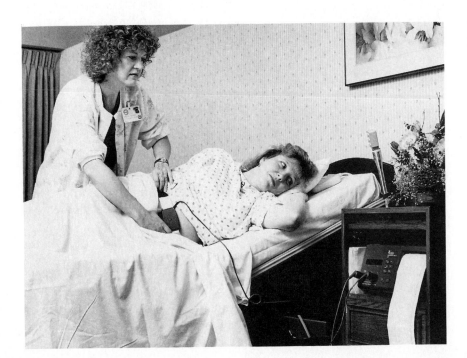

FIGURE 13-3

Electronic Fetal Monitoring. External electronic fetal monitoring can be done using either the ultrasound transducer or the tocotransducer or both. The ultrasound transducer records fetal heart rate. The tocotransducer records uterine activity.
Courtesy St. Elizabeth's Medical Center, Edgewood, Kentucky.

FIGURE 13-4

Electronic Monitor. A, Monitor displays a digital readout of the fetal heart rate (FHR) and a continuous graphic tracing of the FHR pattern and contraction pattern. **B,** The top line of the tracing shows the FHR pattern in beats per minute. The bottom line shows the uterine contraction pattern as determined by measuring the extrauterine pressure in mm Hg when an intrauterine pressure catheter is used. Having both tracings allows observation of changes in FHR in response to uterine activity.

Courtesy St. Elizabeth's Medical Center, Edgewood, Kentucky.

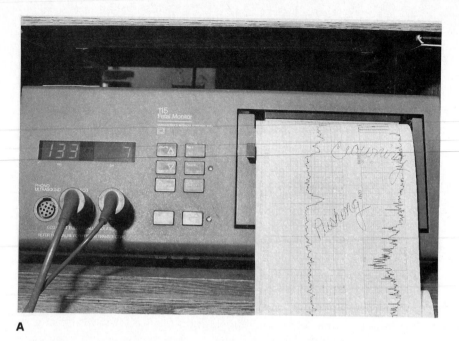

A

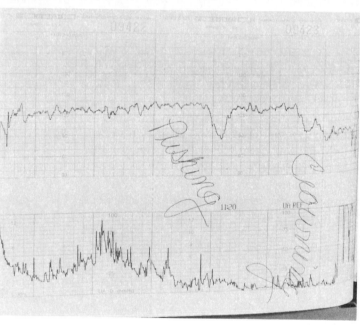

B

are printed on monitor paper and appear on a digital display that is part of the monitoring equipment (Fig. 13-4).

Uterine activity can be monitored externally using a tocotransducer (*toco* is Greek for contraction). This pressure-sensitive instrument records uterine activity as the uterus contracts and presses against the instrument. The changes in pressure produce a pattern that is also printed on monitor paper. Contraction frequency, duration, and shape can be recorded with this device, but contraction intensity and resting tone cannot be recorded accurately because of inability to apply the securing belt tightly to the abdomen (it is uncomfortable for the client), the amount of subcutaneous tissue present, and the position of the mother. Contraction intensity and uterine resting tone must be assessed by manual palpation.

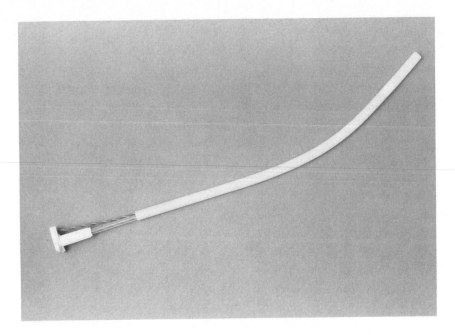

FIGURE 13-5
Spiral Electrode.
for invasive monitoring of the FHR and is the most accurate of the invasive monitoring methods.
Courtesy St. Elizabeth's Medical Center, Edgewood, Kentucky.

Internal Monitoring (Invasive)

After the membranes have ruptured or have been artificially ruptured, a vaginal examination is performed to determine dilatation, effacement, station, and position of the presenting part. If the cervix is 1 cm dilated, a spiral electrode can be attached to a fetal bony prominence to record FHR directly (Fig. 13-5). The electrode is attached by inserting it under the skin of the fetal presenting part (caput, hip, or sacrum). The attached electrode directly conveys the electrical activity of the fetal heart. This method of direct fetal heart monitoring is more exact than the noninvasive ultrasound method.

Contraction data is obtained through a pressure-sensing catheter placed inside the uterine cavity. The catheter is inserted through the dilated cervix alongside the fetus into the body of the uterus to record intrauterine pressure. This device continuously records uterine contraction strength and resting tonus (Fig. 13-6).

When an electronic fetal heart monitor is applied, the nurse can assess three parameters of the FHR: baseline rate, periodic changes, and variability.

BASELINE FHR. **Baseline FHR** is obtained by assessing a 10-minute FHR tracing to determine the one number that occurs most often. At 40 weeks the average FHR is 140 beats/minute.

PERIODIC FHR CHANGES. The second parameter assessed is periodic FHR changes. The FHR occuring during contractions is monitored to note any accelerations or decelerations (see display on p. 318). Periodic FHR **decelerations (bradycardia)** and accelerations **(tachycardia)** from the baseline average may occur in response to uterine contractions.

The four periodic fetal heart responses to contractions of the uterus are acceleration, early deceleration, variable deceleration, and late deceleration.

FIGURE 13-6

Pressure-Sensing Catheter. This invasive monitoring device assists in detecting hypertonic labor or hypotonic uterine dysfunction by recording the contraction amplitude.

Courtesy St. Elizabeth's Medical Center, Edgewood, Kentucky.

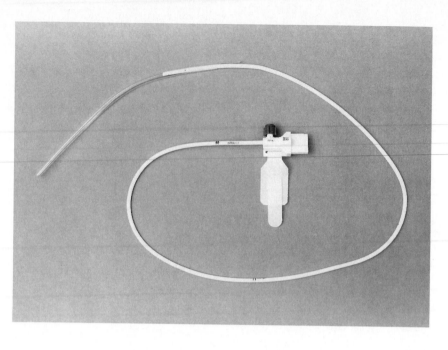

Periodic Fetal Heart Rate Changes

Accelerations: Caused by umbilical vein compression
Early decelerations: Caused by fetal head compression
Late decelerations: Caused by uteroplacental insufficiency
Variable decelerations: Caused by complete cord compression

Acceleration. When the fetal trunk or the umbilical vein (partial cord compression) are compressed, the fetus becomes mildly hypoxic as a result of decreased blood and oxygen to the fetal heart. These accelerations are seen as a sign of health, reflecting an appropriate response to the mild hypoxia.

Early deceleration. Contractions occuring during the end of labor can result in increasing pressure on the fetal head as it passes through the completely dilated cervix or is pushed against a tight perineal floor. This fetal head pressure produces an early deceleration in the FHR (see display below).

Physiology of Variable Deceleration

Pressure on cord
↓
Compression of umbilical vein and arteries
↓
Stimulatation of vagus nerve
↓
Abrupt drop in FHR

Physiology of Early Deceleration

Pressure on head increases intracranial pressure
↓
Decreases cerebral blood flow
↓
Activates central vagus nerve
↓
Produces decrease in FHR with
↓
Recovery occurring as pressure relieved

Variable deceleration. Cord compression causes decreased blood flow and oxygenation to the fetus, resulting in FHR deceleration that are variable in shape. The decreased fetal O_2 flow stimulates the vagus nerve, which in turn causes sudden fetal bradycardia (see display above).

Late deceleration. A uterine contraction slowly decreases flow of blood to the placenta as the contraction increases in intensity. By the peak of the contraction blood flow into the placenta ceases. As long as there is no other underlying pathology and contractions are no closer than 2 minutes apart, the fetus has no problem. However, if pathology exists—either chronic (e.g., pregnancy-induced hypertension) or acute (e.g., too many contractions), blood flow can be significantly interrupted during a contraction, decreasing oxygen flow to the fetus. The fetus could be neurologically damaged or could die during labor. Bradycardia will occur if there is a significant decrease in oxygenation of the fetus (Table 13-2).

Labor can cause stress or distress to the fetus if significant hypoxia occurs. Additional information about assessment of FHR patterns allows recognition of reassuring and nonreassuring FHR signs. A reassuring FHR pattern is as follows:

- Normal and stable FHR baseline (110-160): indicates no bradycardia or tachycardia
- No specific decelerations (lates or variables)
- Normal variability: 5-15 beats/minute (long term with external monitor); 6-15 beats/minute (short term with internal monitor)
- Spontaneous accelerations of FHR in baseline or with contractions ($\geq$5 bpm is indicative of reactivity)

TABLE 13-2

Physiology of Late Decelerations

Acute	Chronic
Uterine hyperactivity or placental separation ↓	True placental dysfunction ↓
Decreased blood flow during contractions ↓	Increasing lack of O_2
Decreased maternal fetal O_2 transfer ↓	
Fetal hypoxia and fetal myocardial depression ↓	↓
Activation of vagal response ↓	Anaerobic metabolism ↓
Late deceleration ←———————	Lactic acidosis

A nonreassuring FHR pattern is as follows:
- Unstable (wandering) FHR baseline
- Persistent tachycardia (>160 beats/minute) or bradycardia (<120 beats/minute)
- Absence of variability
- Late decelerations with decreasing variability
- Severe variable decelerations (drop to 60 beats/minute or less, drop of 60 beats/minute, duration of 60 seconds or more)
- Atypical variable decelerations: loss of initial and secondary accelerations, slow recovery to baseline, return to higher or lower baseline, prolonged secondary acceleration, W-shaped variable
- Deep late decelerations
- Prolonged deceleration or bradycardia
- True sine wave (sinusoidal pattern; sine wave is an oscillating fetal heart pattern ∿∿∿).

Intrauterine resuscitation. When the FHR pattern indicates signs of hypoxia, intrauterine resuscitation should be initiated by the nurse (see Nursing Procedure: Intrauterine Resuscitation).

NURSING
PROCEDURE

Intrauterine Resuscitation

Intervention

1. Change position of mother.

2. Turn off oxytocin if running.

3. Hydrate; begin intravenous infusion or increase rate so approximately 200 ml/15 min will infuse.
4. Administer 6-8 L oxygen through snug face mask.
5. If mother is pushing, encourage her to discontinue pushing until FHR improves.
6. Stimulate the fetus; stimulate scalp or use vibroaccoustic stimulator.

7. If hyperstimulation continues, notify primary care provider.

8. Be prepared to assist with scalp sampling if none of above interventions are effective.
9. Notify primary care provider of all interventions and their effects on the fetal heart.
10. Document interventions on tracing as they are done and summarize in nurses' notes in a timely fashion.

Rationale

1. Relieves pressure on compressed inferior vena cava and aorta and relieves pressure on compressed umbilical cord.
2. Decreased uterine activity may increase uteroplacental circulation.
3. Increases maternal circulatory volume so blood and oxygen are optimally perfusing uterus and placenta.
4. Increases oxygen flow to uterus and placenta.
5. After tracing improved, titrate pushing with FHR reading to ensure best oxygenation.
6. If acceleration occurs, fetus is not decompensated (acidotic); if no acceleration occurs, use chain of command to get physician.
7. Anticipate an order for terbutaline sulfate (Brethine), 0.25 ml.
8. Determines whether acidosis is present based on pH of scalp blood sample.
9. Prepares for emergency delivery or cesarean section.
10. Provides accurate current record of occurrences and interventions.

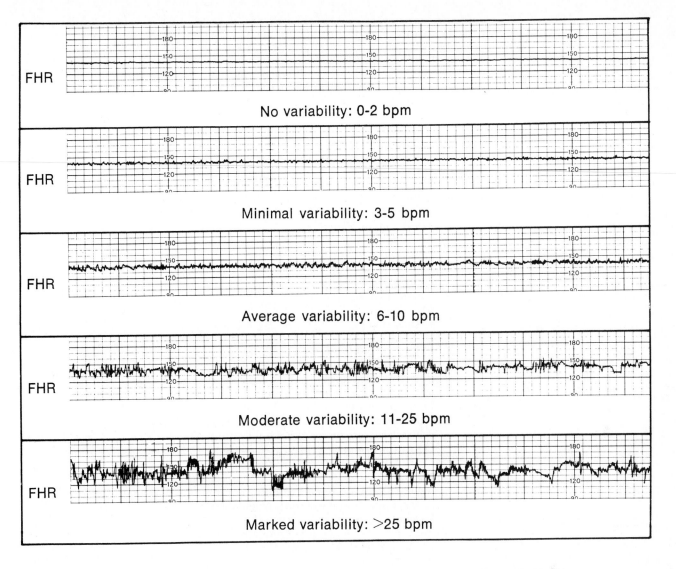

No variability: 0-2 bpm

Minimal variability: 3-5 bpm

Average variability: 6-10 bpm

Moderate variability: 11-25 bpm

Marked variability: >25 bpm

FIGURE 13-7
Fetal Heart Rate Variability. Short- and long-term variability tend to increase and decrease together.

Reproduced with permission of Susan M. Tucker: Fetal Monitoring and Fetal Assessment in High-Risk Pregnancy. St. Louis, CV Mosby, 1978.

VARIABILITY. Finally, variability is assessed. **Baseline variability** represents the range of the FHR occuring above and below the average baseline FHR (Fig. 13-7). The FHR will respond to stimulations and insults but will consistently return to the baseline as long as the fetus is well oxygenated and its central nervous system is intact (see display on p. 322).

Nursing Diagnosis

Potential nursing diagnoses for the second stage of labor are concerned with coping, discomfort, and tissue perfusion (see p. 323).

Planning and Intervention

After the cervix is completely dilated and the fetal head is engaged, the client is asked to push with her contractions to facilitate descent of the fetus.

Clinical Significance of the Fetal Heart Rate

Baseline Fetal Heart Rate (FHR)

Definition: the average FHR when woman is *not* in labor; the average FHR *between* labor contractions (10 min of tracing must be assessed to determine baseline)

Normal FHR: 120–160 beats/min

Tachycardia: >160 beats/min; associated with the following:
  Maternal fever
  Chronic fetal hypoxia
  Fetal immaturity
  Maternal anemia
  Administration of betamimetic drugs for inhibition of preterm labor
  Intrauterine sepsis
  Stress and/or anxiety

Bradycardia: <120 beats/min (more real concern when <100 beats/min; associated with the following:
  Significant interruption of the blood flow carrying O_2 to fetus
  Late fetal hypoxia (terminal event)
  Congenital heart lesions
  Maternal hypotension
  Postdatism

Periodic Change in FHR

Definition: FHR change during the contraction

Early deceleration: begins, peaks, and goes away with contraction shape; associated with the following:
  Increased pressure on head

Late deceleration: uniform; begins at the peak or after the acme of the contraction; associated with the following:
  Decreased maternal-fetal O_2 exchange
  Decreased utero-placental insufficiency
  Maternal hypoxia
  Maternal position (supine), causing compression of inferior vena cava and aorta (may cause maternal hypotension)
  Uterine hyperactivity

Variable deceleration: occurs at any point in the contraction (most common periodic change FHR—an important periodic fetal heart pattern); associated with the following:
  Umbilical cord compression

FHR Variability

Definition: beat-to-beat changes in FHR that vary from the baseline

Short term: beat-to-beat changes occurring within a few heartbeats

Long term: gradual changes in the interval length (range of the FHR over 10 minutes)

Note: Variability has become the most important aspect of the overall clinical evaluation of the fetus in utero.

Many clients are relieved to know that the cervix is finally completely dilated so that they can add their efforts to give birth.

When the cervix is fully dilated, most women cannot resist the urge to push or bear down during a uterine contraction (see Client Self-Care Education: Pushing During Second Stage of Labor). The combined force of the woman's use of her abdominal muscles and the contraction of the uterus helps propel the fetus down the vagina and through the vaginal outlet.

The urge and ability to push occur when the presenting part of the fetus is low enough to trigger the Ferguson reflex. This is a reflex that is

Ineffective Individual Coping—related to physical exhaustion in response to labor

Pain—related to increasing intensity of contractions

Alteration in Tissue Perfusion (utero-placental-fetal)—related to increased frequency, duration, and intensity of contractions

Fear—related to second stage of labor and imminent delivery of the baby (see Nursing Care Plan: Second Stage of Labor.)

Alteration in Cardiac Output—related to compression of inferior vena cava and aorta secondary to supine position of mother

Knowledge Deficit—regarding second stage of labor, pushing, delivery

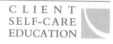

POTENTIAL
NURSING DIAGNOSES

Second Stage of Labor

Pushing During Second Stage of Labor

CLIENT
SELF-CARE
EDUCATION

Intervention	Rationale
1. Examine client to determine if cervix is completely dilated.	1. Pushing should not begin before dilatation is complete.
2. Assist her to achieve position of comfort—more upright (or lateral recumbent).	2. Upright position facilitates descent.
3. Encourage coach to tell client when a contraction is beginning.	3. Prepares client for beginning of contraction.
4. Instruct client to take two or three cleansing breaths until contraction intensity increases.	4. Pushing is more effective nearer acme of contraction.
5. Instruct client to push spontaneously for no longer than 6 sec while emitting grunting or moaning sounds.	5. Gives control to client and negates Valsalva maneuver.
6. Instruct client to rest briefly between pushing efforts (usually takes three breaths or has 2 sec between pushes).	6. Minimizes fall of oxygen tension (PO_2) and rise of carbon dioxide tension (PCO_2).
7. Support client's voluntary pushing efforts.	7. Labor may last longer but also results in fetal, neonatal, and maternal well-being.
8. Assess client for vulvar bulging and for crowning.	8. Indicates imminence of delivery.

initiated when the fetal head presses against and distends the pelvic floor. The urge and ability to push can be eliminated by lack of descent, **analgesia**, or **anesthesia**, thus delaying fetal descent. The nurse uses client positioning to assist with the progress of labor.

Upright positions for second stage labor are more effective than supine positions because gravity aids the descent, aligns the presenting part with the birth canal, and increases the bearing-down reflex. The squatting position is especially helpful in facilitating descent because it enlarges pelvic diameters and increases intraabdominal pressure. However, the position used during labor should be comfortable for the mother. Other positions that can be used during the second stage of labor are upright, squatting, kneeling, and on hands and knees. The nurse works closely with the client to use the best positioning for her and decides with the mother when she should push and how she should push. Each push should last no longer than 6 seconds.

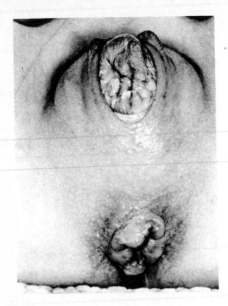

FIGURE 13-8
Perineal Bulging. Extreme bulging of the perineum showing a patulous and inverted anus.

As the second stage of labor progresses, perineal changes occur such as vaginal introitus bulging and anal orifice dilatation (Fig. 13-8). If a fetal scalp electrode is in place, the wire descends as the presenting part descends.

Setting for Delivery

Transfer to the delivery room can be a stressful time for the client. Contributing stress factors include changes in temperature, environment, bed, and nursing staff. Today, maternity centers are changing delivery methods and are using one room (the "LDR room") for labor, delivery, and recovery. This change is called the labor, delivery, recovery concept. In this setting labor, delivery and recovery of both the mother and the infant occur in the same room with the same nurse. This system avoids the need for room transfer and facilitates the family's presence during the entire childbirth process.

Preparation of Delivery Area

The nurse is responsible for preparing the area for delivery (see display on p. 325). The following is a general idea of the equipment and materials used in the typical delivery setting. The delivery bed is designed so that its surface is actually composed of two adjoining sections, each covered with its own mattress (Fig. 13-9). This permits positioning the client in a semi-Fowler's position for delivery. Her legs may or may not be placed in stirrups. The client must be positioned to minimize the risk for compression of the inferior vena cava by the uterus and its contents. A wedge can be placed under the right hip to prevent this compression.

FIGURE 13-9
Deliver Room Bed. To accommodate a range of maternal birthing positions, the standard delivery room bed can be "broken" for use in second stage labor; this position will support the woman in the semisitting position for delivery.
Courtesy Hill-Rom.

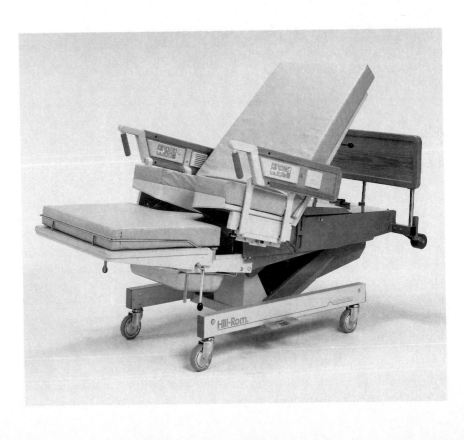

Preparing for Vaginal Delivery

Regardless of the type of delivery system, the nurse makes the necessary preparations for delivery. These preparations include the following:

- Notifying the primary health care provider
- Setting up for the delivery
- Providing a warm environment for the newborn
- Checking to see that infant resuscitation equipment is present and functioning
- Checking that the adult emergency equipment is available
- Preparing for the type of anesthesia the client is requesting
- Assisting the father and other support persons to get ready for the delivery; this may include changing into scrub clothes, washing hands, getting camera or video equipment prepared, and setting out eyeglasses for the client if she needs them for the delivery

Client Preparation

The nurse dons sterile gloves and prepares the client's vulvar area for delivery. The area is cleansed from front to back using a warm antimicrobial solution and is rinsed with warm sterile water (Fig. 13-10). The client is draped and the mirror adjusted so that she can watch the delivery.

To prepare to receive the newborn the nurse washes her hands and sets up the radiant warmer (Fig. 13-11). The infant's bed is turned on, and suction and resuscitation equipment are prepared in case of an emergency.

Asepsis and Antiseptics

Maintaining asepsis and using antiseptics are important during delivery. All hospitals do not use exactly the same techniques. Primary health care providers and nurses do wear scrub clothes and impervious gowns during later labor and delivery. However, caps and masks are worn in some facilities but not in others. It is important to wear a mask or eye protection or both when the mouth, nose, or eyes are at risk of being splashed with body fluids from the mother.

Gloves are worn when it is possible that the hands will be in contact with body substances, i.e., blood, urine, feces, amniotic fluid, bloody show, wound secretions, sputum, or vomitus. Gloves are also worn when

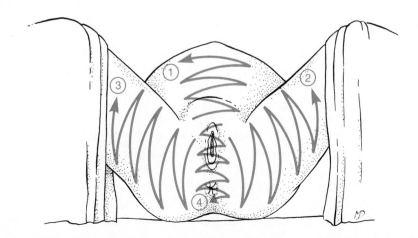

FIGURE 13-10

Perineal Preparation. Recommended method for cleaning the perineum includes (1) using a new sponge for each numbered area; (2) cleaning each area as indicated by the arrow; (3) cleaning rectal area last; (4) rinsing with warm sterile water; and (5) blotting area dry using a sterile towel.

Infant Resuscitation Cart With an Overhead Radiant Warmer for Use in Delivery Room. The overhead radiant heater provides a thermal environment for the infant and allows access to and full visualization of the infant. The lower shelves and metal cabinet to the side of the resuscitation cart are used to store supplies, including equipment and drugs needed in an infant resuscitation.

Courtesy Memorial Medical Center, Long Beach, California.

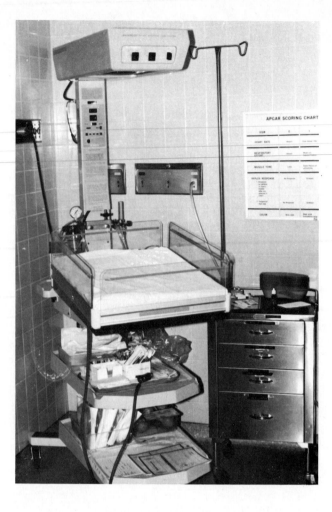

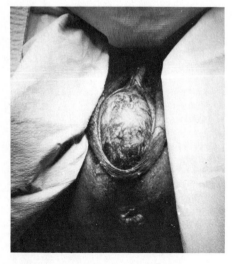

FIGURE 13-12

Crowning. Crowning is encirclement of the largest diameter of the baby's head by the vulvar ring.

handling the newborn after delivery until the initial bath is completed. Bloody linens are handled only when wearing gloves.

Today protection against infection serves a dual purpose. It protects all care providers and support staff as well as the client.

Delivery

As the fetus continues to descend, pressure against the rectum may cause fecal material to be expelled. Moistened sponges are used to keep the area clean.

As soon as the head distends the perineum to a diameter of 6 to 8 cm (Fig. 13-12), the primary health care provider institutes the Ritgen's maneuver (Fig. 13-13). It controls the head to ensure its smallest diameter presents and helps prevent maternal perineal lacerations.

As soon as the infant's head has been delivered, its mouth and nose are suctioned with the bulb syringe to clear the airway (Fig. 13-14). The primary health care provider uses a finger to feel if there is a loop of cord around the neck. If the cord is felt, it is slipped over the neonate's head before delivery resumes. If the cord is too tight to slip over the head, it may be clamped and cut before delivery of the infant's shoulders. Once the cord is cut, the infant must be delivered quickly before asphyxiation results. The anterior shoulder is brought under the symphysis pubis first,

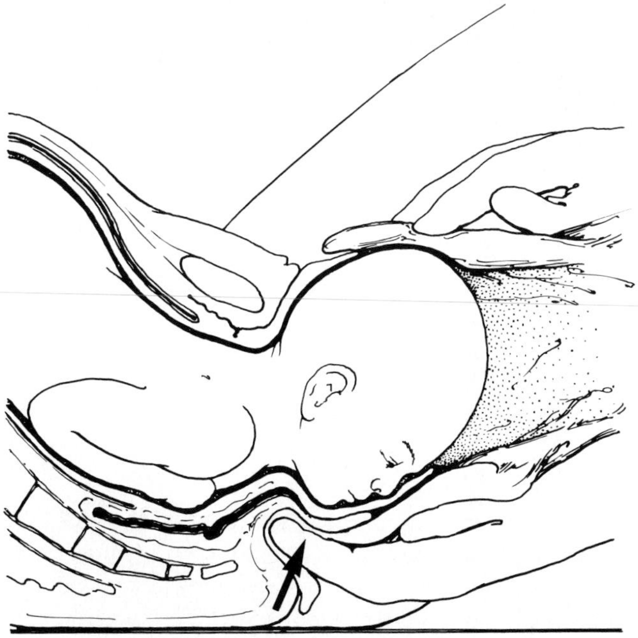

FIGURE 13-13
Ritgen's Maneuver. A towel is placed over the mother's rectum (to prevent contamination of gloved hand), and forward pressure is applied to the chin while downward pressure is applied to the occiput with the other hand. This maneuver provides control of the head and ensures the smallest diameter of the head is presenting.

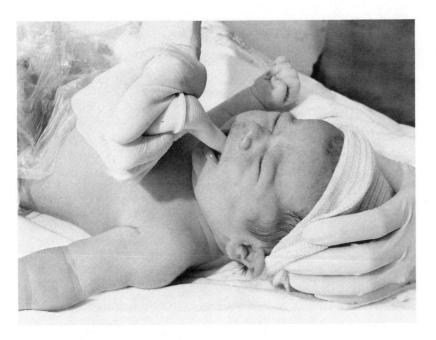

FIGURE 13-14
Procedure for Oropharyngeal or Nasal Suctioning with Bulb Syringe.
(1) Hold bulb syringe tip securely between first and second fingers with thumbs on top of bulb. (2) Compress bulb with the thumbs. (3) Insert syringe tip in the mouth or nostril approximately ½ inch. (4) Remove thumb from bulb so it can reexpand. (5) Remove syringe from nose or mouth. (6) Compress bulb again with tip on tissues to remove secretions from bulb syringe tip. Note: The oral airway is always suctioned first. Suctioning the nares first could cause infant to gasp and aspirate.

and then the posterior shoulder is delivered. The remainder of the body follows (Fig. 13-15).

The nurse notes the exact time of the baby's birth. The infant usually cries immediately, and the lungs expand. Pulsations in the umbilical cord begin to diminish.

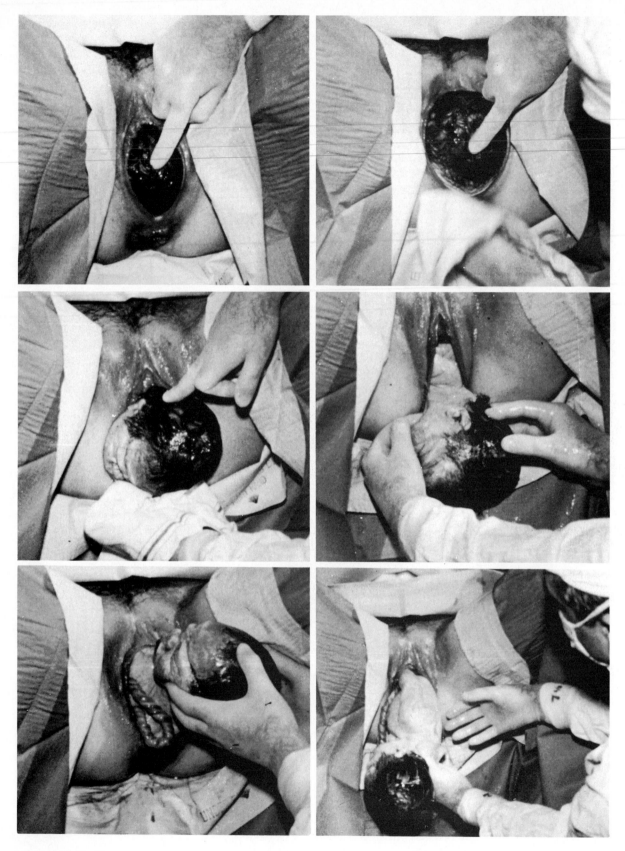

FIGURE 13-15
Normal Birth Process.

From the film Human Birth. Philadelphia, JB
Lippincott.

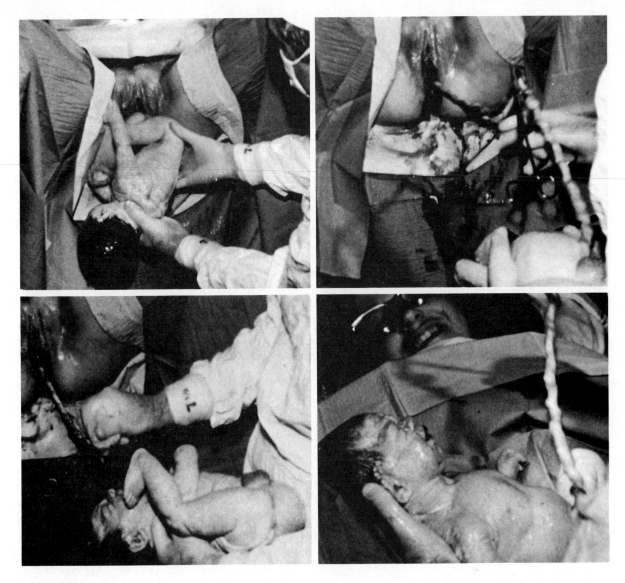

FIGURE 13-15
Normal Birth Process—continued

Clamping the Cord

Within 30 to 60 seconds after delivery the newborn is held on the same
level as the placenta, and a No. 1 Kelly clamp and a cord clamp are used
to clamp the umbilical cord. Figure 13-16 shows a cord clamp, and Figure
13-17 demonstrates its application. This procedure prevents transfusion
from the placenta, which would increase the infant's red blood cell count,
and transfusion to the placenta, which would decrease the infant's red
blood cell count, causing anemia and, potentially, hypovolemic shock.
The primary health care provider may cut the cord or give the scissors
to the father and instruct him to cut between the two clamps.

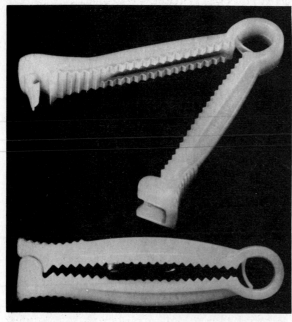

FIGURE 13-16
Umbilical Cord Clamp. A double-grip cord clamp is shown in the opened and closed positions.
Courtesy Hollister, Inc., Chicago, Illinois.

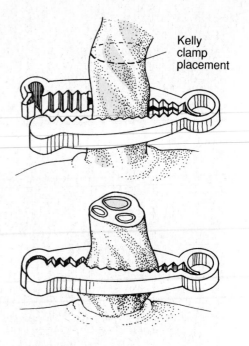

Kelly clamp placement

FIGURE 13-17
Cord Clamping. The umbilical cord is cut between two Kelly clamps that have been placed a few inches from the umbilicus.

Psychosocial Considerations

After delivery the infant is placed on the mother's abdomen. The mother and father are told to touch and handle the infant so the family can share this momentous time. It is important to dry the infant and wrap it in warm blankets to minimize heat loss from evaporation. The infant can continue to bond with the family as long as respirations are regular and easy (rate of 40 to 50), the heart rate is >100 beats/min, and the infant is centrally pink.

Evaluation

Detailed evaluation is noted in Nursing Care Plan: Second Stage of Labor.

NURSING
CARE
PLAN

Second Stage of Labor

Goals (Expected Outcomes)	Interventions	Rationale	Evaluation
Ineffective Individual Coping—Related to Physical Exhaustion in Response to Labor			
Client will proceed through second stage of labor with minimum exhaustion and will feel she has done a good job.	Promote relaxation and rest between contractions.	Conserves strength and decreases exhaustion.	Client is rested and relaxed between contractions.
	Provide quiet environment.	Promotes maximum rest.	Same as above.
	Encourage active participation of support system.	Enhances their working effectiveness and team effort.	Client and support person state they feel good about their team effort.
	Praise client's pushing efforts.	Promotes continued pushing efforts.	Client verbalizes positions she prefers for pushing.
	Praise support person for doing good coaching.	Increases feelings of worth and helping.	
	Suggest alternative positions for pushing (upright, squatting, knee chest, lateral recumbent).	Increases alignment of fetus to pelvis; uses forces of gravity.	Client states she has increased urge to push; pushing feels more effective.
	Assist in promoting constructive behaviors.	Helps client feel positive about her role (clients need firm, but kind coaching).	Client is pleased with her behavior during labor.
Pain—Related to Increasing Intensity of Contractions			
Client will understand the alterations available for pain control and make decisions to manage her pain or discomfort.	Assess response to pain; give encouragement and suggestions to help cope.	Accents the positive and helps client cope.	Client appears in control and uses suggestions.
	Review tools that provide most help to client: deep ventilation before and after contraction; use of breathing technique and pushing with contractions; short pushes rather than sustained ones; relaxation between contractions.	Assists client's remembering the tools (using familiar tools may be helpful).	Client uses tools that help the most.
	Continue coaching to push.	Increases descent.	Fetus is descending 1 cm/hr primigravida, 2 cm/hr multipara.
	Monitor maternal and fetal vital signs with every contraction during push and after contraction.	More potential for problems as labor progresses.	Client has normal vital signs; fetus has normal baseline FHR and no decelerations.
	Assist with positioning for induction of anesthesia.	Difficult to curl around baby with close, hard contractions.	Anesthesia was given with no difficulty.
	Continue helping to coach during pushing.	Ensures client and fetus are OK.	Client's vital signs are normal; fetus has normal baseline FHR and no decelerations.

Continued

NURSING
CARE
PLAN

Second Stage of Labor—*continued*

Goals (Expected Outcomes)	Interventions	Rationale	Evaluation
Alteration in Perfusion (Utero-Placental-Fetal)—Related to Increased Frequency, Duration, Intensity of Contractions			
Client and fetus will progress through second stage without problems.	Maintain client's upright, or side-lying position.	Maximizes utero-placental fetal blood flow and assists with normal contraction pattern.	Client maintains appropriate positions.
	Coach pushing efforts: no closed glottis pushing; no push greater than 6 sec.	Maintains normal maternal acid-base balance.	Client and fetus are well oxygenated.
	Assess maternal vital signs and FHR.	Assesses maternal and fetal well-being and recognizes if problems occur.	Client's vital signs are normal; fetus has reassuring FHR pattern.
	Record on strip and chart every intervention, client's response, presence or absence of pain, fetal responses.	Provides legal record of nursing assessment and interventions.	All documentation is complete and up-to-date.
Fear—Related to Second Stage of Labor and Imminent Delivery of the Fetus			
Couple will fulfill birth plan through constant support for and confidence in their abilities.	Explain what is happening as it happens.	Helps dispel fear and increases understanding; promotes compliance.	Couple verbalizes understanding of pushing and delivery and appears more relaxed.
	Continuously encourage and reinforce couple's efforts and coping strategies and keep them informed of progress.	Perpetuates the positive efforts; gives positive strokes.	Couple participates, is effectively compliant, and is pleased with their experience.
	Provide environment conducive to couple's work. Ask what will make environment more comfortable.	Enables couple to work and cope their best.	Couple participates effectively.
	Encourage client to push according to perceived urge; add tips that will enhance the pushing.	Allows mother to push when it feels most effective and natural for her to do so; nurse's tips assist.	Fetus descends progressively.
	Notify anesthesiologist and primary care giver when delivery is imminent.	Ensures appropriate medical assistance available for delivery.	Delivery occurs with no problems.
	Prepare for delivery.	Ensures enough time for setting up so that everything needed is available and working.	All delivery equipment is prepared in time for safe, expeditious delivery.

SUGGESTED READINGS

Bean CA: Methods of Childbirth. New York, Dolphin Books, 1982

Bing E: Six Practical Lessons for Easier Childbirth. New York, Grosset & Dunlap, 1982

Bowes WA: Clinical aspects of normal and abnormal labor. In Creasy RK, Resnik R (eds): Maternal-Fetal Medicine: Principles and Practice. Philadelphia, WB Saunders, 1989

Chez BF, Verklan MT: Documentation and electronic fetal monitoring: How, where and what? J Perinat Neonatal Nurs July, 1987

Cunningham FG, MacDonald PC, Gant NF: Williams' Obstetrics. Norwalk, Conn, Appleton & Lange, 1989

Fenwick L, Simkin P: Maternal positioning to prevent or alleviate dystocia in labor. Clin Obstet Gynecol 30:1, March 1987

Grossman SZ, Spence JB: The nature of lawsuits related to obstetric care. In Knuppel RA, Drukker JE (eds): High Risk Pregnancy: A Team Approach. Philadelphia, WB Saunders, 1986

Gulanick M, Klopp A, Galanes S: Nursing Care Plans: Nursing Diagnosis and Intervention. St. Louis, CV Mosby, 1986

Hanson-Smith B: Nursing Care Planning Guide for Childbearing Families. Baltimore, Williams & Wilkins, 1989

Ho EH: An introduction to fetal heart rate monitoring, Post Graduate Division, Los Angeles, University of Southern California, School of Medicine, 1975

Howe CL: Physiologic and psychosocial assessment in labor. Nurs Clin North Am 17(1):49-56, March, 1982

Kilpatric SJ, Laros RK: Characteristics of normal labor. Obstet Gynecol 74:1, July 1989

Kintz DL: Nursing support in labor. JOGN, March/April, 1987, pp 203-208

Malinowski JS, Pedigo CG, Phillips CR: Nursing Care During the Labor Process. Philadelphia, FA Davis, 1989

Murray M: Essentials of Fetal Monitoring: Antepartal and Intrapartal Monitoring. NAACOG, 1989

NAACOG: Stagement: Nurses' responsibilities in Implementing Intrapartum Fetal Heart Rate Monitoring. October 1988

Nelson JD: Clinical Manual of Maternity Nursing. Philadelphia, JB Lippincott, 1987

Petrie RH, Williams AM: Labor. In Knuppel RA, Drukker J (eds): High Risk Pregnancy: A Team Approach. Philadelphia, WB Saunders, 1986

Roberts J, van Lier D: Debate: Which position for the second stage. Childbirth Educator/Spring, 1984

Rossi MA, Lindell SG: Maternal positions and pushing techniques in a nonprescriptive environment. JOGN, May/June, 1986, pp 203-208

Russell KP: The course and conduct of normal labor and delivery. In Pernall ML, Benson RC (eds): Current obstetrics and gynecologic disorders. New York, Appleton & Lange, 1987

Varney H: Nurse-Midwifery. Boston, Blackwell Scientific, 1987

Zlatnik FJ: Normal labor and delivery and its conduct. In Scot JR et al (eds): Danforth's Obstetrics and Gynecology. Philadelphia, JB Lippincott, 1990

Operative Obstetrics

IMPORTANT TERMINOLOGY

amniotomy Artificial rupture of the amniotic membranes or bag of waters

breech birth Birth in which the buttocks or feet present first

cesarean section delivery Extraction of the fetus, placenta, and membranes through an abdominal incision

external version Abdominal manipulation of the fetus to alter position from breech or transverse to cephalic presentation

forceps Two-bladed instrument used to facilitate delivery of the fetal head after complete dilatation of the cervix

induction of labor Deliberate initiation of uterine contractions before they begin spontaneously

internal version Internal manual turning by grasping the feet (inside the uterus) and converting the fetus into a footling breech position for delivery by extraction

VBAC Vaginal birth after prior cesarean delivery

vacuum extraction Application of a plastic (or metal) cup to the fetal head by creating a vacuum (between the cup and the head) to assist in delivery of the fetus

There are several special procedures that the physician may use to assist the mother in labor and delivery. They come under the heading of operative obstetrics. These include version, induction of labor, the application of forceps or a vacuum extractor, repair of lacerations, and cesarean birth.

Version

Version consists of turning the fetus in the uterus from an undesirable position to a desirable position. There are two types of version, external and internal.

External (Cephalic) Version

When a breech presentation is recognized during the third trimester, an attempt may be made to perform an **external version.** External version

External Version

Intervention

1. Obtain informed consent.

2. Explain the procedure before and during each step.
3. An ultrasound scan is performed.

4. A nonstress test is done.

5. Blood is drawn for Kleihauer-Betke test (to detect fetal red blood cells in maternal circulation).
6. Start intravenous infusion with ritodrine added (0.15 mg/min for 15 minutes prior to version).
7. Inform the mother that no analgesia or anesthesia will be given and she is to inform staff if maneuvers are too painful.

8. An ultrasound scan will be done continuously throughout the version.
9. Repeat Kleihauer-Betke test.

10. Repeat nonstress test.

Rationale

1. Ensures client understanding of the procedure to be done.
2. Minimizes client anxiety and fear.
3. Verifies breech presentation and rules out fetal and uterine abnormalities.

4. Ensures fetal well-being prior to attempting the version.
5. Rules out evidence of fetomaternal transplacental hemorrhage prior to version.

6. Relaxes uterine muscle and prevents contractions and irritability.
7. Allows the mother to cooperate and communicate if procedure is too painful and describe how and where it hurts as turn is being done.
8. Determines fetal well-being and documents the version.

9. If mother is Rh negative and infant is Rh positive, Rh_o D immune globulin (RhoGAM) is given to prevent sensitization.
10. Determines fetal well-being in vertex presentation. No ill effects due to version.

is most successful in multiparous clients with lax abdominal walls than in nulliparous women.

External version is a procedure done to turn the fetus from a breech to vertex (cephalic) presentation. Versions are performed near term (37-42 weeks). Prerequisites for the procedure are (1) breech or footling breech presentation that is not engaged at the pelvic inlet and (2) an adequate amount of amniotic fluid, which assists in turning the fetus (see Client Self-Care Education: External Version). Contraindications for external version include oligohydramnios, placenta previa, premature rupture of membranes, previous uterine surgery, and any high-risk problems with the mother or fetus.

Internal (Podalic) Version

Internal podalic **version** is a rarely performed fetal life-saving procedure used to convert the malpositioned fetus to a breech position for delivery (Fig. 14-1).

When cervical dilatation is complete, the whole hand of the physician is introduced high into the uterus and one or both of the fetus' feet are grasped and pulled downward in the direction of the birth canal. With

FIGURE 14-1

Internal Podalic Version. If the bag of water is still intact, it is ruptured. Physician inserts hand through a completely dilated cervix and grasps feet of fetus. Fetus is turned and delivered (extracted) feet first.

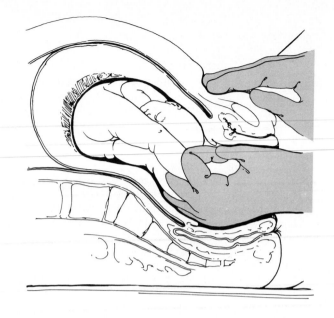

the external hand, the physician may expedite the turning by pushing the head upward. The version is followed by breech extraction.

Internal version is most useful in cases of multiple pregnancy in which the birth of the second twin is delayed or when the second twin is in a transverse lie. It is now almost never used in other circumstances.

Induction of Labor

Induction of labor is an artificial initiation of labor after the period of viability. Induction of labor is indicated when continuation of pregnancy would adversely affect maternal health or when there are conditions that would affect fetal well-being. Complications of pregnancy that may require induction include hypertensive disease of pregnancy, diabetes, hemolytic disease, and postmaturity.

Before induction is attempted the physiologic readiness of both the mother and the fetus are evaluated. Tests of fetal maturity and fetal well-being are usually done before the decision is made to induce labor. Maternal readiness refers to the condition of the cervix and the likelihood that induction will be successful.

There are several numerical scoring systems that assess readiness of the cervix. They are based on the physical characteristics of the cervix as determined by vaginal examination (Table 14-1).

Oxytocin Administration and Monitoring

Overview

Oxytocin is perhaps the most commonly used medication to induce labor. Oxytocin is administered by the intravenous route only and always through an infusion controller or pump that ensures a precise flow rate (Fig. 14-2). When oxytocin stimulation is ordered, the mother must be continuously assessed and monitored during the infusion. Only a phy-

TABLE 14-1

Bishop Method of Pelvic Scoring for Induction of Labor★

| | Points | | |
Examination	1	2	3
Cervical dilatation (cm)	1-2	3-4	5-6
Cervical effacement (%)	40-50	60-70	80
Station of presenting part	−1, −2	0	+1, +2
Consistency of cervix	Medium	Soft	—
Position of cervix	Middle	Anterior	—

Adapted from Bishop EH: Pelvic scoring for elective induction. Obstet Gynecol 24:66, 1964.
★Successful induction of labor is greater when score is 9 or more.

sician who has privileges to perform a cesarean section is permitted to order this procedure.

While the oxytocin is being administered, an electronic fetal monitor and intrauterine pressure monitor must be used to continuously record the fetal heart rate and uterine contractions (see Legal and Ethical Considerations: Oxytocin Administration). The nurse caring for the mother must (1) be familiar with the effects of oxytocin, (2) provide continuous assessment, (3) be prepared to implement emergency interventions based on potential or actual nursing diagnoses, and (4) evaluate and document every change in maternal or fetal status.

LEGAL AND ETHICAL
CONSIDERATIONS

Oxytocin Administration

The American College of Obstetrics and Gynecology recommends the continuous use of electronic fetal monitoring when labor is induced by intravenous oxytocin. Plaintiff's attorneys now equate the failure to use electronic fetal heart rate monitoring with negligence.

From Northrup C, Kelly ME: Legal Issues in Nursing. St. Louis, CV Mosby, 1987.

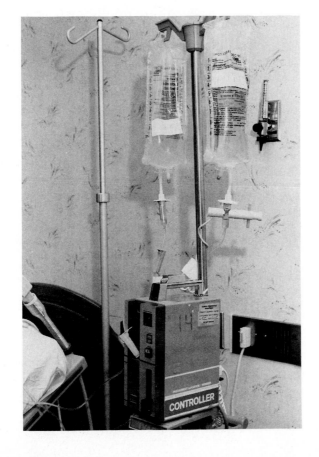

FIGURE 14-2

Oxytocin Infusion for Induction of Labor. Intravenous infusion (primary line) is started by nurse. Second intravenous solution with the prescribed amount of oxytocin added is prepared. IV tubing is inserted into infusion controller or pump and then "piggybacked" into primary infusion line at port nearest needle insertion site. Controller or pump is then set for volume to be infused and controller turned on.

Administration Procedure

The only agent approved for the induction of term labor is oxytocin. Before the procedure can be initiated the fetal heart rate (FHR) is monitored to ensure reactivity indicating well-being of the fetus.

Oxytocin (Pitocin) is always given intravenously and by a controlled infusion device such as an IVAC to precisely control the amount of medication administered. A piggyback setup—two intravenous (IV) lines of the same solution—is prepared, one without oxytocin (primary line) and the second (secondary line) with oxytocin 10 U added. After the primary line is established, the secondary line is attached to the infusion pump and then piggybacked into the primary line through the port closest to the client. When the oxytocin infusion is started, it is administered 0.5 to 1 mU/min and increased in increments of 1 to 2 mU/min every 30 to 60 minutes until a stable contraction pattern has been established.

Ideally a stable contraction pattern will be achieved when the oxytocin is at 4 to 8 mU/min. Seldom is more than 20 to 40 mU required to achieve a progressive dilatation. As soon as a stable contraction pattern is achieved and cervix is dilated 5 to 6 cm, the oxytocin rate can reduced.[1] If frequency of contractions is less than 2 minutes apart or longer than 90 seconds in duration, there is loss of resting tone between contractions, or the FHR tracing indicates stress or distress of the fetus, the oxytocin infusion must be turned off.

Discontinuation Procedure

Interventions required after the discontinuation of oxytocin are increase the mainline infusion, have the mother turn on her side (preferably the left), administer oxygen 6 to 8 L by snug face mask, notify the charge nurse and physician, and then evaluate to determine effectiveness of interventions and document.

Additional assessment includes maternal blood pressure, pulse, and respirations. A vaginal examination is done to assess changes in the cervix, i.e., softening, effacement, and dilatation. It is also important to measure intake and output to ensure proper hydration and to rule out fluid retention caused by the antidiuretic action of oxytocin. The laboring client and her support person are kept informed of progress and measures that can and will be used to assist her to cope with the laboring process.

FHR and Contraction Assessment

When the oxytocin is started, it should be noted on the fetal heart tracing. Also each time the drip rate is increased or stopped it is noted on the tracing.

Before increasing the oxytocin drip rate the nurse assesses maternal contractions and the FHR tracing. Contractions are assessed for frequency, duration, intensity, and uterine resting tone by manually palpating if using an external monitor or noting the pressures recorded on the tracing if using internal monitor (see display on p. 339).

Tips About Contractions (With or Without Use of Oxytocin)

There is a relationship between *frequency* of contractions and *intensity* of contractions.

As contraction *frequency* increases, contraction *intensity* decreases.

OR

As contraction *intensity* increases, contraction *frequency* decreases.

Pharmacologic Response of Uterus to Oxytocin

Contractions should not be more frequent than every 2 minutes and should not last longer than 90 seconds, and resting tone of the uterus should not increase (see below). Assessment of the FHR includes baseline rate and variability and presence or absence of periodic FHR, i.e., no late or variable decelerations (Fig. 14-3). (See Assessment Tool: Oxytocin Infusion: Signs of Hyperstimulation of the Uterus on p. 340.)

Pharmacologic Response of Uterus to Oxytocin

Incremental phase—as oxytocin is increased, uterine activity increases.

Stable phase—uterine activity continues to increase until a stable phase of contractions is established, i.e., frequency, duration, quality, shape, and resting tone. Contraction pattern no longer requires stimulation with oxytocin.

If oxytocin is increased, contractions become too frequent and resting tone of uterus will increase, resulting in tetany.

FIGURE 14-3

Fetal Heart Rate and Uterine Contractions. Monitor tracing for client with oxytocin infusion. Note hyperstimulation. Oxytocin was turned off due to tachycardia, late decelerations.

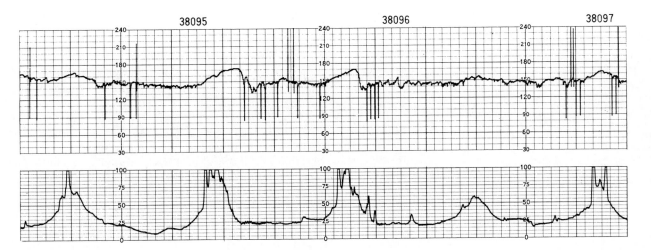

Oxytocin Infusion: Signs of Hyperstimulation of the Uterus

Maternal

1. Contractions occur more frequently than every 2 minutes.
2. Duration of contraction is longer than 90 seconds.
3. Elevation of resting tone of uterus (hypertonus) is greater than 15 to 20 mm Hg by intrauterine pressure catheter. Uterine palpation reveals loss of complete relaxation between contractions.
4. Blood pressure increases when contractions increase in frequency, duration, and intensity because of decrease in uteroplacental circulation.
5. Client experiences increasing pain because of increased frequency, duration, and intensity of contractions.
6. Sustained tetanic contractions occur.

Fetal

1. Tachycardia or bradycardia.
2. Late decelerations, variable decelerations, or prolonged deceleration.
3. Loss of variability.
4. Increased fetal activity due to decreased oxygenation.

Sample Narrative Charting: Contractions are 1½ to 4½ minutes apart, duration 40 to 45 seconds, intensity 50 to 70 mm Hg, and resting tone is 5 to 15 mm Hg. Baseline FHR 155. Decreased long- and short-term variability. Repetitive late decelerations are occurring. Positioned on left side. Pitocin discontinued. Mainline infusion increased. Oxygen started at 8 L/min by face mask. Cervix is 5 to 6 cm, 90% effaced, station is 0. Moderate amount of fresh bloody show. Leaking meconium-stained fluid. Relaxing well between contractions. Husband helping with breathing during contractions. Explained interventions initiated and that physician is coming in to assess situation. Concerned but state they are glad physician is coming.

Potential Side Effects or Complications of Oxytocin

A high concentration of oxytocin can cause hypertension accompanied by a frontal headache, which disappears when the drug is discontinued.

Oxytocin has antidiuretic properties that can lead to water intoxication when used in large amounts. Signs and symptoms of water intoxication include nausea, vomiting, hypotension, tachycardia, and cardiac arrhythmia. This risk can be decreased by using an electrolyte solution for the oxytocin infusion and by avoiding infusion of a large volume of fluid.

Nursing Interventions

Since the nurse is with the couple continuously during oxytocin stimulation, a good rapport can be quickly established. Minute-to-minute explanations and reassurance are provided. The nurse provides assistance with relaxation, breathing (if it is a useful tool), and changes in position that can improve the contraction pattern, increase uteroplacental perfusion, and improve fetal oxygenation.

The nurse must also be familiar with indications for induction or augmentation of labor (Table 14-2), oxytocin drug information (see Drug Guide on p. 342), and the procedure for preparing and administering an oxytocin infusion (see Nursing Procedure on pp. 344–345).

TABLE 14-2

Some Indications and Contraindications for Induction of Labor

Indications	Contraindications
Pregnancy-induced hypertension	Placenta previa
Premature rupture of membranes	Abnormal fetal presentation
Choriamnionitis	Cord presentation
Suspected fetal jeopardy as evidenced by biochemical or biophysical indications, e.g., fetal growth retardation, postterm gestation, isoimmunization	Presenting part above the pelvic inlet
	Prior classic uterine incision
	Active genital herpes infection
Maternal medical problems, e.g., diabetes mellitus, renal disease, chronic obstructive pulmonary disease	Pelvic structural deformities
	Invasive cervical carcinoma
Fetal demise	
Logistic factors, e.g., risk of rapid labor, distance from hospital	
Postterm gestation	

From NAACOG: The nurse's role in induction/augmentation of labor. OGN Nurs Pract Resource, January 1988.

Cervical Ripening Agents

Currently no cervical ripening agents have been approved for use by the U.S. Food and Drug Administration. However, investigation of prostaglandin E_2 (PGE_2) gel and laminaria tents have shown promise as ripening agents.

Prostaglandins

The uterus is sensitive to the uterotonic effects of PGE_2 and PGF_{2a} before, during, and after pregnancy. Prostaglandins in the form of a suppository or gel ripen the cervix so induction of labor using oxytocin is more likely to succeed.

Laminaria Tents

Laminaria tents are used to ripen the unfavorable cervix prior to induced abortion or induction of labor. *Laminaria digitata* is a specific type of seaweed that is dried and sterilized. When inserted in the cervical os, the smooth, rounded stem absorbs moisture and swells to three to five times its original diameter. Insertion of the laminaria the night before induction is planned usually causes gradual softening, and dilatation of the cervix begins by morning. Induction by **amniotomy** or intravenous oxytocin infusion can then be instituted with an increased chance of success.

Nonpharmacologic Methods of Labor Induction

Enema

If the client's cervix is ready (ripe) for labor, an enema may be enough to start labor. The stimulation of the enema solution on the intestines

Oxytocin (Pitocin): Synthetic hormone that stimulates rhythmic contractions of the uterine muscle. The onset of action is immediate. When properly administered, oxytocin should stimulate contractions comparable to those seen in normal spontaneous labor.

Obstetric Action: Exerts a selective stimulatory effect on the smooth muscle of the uterus and of the blood vessels. It affects the myometrial cells by increasing the excitability of the muscle cell, which increases the strength of the muscle contraction and supports propagation of the contraction, i.e., movement of the contraction from one myometrial cell to the next.

Uterine sensitivity to oxytocin increases gradually as gestation continues toward term and increases sharply before parturition. Oxytocin is used for the initiation or improvement of uterine contractions for clients with medical indications, when birth is in the best interest of both mother and fetus, for uterine inertia, for afterbirth of the placenta, to control postpartum hemorrhage, and in inevitable or incomplete abortion.

Administration for Induction or Augmentation of Labor: Average dosage is usually 10 U (1 ml) added to 1000 ml of IV electrolyte solution delivered to the mainline through a secondary line.

Maternal Contraindications: Hypersensitivity, significant cephalopelvic disproportion, prolonged use in uterine inertia or severe toxemia, abnormal fetal presentation or position, where surgical interventions are favored for the maternal client and fetus, elective induction, prior classic cesarean section; active genital herpes, rigid unripe cervix, presence of fetal stress and/or distress.

Potential Side Effects and Complications: Hyperstimulation of the uterus results in hypercontractibility, which in turn may cause (1) abruptio placentae; (2) decreased uterine blood flow, which can cause fetal hypoxia; (3) rapid labor and delivery, which can result in lacerations of cervix, vagina, and perineum and uterine atony, fetal trauma; (4) uterine rupture; or (5) water intoxication, i.e., nausea, vomiting, hypotension, tachycardia, or cardiac arrhythmia, if oxytocin is given in electrolyte-free solution.

Nursing Implications:
1. Assess client's medical, prenatal, labor history, and fetal monitor to identify reasons for administration and potential contraindications.
2. Prepare and begin infusion as ordered by physician.
3. Monitor uterine activity before increasing oxytocin infusion for frequency, duration, intensity, and shape of contractions and resting tone of uterus.
4. Assess FHR for tachycardia, bradycardia, late and severe variable decelerations.

Note: If there is excessive uterine activity (contractions closer than 2 minutes and lasting longer than 90 seconds) or a nonreassuring fetal heart tracing, turn the oxytocin infusion OFF, begin intrauterine resuscitation, and notify the physician immediately (see Nursing Procedure: Intrauterine Resuscitation on p. 343).

5. Monitor maternal blood pressure and pulse each time before increasing oxytocin infusion drip rate.
6. Document all maternal and fetal observations on the monitor tracing and in the nurses' notes.
7. Monitor and document intake and output.
8. Be alert for signs of uterine rupture which occurs infrequently, including excruciating pain, cessation of contractions, vaginal hemorrhage (may occur), signs of hypovolemic shock, and loss of FHR.

Note: Oxytocin has an antidiuretic effect; therefore, large volumes of nonelectrolyte solutions are avoided. This eliminates the risk of water intoxication.

---

may cause reflex stimulation to the uterus. However, this method is not often successful.

Artificial Rupture of the Membranes

Amniotomy, or artificial rupture of the membranes, is a common method of enhancing labor, and has been used to induce labor. When the client is near term and the cervix is favorable, amniotomy is almost always followed by labor within a few hours.

The intact membranes serve as a barrier against bacterial invasion. For this reason, delivery should be accomplished expeditiously once this barrier has been eliminated by amniotomy. Many obstetricians now feel that

Intrauterine Resuscitation

The following steps are recorded on the fetal monitor tracing as they are performed:

Intervention	Rationale
1. Turn off oxytocin infusion.	1. Decreases uterine activity.
2. Increase mainline IV.	2. Increases circulatory volume and increases blood flow (containing O_2) to uterus.
3. Change client's position.	3. Left lateral or side-side position keeps fetus off vena cava to ensure maximum uteroplacental circulation and keeps fetus off umbilical cord to maximize umbilical cord blood flow.
4. Start O_2 at 6 to 8L by tight face mask.	4. Increases oxygenation.
5. Reevaluate client's condition.	5. Determines effectiveness of intervention.
6. Report significant findings to physician.	6. Ensures physician is up to date on progress and problems and is alerted to come to hospital when needed.
7. Chart in nurses' notes.	7. Documents events and interventions as they occur.

the procedure should be delayed until after the initiation of good contractions with intravenous oxytocin. Besides the danger of infection, amniotomy also increases the risk of cord prolapse and fetal head compression. Amniotomy is contraindicated when the presenting part is high or there is an abnormal presentation such as breech or transverse lie.

To perform an amniotomy the obstetrician inserts the first two fingers of one hand into the cervix until the membranes are encountered. A long hook, usually an Allis clamp or a plastic Amnihook, is inserted into the vagina and the membranes are simply hooked and torn by the tip of the sharp instrument. The fluid may initially come out with a gush or leak out slowly. Leaking of amniotic fluid from the vagina usually continues throughout labor. The color, odor, and consistency of the amniotic fluid should be noted. It is usually clear and almost odorless, and deviations can indicate problems. For example, brownish and greenish discoloration is a sign that the infant has passed meconium in utero, and a foul odor is a sign of infection.

NURSING PROCESS IN AMNIOTOMY. Assessment is an ongoing part of the nurse's responsibility when an amniotomy is performed. The condition of mother and fetus are assessed before, during, and after the procedure, and any changes are reported to the physician. Possible nursing diagnoses might include potential for infection related to rupture of membranes, pain related to increasing strength of uterine contractions, or anxiety or fear related to an unfamiliar procedure.

Nursing planning and intervention involve preparing the client for the procedure and carrying out the necessary assessments. The nurse should explain the procedure to the client, reassure her that it is no more un-

Preparing and Administering Oxytocin Infusion

Intervention

1. Explain procedure and rationale to client.
2. Apply fetal monitor and monitor the FHR to establish a baseline tracing.
3. Start an electrolytes solution IV infusion, called the primary line.
4. Prepare a second IV (secondary line) and add the prescribed amount of oxytocin (usually 10 U/1000 ml). The IV tubing is inserted into the infusion controller (or pump) and primed to clear air from the line.
5. "Piggyback" the secondary line into the primary line at the port closest to the needle insertion site and then turn on at the prescribed rate of infusion.
6. Turn on oxytocin infusion pump at prescribed rate.
7. Monitor FHR, uterine resting tone, frequency, duration and intensity of contractions, blood pressure, and pulse and record at intervals comparable to the *dosage regimen,* i.e., at 30- to 60-minute intervals, when the dosage is evaluated for maintenance, increase, or decrease. Evidence of maternal and fetal surveillance should be documented. All observations and increases or decreases in oxytocin are documented on the fetal heart tracing and the mother's chart.
8. Once the desired frequency of contractions has been reached and labor has progressed to 5 to 6 cm dilatation, oxytocin may be reduced by similar increments (or as prescribed by physician).

Rationale

1. An informed client is less anxious and fearful.
2. Ensures fetal reactivity.
3. An electrolyte solution minimizes the risk of water intoxication.
4. Oxytocin must be administered with an infusion pump (or controller) to ensure accurate dose administration.
5. The secondary line contains the oxytocin. If there is an indication to stop the oxytocin infusion, it can be done without affecting the infusion of the primary line, and fluid volume can be maintained.
6. No other medications should be given through the oxytocin (secondary) line, since it will be given at prescribed rates and may be turned off if contractions are too close, hypertonus occurs, or the FHR pattern indicates fetal distress.
7. If uterus becomes hyper-stimulated, blood flow to uteroplacental site will be decreased and fetus will suffer from hypoxia.
8. Sensitivity to oxytocin increases as labor progresses. If stable pattern is achieved, need for oxytocin decreases.

Adapted from NAACOG: The nurse's role in the induction/augmentation of labor. OGN Nurs Pract Resource, January 1988.

Preparing and Administering Oxytocin Infusion—continued

Intervention

9. If hyperstimulation of the uterus occurs (less than 2 minutes between contractions and lasting longer than 60 seconds) or a nonreassuring fetal heart rate pattern occurs, the following actions are taken:
   a. Turn off oxytocin infusion
   b. Speed up primary infusion
   c. Change position, may turn to left side
   d. Give oxygen 6 to 8 L/min by face mask
   e. Notify charge nurse (supervisor) and physician STAT
   f. Provide support to parents
   g. Document on monitor strip and client's chart
   h. Document effectiveness of interventions

10. Notify the physician of hypertonic/hyptonic contractions or failure to progress.

11. Continue to assess client's progress, both physically and emotionally (care is for the client, not the monitor).

12. Notify the physician to evaluate client when oxytocin infusion is 10 mU/min.
    Note: A client seldom requires more than 20 to 40 mU/min of oxytocin to achieve progressive cervical dilation; 90% of clients will respond to 16 mU or less.

13. Accurately record fluid intake and output every 2 hours.

Rationale

9. Intrauterine resuscitation is initiated when there is significant interruption of oxygenation due to decrease or cessation of utero-placental perfusion.

10. Clients may vary in their individual responsiveness to oxytocin. Some may require more; some less.

11. Induced or augmented labor is stressful to couple. The nurse is attuned to their responses and intervenes as indicated. They need to know that progress is occurring.

12. Assesses client's response to oxytocin.

13. Ensures proper hydration and to rule out fluid retention due to antidiuretic action of oxytocin.

comfortable than a vaginal examination, and describe the warm, wet sensations that she will probably experience. Expectations for increased strength of uterine contractions should also be explained.

Prior to the procedure the nurse can assist the client in assuming a position on her back with her knees flexed and separated. Antiseptic preparation of the vulva is carried out according to hospital policy. Fetal heart tones should be checked before and immediately after the amniotomy for possible changes indicating prolapse of the cord. They should continue to be checked frequently because of the increased possibility of cord prolapse. The time of the amniotomy and the color, amount, and odor of the fluid should be recorded on the chart. If an electronic fetal monitor is in use, the time of the amniotomy should also be recorded on the graph. The bed linens should be changed as often as necessary to keep the client comfortable.

Breast Stimulation

Breast stimulation is another method used to induce or augment labor. The mother is instructed to stimulate her nipples by rolling and pulling or applying moist heat with a warm moist wash cloth to initiate uterine contractions. It is not clear why this method causes contractions of the uterus.

Mechanical Aids That Assist With Delivery
Forceps Delivery

Obstetric **forceps** are surgical instruments designed to aid in delivering the fetus. Forceps function to provide traction on the fetal head or to rotate the head into a more favorable position.

A forceps delivery is a procedure for extracting the fetal head. Indications for using forceps include those conditions that require a shortened second stage labor either because the mother is unable to push or the fetus is in jeopardy. The mother's inability to push can be due to conduction anesthesia, exhaustion, heart disease, acute pulmonary edema, or infection. Fetal jeopardy is suggested by repetitive late decelerations, severe variable decelerations, tachycardia, prolonged bradycardia, loss of variability, and loss of reactivity.

The following conditions are prerequisites for safe forceps delivery:
- Ruptured membranes
- Complete dilatation of cervix
- Fetal head engaged
- Confirmed vertex or breech fetal positions, adequate inlet, midpelvis, and outlet pelvic measurements
- Adequate regional or general anesthesia

In the vast majority of instances today, the forceps delivery is carried out at a time when the fetal head is on the perineal floor (visible or almost so) and internal rotation may have already occurred, so that the fetal head lies in a direct anteroposterior position (Figs. 14-4 to 14-6). This is called

FIGURE 14-4

Forceps Extraction. Application of blades for forceps occiput anterior outlet delivery.

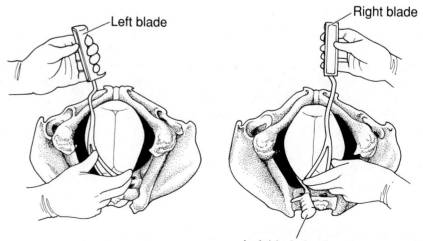

Left blade

Right blade

Left blade in place

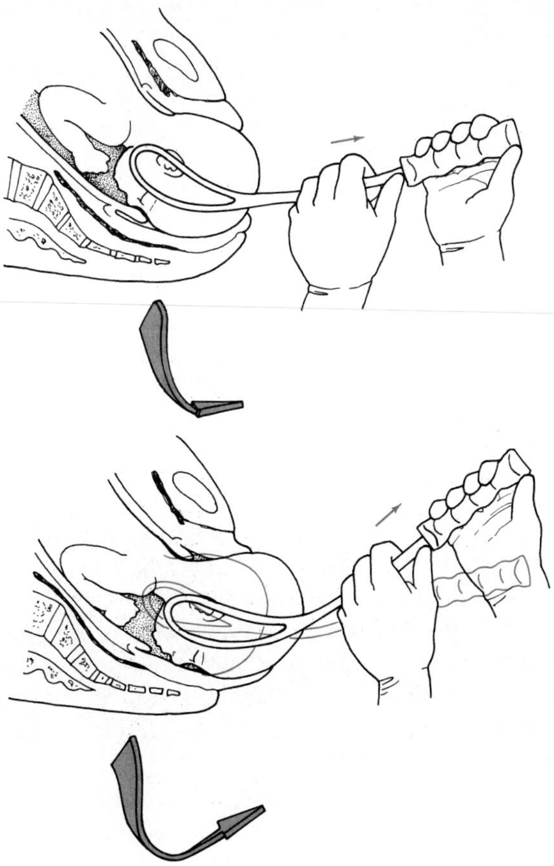

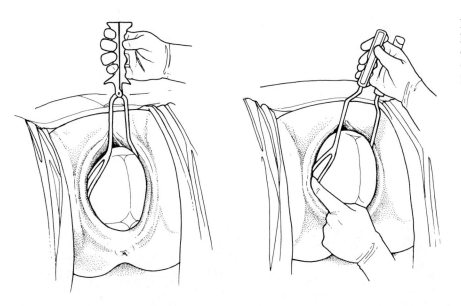

FIGURE 14-5
Forceps Delivery. Gentle downward traction with forceps to produce extension of fetal head (extension is the fourth mechanism of labor) until occiput appears beneath pubic arch.

FIGURE 14-6
Forceps Delivery. When largest diameter of fetal head is encircled in vulvar ring, forceps are removed and head delivered over perineum when extension is complete.

low forceps, or "outlet forceps." When the head is higher in the pelvis but engaged and its greatest diameter has passed the inlet, the operation is called *midforceps*. "Under no circumstances should forceps be applied to an unengaged presenting part or when the cervix is not completely dilated"[2] (see display p. 348).

Disadvantages of Using Forceps

Disadvantages related to maternal and neonatal trauma:

Lateral vaginal tears

Cervical tears

Extension of episiotomy

Uterine rupture

Bladder trauma

Increased risk of uterine atony and vaginal bleeding

Fracture of coccyx

Increased risk for infection

Potential trauma and bruising of neonate's head

Vacuum Extraction

Some physicians use vacuum extractors instead of forceps (Fig. 14-7). The vacuum extractor consists of a cup that is applied to the fetal head and tightly affixed there by creating a vacuum in the cup through withdrawal of the air by a pump. Cups are supplied in various sizes. The largest cup that can be applied with ease is selected for use. Vacuum is built up slowly, and the suction creates an artificial caput within the cup, providing a firm attachment to the fetal scalp. Traction can then be exerted by means of a short chain attached to the cup, with a handle at its far end.

The indications for using the vacuum extractors are the same as for using forceps. The vacuum extractor is more popular in Europe and Asia than in the United States. Previously the most commonly used vacuum extractor (Malmström) was associated with specific scalp and cranial injuries.[3] In 1973 a silastic obstetric vacuum cup was introduced. The University of Texas Health Science Center did a study on the silastic vacuum extractor and found it to be less traumatic than forceps delivery for the mother and as safe as forceps for the infant.

Nursing Care

The nurse should briefly explain the procedure and its necessity to the mother and support person. The mother will feel pressure and pulling sensations but will not feel pain with adequate regional or spinal anesthesia. Breathing techniques to prevent tensing and pushing are encour-

FIGURE 14-7

Vacuum Extraction With Suction Cup Applied to Scalp. Vacuum extraction, used when there is a prolonged first stage of labor, assists the descent of the fetal head through the birth canal. Suction bottle (pump) creates negative pressure (suction) in the cup.

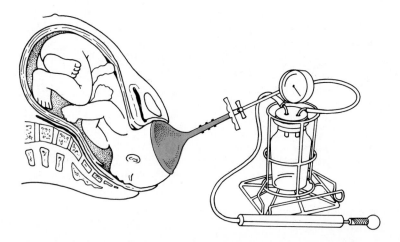

aged during application of the vacuum extraction cup. The mother is kept informed by the nurse during the procedure.

The nurse provides the physician with the vacuum extraction equipment, including the size cup requested and sterile tubing. After the physician assembles the cup and tubing, the nurse attaches the distal end to suction. With the cup applied to the fetal head, the nurse activates the suction. To avoid damaging vaginal tissues, suction must be released if the cup slips off the fetal head. The nurse encourages the mother to push during contractions to aid birth, while traction is applied by the physician.

The fetal heart rate should be monitored frequently by the nurse during the procedure. Infant resuscitation equipment should be available, and the pediatrician should be called if complications are expected with the infant. Parents are informed that the baby's head will have a caput (chignon) where the cup was applied, but that this will disappear in a few hours.

Cesarean Delivery

Definition and Incidence

Cesarean section is the transabdominal delivery of an intrauterine fetus (or fetuses) weighing 500 g or more through an incision made in the abdominal wall and the uterus. The first cesarean delivery performed on a client is a primary cesarean delivery and subsequent ones are referred to as repeat cesarean deliveries. The current indications for cesarean delivery are noted in the display below.

Cesarean delivery rates continue to rise. Of the more than 3.7 million infants born each year in the United States, approximately 24% are delivered by cesarean section.[4]

Types of Cesarean Delivery

There are four types of cesarean delivery: low segment section, classic section, extraperitoneal section, and cesarean section–hysterectomy (Fig. 14-8). The low segment section is the most common. The uterus is entered through a transverse incision in the lowest, thinnest portion of the uterus, resulting in minimal blood loss.

In the classic section a vertical incision is made directly into the wall of the body of the uterus. Because large vessels are present, more blood is lost than with other types of cesarean section. The risk of rupture with subsequent labors is slightly increased.

Current Reasons for Cesarean Delivery

Breech presentation
Macrosmia (fetus greater than 4000 g)
Herpes genitalis
Placental insufficiency
Severe preeclampsia or eclampsia with unripe cervix
Multiple gestation
Failure to progress in labor
Fetal distress as indicated by fetal heart rate pattern, acid base balance
Hydrocephaly

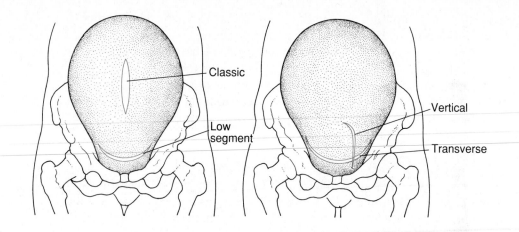

FIGURE 14-8

Types of Cesarean Incisions. *Left,* Low segment section and classic incision section. The low segment type of cesarean delivery is usually the operation of choice and employs a transverse incision into the thinnest part (lower segment) of the uterus. There is minimum blood loss, and the incision is easy to repair. This type of delivery section decreases the potential for both infection and uterine rupture in subsequent pregnancies. The classic incision section type of cesarean delivery employs an incision in the uterine fundus. While rarely used today, the advantage of this type of section delivery is rapid delivery of the infant. However, the disadvantages are far reaching and include increased risk for infection and uterine rupture and greater blood loss during the procedure. *Right,* Extraperitoneal section (vertical or transverse incision). This type of cesarean delivery is rarely done because it technically is very difficult to perform and requires increased anesthesia time. The procedure difficulty is due to the need to dissect the tissues around the bladder to enter the lower uterine segment without entering the peritoneal cavity.

The extraperitoneal section employs either a transverse or vertical incision made low in the uterus. The incision is made into the uterus without entering the peritoneal cavity. This type of delivery prevents pus or infected amniotic fluid from reaching the peritoneal surface.

Cesarean section–hysterectomy includes a hysterectomy after the cesarean delivery.

Operative Overview

After the abdominal cavity has been opened, the initial incision is made transversely across the uterine peritoneum, where it is attached loosely just above the bladder. The lower peritoneal flap and the bladder are now dissected from the uterus, and the uterine muscle is incised either vertically or transversely (Fig. 14-9 *A* through *D*). The membranes are ruptured, and the infant is delivered (Fig. 14-9 *E* through *L*). The placenta is extracted (Fig. 14-10), and intravenous oxytocin (Pitocin) is administered to contract the uterus. The uterine incision is sutured, and the lower flap is imbricated over the uterine incision. This two-flap arrangement seals off the uterine incision and is believed to prevent the egress of infectious lochia into the peritoneal cavity.

Factors Contributing to Increased Cesarean Births

Numerous factors are involved in the rising cesarean rate, and understanding their interrelations and relative importance is a complex task. Standards of obstetric practice in managing certain labor complications contribute significantly to the increased cesarean birth rate. Four diagnostic categories account for about 80% of all cesareans and for 80% to 90% of the rise in the rate: repeat cesareans, dystocia, breech presentation, and fetal distress.

By and large, the increase in the incidence of cesarean birth is attributable to fetal indications. Fetal monitoring has permitted earlier diagnosis of fetal distress, and modern methods for assessment of fetal well-being during the course of pregnancy also provide a basis for early delivery. In the latter circumstances, cesarean delivery is a justifiable substitute for prolonged and difficult medical induction. Cesarean birth is a less traumatic substitute for some previously preferred operative procedures, such as difficult midforceps and vaginal breech delivery in the primigravida or mother in preterm labor, to avoid trauma to the aftercoming head.

The purpose of operative intervention in cases of maternal disease or

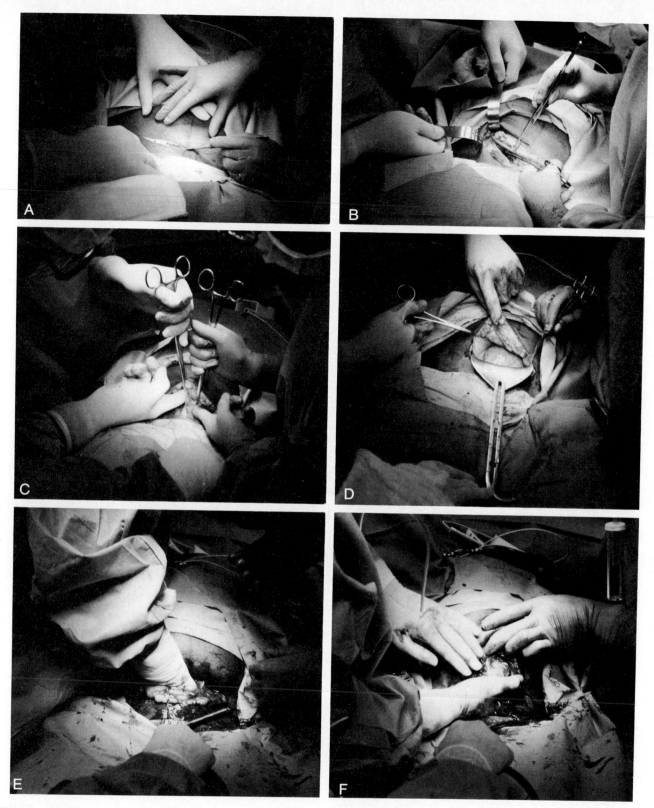

FIGURE 14-9

Cesarean Birth. **A,** Pfannenstiel's incision through skin at start of operation. **B,** Fascia has been nicked at the midline and is being opened in smiling fashion with heavy scissors. **C,** Fascia is separated from underlying rectus muscle in combination of blunt (shown in picture) and sharp dissection. **D,** Peritoneum has been opened (hemostats on edges), and bladder blade has been positioned. Lower uterine segment is visible through incision. **E,** Bladder flap has been created; low transverse uterine incision has been made, and operator's hand is introduced in lower uterine segment to facilitate delivery of fetal head. **F,** Vertex has been brought to site of uterine incision, and operator's right hand is guiding delivery of head. Fundal pressure from right hand of surgical assistant is facilitating process.

Continued

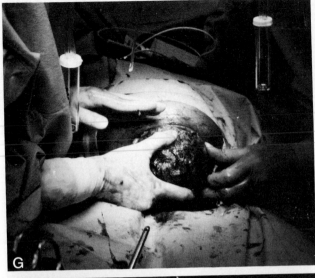

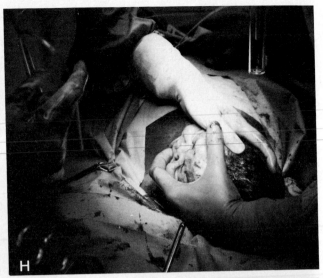

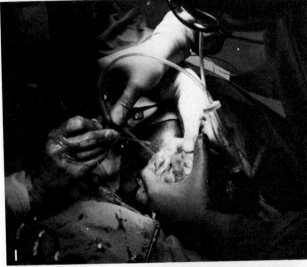

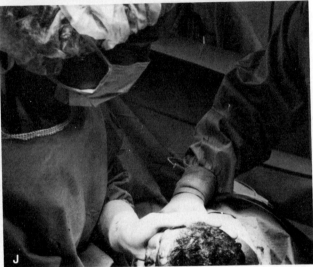

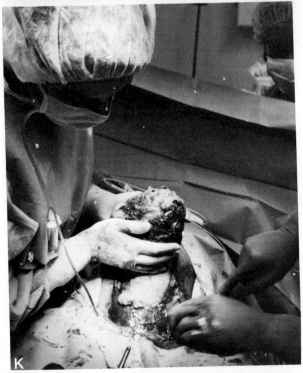

FIGURE 14-9—cont'd
G, Fetal head is gently being delivered through uterine and abdominal incisions. H, Fetal head has been delivered; index finger of assistant is being introduced into infant's mouth to facilitate oropharyngeal suctioning of amniotic fluid and secretions prior to neonate's first breath. I, Nasopharyngeal and oropharyngeal suctioning are being performed by both operator and assistant using DeLee catheters. J, Delivery *first* of posterior shoulder through uterine and abdominal incisions by gentle upward traction. K, Delivery of anterior shoulder by gentle downward traction. L, Neonate has been delivered, and umbilical cord has been clamped with Kelly clamps and cut.

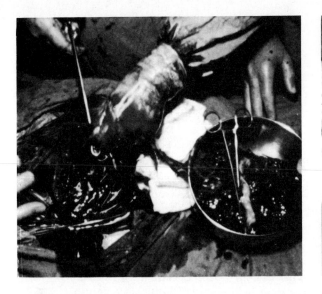

FIGURE 14-10
Placental Extraction. Placenta is extracted through abdominal incision.
From the film, Human Birth, published by JB Lippincott, Philadelphia.

labor complications is to improve the fetal outcome. A virtual explosion of obstetric technology has occurred to assist physicians in monitoring the condition of the fetus and diagnosing the presence of a dangerous situation.

Previous Cesarean Birth

About 98% of women in the United States with a previous cesarean birth had, until recently, operative deliveries with subsequent births. Almost one third of all cesarean births are done for this indication, and it accounts for 25% to 30% of the rise in the cesarean rate. Because of the increasing rate of primary cesareans, this category multiplies the overall rate increase. Increasingly, the client is offered the option of attempting labor and vaginal delivery, especially when the previous cesarean birth occurred for reasons other than cephalopelvic disproportion (CPD).

Dystocia

Dystocia includes such diagnoses as CPD, prolonged labor, uterine dysfunction, and failure to progress in labor. It accounts for 30% of the rise in the cesarean rate, the largest single category for primary operations.

Breech Presentation

It is now generally accepted that the small premature breech does best when delivered by cesarean section, although there is still some controversy due to absence of well-controlled studies. One reason is the concern about hypoxia. Hypoxia might occur during vaginal delivery as a result of cord compression as the small body is delivered through an incompletely dilated cervix. The head can become trapped behind the cervix, which results in trauma and more hypoxia.

Large Fetus

As the weight of the fetus increases, the risk of trauma during vaginal delivery increases. It is recommended that fetuses weighing over 4000 g be delivered by cesarean section.

Fetal Distress

Before introduction of electronic fetal monitoring, fetal distress was diagnosed on the basis of bradycardia or irregularity in the FHR, particularly if there was meconium in the amniotic fluid or a prolapsed cord. Today because electronic fetal monitoring technology readily identifies non-reassuring FHR patterns, there has been an increase in the number of cesarean deliveries performed for fetal distress.

Scalp pH is also used in some hospitals to assist in identifying fetal distress. However, the results of scalp pH can be inaccurate, depending when during a contraction the sample is obtained and the position of the mother while the sample is being obtained.

Medicolegal Factors

Because of the medicolegal climate, obstetricians more readily perform operative deliveries today than in the past. Childbearing families expect to have a perfect infant, and anything less is unacceptable. If a less than perfect infant is born, there is the potential for lawsuit.

Education to Avoid Cesarean Delivery

Women and their partners can benefit from understanding how they can avoid unnecessary cesarean birth. Often a series of occurrences from early pregnancy through the labor process leads to the decision for surgical delivery. Different choices by parents, or different actions in relation to health providers, might lead to a different outcome. Choice of birth attendant, locale for delivery, health practices, level of knowledge about childbearing, and participation in childbirth preparation can all affect the type of delivery (see Client Self-Care Education: Avoiding Unnecessary Cesarean Birth).

Disadvantages of Cesarean Delivery

There are, of course, disadvantages to delivering by cesarean. Maternal mortality and morbidity are involved along with the discomforts occurring following any surgery. Maternal-infant bonding may be affected, including development of mothering skills and breast-feeding (see display p. 356).

Unanticipated Cesarean Delivery

Emergency cesarean deliveries are performed when fetal or maternal complications pose serious risks. Complications may arise at any stage of labor, but often the decision for surgery is made after hours of nonprogressive labor or as a result of abnormal fetal heart monitor tracings. The woman is often discouraged, exhausted, very worried about her own or the infant's condition, and possibly dehydrated with low glycogen reserves. Preoperative preparations usually must be done rapidly, leaving little time for explanations.

The nurse provides short, simple, and very concise explanations of reasons for the surgery and procedures that must be done. It is important that the nurse offer as much reassurance about the mother's and baby's

Avoiding Unnecessary Cesarean Birth

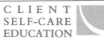

Action

1. Choose birth attendant carefully (nurse-midwife vs. obstetrician vs. family practice physician).
2. Select the birth environment carefully.

3. Become informed about the childbearing process and the available alternatives. Become familar with the pregnancy bill of rights.
4. Attend and actively participate in childbirth education classes.

5. Eat a nutritious diet. Follow recommended weight gain. Exercise every day. Avoid unhealthy practices, e.g., smoking, drinking, or nonprescription drug use.
6. Discuss care provider's philosophy regarding labor, birth, cesarean section, induction or augmentation of labor.
7. Tour hospital and gather information regarding cesarean deliveries and fetal monitoring.

Rationale

1. Ensures the care provider selected is supportive of client's needs and desires for the birth experience.
2. Ensures the setting best suited for chosen style of birth (alternative birth center vs. hospital).
3. There are many choices available. Each client must find what is best suited for them.

4. Increases knowledge and reduces fear. Provides tools for positive management of labor and delivery. Assists mother attain optimum and realistic physical and emotional condition for labor and birth.
5. Maintains general health. Provides optimum environment for fetal growth and development.

6. Determines if philosophies are congruent and birth experience will be positive.

7. Ensures understanding of alternatives for labor, delivery, and post partum.

conditions as can reasonably be given. However, the client's and her partner's anxiety level will be high, and they may not recall much or may misunderstand. After the operation, the nurse should spend time reviewing events leading up to the surgery, what occurred in the operating room, and the newborn's status to allow the parents to understand and integrate their experiences.

Often there is actual grieving over loss of planned childbearing experience, which continues for up to a year after delivery. Follow-up grief counseling by the nurse or a support group is helpful in assisting the mother to resolve her feelings (depression) about the unfulfilled birth experience.

Vaginal Birth After Cesarean Birth

The practice of "once a cesarean always a cesarean" birth has been standard in American obstetrics since 1916, although in Europe vaginal delivery after cesarean birth is not uncommon. Fear of uterine rupture deterred physicians from allowing a woman to deliver vaginally after a cesarean birth in what is called trial of labor or vaginal birth after cesarean (**VBAC**).

Maternal Risks in Cesarean Birth

Maternal mortality, although rare, is four times higher with cesarean delivery than with vaginal delivery. Half of this increased mortality is due to complications leading to the cesarean or to maternal disease. The other half is due to the surgery itself.

Maternal mortality in repeat cesarean is about twice that in vaginal deliveries.

Maternal morbidity is much greater after cesarean; the major risks are from:
Infection of uterus and other genital tract structures
Infection of respiratory or urinary tract
Hemorrhage

Postoperative discomforts occur frequently, including incisional pain, gas, weakness, and difficulty in movement.

Maternal–infant bonding is interfered with through common hospital practices such as:
General anesthesia during surgery
Separation of mother and infant during recovery and first day
Analgesics given the mother for pain relief
Isolation necessary for infections

Development of mothering skills is interfered with because of
Disorientation following anesthesia and surgery
Pain limiting activities and requiring sedation
Weakness, which limits the energy the mother can give to infant caretaking
Postoperative complications further reducing mother–infant contact
Emotional turmoil and the need to process feelings (anger, loss, confusion, fear, inadequacy, etc.) associated with undergoing cesarean birth and operative procedures
Delay and increased difficulty gaining a sense of mastery over the mother's body

Breast-feeding is more difficult or impossible because of
Pain, weakness, limited activities
Infections or other serious complications
Medications that may be excreted in breast milk
Sense of inadequacy related to childbearing capabilities

In 1980 the National Institute of Child Health and Human Development of Childbirth concluded that vaginal delivery after cesarean birth is an appropriate option. It has been suggested that even women who have had more than one prior cesarean delivery can be safely allowed to have a trial of labor. Data reveals there are probably no greater risks for these women than for women who have only had one cesarean section. Note the guidelines for VBAC in the display on page 357.

Preparation for Cesarean Delivery

Cesarean delivery childbirth preparation classes are increasing in number. Some educators feel all childbirth classes should present information about cesarean birth, even when vaginal delivery is anticipated.

Psychoemotional factors are very important for couples experiencing cesarean birth. Many describe feelings of fear, disappointment, frustration over loss of control, grief over losing their ideal birth experience, anger or victimization, or confusion over the necessity for the procedure. Mothers are particularly susceptible to decreased self-esteem.

The nurse must be prepared to deal with these feelings, fears, and uncertainties. Opportunity for exploration and expression of feelings and clarification of uncertainties and misunderstandings must be provided either in group or individual discussions. Emphasizing that cesarean birth can be a satisfying and fulfilling experience creates a positive context.

Guidelines for Vaginal Delivery After Previous Cesarean Birth

1. Clients who have had one previous cesarean delivery with a low transverse incision should be counseled and encouraged to have a trial of labor if there are no contraindications.
2. Clients with two or more previous cesarean deliveries, with low transverse incisions who wish to attempt vaginal birth should not be discouraged if there are no complications.
3. If no specific data on risk are available, the decision to permit a trial of labor should be assessed on an individual basis.
4. A previous classic uterine incision is a contraindication to labor.
5. Professional and institutional resources must be able to respond to acute obstetric emergencies such as performing a cesarean delivery within 30 minutes from time of decision to actual beginning of the operation.
6. Normal activity should be encouraged during latent phase of labor.
7. A physician who is capable of evaluating labor and performing a cesarean delivery must be readily available.
8. Use of oxytocin (Pitocin) for augmentation of labor for clients who have had a previous cesarean section with a low transverse incision causes no greater risk than for the general population.
9. There is no evidence that epidural anesthesia is contraindicated in these clients.

From ACOG Committee Opinion No. 64, October 1988.

Assessment

The woman who has had a cesarean delivery has undergone both abdominal surgery and a birth. Postoperative care includes the same procedures as for any abdominal surgery with the added dimension of postpartum care.

Vaginal bleeding is assessed as in any delivery. The mother must be observed for hemorrhage by frequently inspecting the perineal pad and checking the fundus. The incision is also checked for intactness, signs of hematoma, or infection. Vital signs are assessed as well as intravenous intake and output through Foley catheter.

Nursing Diagnosis

Nursing diagnoses are developed to guide nursing interventions for the woman experiencing cesarean delivery (see Potential Nursing Diagnoses).

Planning and Intervention
Preoperative Preparation

Cesarean birth involves preparation both for surgery and for the infant. The scrub nurse prepares the operating room for surgery. The warmed bed and necessary equipment for the initial care of the infant are set up before scrubbing for the surgery. The anesthesiologist (or anesthetist) administers the anesthesia with the assistance of the circulating nurse (see Nursing Procedure: Preoperative Preparation and the display on p. 359).

◻◻ POTENTIAL
NURSING DIAGNOSES

Cesarean Delivery

Anxiety, Fear—related to unexpected need for cesarean delivery, pain, concern about maternal and fetal outcome, lack of knowledge about preoperative procedures
Knowledge Deficit—regarding reasons for cesarean delivery, preoperative procedures, pain relief
Self-Esteem Disturbance—related to self-perceived "failure" to have anticipated vaginal birth, insufficient personal "control" over childbearing, altered body image (incision), and time required for recovery

Focus Assessment

Observe couple's response to being informed of the need for cesarean delivery.

Note nonverbal signs of emotional stress and level of coping.

Determine level of understanding of the reasons for the physician's decision to operate, e.g., fetal hazard, expectations for the surgery itself, and the outcomes.

Identify current level of knowledge regarding expected preoperative procedures, e.g., insertion of indwelling catheter, intravenous infusion, anesthesia.

Explore individual concerns.

Explore nonverbal indicators of feelings towards self, e.g., affect, mood, appearance, body language.

Elicit information regarding client's perception of the event, i.e., surgery, and its outcome, her self-care and infant care abilities, and future childbearing options.

Note interactions with infant, family, and visitors.

NURSING
PROCEDURE

Preoperative Preparation

Intervention

1. When client reports to the hospital the day before surgery for preadmission testing, obtain complete blood count, type, and screen and perform initial data base assessment. Anesthesiologist performs anesthesia assessment.
2. Instruct client to take nothing by mouth after 12 midnight.
3. Remind client to report to hospital 2 hours prior to scheduled surgery time for cesarean section.
4. Assist into bed; assess vital signs.
5. Shave abdomen.
6. Insert indwelling catheter and attach to drainage bag.
7. Start intravenous fluid.

8. Remove client's jewelry for safe keeping.
9. Have client remove fingernail polish, dentures, glasses, and contact lenses.

10. Apply fetal monitor for a brief time.

11. Administer regional anesthesia (spinal or epidural).
12. Check blood pressure.

13. Assist client on to operating table so there is displacement of uterus from left to right.

14. Seat husband or significant other at head of client.

Rationale

1. Completion prior to admission permits the mother to be at home with her family the night before surgery, which may increase her comfort.

2. Decreases potential for aspiration pneumonia during surgery.
3. Permits time to prepare.

4. Ensures vital signs are normal.

5. Minimizes risk of infection.
6. Keep bladder empty due to close proximity of incision.
7. Hydrates and increases maternal circulatory volume.
8. Avoids being lost.

9. Nail polish is removed so nail beds can be assessed for color. Prostheses are removed to avoid client injury.
10. Ensures that baseline FHR is normal and no decelerations are noted indicating fetal well-being.
11. Ensures no pain is experienced.

12. Ensures no hypotension is present.
13. Minimizes risk of maternal hypotension resulting in decreased uteroplacental perfusion and fetal hypoxia.
14. Provides support and sharing of childbearing experience.

Options to Facilitate Family-Centered Cesarean Births ★

1. Admission to the hospital on the morning of the birth for elective cesareans so that parents can spend the previous night together (provided they have had previous orientation)
2. Father to remain with the mother during the physical preparation, e.g., shave, catheterization
3. The choice of regional anesthesia where possible, and explanation of the difference between regional and general anesthesia
4. Father in the delivery room when either regional or general anesthesia is the choice
5. Mirror or ongoing commentary from a staff member for mother or father
6. Photographs or video taken in the delivery room—if even one parent is unable to witness the birth
7. Mother's hand freed from restraint for contact with husband and infant
8. Opportunity for both parents to interact with the infant in the delivery room or postanesthetic recovery room
9. Opportunity for breast-feeding in the delivery room or postanesthetic recovery room
10. Modified Leboyer practices, for example, father to submerge infant in warm water until relaxed and alert in the delivery room or in the nursery, if available for vaginal delivery
11. Delayed antimicrobials in infant's eyes
12. If father chooses not to be in the delivery room:
    (a) A support person should replace him at the mother's side
    (b) Father to be given infant to hold en route to nursery
    (c) Father to have the birth experience relayed to him by a staff member
13. Father to accompany infant to the nursery and remain with infant until both are reunited with the mother
14. Family reunited in postanesthetic recovery room if possible
15. Father to be in postanesthetic recovery room to tell his wife about the birth if she has had a general anesthetic
16. If it is difficult to reunite the family in postanesthetic delivery room, the mother's condition should be judged individually to allow the family to be reunited as soon as possible
17. Infant's condition to be judged individually so that time alone in an incubator in the nursery can be avoided if possible
18. Provision of time alone for the family in those first critical hours
19. Mother-infant nursing as soon as possible, that is, if mother feels well enough she may be able to have mother-infant nursing on the first day
20. Father to be included in the teaching of caretaking skills
21. Siblings to be included where possible

Adapted from Leach L, Sproule V: Meeting the challenge of cesarean births. JOGN 13(3):193, 1984.
★In an effort to make the cesarean delivery more family centered, the above options should be available where safety permits.

Care During Surgery

Many cesarean deliveries are done under conduction anesthesia, so the woman is aware of events. The father, gowned appropriately, may also be in the room, sitting close to the mother's head. The nurse has a special role in keeping parents informed about what is occurring, providing calm reassurance, and interpreting events.

The birth can be exciting, as parents hear the infant's first cries and are able to see him shortly after delivery.

Care of the Infant

A nurse or pediatrician is present at cesarean birth to give the infant initial care and to resuscitate if necessary. In many hospitals it is customary to have a pediatrician present to take over the care of the infant as soon as it is born.

The nurse encourages and fosters the parent-infant bonding process by providing the mother (when she is awake) and the father the opportunity to touch and hold the newborn.

Immediate transport to the NICU must be available, in case the infant is compromised at birth. Depending on the infant's condition and hospital policies, newborn care and evaluation may be done in the operating room. The father may be given the newborn to hold and show to the mother, or they may be united in the recovery room.

Evaluation

Parents are well-prepared and there is a family-centered approach to care following the cesarean section. This birth is a satisfying experience and both parents integrate the experience quickly. Parents express their feelings and are supportive of each other. The experience helps them to grow together as a family.

NURSING
CARE
PLAN

Cesarean Delivery

Goals (Expected Outcomes)	Interventions	Rationale	Evaluation
Anxiety, Fear—Related to Concern About Maternal and Fetal Outcome, Pain, Lack of Knowledge About Preoperative Procedures			
Client/couple will verbalize her/their fears and concerns, use effective coping mechanisms to manage anxiety, and demonstrate increasing psychologic comfort.	Encourage father to remain with client as long as possible.	Provides emotional support for mother.	Father is present; couple demonstrates effective coping patterns throughout preparation and wait for surgery.
	Encourage or reinforce use of relaxation and breathing techniques to cope with preparation for surgery.	Facilitates pain management and supports effective coping with stress.	Client is relaxed and cooperative during preoperative preparations.
	Reassure regarding fetal status as possible.	Reduces anxiety for safety of fetus.	Couple verbalizes minimum anxiety and concern.
	Describe and explain the what, when, why, and how for all procedures as needed.	Ensures understanding of what is happening and the benefits of the procedures to reduce anxiety.	Couple verbalizes understanding of procedures.
	Describe personnel who will be present during the surgery and their roles.	Reduces anxiety at sight of unknown persons; increases confidence in care and safety.	Couple displays minimum anxiety.
	Encourage prepared father's presence during surgery.	Provides emotional support for mother. Reassures father of her safety and that of the infant. Permits sharing of the childbearing experience.	Father is present during surgery. Couple exhibits effective coping patterns throughout the procedure.
	Request escort for father.	Provides emotional support for him; minimizes risk of potential injury.	

Cesarean Delivery—continued

Goals (Expected Outcomes)	Interventions	Rationale	Evaluation
Knowledge Deficit—Regarding Reasons for Surgical Delivery, Preoperative Procedures, Pain Relief			
Client/couple will verbalize understanding of reasons for surgery and expected effects and benefits of preoperative procedures and anesthesia.	Review information discussed in childbirth education classes.	Revives and reinforces previous discussions.	Client/couple asks questions as necessary for clarification.
	Explain all procedures and sensations client may experience.	Increases understanding and reduces anxiety.	Client/couple verbalizes understanding regarding reasons for surgical delivery, preoperative procedures, and method of pain management.
	Emphasize benefits to mother and fetus.	Promotes perceptions of positive aspects of care procedures.	
	Introduce other personnel, e.g., nurses, technicians, anesthesiologist and their roles.	Enables understanding of actions observed before and during surgery. Increases confidence in care and reduces anxiety.	Couple is calm and cooperative throughout preparation for surgery. Couple appears comfortable with decision.
	Inform couple that infant will remain with them for bonding as long as status permits.	Reassures against any unnecessary interference with bonding behaviors.	
Self-Esteem Disturbance—Related to Self-Perceived "Failure" to Have Anticipated Vaginal Birth, Lack of Personal "Control" Over Childbearing and Time Required for Recovery, Altered Body Image			
Client will identify positive aspects of self. Client will verbalize comfort with decision for surgery and satisfaction with outcome.	Avoid using terms that suggest any "failure."	Client may perceive terms such as "failure to progress" as inferring her personal control over the ability to deliver vaginally.	When expressing disappointment at change in birthing plans, client also verbalizes understanding that reasons for surgical delivery were beyond her personal control.
	Demonstrate acceptance, reassurance, and a nonjudgmental attitude about comments and behaviors that indicate disappointment over having to change childbirth plans. Include father in discussions.	Communciates understanding and acceptance of her/their feelings as normal and expected. Reassures that they have not failed.	Client verbalizes the potential for vaginal birth with subsequent pregnancies.
	Reassure client/couple that they managed the labor appropriately and effectively.	Provides an objective measure of their behaviors.	Couple expresses positive feelings about the care and management of the labor and delivery and satisfaction with the outcome.
	Comment on their effective coping with unexpected stress.	Supports positive self-concept.	
	Discuss potential for later transient depression over unfulfilled birth plans.	Anticipatory guidance enables recognition and understanding of "baby blues" as a normal phenomenon that may precipitate grieving over the inability to achieve their goal. Facilitates coping with feelings.	Client experiences minimal depression over change in birth plans and copes effectively if it occurs and recovers rapidly. Father recognizes and understands her behavior and provides needed support.

REFERENCES

1. NAACOG: The nurses' role in the induction/augmentation of labor. OGN Nurs Pract Resource, January 1988
2. ACOG Committee opinion: Guidelines for vaginal delivery after a Cesarean birth, No. 64, October 1988
3. Berkus MD et al: Cohort study of sclastic obstetric vacuum cup deliveries: I. Safety of the instrument. Obstet Gynecol 66:4, 1985
4. Placek PJ, Taffel SM, Moien M: 1986 c-sections rise; VBAC's inch upward. Am J Public Health 78(5): 562-563, 1988

SUGGESTED READINGS

Bowes WA: Clinical aspects of normal and abnormal labor. In Creasy RK and Resnik R (eds): Maternal-fetal medicine: principles and practice, WB Saunders, 1989

Cain RL et al: Effects of the father's presence or absence during a cesarean delivery. Birth 11(1):10-15, Spring 1984

Dell DL et al: Soft cup vacuum extraction: a comparison of outlet delivery. Obstet Gynecol 66:5, 1985

Grossman SZ and Spence JB: The nature of lawsuits related to obstetric care. In Knuppel RA and Drukker JE (eds): High risk pregnancy: a team approach, WB Saunders, 1986

Gulanick M, Klopp A, Galanes S: Nursing care plans: nursing diagnosis and intervention, St. Louis, CV Mosby, 1986

Hanson-Smith B: Nursing care planning guide for childbearing families, Baltimore, Williams & Wilkins, 1989

O'Driscoll K, Foley M, MacDonald D: Active management of labor as an alternative to cesarean section for dystocia. Obstet Gynecol 63(4):485-490, April 1984

Paul RH, Phelan P, Yeh S: Trial of labor in a patient with a prior cesarean birth. Am J Obstet Gynecol 151: 297, 1985

Porreco RD: High cesarean rate: A new perspective. Obstet Gynecol 65:307, 1985

Prichard JA, MacDonald PC, Gant MF: William's Obstetrics, 18th ed. New York, Appleton-Century-Crofts, 1989

Third and Fourth Stages of Labor

IMPORTANT TERMINOLOGY

acrocyanosis Cyanosis of extremities, particularly hands and feet; may be noted particularly in first few hours after birth

Apgar scoring system System of scrutinizing the condition of the newborn at 1 and 5 minutes after birth on basis of heart rate, respiratory effort, muscle tone, reflex irritability, and color; maximum score is 10

bonding Process by which newborn and parents become attached

episiotomy An incision of the perineum made to facilitate delivery

oxytocin A hormone produced by the hypothalamus that stimulates contractions of the uterus

resuscitation Restoring life to an infant who is severely depressed, dead, or dying

The third stage of labor begins when the infant is delivered and ends with the complete delivery of the placenta. The major tasks during the third stage are delivery of the placenta, monitoring status of both the mother and the neonate, and encouraging the parents to interact with the newborn.

The fourth stage begins after the placenta is delivered and ends when the mother's physical status has stabilized. The major tasks during the fourth stage are continued monitoring of both the mother and the newborn to ensure that body systems stabilize. This stage is a transitional period for the new parents, and many important physical and psychosocial tasks begin at this time.

Third Stage of Labor

There are two phases to delivery of the placenta: placental separation and placenta expulsion (delivery). These processes are brought about by contractions, which begin again after a brief pause following the delivery.

Immediately after delivery of the infant, the height of the uterine fundus and its consistency are ascertained by palpating the uterus through a sterile towel placed on the lower abdomen. The primary care provider places a hand on top of the sterile drape and holds the uterus very gently, with the fingers behind the fundus and the thumb in front. So long as the uterus remains hard and there is no bleeding, the policy is ordinarily one of watchful waiting until the placenta is separated. No massage is done; the hand simply rests on the fundus to ensure that the organ does not balloon out with blood.

Placental Separation

After delivering the infant the uterus undergoes a sudden decrease in size, and the placenta begins to separate from its site of uterine attachment.

Separation is aided by strong uterine contractions (Fig. 15-1), maternal pushing, and gravity. These uterine pressures also compress the spiral arteries in the myometrium to ensure that excessive bleeding does not occur. The placenta usually separates from the uterus and is delivered within 5 to 30 minutes after delivery.

Signs of placental separation are lengthening of the umbilical cord from the vagina, the uterus rising upward in the abdomen and becoming firmer and more globular in shape, and a sudden brief spurt of blood from the vagina. The brief spurt of blood indicates the placenta has separated and that the contracting uterus is compressing the blood vessels. See display on page 365 for signs of placental separation.

FIGURE 15-1
Decrease in Size of Placenta Attachment Site After Birth. After fetus is delivered, uterus contracts and sudden decrease in size results in separation of placenta.

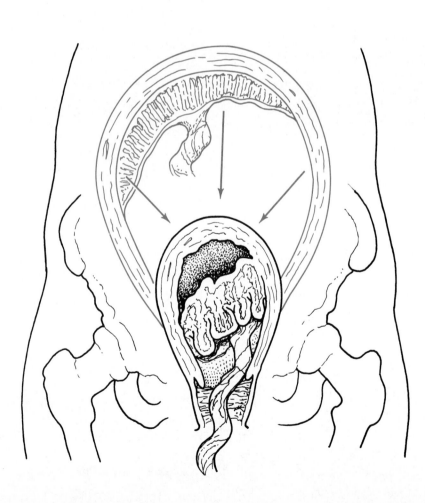

Signs of Placental Separation

1. The uterus becomes globular and firmer.
2. The uterus rises upward in the abdomen.
3. The umbilical cord descends 3 inches or more farther out of the vagina.
4. A sudden gush of blood often occurs.

These signs usually occur within 5 minutes after the delivery of the infant.

Placental Expulsion

When signs indicate the placenta has separated and a uterine contraction occurs, the client is asked to push to aid expulsion (delivery) of the placenta (Fig. 15-2). If additional assistance is needed to deliver the placenta, the primary care provider may apply gentle pressure to the fundus. This procedure is never attempted unless the uterus is well-contracted or the uterus may be turned inside out (inversion). Figure 15-2 illustrates delivery and inspection of the placenta. The placenta is inspected to determine if all the cotyledons (rounded portions of chorionic villi that comprise the placenta's surface) are present and intact. Placental remnants left in the uterus prevent firm contraction and can cause hemorrhage. If all cotyledons are not present, the primary care provider explores the uterus by wrapping a sponge around the first two to three fingers of the hand and wiping the inside of the uterus at the placental site. The nurse documents the time of placental expulsion and if it appeared to be intact. A sample of delivery information to be documented is shown in the display below.

Achieving Homeostatis

After separation and delivery of the placenta, homeostasis is achieved at the placental site by involuntary uterine contractions. Gentle massage of the fundus helps to ensure its contractility. Oxytocic drugs are utilized in most instances as well, since they stimulate uterine contractions and minimize blood loss. **Oxytocin** (Pitocin, Syntocinon) 10 to 20 U is usually given as soon as the placenta is delivered (see Drug Guide: Oxytocin on p. 367). It is given into the intravenous (IV) infusion or intramuscularly.

Summary of Delivery Information to Be Documented

The following information is noted and documented on the delivery record:

1. Date and time of delivery.
2. Presence of nuchal cord (cord around the neck or shoulder).
3. Position at delivery (OA is most common).
4. Episiotomy (type or extension, lacerations).
5. Sex of newborn.
6. Apgar scores at 1 and 5 minutes of age.
7. Response of newborn during initial care.
8. Time of placenta delivery (method, spontaneous, expressed).
9. Appearance and intactness of placenta.
10. Number of vessels in cord.
11. Any medications given to mother, i.e., oxytocin (Pitocin).
12. General condition of mother and newborn.
13. Medication given to the infant, i.e., erythromycin (Ilotycin) eye ointment.

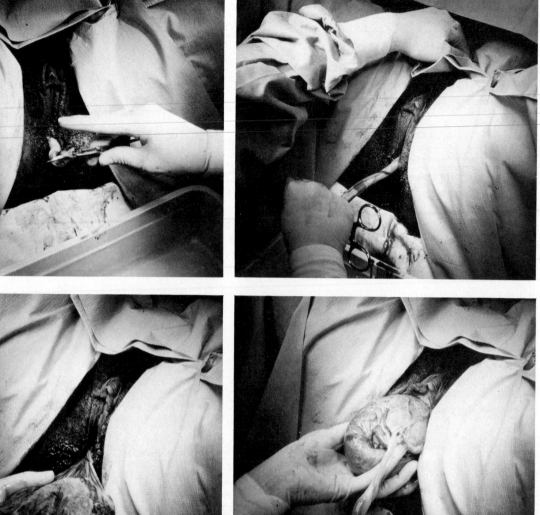

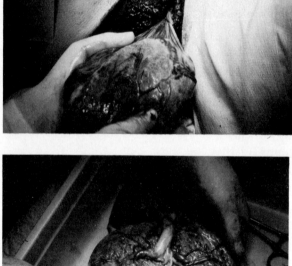

FIGURE 15-2

Placental Delivery and Inspection. **A,** Waiting for placenta to separate from uterine wall. **B,** Cord visually lengthens, indicating placental separation. **C,** Client is asked to give another push to facilitate placental expulsion. **D,** Placenta is delivered. **E,** Inspection of fetal surface of placenta to ensure it has been delivered intact.

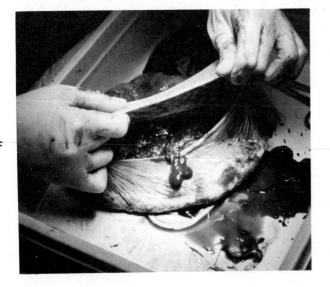
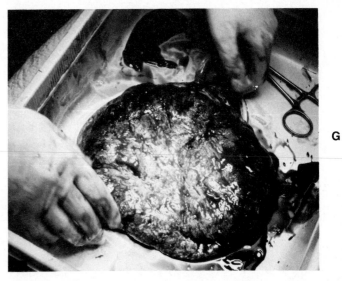

F

G

FIGURE 15-2—cont'd
F, Placenta is carefully turned inside out. **G,** Maternal surface is inspected.

⊖ DRUG
  GUIDE

Oxytocin: The oxytocic principle of the posterior pituitary hormone. Pitocin or Syntocinon are highly purified synthetic oxytocin.

Note: This drug guide is specific for oxytocin given during the immediate recovery period after delivery.

Obstetric Action: Appears to act on uterine muscle activity increasing the effectiveness of contractions; uterine sensitivity is increased after delivery; causes sustained contraction for 5 to 10 minutes, then contractions are intermittent.

Postpartum Administration: 10 to 20 U/L of intravenous fluid intramuscularly—usually 10 U if the client has no intravenous infusion.

Maternal Contraindications: Hypersensitivity.

Potential Side-Effects and Complications: Nausea and vomiting, cardiac arrhythmias, water intoxication if given too rapidly.

Nursing Implications:
1. Assess fundus of uterus for size, height, and consistency (firmness).
2. Assess bleeding for amount, color, clots, and odor.
3. Monitor fluid intake and output.

Many Level I hospitals do not use IVs during delivery, so oxytocin is given intramuscularly in those facilities. If the uterus fails to contract sufficiently, ergonovine maleate (Ergotrate) or methylergonovine maleate (Methergine) may be ordered by the physician to sustain uterine contractions and control bleeding (see Drug Guides: Ergotrate Maleate and Methylergonovine Maleate on p. 368).

Fourth Stage of Labor

The fourth stage or the immediate postpartum recovery period begins after the placenta is delivered and ends when the mother has stabilized and can be transferred to the postpartum nursing unit. After delivery the

⊖ DRUG
  GUIDE

Ergonovine maleate (Ergotrate): Obtained from ergot and has all the properties of oxytocic activity.

Obstetric Action: Produces a firm sustained contraction of the uterus; indicated for the prevention and treatment of postpartum hemorrhage; produces a contraction within minutes.

Postpartum Administration: Ergonovine maleate is indicated for the prevention and treatment of postpartum hemorrhage. It is intended for intramuscular injection 0.2 mg / ampule. Intravenous use is reserved for emergencies, 0.2 mg (1 / 320 gr). It is given orally when the mother is permitted to take fluids.

Maternal Contraindications: Clients who are allergic or have a reaction to ergonovine maleate; contraindicated for induction of labor.

Potential Side Effects and Complications: Rarely nausea and vomiting. Use with caution if client is hypertensive.

Nursing Implications:
1. Assess fundus of the uterus for level (height), size, and firmness.
2. Assess bleeding for amount, color, clots, and odor.
3. Monitor blood pressure and pulse before giving the drug.

⊖ DRUG
  GUIDE

Methylergonovine maleate (Methergine): Semisynthetic ergot alkaloid for prevention and control of postpartum hemorrhage.

Obstetric Action: Induces rapid and sustained contractions, which can shorten the third stage of labor and reduces blood loss.

Postpartum Administration: 0.2 mg (1 / 320 gr) intramuscularly (IM) or orally after delivery of the placenta or during the puerperium; may be repeated every 2 to 4 hours for 24 hours; used intravenously as a lifesaving measure; used to hasten postpartum involution.

Maternal Contraindications: Hypertension, toxemia (pregnancy-induced hypertension); contraindicated for the induction of labor.

Potential Side Effects and Complications: Nausea, vomiting, transient hypertension, dizziness, headache, tinnitus, diphoresis, and palpation; temporary chest pain and dyspnea. Onset of side effects if administered to IM is 2 to 5 minutes; orally, 5 to 10 minutes.

Nursing Implications:
1. Assess fundus of the uterus for height, size, and firmness.
2. Assess bleeding for amount, color, clots, and odor.
3. Monitor blood pressure and pulse.
4. Assess for nausea, vomiting, and other subjective signs.

immediate needs of both the newborn and the mother are being provided for simultaneously. But for the discussion in this chapter the mother's care is presented separately from the care of the newborn.

After the delivery has been completed and the **episiotomy** (if needed) repaired, the mother's legs are lowered simultaneously to prevent cramping or twisting of the extremities. A sterile perineal pad is applied, and the mother is given a clean gown and covered with a warm blanket.

The family now enters the recovery phase. This phase can be defined as starting after the delivery of the placenta and ending when the physical status of both the mother and newborn have stabilized. This usually occurs within 1 to 2 hours after delivery.

This phase is a transitional period for the new parents, and many important physical and psychosocial tasks begin at this time. A couple making the transition to a three-member family is shown in Figure 15-3.

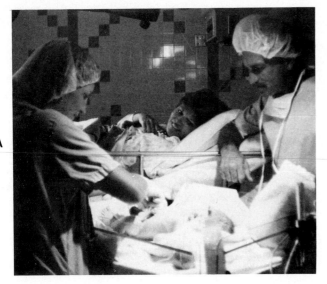

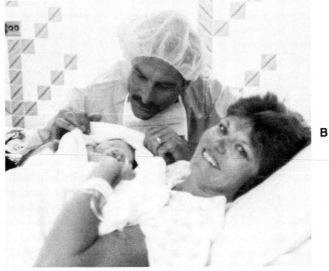

FIGURE 15-3
Psychosocial Tasks Begin After Birth.
A, Both parents watch intently as nurse cares for newborn. **B**, Father gazes fondly at newborn while mother shows pride in her accomplishment.

Repair of Episiotomy and Lacerations

An episiotomy is an incision of the perineum made to facilitate delivery (Fig. 15-4). As the fetal head crowns and is about to be born or if a laceration seems inevitable as the infant's head distends the vulva, the physician incises the perineum rather than allow that structure to sustain a traumatic tear. The display on page 370 lists the advantages and disadvantages of an episiotomy.

The incision is made with blunt-pointed straight scissors when the head distends the vulva and is visible to a diameter of several centimeters. After delivery the physician inspects the vagina and cervix for lacerations and then repairs the episiotomy (and lacerations).

Some clients wish to deliver without an episiotomy and request interventions that decrease the need for one. Measures that can decrease the need for an episiotomy include applying hot compresses to the per-

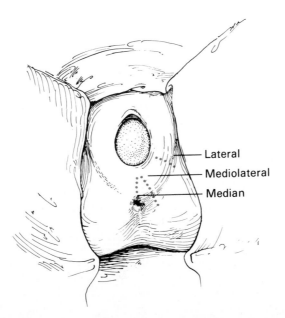

Lateral
Mediolateral
Median

FIGURE 15-4
Types of Episiotomies. There are two types of episiotomies. **A**, Midline (median) incision in midline of perineum and, **B**, Mediolateral in which the incision begins in midline and is directed downward but laterally (to the right or left) away from rectum. Mediolateral is chosen to increase diameter of outlet.

Episiotomy

Advantages

1. Ensures a straight, clean-cut surgical incision and allows easier repair and better healing.
2. Direction of opening can be controlled.
3. Avoids undue stretching and tearing of perineal musculature.
4. Shortens duration of second stage of labor.
5. Can minimize potential for later relaxed pelvic floor.
6. Heals more rapidly than a laceration.
7. Facilitates delivery of a distressed infant.

Disadvantages

1. Pain.
2. Increased risk of infection.
3. Inability to void and defecate after delivery because of pain and edema.
4. Increased risk for dyspareunia (may last 6 months or more).

ineum, using a lubricant to massage the perineum, encouraging the client to avoid bearing down during crowning, and utilizing sidelying or semisitting maternal positions, which can increase the perineum's ability to distend.[1]

Birth canal lacerations can involve the uterus, cervix, vagina, or vulva. They usually result from a precipitate and uncontrolled delivery, malpresentation, or operative delivery of a large infant. However, lacerations can occur during any delivery. The classifications of perineal lacerations are outlined in the display below.

Maternal Assessment

Postpartum assessment begins immediately after delivery as the mother makes numerous physical and psychologic adjustments. Any problems that arise during this period need to be addressed promptly to assure well-being.

The initial postpartum assessment (see Assessment Tool: Initial Maternal Postpartum Assessment) includes blood pressure, pulse, and respiration. Also assessed is vaginal bleeding, fundal status, and condition of the perineum. Intravenous solutions and recovery from anesthesia are monitored. Condition of the bladder is assessed and catheterization corrects distention (see Focus Assessment).

Classification of Perineal Lacerations

First Degree Laceration: Involves the fourchette, perineal skin, and vaginal mucous membrane without involving the muscles.

Second Degree Laceration: Involves (in addition to skin and mucous membrane) the muscles of the perineal body but not the rectal spincter. These tears usually extend upward on one or both sides of the vagina.

Third Degree Laceration: Extends completely through the skin, mucous membrane, and rectal spincter.

Fourth Degree Laceration: Extends through the rectal mucosa into the rectum.

Initial Maternal Postpartum Assessment

1. Vital signs
   Blood pressure
   Pulse
   Respiration
2. Fundus
   Height
   Size
   Location
   Consistency
   Massage initiated if relaxation
     occurs
3. Lochia
   Amount
   Consistency
   Color
   Odor
4. Perineal status
   Episiotomy
   Tears
   Edema
   Discoloration
   Bleeding
   Hematoma present
5. Bladder status
   Distention
   Foley in place if cesarean delivery
6. Intravenous fluid
   Site
   Type
   Bottle number
   Amount infused
   Medication(s) added to IV (e.g.,
     Pitocin)
   Amount remaining in bottle or
     bag
7. Anesthesia
   Type
   Motor or sensory residual
   remaining
8. Parents' reactions and responses
     to the newborn
   Do they look at or away
   What do they say
   Do they reach for or push away
9. Pain
   Source (episiotomy, afterpains,
     cesarean delivery incision)

Sample Narrative Charting: T 98.2 (F) BP 100/70, pulse 80 and respirations 18. Fundus at the U, firm, midline. Massaged, no blood or clots expressed. Bleeding moderate, presently bright red. Perineum intact, no edema or bruising noted. Ice pack in place. No bladder distention palpable. #3 IV (1000 ml Normasol with 10U Pitocin added) infusing at 125 ml/hr. States, "My bottom is beginning to burn a little but I still want to breast-feed my baby." Both parents are inspecting infant carefully, exclaiming how beautiful and alert it is. Infant smacking lips and sucking on fingers and fists. Is holding one of father's fingers.

Focus Assessment

Monitor pulse, respirations, and blood pressure closely.
Monitor consistency and height of fundus, amount and character of lochia every 15 minutes for 1 hour, then every 30 minutes for 1 hour.
Note verbal and nonverbal signs of pain.
Identify signs and symptoms of fatigue.
Monitor intake and output.
Elicit verbalization of perception of birth experience.
Observe interaction with newborn and significant other.
Identify individual teaching or learning needs.

Ongoing assessments (see Assessment Tool: Ongoing Assessment During Fourth Stage on p. 372) are done every 15 minutes during the first hours and every 30 minutes during the second hour after delivery. Temperature is taken once within the first postpartum hour. Vaginal bleeding is assessed for amount, color, consistency, and presence of clots or foul odor. The amount of bleeding is recorded as scant, light, moderate, or heavy (see display on p. 372). During each assessment the fundus is

Ongoing Assessment During Fourth Stage

1. Vital signs
   Temperature
   Blood pressure
   Pulse
   Respirations
2. Fundus
   Height
   Location
   Consistency
3. Lochia
   Amount
   Consistency
   Odor
4. Perineal status
   Episiotomy
   Tears
   Edema
   Discoloration
   Bleeding
   Hematoma
5. Bladder status
   Distention
   Foley patent (if used)
   Output
   Urine color
6. Pain
   Source
7. Intravenous fluids
   Type
   Bottle or bag number
   Amount infused
   Medication(s) added
   Amount remaining in bottle or
     bag
   IV site
8. Residual effects of anesthesia
   Motor or sensory
9. Parental responses to newborn
   Success with breast-feeding (if
     chosen feeding method)
   Face-to-face interaction

Standardized Recording of Vaginal Flow

1. **Scant**—blood noted on tissue after wiping or less than 1-inch stain on peripad
2. **Light**—less than 4-inch stain on peripad
3. **Moderate**—less than 6-inch stain on peripad
4. **Heavy**—peripad saturated within 1 hour; bleeding is bright red and clots may be present

Deviations From Expected Patterns

The following assessment findings should be reported to the physician immediately:
1. Uterine atony
2. Excessive bleeding
3. Hypotension or tachycardia
4. Hypertension
5. Headache or visual disturbance
6. Elevated temperature

massaged to ensure that bleeding is not excessive (Fig. 15-5), and its location, height, and consistency are documented. See Deviations from Expected Patterns in the display above.

The first hour or two after delivery are a time of integration for the family. This time of openness provides the nurse with an opportunity to assess the responses of the family. The nurse assists them in interacting with the infant while assessing parenting behaviors (see display on p. 373).

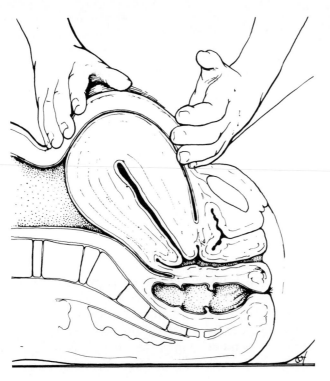

FIGURE 15-5
Fundal Palpation. This is proper method of palpating fundus of uterus during first hour after delivery to guard against relaxation and hemorrhage. Left hand is placed just above symphysis pubis to act as guard. Meanwhile other hand is cupped around fundus of uterus, and massage is carried out if any uterine relaxation is noted.

Positive Verbal and Nonverbal Responses

Calls infant by name.
Comments on beauty of infant.
Talks about infant.
Reaches for infant.
Touching progresses from fingertips on infant's extremities to caressing with
hand on infant's trunk and face to making and maintaining eye contact.

Nursing Diagnosis

During the immediate postpartum period the nursing goal is to maintain maternal and newborn well-being and support the parents in becoming acquainted with the infant. Potential nursing diagnoses guide the continuing care of the new mother and assist in preparing the parents for the parenting role (see Potential Nursing Diagnoses: Fourth Stage of Labor on p. 374).

Planning and Intervention

Frequently the mother has episodes of uncontrollable chilling during this early recovery period. Provide a warm blanket. The exact etiology of these episodes is not known, but it is upsetting to the client and may cause concern for her family. Explanations that have been suggested for the chilling are sudden release of intraabdominal pressure after delivery, nervous and exhaustion responses related to the stress of childbirth, disequilibrium in body temperature, minute circulatory amniotic fluid emboli, and previous maternal sensitization to elements of fetal blood.

POTENTIAL NURSING DIAGNOSES
Fourth Stage of Labor

Fluid Volume Deficit (2)—related to excessive bleeding secondary to uterine atony

Potential for Infection—related to bacterial invasion of vagina and perineum secondary to trauma of labor, delivery, episiotomy

Urinary Retention—related to edema of bladder sphincter and perineal discomfort secondary to birth process or episiotomy

Pain—related to uterine involution (afterpains) or episiotomy

Sleep Pattern Disturbance—related to excessive stimulation and energy expenditure during labor

Altered Nutrition: Less Than Body Requirements—related to enforced fasting during labor

Self-Esteem Disturbance—related to unfulfilled personal expectations for labor and delivery

Knowledge Deficit—regarding self-care, physiologic changes of the post partum, infant care, and newborn behaviors

Altered Parenting—related to inexperience and lack of role models

---

The mother may be emotional as a result of the psychologic tension that occurred during the preceding hours of labor and delivery. She is beginning the new role of motherhood. She must begin a new relationship with her infant as a real entity outside her body. The nurse encourages the mother and her coach to interact with the infant. This initial opportunity for **bonding** is important for both the parent(s) and infant. If the mother has chosen to breast-feed, the nurse assists with the process.

Evaluation

Evaluation of the immediate postpartum period includes stabilization of maternal blood pressure, vital signs, uterus is consistently firm with no excessive bleeding, and initial parent-child interactions are positive experiences. The couple holds, touches, and examines their infant's appearance and behavior. The mother breast-feeds (if desired). The couple state they are satisfied with the way they handled labor.

LEGAL AND ETHICAL CONSIDERATIONS

Abandonment has been defined as the unilateral severance of the professional relationship with the client without adequate notice and while the necessity for attention still exists. Failure to attend to the client in labor is a form of abandonment.

Overview of Initial Postdelivery Care of the Neonate

As stated earlier, the immediate care of the newborn is being carried out simultaneously with the immediate postpartum care of the mother. For purposes of clarity they are presented separately here.

The initial care of the newborn consists of four components: (1) preventing heat loss, (2) maintaining a patent airway, (3) establishing and maintaining respirations, and (4) physical evaluation. Figure 15-6 is a summary of initial care of the newborn after delivery.

When delivery is imminent the radiant warmer is turned on and equipment made ready (see display p. 376) As soon as the head is born, a bulb syringe is used to suction the infant's mouth and nose (Fig. 15-7). When expulsion of the infant is complete, the nurse notes and records the time of birth, the sex of the infant, and sets the 1-minute timer to indicate when the one-minute Apgar should be determined. The primary health care provider holds the infant at the same level as the uterus, with the head slightly dependent, to facilitate drainage of fluid and mucus from the infant's nose and mouth. Two clamps, a Kelly and a cord clamp, are placed on the cord, and then scissors are used to cut between them (Fig. 15-8). Sometimes the father is asked if he would like to cut the cord.

By this time the infant usually is breathing and may be crying vigorously. The infant is cleaned up and handed to the parents or placed in the warmed bed. When the timer sounds, the nurse determines the 1-minute Apgar score and then resets the timer for the 5-minute score.

It is important to minimize the newborn's evaporative heat loss. This can be accomplished by quickly drying and wrapping the infant in a warm dry blanket. A hat may be placed on the infant's head to prevent heat loss.   *Text continued on page 378.*

NURSING
CARE
PLAN

Fourth Stage of Labor

Goals (Expected Outcomes)	Interventions	Rationale	Evaluation
Pain—Related to Episiotomy			
Client will experience minimum pain.	Apply ice (in bag or glove) to perineum.	Ice numbs area.	Client verbalizes she is more comfortable.
	Administer analgesia for episiotomy pain and afterpains as needed.	Medication should minimize pain so that family interaction can occur.	
Sleep Pattern Disturbance—Related to Exhaustive Work of Labor			
Client will be rested and sleep after bonding time with infant.	Assist to position of comfort.	Promotes rest and facilitates interaction with infant.	Family displays positive interactions with infant.
	Provide quiet, relaxing environment conducive to rest and bonding; ensure privacy.	Promotes rest and facilitates interaction with infant.	Client is quiet and relaxed as she interacts with her "new" family.
			Client sleeps after bonding time.
Altered Nutrition—Related to Fasting of Labor			
Client will tolerate fluids and have a healthy appetite.	Encourage fluids (cold or warm if desired).	Labor requires great energy expenditure. Mother usually very thirsty. Fluids should be given initially to ensure no gastric upset.	Client is tolerating fluids well. Intake 500 ml warm sweetened tea. Client eats 80% of regular diet and verbalizes relief of hunger and thirst.
Fluid Volume Deficit—Related to Excessive Blood Loss Secondary to Uterine Atony, Cervical and/or Vaginal Lacerations			
Client will exhibit moderate amount of lochia rubra.	Massage fundus as needed to maintain firmness and expel clots.	Stimulates uterine contractions, which compress vessels in placenta site. Minimizes blood loss. Clots may interfere with firmness and contribute to increase in size of uterus leading to relaxation.	Uterus well contracted, midline in position, at level of umbilicus. No clots present. Moderate amount of lochia rubra.
	Encourage to void.	Full bladder contributes to uterine relaxation.	Bladder not distended.
	Change pads after every fundal check.	Allows estimation of blood loss.	Blood (lochia) loss is minimal to moderate. Vital signs are normal (compared to prenatal and labor and delivery).

Continued

NURSING
CARE
PLAN

Fourth Stage of Labor—*continued*

Goals (Expected Outcomes)	Interventions	Rationale	Evaluation
Self-Esteem Disturbance—Related to Unfulfilled Birth Plans			
Client will integrate a positive birthing experience.	Encourage verbalization of labor and delivery experience. Reinforce positive view of performance.	Time of openness and nurse can reinforce positive interactions and give explanations when needed.	Family is communicating openly about their birth experience.
	Answer anticipated as well as verbalized questions about labor and delivery.	Minimizes memory gaps (missing part of experiences).	Client discusses the labor and delivery experience and asks questions about areas that are unclear or cannot be remembered.
	Facilitate family interactions.		Family talking about the experience. Include nurse as integral part of experience.
	Praise the couple on how well they managed.	Accentuate the positive— "Did a good job." Parents need to feel supported and comfortable about the experience.	Couple emphasizes their strengths and minimizes their perceived weaknesses or disappointments.
	Encourage verbalization of negative perceptions.	Allows nurse to clarify and minimize the negative or misconception.	Open-mindedness of present may minimize negative feelings and clear up misconceptions.
Altered Parenting—Related to Inexperience and Feelings of Inadequacy			
Client will display readiness to begin to parent.	Encourage family interactions after delivery.	Parents need to begin to develop confidence in their new parenting role.	Couple expresses their lack of parenting skills but verbalizes their desire and readiness to parent and work on acquired skills.
	Note and communicate reciprocal responses with newborn.	Important cues of parenting role.	Bonding evidenced by eye contact, cuddling, stroking. Calls infant by name.

Items to Be Available When Delivery Is Imminent

1. Preheated radiant warmer
2. Warm sterile towels, blankets, and newborn hat
3. Oxygen, suction, resuscitation equipment
4. Identification bracelets
5. Erythromycin eye ointment
6. Neonatal vitamin K (phytonadione); protect drug from light
7. Birth record, foot printer, alcohol sponges
8. Chart materials

Note: Precheck equipment to ensure everything works properly.

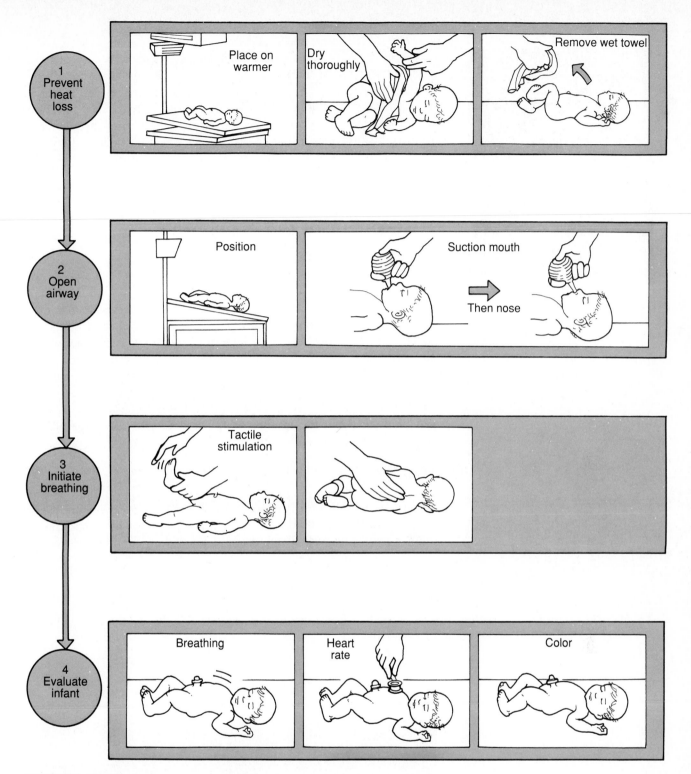

FIGURE 15-6

Summary of the Initial Care of the Newborn. *1,* First step in initial care of newborn is to prevent heat loss by using radiant warmer, drying the infant, and discarding wet linen. *2,* Second step is to ensure patent airway. Infant is placed in recumbent position in slight Trendelenburg position. Neck is slightly extended and straight, neither underextended nor hyperextended. Neonate is suctioned with bulb syringe first in mouth and then in both nostrils. Mechanical suction may also be used. *3,* If steps *1* and *2* do not induce spontaneous respirations, additional tactile stimulation may be done. Gentle flicking or tapping soles of feet or rubbing back once or twice usually stimulates respirations. *4,* Fourth step is to physically evaluate infant. Observe and evaluate neonate's respirations, heart rate, and color. To complete the Apgar scoring assess reflexes and muscle tone.

Adapted from Bloom RS, Cropley C: Textbook of Neonatal Resuscitation. American Heart Association and American Academy of Pediatrics, 1987.

A quick assessment is done to determine if there are any observable abnormalities. Two identification bands and a security sensor (if used in the facility) are placed on the infant's wrists or ankles and a matching identification band is attached to the mother's wrist. An injection of vitamin K may be administered during the postpartum recovery period or may be delayed until after the newborn is admitted to the nursery. Erythromycin ointment is put in the infant's eyes during this time, or it may also be deferred until the infant is transferred to the nursery.

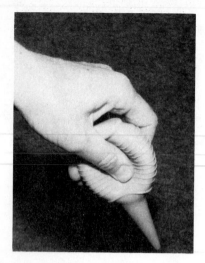

FIGURE 15-7
Suctioning With Bulb Syringe. To prevent mucus from being forced into bronchi and lungs, bulb syringe is collapsed before it is inserted into newborn's mouth and nostrils.

Assessment of the Newborn
Apgar Scoring System

The **Apgar scoring system** (Table 15-1) is universally used for 1- and 5-minute physical assessment of the newborn. It focuses attention on five signs: heart rate, respiratory effort, muscle tone, reflex irritability, and color. Each sign is evaluated and given a score of 0, 1, or 2 according to the established criteria (see Table 15-1). Each of the five criteria scores are then added to give a total score, with 10 being the maximum. If the 5-minute score is less than 7, the newborn is reassessed every 5 minutes until two consecutive scores are greater than 7. The Apgar assessment can be done while the mother or father holds the infant or while the neonate is under the radiant warmer.

Heart Rate

Heart rate is evaluated by palpating the umbilical cord (where it enters the abdomen) with the thumb and first finger or by auscultation of the infant's heart rate with a stethoscope. The rate is counted for 6 seconds

FIGURE 15-8
Clamping and Cutting Cord.
clamp is attached to umbilical cord about 1½ to 2 inches from it's abdominal attachment. Kelly clamp is attached to umbilical cord about 1 to 1½ inches below cord clamp. Cord is then cut with scissors between two attached clamps.

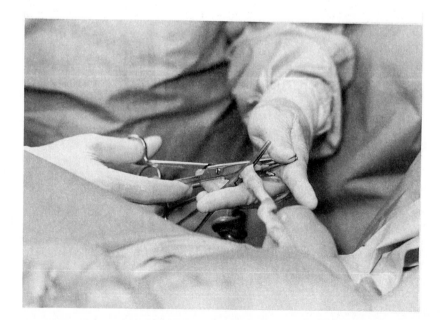

TABLE 15-1

The Apgar Scoring Chart

Sign	0	1	2
Heart rate	Absent	Slow (less than 100)	Over 100
Respiratory effort	Absent	Slow, irregular	Good, crying
Muscle tone	Flaccid	Some flexion of extremities	Active motion
Reflex irritability	No response	Weak cry or grimace	Vigorous cry
Color	Blue, pale	Body pink, extremities blue	Completely pink

Each of the five signs are evaluated and given a score of 0, 1, or 2 at 1 minute and 5 minutes of age. The highest possible score is 10.

and multiplied by 10. The rate should be greater than 100; if lower, asphyxia is possible.

Respiratory Effort

If the infant breathes and cries vigorously at birth, regular respirations usually are established in about 1 minute. Respirations that are slow, irregular, or apneic indicate respiratory difficulty or depression. This infant may require resuscitative measures.

Reflex Irritability

The easiest way to elicit this response is to observe the infant during suction or touch the cheek and note the infant's rooting response.

Muscle Tone

The infant should assume a flexed posture, resist efforts to straighten extremities, and have active motion.

Color

With regular respirations and heart rate greater than 100 the infant's body usually attains a pink color quickly (unless the infant is cold). **Acrocyanosis** (cyanotic hands and feet) is a sign the infant is cold.

Physical and Gestational Age Assessments

Physical and gestational age assessments of the newborn are done after airway patency and respirations are established and stable. The physical assessment is outlined in Table 15-2. A rapid estimation of newborn gestational age is outlined in Table 15-3.

Nursing Diagnosis

Assessment assists the nurse to identify problems or potential problems that require early intervention (see Potential Nursing Diagnoses: Newborn on p. 381).

TABLE 15-2

Immediate Postdelivery Assessment of the Newborn★

	Assessment	Significant Findings
Inspection		
Head	Molding Caput seccedaneum Cephalohematoma	Significant head trauma predisposes neonate for development of hyperbilirubinenemia.
Eyes	Placement on face Clear or clouded Drainage	Cloudiness could indicate presence of cataracts. Drainage could be a symptom of inflammation or infection.
Nostrils	Patency (check with #8 French catheter or close off one side at a time with finger and assess for color change)	Inadequate patency could cause respiratory distress. Deviated septum could be cause for inadequate patency.
Mouth	Asymmetry with sucking or crying Palate intact Rooting Sucking, rooting, swallowing, gag reflexes	Rules out cleft lip or cleft palate. Deviation or absence could indicate nerve injury or other neurologic problems.
Ears	Normal placement vs. low set	Low-set ears are associated with chromosome abnormalities.
Chest	Tachypnea, retractions, abdomen for distention	Retractions, tachypnea, and grunting are signs of respiratory distress or difficulty.
Back	Pilonidal dimple or sinus meninogomyelocele	Pilonidal dimple or meningomyelocele are central nervous system (CNS) anomalies.
Extremities	Obvious defects or asymmetry of movement Presence or absence of grasp Simian crease Polydactyly or syndactyly	Movement asymmetry or absence of grasp could indicate CNS injury, fracture, or brachial injury. A single palmar crease (Simian) is seen in infants with Down's syndrome.
Skin	Color, staining (meconium), peeling	Staining of skin from meconium indicates previous fetal distress. Dry, peeling, parchmentlike skin usually indicates placental dysfunction often due to postmaturity.
Genitalia	Sex determination Ambiguous genitalia	Ambiguous genitalia can indicate genetic problems.
Anus	Present and patent	Meconium passage ensures patency. If not patent, emergency surgery is required.
Cord	Presence of three vessels	A two-vessel cord may be accompanied by other abnormalities.
Auscultation		
Heart	Rate, quality, and location of sounds	If sounds are not heard easily and clearly to left of midline, it could indicate cardiac problems or anomalies. Tachycardia, bradycardia, murmurs, and arrhythmias also indicate possible cardiac dysfunction.
Palpation		
Chest	Location of maximal heart impulse	Maximum impulse area other than to left of midline could indicate cardiac abnormality.

★Note: Gloves should be worn during newborn care until infant is bathed because of concern about potential infection of hospital personnel with blood-borne pathogens such as hepatitis B and AIDS.

TABLE 15-3

Rapid Estimation of Gestational Age of the Newborn

Sites	Gestational Age		
	36 Wk or Less	37-38 Wk	39 Wk or More
Sole creases	Anterior transverse crease only	Occasional creases anterior two thirds	Sole covered with creases
Breast nodule diameter	2 mm	4 mm	7 mm
Scalp hair	Fine and fuzzy	Fine and fuzzy	Coarse and silky
Earlobe	Pliable, no cartilage	Some cartilage	Stiffened by thick cartilage
Testes and scrotum	Testes in lower canal, scrotum small, few rugae	Intermediate	Testes pendulous, scrotum full, extensive rugae

From Cunningham FG, MacDonald PC, Gant NF: Williams Obstetrics, 17th ed. Norwalk, Conn, Appleton & Lange, 1989.

Focus Assessment

Observe for signs of cyanosis, gagging, nasal flaring, costal breathing, and sternal retractions, respiratory rate less than 60 breaths per minute or more than 30 breaths per minute.

Identify signs of cold stress, e.g., pallor, jitteriness, tremors.

Monitor body temperature.

Observe parent-infant interaction, signs of bonding (e.g., eye contact, cuddling, calling by name).

POTENTIAL
NURSING DIAGNOSES

Newborn

Ineffective Airway Clearance—related to excessive oropharyngeal mucus
Ineffective Breathing Patterns—related to hypoxia or respiratory depression before or during birth
Ineffective Thermoregulation—related to sudden change in environmental temperature
Altered Peripheral Tissue Perfusion—related to hypothermia
Potential for Infection—related to immature immune system
Knowledge Deficit—regarding newborn care and behavior
Altered Parenting—related to lack of knowledge regarding infant care

Planning and Intervention

Initial care of the newborn during transition from intrauterine to extrauterine life ensures a patent airway and maintains respirations, prevents cold stress, provides a safe environment, and ensures infant identification (see below).

Maintaining Patent Airway and Respirations

At birth the neonate undergoes profound and rapid physiologic changes as the fetoplacental circulation ceases to function. The fluid-filled alveoli of the infant's lungs must fill with air, and respiratory motion must occur for air to be exchanged.

As soon as the infant is born, measures are taken to promote a clear air passage. As the head is delivered, the mucus and fluid are wiped or suctioned from the infant's mouth and then nose with a bulb syringe or mechanical suction to establish an airway (see Nursing Procedure: Mechanical Suctioning of Newborn on p. 382). Drying the infant with a towel or blanket usually provides sufficient stimulus to initiate crying.

If the bulb syringe is not adequate to remove the mucus, mechanical suction may be used. If the DeLee mucus trap is used, it must have an attachment to hook into the mechanical suction or an additional safeguard

Goals of Immediate Care

1. Ensure an airway and maintain respirations.
2. Prevent cold stress (hypothermia).
3. Provide a safe environment.
4. Identify actual or potential problems that might require immediate attention.
5. Ensure infant identification.

Mechanical Suctioning of Newborn

Intervention	Rationale
1. Attach a #10 French catheter to suction tubing.	1. #10 French catheter is correct size for average-sized newborn. Note: If catheter is used to check nasal patency, #8 should be used to prevent trauma to mucous membrane of nares.
2. Turn on suction, place finger over finger-tip control to check negative pressure.	2. Negative pressure used is 80 to 100 cm H_2O. Suction should always be checked to be sure that pressure is within this range. (If thick meconium is present, intubation and endotracheal suction are necessary.)
3. Place the end of the catheter into newborn's mouth first (approximately 3 to 5 inches). Place finger over finger-tip control and suction secretions from oropharynx.	3. No suctioning episode should be greater than 6 seconds so that newborn respiratory depression does not occur.
4. Rotate suction catheter gently and covering finger-tip control as it is being withdrawn to suction.	4. Prevents trauma to mucous membranes.
5. Suctioning of oropharynx may be repeated if necessary to clear secretions.	5. Note color of infant. Give blow-by oxygen (5L of 100%) if central cyanosis (lips, perioral and mucus membrane) occurs. Repeated suctioning must provide intervals of 10 to 15 seconds recovery time to prevent respiratory depression.
6. Avoid deep suction during early minutes following delivery.	6. Deep suction (suction catheter passing down newborn's throat) can stimulate the vagus nerve causing decrease in heart rate.
7. Do minimum nasopharynx suctioning.	7. Oversuctioning of nares and nasopharynx can traumatize mucous membranes causing edema and respiratory distress.
8. Pass a #8 catheter into nasopharynx to determine patency.	8. Newborns are obligatory nasal breathers so patency should be determined. Larger catheter may cause trauma.
9. After the initial minutes following delivery, some primary health care givers pass a suction catheter through the mouth into the stomach to empty gastric contents.	9. Suctioning episode should not be greater than 6 seconds. Gastric contents that are acidic are removed to prevent aspiration, which could cause a chemical pneumonitis.

to ensure the secretions of the infant are not suctioned into the mouth of the person doing the suctioning. It is no longer considered safe to use the mouth for suction. Deep, prolonged suctioning should not be done, since it can cause vagal stimulation, which can result in fetal bradycardia. Further suctioning may be required when the infant is placed under the radiant warmer in a slight Trendelenberg position. The infant is observed to ensure respirations are maintained.

Resuscitation

The majority of normal newborns have little need for ventilation assistance measures beyond clearing the airway. A small percentage of newborns, however, do require some additional respiratory assistance. Figure 15-9 is an overview of **resuscitation** in the delivery room. Decisions for resuscitation are based on respirations, heart rate, and color.

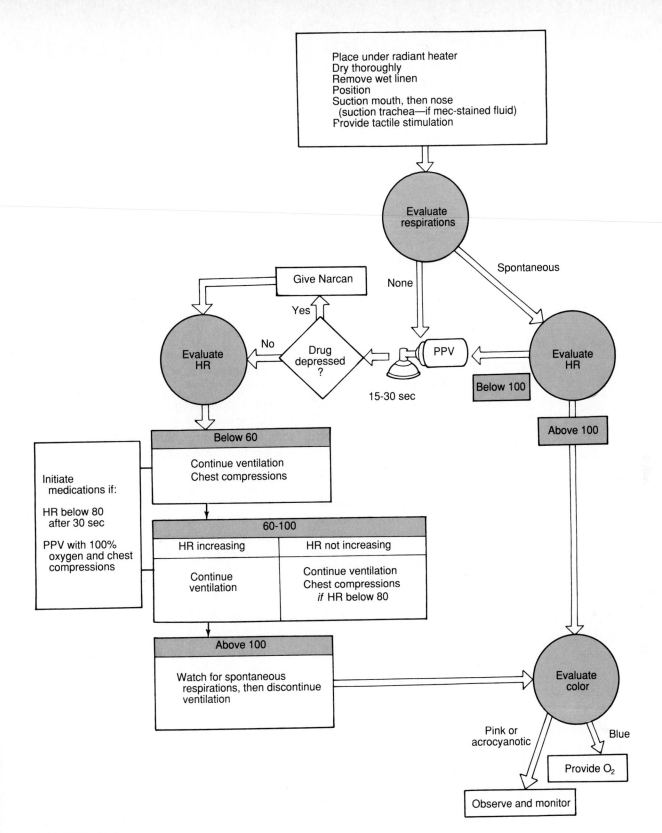

FIGURE 15-9

Overview of Resuscitation in Delivery Room. Before beginning resuscitative efforts with positive pressure oxygen, the airway must be cleared well by suctioning because oxygen delivered under pressure may force any foreign material present in the airway deep into the infant's lungs. A well-fitting mask is placed over the infant's mouth and nose, and oxygen is administered by bag and mask ventilation at a rate of 40-60 breaths per minute to deliver the oxygen into the bronchi. If this procedure (called "bagging") does not stimulate breathing and correct the evidence of hypoxia, endotracheal intubation will be necessary under direct visualization with a laryngoscope.

FIGURE 15-10

Artificial Ventilation of Newborn with Bag and Mask. Before beginning resuscitative efforts with positive-pressure oxygen, airway must be cleared well by suctioning, because oxygen delivered under pressure may force any foreign material present in airway deep into infant's lungs. Well-fitting mask is placed over infant's mouth and nose, and oxygen is adminstered by bag and mask ventilation at rate of 40 to 60 breaths per minute to deliver oxygen into the bronchi. If this procedure (called "bagging") does not promptly stimulate breathing and correct evidence of hypoxia, endotracheal intubation will be necessary under direct visualization with laryngoscope.

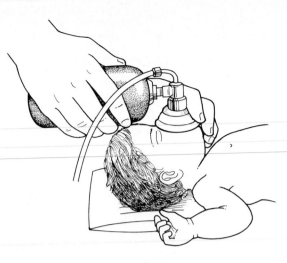

Patency

If the infant does not establish spontaneous respirations, brief tactile stimulation can be done (rubbing the back twice or flicking the feet twice, no more). If respirations do not begin, positive pressure ventilations with bag and mask and 100% oxygen are initiated for 15 to 30 seconds (Fig. 15-10). Then respirations and heart rate are evaluated. If there are no respirations and heart rate is still below 100, positive pressure ventilation is continued for 30 additional seconds. Then respirations and heart rate are reevaluated. When the heart rate is greater than 100 beats per minute and the infant is breathing, positive pressure ventilation can be discontinued. Blow-by oxygen at 5 L/min at 100% will be given following bag and mask ventilations. The mask will continue to be lightly applied to the infant's face. As the condition of the infant continues to improve, the mask will be held over (but not touching) the face and is gradually weaned away. If the infant's heart rate falls below 80 beat per minute, chest compressions are initiated.

Decisions regarding resuscitation are made every 15 to 30 seconds. Respirations, heart rate, and color are evaluated to determine if there is need for blow-by oxygen or positive pressure with bag and mask with 100% oxygen or chest compressions. Finally, if no improvement occurs and the infant's condition worsens, medications may be added to the resuscitative efforts.

Preventing Cold Stress (Hypothermia)

One of the principles in the immediate postpartum care of the newborn is the prevention of "cold stress" or hypothermia. The four mechanisms that cool the infant and methods to prevent heat loss are noted in Table 15-4. The fetus in the uterus has a temperature of about 99.5° F or about 0.5° C above the mother's core temperature. Conditions such as cold delivery room temperatures and the wet infant are instrumental in producing "cold stress" in the newborn. Drying, removing wet linen, wrapping the newborn in warm dry blankets, and placing the infant in one of the parent's arms or under the radiant warmer assist in stabilizing the infant's body temperature. When the infant is placed under the radiant warmer, blankets are removed as most of the infant's skin is exposed to the radiant heat. A temperature probe is attached with tape midway

TABLE 15-4

Controlling Mechanisms of Heat Loss

Mechanisms of Heat Loss	Preventing Heat Loss
Evaporation: Loss of heat when water on the skin is converted to vapor	First step in newborn care is to immediately dry infant and remove wet linen.
Conduction: Loss of heat to a cooler surface (unwarmed bed, cool scale, cold stethoscope, cold hands) by direct skin contact	Place on prewarmed bed under radiant heat source for care. Cover scale with blanket before weighing infant, warm bell of stethoscope in hands before auscultating infant's chest, and warm hands before handling neonate (rub together under warm water).
Convection: Loss of heat from warm body surface to cooler air currents such as air-conditioned rooms, unwarmed oxygen, or not using radiant warmer for care	Check placement of warmed bed or radiant warmer to ensure the area is free from drafts and is away from air vents. Use warmed humified oxygen if needed for oxygenation and keep newborn wrapped when not skin-to-skin or under radiant warmer with temperature probe attached.
Radiation: Loss of heat from body surfaces to cooler surfaces and objects not in direct contact with the body, (e.g., walls of a room or window)	Use temperature probe to help maintain stable skin temperature, avoid placing warmed bed or radiant warmer next to outside wall or windows that are not well insulated. Turn up thermostat in room prior to delivery.

between lower border of the sternum and the umbilicus (see Table 15-4). The probe causes the bed heating unit to shut off when the indicated temperature set point is reached. The probe acts as a thermostat to regulate the radiant warmer temperature.

It is important to reduce caloric loss due to cold stress, since no calories are taken in until breast-feeding or formula feeding is initiated (see Consequences of Cold Stress, Neonatal Mechanisms to Maintain Temperature, and Signs of Hypothermia in the Newborn on p. 386).

Providing a Safe Environment

The newborn is vulnerable to environmental hazards, including infection and trauma. A safe environment must be provided and frequent assessment done by the nurse to note any change in condition. Handwashing is important in assuring a safe environment. The primary care provider and nurse wear gloves while handling the newborn until the initial bath is given and the amniotic fluid and blood are removed from the infant's skin.

The umbilical cord stump is a potential portal of entry for infection, particularly while it is moist. It is wiped with alcohol (or another antiseptic) and left exposed to enhance drying and to minimize invasion by bacteria.

Consequence of Cold Stress (Hypothermia)

1. Hypoglycemia: Metabolism increases to maintain or produce heat, which depletes glycogen stores.
2. Hypoxia: O_2 consumption increases to produce more body heat, which can lead to metabolic acidosis due to anaerobic metabolism.
3. Inhibition of surfactant production: Creates potential for development of severe respiratory distress.

Neonatal Mechanisms to Maintain Temperature

1. Flexed position
2. Crying
3. Increased respiratory rate
4. Increased motor activity

Signs of Hypothermia in the Newborn

1. Skin feels cool to touch
2. Acrocyanosis (hands and feet are blue) or mottling of skin particularly in extremities due to vasoconstriction; may become centrally cyanotic
3. Quiet, less responsive
4. Jitteriness possibly indicative of hypoglycemia
5. Increased respiratory rate (tachypnea) and development of respiratory distress and acidosis

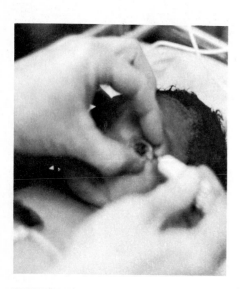

FIGURE 15-11
Eye Prophylaxis. Ointment is applied to eyes to prevent infection.

Care of the Eyes

The eyes of the newborn are at risk for infection by a variety of organisms that are present in the mothers' vagina. In the United States the use of some form of prophylaxis against eye infection is required by law. Although silver nitrate was used almost exclusively for years, it is not effective against chlamydia and has been replaced with tetracycline or erythromycin ophthalmic ointment. These prophylactic eye medications prevent both gonococcal and chlamydial infection. Erythromycin ointment is less expensive and more effective against chlamydia and is usually the drug of choice. Figure 15-11 shows instillation of erythromycin eye ointment.

It is recommended that eye prophylaxis be done within 1 hour of delivery (see Nursing Procedure: Eye Prophylaxis). By delaying the eye prophylaxis for up to 1 hour, the parents can intereact with the infant when the eyes are open. See the Drug Guide for further information about erythromycin antibiotic eye ointment. Delaying the eye prophylaxis until after the infant has been transferred to the nursery provides the parents an opportunity to interact with the infant when the eyes are open.

Infant Identification

While the newborn is still in the delivery room, it is the nurse's responsibility to prepare and apply some means of identification. Most hospitals

Eye Prophylaxis

Intervention	Rationale
1. Lay out tube of erythromycin ophthalmic ointment and sterile cotton balls. Note: Do not place under radiant warmer.	1. To have available for eye prophylaxis. Infection control principle is that each infant will have his own ointment and cotton balls.
2. Gently clean the skin around the eyes with sterile cotton (cotton may be moistened with sterile water).	2. Clears debris of blood and vernix away from eyes and provides traction for the fingers when gently opening the eye to instill the ointment.
3. Using the first finger and thumb (in the same position as holding a pencil) gently open the infant's eyelids.	3. This must be done gently to minimize trauma to the soft tissues around the eye.
4. Instill a thin line of ointment (at least ½ inch or 1 to 2 cm) along the lower conjunctival area from the inner aspect of the eye outward. (Be careful not to touch another part of the eye with the tube.)	4. The normal lubrication of the eye will distribute the ointment. Touching the eye with the tube could cause trauma and be a source of infection.
5. Carefully manipulate lids to spread and distribute ointment.	5. This should also be done gently to assist spread of ointment and prevent trauma.
6. After about 1 minute, gently wipe off any excess ointment from eyelids and surrounding skin with sterile cotton ball. (May be moistened with sterile water.)	6. Do not irrigate the eye after instillation because it may wash away the effectiveness of the prophylaxis.

DRUG GUIDE

Erythromycin (Ilotycin) Ophthalmic Ointment: Provides bacterocidal or bacterostatic protection, depending on the organisms and the concentration of the drug.

Neonatal Action: A single dose (about ½ inch [2 cm] long strand of ointment) is placed along the lower conjunctival sac of each eye (from inner canthus outward). It is preferable that the newborn have some time to attach with the family before the ointment is instilled.

Neonatal Contraindications: Contraindicated if there is known history of hypersensitivity.

Potential Side Effects and Complications: Chemical conjunctivitis occurs in approximately 20% of neonates; may interfere with ability to focus and may cause edema and inflammation. Side effects usually disappear within 24 to 48 hours.

Nursing Implications:
1. Wash hands before instilling eye ointment.
2. Wear gloves if initial bath has not been given.
3. Gently open eyelids to prevent undue trauma.
4. Do not irrigate eyes after instillation.
5. Observe for hypersensitivity.

use flexible plastic bands that come in sets of three with identical numbers on them. The mother's name and admission number, the physician's name, the date, the time of birth, and the sex of the baby are written on a special insert, which is put into each band. Two bands are placed on the infant, usually one on a wrist and one on an ankle (or both wrists or ankles), and the third band is placed on the mother's wrist (Fig. 15-12). These bands are checked carefully when the infant is admitted to the nursery, each time the infant is taken to its mother, and at discharge.

Some hospitals are employing more sophisticated surveillance systems to prevent unauthorized individuals from leaving the maternity unit or hospital with a newborn. An additional tag or disc is added to the identification bracelet; if an infant is taken outside the established parameters of the maternity unit, an alarm will sound to alert the nursing station and the security department.

Many hospitals continue to get footprints of the infant and fingerprints of the mother, even though they are no longer recommended as universal practice.

Prophylaxis Against Hypoprothrombinemia

A single 0.5 mg to 1.0 mg dose of phytonadione solution (Aquamephyton) is administered intramuscularly to the newborn in the delivery room or on admission to the nursery. This water-soluble form of vitamin K acts as a preventive measure against neonatal hemorrhagic disease (see Drug Guide: Phytonadione).

Promotion of Early Maternal-Infant Attachment

It is important for the new mother and father to see and hold the infant as soon as possible after birth. When desired, and the condition of mother and infant are favorable, allowing the mother to breast-feed or have skin-

FIGURE 15-12

Newborn Identification. The newborn wears a medallion (disc) which is attached to the ID bracelet on the ankle. The newborn cannot be taken out of the postpartum nursery area until the disc is removed or the alarm system is activated alerting nursing staff, security, and other designated individuals.

Courtesy St. Elizabeth's Medical Center, Edgewood, Kentucky.

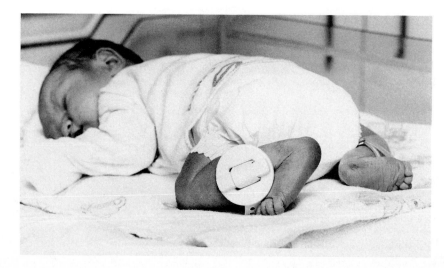

Phytonadione (Aquamephyton): Aqueous colloidal solution of vitamin K. Possesses the same type and degree of activity as naturally occurring vitamin K. Necessary for blood clotting.

Neonatal Action: Used as prophylaxis and treatment of hemorrhagic disease of the newborn. Promotes liver formation of several clotting factors. At birth, the newborn does not have the bacteria in the colon necessary for synthesizing fat-soluble vitamin K, so prothrombin levels are decreased for 5 to 8 days of life.

Neonatal Administration: A one-time prophylactic dosage of 0.5 to 1.0 mg is administered intramuscularly into the anterior or lateral thigh. May be given after delivery as a part of the initial care or a little later during the assessment process done by the mother-infant nurse or nursery nurse. May need repeat dose in 6 to 8 hours if mother was on anticoagulants.

Neonatal Contraindications: Hypersensitivity to any component of this medication.

Potential Side Effects and Contraindications: Pain and edema may occur at the site of injection. There may be allergic reaction (rash and urticaria). Some newborns may develop hyperbilirubinemia and jaundice if a larger dose is given.

Nursing Implications:
1. Store in a dark place to protect vitamin K from light before use. The drug is photosensitive and decomposes with loss of potency on exposure to light.
2. Wash hands prior to administering.
3. Wear gloves if initial newborn bath not yet given.
4. Observe for signs of local inflammation.
5. Assess for bleeding, which may occur as generalized ecchymoses or as bleeding from cord, nose, or gastrointestinal tract.
6. Assess for jaundice.

to-skin contact with the infant in the delivery room is an excellent way to promote attachment. Provision for warmth is made by using a radiant warmer or warm blankets. Allowing time for parents and infant to be alone together, with the nurse near enough to provide assistance if needed, is another way of getting the new family off to a good start.

When there are physical problems with mother or infant and early contact is not possible, it is important that the infant be shown to the mother before being taken from the delivery room. The mother is given continuing information about the infant's condition. The display on page 390 provides a summary of postdelivery care of the newborn.

Baptism of the Infant

If the infant seems in imminent danger and may not live, baptism should be considered if the family is Roman Catholic. This also applies to some of the other denominations of the Protestant church.

The following simple instructions, issued by a member of the clergy, may be followed.

The Catholic church and the Protestant Episcopal churches teach that in case of emergency, anyone may and should baptize. As water is poured on the child (preferably the head), these words are spoken, "I baptize thee in the name of the Father and of the Son and of the Holy Ghost." The water may be warmed if necessary, and care should be taken to make it flow. If there is any doubt whether the child is alive or dead, it should be baptized but conditionally (i.e., "If thou art alive, I baptize thee. . .").

Evaluation

For specific evaluation criteria refer to Nursing Care Plan: Immediate Care of the Newborn. *Text continued on p. 393.*

Summary of Postdelivery Care of the Neonate

1. Wash hands and don gloves.
2. Note time of delivery.
3. Receive newborn in warmed blankets and place under radiant warmer. Dry briefly and discard wet blankets.
4. Attach temperature probe (tape in place) to newborn's abdomen. Set temperature set point at 36 to 36.5°C.
5. Briefly suction oropharyngeal to ensure patent airway. Nasopharynx can be suctioned or each nostril can be blocked one at a time to assess patency.
6. Complete 1-minute Apgar.
7. Blow-by oxygen may be given for central cyanosis.
8. Check capillary refill time. Blanche skin over chest and assess how quickly the blood returns.
9. Assess respirations and auscultate chest for heart and breath sounds.
10. Complete the 5-minute Apgar score.
11. Count number of cord vessels present.
12. Evaluate for obvious gross abnormalities of infant.
13. Place identification bracelets and security disc on wrists or ankles.
14. Administer vitamin K (phytonadione) 0.5 to 1 mg IM. May be given in the delivery area or after admitted to nursery.
15. Place erythromycin ophthalmic ointment in each eye. May be done in the delivery area or after admitted to nursery.
16. Wipe off newborn's feet and take footprints.
17. Wrap infant and give to parents to hold.
18. Assess and record parent's initial reaction and responses to the newborn.
19. Assist mother to breast-feed if she desires.
20. Evaluate infant's respirations, color, heart rate, and temperature and note any changes that are indicative of problems.
21. Document all care.

NURSING
CARE
PLAN

Immediate Care of the Newborn

Goals

(Expected Outcomes)	Interventions	Rationale	Evaluation
Ineffective Thermoregulation—Related to Extreme Sudden Change in Environmental Temperature and Newborn Status			
Infant will maintain normal temperature.	Wrap infant in warmed blankets or place on warmed bed (if given to mother for skin-to-skin contact place warmed blankets over mother and infant).	Minimizes heat loss by conduction, convection, and radiation.	Infant's temperature is 97.7 to 98.6°F (axillary) or 97.8 to 99°F (rectally).
	Dry briefly and quickly discard wet linens. Apply warm, dry blankets. Put a hat on infant's head. (Some hospitals place the infant in a plastic bag that comes up under the arms.)	Minimizes or prevents unnecessary evaporative loss. Heat loss increases metabolism and O_2 consumption.	
	If on heated bed, attach temperature probe to abdomen about midway between umbilicus and lower border of the sternum.	Monitors body temperature.	Infant maintains skin temperature at 97.7 to 98.6°F.

NURSING
CARE
PLAN

Immediate Care of the Newborn—*continued*

Goals (Expected Outcomes)	Interventions	Rationale	Evaluation
Ineffective Airway Clearance—Related to Oropharyngeal Secretions			
Infant will begin to breathe and cry lustily.	Mouth and then nose suctioned with bulb syringe when head delivered.	Removes oropharyngeal secretions. Mouth always suctioned first. When nares are suctioned it could cause a reflex gasp, causing possibility of aspiration.	Newborn requires minimal suctioning and establishes respiratory activity.
	Place infant on radiant warmer in supine position with neck slightly extended (so that neck is straight).	Ensures patent airway.	Newborn exhibits 40 to 60 unlabored respirations per minute.
	Suction mouth and then nose (with bulb, mechanical or DeLee) if needed.	Removes secretions and ensures patent airway.	
	Initiate tracheal suctioning if meconium present.	Clears airway to prevent meconium aspiration or pneumonia.	Lungs are clear to auscultation. Newborn exhibits no signs of respiratory distress.
Ineffective Breathing Patterns—Related to Intrapartum Hypoxia			
Newborn will establish successful gas exchange with regular pattern of breathing at respiratory rate of 40 to 60.	Provide brief stimulation to initiate respirations if necessary (rub back twice or flick soles twice—no more.	Stimulates breathing.	Newborn spontaneously initiates regular pattern of breathing at respiratory rate of 40 to 60.
	Initiate resuscitation if still not breathing—positive pressure ventilation with 100% oxygen at 5L with bag and mask for 30 seconds and then reevaluate respirations, then heart rate and then color.	Initiates respirations, maintain oxygenation to prevent further hypoxic depression.	Newborn responds to resuscitation. Establishes normal newborn breathing pattern.
	Initiate tracheal suctioning if meconium present.	Clears airway so breathing occurs and hypoxia and aspiration prevented.	Newborn is breathing freely, color is pink; and is active and responsive.
	Auscultate breathing sounds.	Determines need for further suctioning.	Normal breath sounds auscultated.
Altered Tissue Perfusion—Related to Hypothermia			
Color will be pink by time of 1-minute Apgar score (some acrocyanosis may be present).	Place on warm bed, dry, remove wet linen, wrap in warm blankets, and place hat on head.	Prevents heat loss.	Apgar score of 7 to 10 at 1 and 5 minutes of age. Temperature 97.7 to 98.8°F. Apical pulse 120 to 160. Infant exhibits rapid capillary refill.
	Administer 5L of free flow oxygen if infant exhibits central cyanosis.	Ensures breathing is satisfactory rate of 40 to 60 and heart rate is greater than 100. Assess perfusion. Ensures no cold stress. Ensures adequate oxygenation and perfusion.	

Continued

NURSING
CARE
PLAN

Immediate Care of the Newborn—*continued*

Goals (Expected Outcomes)	Interventions	Rationale	Evaluation
Potential for Infection—Related to Immaturity of Immune System			
Normal infection-free infant will leave hospital.	Wash hands and apply gloves to prepare for initial care.	Universal precautions for self-protection from body fluids and secretions.	Infant displays no signs or symptoms of infection.
	Ask all who will observe delivery to wash hands and wear a gown.	Ensure infection control and maintains cleanliness. Some hospitals do not require gowning but do ask all observers to wash their hands prior to handling or touching the infant.	
	Gently open eyes and apply prophylactic erythromycin eye ointment.	Minimizes trauma to soft tissues around the eyes. Antibiotic ointment prevents ophthalmia neonatorium, chlamydia, and other infections.	Infant has no trauma of the eyes and is free of conjunctivitis and eye infection.
Altered Parenting—Related to Recent Birth of Infant			
Family is excited about being together.	Encourage family interaction before, during, and after birth.	Encourages family attachment in atmosphere of openness just after birth. Nurse can assist with getting reciprocal interactions to occur between parents and infant.	Family interacts spontaneously and favorably.
	Allow couple to hold and get to know newborn as soon as possible after birth.	Bonding occurs from conception through birth and beyond, but immediately after birth is a sensitive period for attaching and additional bonding.	
	Point out features and try to make the first interaction as positive as possible.	If the infant responds in a positive way, it causes a positive response from the parents and reciprocal relationship gives a boost to the process of attaching.	

Immediate Care of the Newborn—continued

Goals (Expected Outcomes)	Interventions	Rationale	Evaluation
Knowledge Deficit—Related to Care and Behavior of the Newborn			
Family has positive attitude about their birth experience and are comfortable about asking questions.	Promote rooming in (if available).	Every interaction the nurse has with the family should include as much teaching as they can handle at a time. Again this enhances the attachment process.	Family can verbalize how to use resources and knows to ask the nurse or physician if they have questions.
	Point out reflexes, how to get infant to open eyes by tilting back and then upright.		
	Describe some of the obvious characteristics.	Pointing out characteristics helps the couple to learn about their infant and enhance attachment.	Infant is quiet, alert, looking around, and responsive to parents.
	Assist the mother to breast-feed in the delivery area if she has decided to breast-feed.	After delivery most newborns are in an alert state and ready to suck and breast-feed.	Infant goes to breast eagerly, and mother and infant have a successful new experience. Colostrum is very nutritious.
	Encourage couple to talk to infant.	Talking, stroking, making eye contact are a part of "falling in love" with their infant and the infant is capable of responding.	Parents and infant enjoy a reciprocal getting acquainted period.
	Describe resources available for teaching—videos, booklets, phone numbers.	Couple can be introduced to teaching that is and will be available to assist them in their parenting role.	Parents are asking questions about resources for learning about parenting.

Transfer to Mother-Infant Care

After both the mother and infant's physical conditions have stabilized, they will be transferred to a postpartum nursing unit. The nurse transferring the newborn to the nursery also takes the completed delivery record. The transferring labor and delivery nurse provides a complete report about both the mother and infant to the receiving postpartum unit nurse (see displays p. 394). This ensures continuity of care. Identification bands are checked with the record by the nursery nurse receiving the infant.

Transferring Mother to Postpartum Care

The postpartum unit is notified that the client is ready to be transferred. The mother is transported to the postpartum unit by bed or wheelchair.

The following information is to be communicated by the transferring recovery (labor and delivery) nurse to the receiving postpartum unit nurse when the mother is transferred from the recovery area to the postpartum unit.

Report Information

1. Review prenatal history relevant to postpartum care:
   Any known allergies
   Mother's Rh status
   Any problems during pregnancy
   If mother was term
2. Review events of labor and delivery:
   Normal or abnormal length of labor
   Mother's response to labor
   FHR response during labor
   Analgesia or anesthesia
   Vaginal or cesarean delivery
   Spontaneous or forceps delivery
3. Review recovery events:
   Fundal location and status
   Lochia description
   Vital signs
   Bladder status
   Perineal trauma (if any)
   Bonding events

Transferring Newborn to Nursery Care

1. The newborn is transported to the nursery in the mother's arms or in a baby bed.
2. On arrival in the nursery both the transferring labor and delivery nurse and the receiving nursery nurse
   a. Check the identification bracelets to verify name and identification number with information noted in the chart
   b. Verify the sex of the newborn
   c. Verify the official newborn's weight
3. The newborn is placed under a radiant warmer.
4. The following report information is communicated by the transferring labor and delivery nurse to the receiving nursery nurse:
   a. Maternal prenatal history
      (1) Last menstrual period and expected date of confinement
      (2) Medical or obstetric complications
   b. Maternal blood type and Rh factor
      (1) Tests done if mother is Rh negative
   c. Maternal screening for infection
      (1) Rubella titer
      (2) VDRL
      (3) Herpes
   d. Labor history
      (1) Onset and length of labor
      (2) When membranes ruptured
      (3) Nature of amniotic fluid
      (4) Medications received by mother
      (5) Anesthesia used during labor and delivery
   e. Fetal monitor tracing
   f. Delivery information
      (1) Length of second stage
      (2) Medications administered in delivery room
      (3) Type of delivery
      (4) Operative obstetric procedures used
   g. Post delivery care
      (1) Apgar score
      (2) If resuscitation was required, medications administered
      (3) Evidence of birth injury
      (4) Passage of urine or stool
      (5) Parent-infant interaction
      (6) If newborn was breast-fed

REFERENCE

1. Neeson JD: Clinical Manual of Maternity Nursing. Philadelphia, JB Lippincott, 1987

SUGGESTED READINGS

Bloom RS, Cropley C: Textbook of Neonatal Resuscitation. American Heart Association and American Academy of Pediatrics, 1987

Bryant BG: Unit dose erythromycin ophthalmic ointment for neonatal ocular prophylaxis. JOGN 13(2):83-87, March/April 1984

Committee on Ophthalmia Neonatorum: Prevention and treatment of ophthalmia neonatorum. New York, National Society to Prevent Blindness, 1981

Cunningham FG, MacDonald PC, Gant NF: Williams Obstetrics. Norwalk, Conn, Appleton-Century & Crofts, 1989

Ehrenkranz RA: Delivery room emergencies and resuscitation. In Warshaw JB, Hobbins JC (eds): Principles and Practice of Perinatal Medicine. Menlo Park, Calif, Addison-Wesley, 1983

Gill WL: Essentials of normal newborn assessment and care. In Pernoll ML and Benson RC (eds): Current Obstetric and Gynecologic Diagnosis and Treatment. Norwalk, Conn, Appleton & Lange, 1987

Gulanick M, Klopp A, and Galanes S: Nursing Care Plans: Nursing Diagnosis and Intervention. St. Louis, CV Mosby, 1986

Hanson-Smith B: Nursing Care Planning Guides for Childbearing Families. Baltimore, Williams & Wilkins, 1989

James LS: Emergencies in the delivery room. In Fanaroff AA, Martin RJ (eds): Behrman's Neonatal-Perinatal Medicine. St. Louis, CV Mosby, 1983

Jacobson H: A standard for assessing lochia volume. Maternal Child Nurs J 10(3):174, 1985

Klaus MH, Kennell JH: Care of the mother, father, and infant. In Fanaroff AC, Martin RJ (eds): Behrman's Neonatal-Perinatal Medicine. St. Louis, CV Mosby, 1983

Malinowski JS, Pedigo CG, Phillips CR: Nursing Care During the Labor Process. Philadelphia, FA Daves, 1989

Russell KP: The course and conduct in normal delivery. In Pernoll ML, Benson RC (eds): Current Obstetric and Gynecologic Diagnosis and Treatment. Norwalk, Conn, Appleton & Lange, 1987

Varney H: Nurse-Midwifery. Boston, Blackwell Scientific, 1987

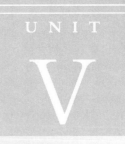

The Family in the Postpartum Period

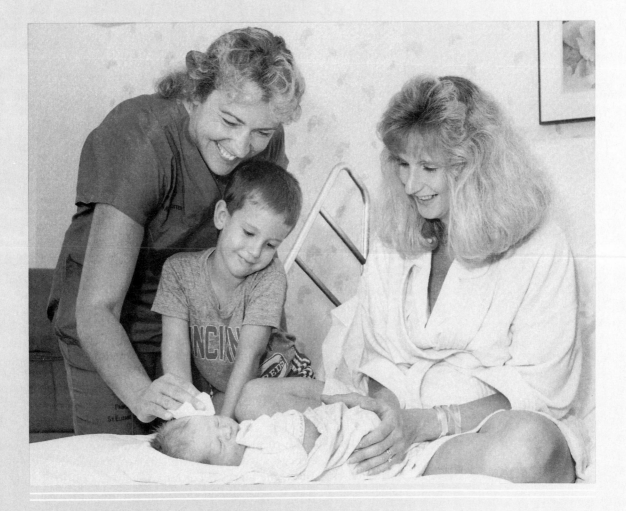

Biophysical Aspects of the Postpartum Period

IMPORTANT TERMINOLOGY

autolysis Cellular self-digestion resulting from enzyme actions

fundus Rounded "crown" area of the uterus between the fallopian tubes

introitus Opening into the vaginal canal

involution Return of the uterus to normal nonpregnant size, shape, and consistency; accomplished by uterine contractions and autolysis

lochia Postpartum vaginal discharge, which lasts 1 to 3 weeks after delivery

parturition Childbirth

puerperium Six-week period following childbirth; begins with fourth stage of labor

This chapter focuses on the physical changes a woman's body goes through immediately (2 to 5 days) after the birth of her child. The nursing process emphasizes assessment of these changes that influence the mother's recovery.

Reproductive System and Accessory Organs

Marked anatomic and physiologic changes occur during the **puerperium** as the alterations in structure and function that occurred during pregnancy are reversed. Table 16-1 summarizes clinical aspects of the normal biophysical responses to the process of childbearing; focused assessments assist the nurse in differentiating between physiologic and pathophysiologic responses to **parturition.**

Uterus

Involution, the return of the uterus to normal shape, size, and position after childbirth, begins with the fourth stage of labor. Immediately after placental expulsion, the uterus becomes a solid mass of tissue. The thick anterior and posterior walls lie in close opposition, flattening the central

TABLE 16-1

Clinical Aspects of Physiologic Responses to Parturition

Physiologic Response	Clinical Aspects
Vital signs	
Temperature	Temperature elevations that occur during the first 24 hours may be due to dehydration, excessive blood loss, or infection. Temperature elevation does *not* accompany breast engorgement.
Pulse	Physiologic bradycardia is common during the immediate and early postpartum period due to hemodynamic changes and vagal responses. Tachycardia may indicate pain, anxiety, excessive blood loss (hemorrhage), infection.
Respirations	Respiratory rate usually remains within expected limits post partum. Transient elevations may occur in response to fear, pain, excessive blood loss.
Blood pressure (BP)	BP undergoes little change under normal conditions. Drop in BP is associated with excessive blood loss; elevations in the first 48 hours post partum may signal preeclampsia.
Blood values	Elevated hematocrit and red blood cell levels immediately post partum may reflect excessive blood loss. Normal leukocytosis (12,000 to 30,000 white blood cells) and high sedimentation rate (50 to 60 mm/hr) may confuse interpretation of infection.[2]
Breast status	In women who have not received medication to inhibit lactation, milk secretion usually is established on postpartum day 3 or 4.
Involution	
Fundal consistency and height	The postpartum uterine fundus should be firm; fundal height in relation to the umbilicus reflects the progress of involution. Deviations in consistency and height may be related to (1) displacement and uterine inability to contract effectively because of bladder distention, (2) uterine atony, (3) retained placental fragments, or (4) infection.
Lochia	The quantity and character of lochia reflect the healing process of the uterine endometrium. Excessive lochia is associated with uterine atony. During the immediate postpartum period bright red vaginal bleeding in the presence of a well-contracted (firm) uterine fundus may indicate cervical or vaginal lacerations. Deviations from the normal lochial progression (rubra to serosa to alba) may be associated with infection and retained placental fragments.
Bladder status	
Amount and frequency of voiding	Decreased bladder tone and diminished sensitivity to distention increase potential for overdistention and may result in overflow voiding. Overdistention retards return of bladder tone, further impairs bladder function, and may contribute to development of an ascending urinary tract infection.[1]
Perineum	Marked edema or discomfort may inhibit voiding and defecation. Pain, distention, ecchymosis may indicate hematoma.
Bowel status	Decreased gastrointestinal motility contributes to constipation.

cavity (Fig. 16-1). The uterine **fundus** is approximately midway between the umbilicus and the pubic symphysis or slightly higher.[1] During the immediate postpartum period the fundus rises to the level of the umbilicus.

Decrease in Uterine Size

Two integrated physiologic processes accomplish uterine involution: (1) uterine contractions and (2) **autolysis,** a catabolic process whereby some of the protein in the myometrial cells is broken down into simpler components and is reabsorbed. Strong, frequent contractions cause rapid regression in uterine size. Within 24 hours of delivery the uterus is a firm, globular mass approximately the size of a 20-week gestation.[3] As involution progresses, fundal height in relation to the umbilical landmark recedes approximately one fingerbreadth (1 cm) per day. Assessment of uterine involution is described in Chapter 19.

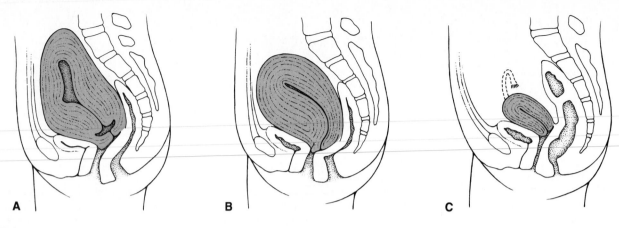

FIGURE 16-1

Changes in Uterine Size and Shape During the Postpartum Period.
A, Immediately after delivery the body of the uterus resembles a deflated balloon with an empty central cavity. **B,** By the end of the first postpartum week the uterus is approximately one-half its size at delivery, and **C,** by the fourth week postpartum the uterus has regained its previous nonpregnant size.

During pregnancy women are in a state of positive nitrogen balance. The retained nitrogen is important for cell growth in the breasts, fetus, uterus, and placenta. After delivery, although the number of uterine myometrial cells remains unchanged, autolytic processes reduce the size of each cell to 10% of that in term pregnancy (Fig. 16-2). The excess protein stored in the uterine muscle cells during pregnancy is broken down and reabsorbed for use in lactation or is excreted in the urine.[4]

Endometrial Changes

During the fourth stage of labor, uterine contractions reduce the placental site to nearly half its predelivery size. Blood loss is controlled by (1) compression of the maternal blood vessels that supply the decidual sinuses, (2) compression of the sinuses themselves, and (3) clot formation in the vessels that supply the decidua.[4] Leukocytes infiltrate the tissue surrounding the site of placental separation, the decidual sinuses, and their blood vessels. By the second postpartum day, tissue necrosis has begun. On the third postpartum day, regeneration of the uterine endometrium

FIGURE 16-2

Changes in Myometrial Cell Size and Shape Occur During Pregnancy and Postpartum. A, During pregnancy the myometrial cells stretch and become elongated; **B,** in the puerperium they are somewhat plumper and shrink rapidly toward the, **C,** nonpregnant state. Catabolic autolytic changes result in rapid reduction in the size and shape of uterine myometrial cells.

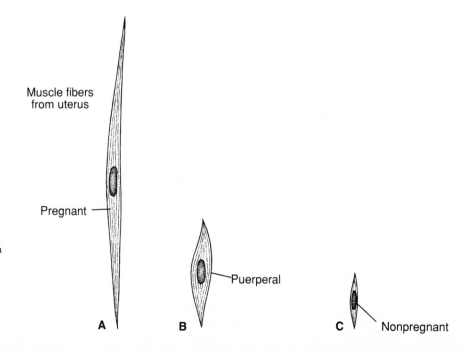

Muscle fibers from uterus

Pregnant

Puerperal

Nonpregnant

A   B   C

begins and progresses rapidly. With the exception of the placental site, the endometrial lining of the uterus has been replaced by the end of the third week. Another 2 to 3 weeks are needed to complete sloughing of the infarcted tissue and reepithelialization of the placental site.[1]

Lochia

Immediately after delivery, the **lochia** is composed almost entirely of blood. As the open sinuses are compressed and clot formation begins in the blood vessels, the blood component diminishes. **Lochia rubra** consists of blood with a small amount of mucus, particles of decidua, and cellular debris that escape from the placental site. For 6 to 24 hours after delivery, the endometrial cavity is sterile. However, the upward migration of vaginal bacteria contaminates the necrotic decidua; bacterial growth and leukocytes contribute to the lochial discharge.[4]

Within 3 to 4 days, as the oozing of blood from the healing surface diminishes, the lochial discharge becomes more serous (watery), gradually changing to a pinkish-tan color. This discharge is called **lochia serosa.** As involution of the placental site progresses, lochial fluid content diminishes, and leukocytes and cellular debris predominate. By postpartum day 10, the **lochia alba** is yellowish-white to white in color.[1]

The quantity of lochia varies among women. Lochial flow often is heavier among multiparous women. Usually lochia is heaviest on postpartum day 3 or 4. Following this peak flow, lochia usually diminishes rapidly. By the end of the third postpartum week, the discharge usually disappears, although a brownish mucoid discharge may persist for a few days longer.[5]

Lochia has a characteristic scent similar to menstrual flow and should never, at any time, have an offensive odor. Odor may indicate either poor hygiene or infection.

Afterpains

Normally, following delivery of the first child, the uterine muscles tend to remain in a state of tonic contraction and retraction. However, if the uterus has been subjected to marked distention such as with a twin pregnancy or excessive amniotic fluid, active contractions restore tone. If tissue or blood clots have been retained in the uterine cavity, active contractions occur in an effort to expel them. These active contractions may be painful.

In multiparas some uterine tone has been lost, and retraction cannot be sustained as easily. Consequently, intermittent muscular contractions give rise to the sensation called afterpains. Afterpains also may occur as a result of posterior pituitary release of oxytocin in response to infant suckling; oxytocin causes contractions of the lacteal ducts and of the uterine muscles.

Cervix

Immediately after delivery, the cervix and lower uterine segment are thin and collapsed and have little tone. The cervix appears soft and edematous, with multiple small lacerations of the external os. It can admit two fingers and is approximately 1 cm thick. Gradually the cervical os closes and thickens, reforming the cervical canal. The external os, however, never returns completely to the prepregnant state (Fig. 16-3).

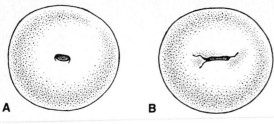

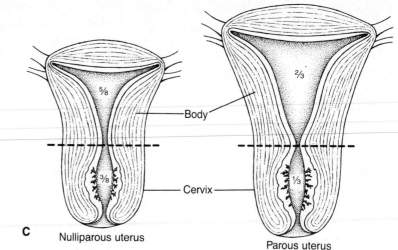

FIGURE 16-3

Permanent Cervical Changes Occur as a Result of Parturition. The perfectly round os of the nulliparous cervix becomes an elongated, slitlike opening. The external os of the multipara may gape if there have been significant lacerations during delivery. **A,** Round nulliparous cervical os. **B,** Transverse slit in parous cervix. **C,** Cervix occupies one-third of the total length of the parous uterus.

Vagina and Introitus

Some damage to the soft tissue and support structures of the birth canal accompanies every delivery.[4] Primiparas, in particular, may sustain numerous small tears in the underlying fascia and musculature of the vagina. These tears occur because the birth canal has not been subjected previously to the pressures and distentions of childbearing and the tissue of the primipara is firmer and offers greater resistance to fetal descent.

The vagina is smooth and swollen and has poor tone after delivery. Normal tone is restored gradually, but the vagina rarely returns to the nulliparous state. The rugae reappear by the third postpartum week.[1,3] Many rugae may remain permanently flattened. Further, the rugae in the parous female are not as thick as in nulliparous women.

By the third or fourth week, on microscopic examination vaginal epithelial cells exhibit atrophy related to estrogen deficiency. The relative estrogen deficiency associated with loss of the placenta contributes to poor vaginal lubrication, decreased vasocongestion, and diminished sexual response. By 6 to 10 weeks post partum, the normal estrogen level has been restored.

Immediately after delivery, the **introitus** is reddened and swollen. If lacerations have occurred or an episiotomy has been performed, redness and edema may be more pronounced in the area repaired. Extensive lacerations or inadequate repairs can later result in a relaxed perineal floor. In the absence of infections or hematomas, the introitus heals rapidly. By 2 weeks after delivery, the introitus has returned to the prepregnant state, and most women are free of perineal pain.

Fallopian Tubes

Microscopic examination of the fallopian tubes reveals additional response to lowered estrogen levels: reduction in size of secretory cells, decreased size and number of ciliated cells, and evident atrophy of the tubal epithelium. A transient nonbacterial inflammation of the tubal lumen appears around postpartum day 4. After 6 to 8 weeks when normal estrogen levels have been restored, the tubal epithelium demonstrates changes consistent with the early follicular phase of the menstrual cycle.[4]

Hormonal Changes: Ovulation and Menstruation

Loss of the hormone-producing placenta results in decreased blood levels of estrogen and progesterone, reactivating the normal hypothalamic-pituitary-ovarian feedback cycle. Levels of follicle-stimulating hormone (FSH) and luteinizing hormone (LH) rise gradually but are lower than those during normal menstrual cycles.[4] Return of normal ovarian function, ovulation, and menstruation is governed principally by whether or not the mother is breast-feeding her infant.

In nonlactating women, FSH and estrogen levels increase to follicular phase concentrations by the third week post partum. Nonlactating women may experience menstruation 6 to 8 weeks after delivery; however, initial menses occurring within the first 6 weeks rarely are ovulatory. In most women initial ovulation occurs approximately 10 weeks post partum. Women who breast-feed for less than 28 days demonstrate a similar ovulation time.[3] By 12 weeks post partum 70% of nonlactating women will have had their first menses; over the next 24 weeks the percentage rises to 80%.

Breast-feeding is associated with delayed ovulation. Menses return more gradually among lactating women; by 12 weeks post partum only 45% have had a menstrual period.[2] By 36 weeks 55% to 75% have resumed menstruation. Most commonly, the first postpartum ovulation is preceded by one or more anovulatory cycles. However, the time of initial ovulation varies widely among both nonlactating and breast-feeding mothers. Investigators have identified secretory endometrium indicative of ovulation in lactating mothers as early as postpartum day 33 and as late as day 422.[1,4]

The cause of postdelivery amenorrhea is not completely understood. The hormone prolactin (associated with lactation) reaches peak concentration around delivery. In nonlactating women the level declines erratically over the next 2 weeks. In women who breast-feed the level increases in the early puerperium, then diminishes. Return to normal estrogen levels is delayed by lactation; however, the return of normal gonadotropins, e.g., FSH, LH, occurs whether or not the woman is lactating. The delay of ovulatory menses suggests that lactation temporarily inhibits the ovarian response to pituitary gonadotropins. Table 16-2 presents average time for initial ovulation and menstruation. The wide variation in time of initial

TABLE 16-2

Return of Menstruation

	Average Time of First Ovulation	Average Time of First Menstruation
Nonlactating women	10.2 weeks	7-9 weeks‡
Lactating women	17.0 weeks*	30-36 weeks§
	28.0 weeks†	

*Lactating for 3 months.
†Lactating for 6 months.
‡First menses usually anovulatory.
§Depends on duration of lactation.

ovulation has prompted authorities to emphasize the importance of avoiding delay in selection and implementation of contraceptive techniques.[1,3,4]

Breasts

During pregnancy progressive changes occur in the breasts in preparation for lactation. Under estrogen and progesterone stimulation, the breast lobules develop, and the lactiferous ducts undergo further branching and elongation. Other hormones that contribute to breast changes during pregnancy include prolactin from the anterior pituitary gland, cortisol from the maternal adrenal gland, human placental lactogen (hPL), and insulin. Prolactin plays a central role in initiation of lactation; however, during pregnancy its actions are inhibited by the high levels of estrogen and progesterone.[3] In the last month of pregnancy the parenchymal cells of the breast alveoli hypertrophy with formation of a thin, yellow fluid, colostrum. The abrupt drop in estrogen and progesterone levels that accompanies loss of the placenta appears to initiate lactation.[1,3]

With delivery, the breasts produce increased amounts of colostrum. It contains more protein and inorganic salts but less fat and carbohydrate than breast milk; thus colostrum has a lower nutritive value. However, colostrum contains demonstrable levels of antibodies, and its immunoglobulin content (IgA) may protect the newborn against enteric infections.[1]

On postpartum day 3 or 4, the breast milk usually "comes in." There is an obvious change in the color of the secretion from the nipples; it becomes bluish white, the usual color of normal breast milk. As lactation is established, the breasts suddenly become larger, firmer, and tender. Engorgement is caused by increased circulation of blood and lymph in the mammary gland, producing tension on the very sensitive surrounding tissues. Pressure from the increased amount of milk distending the lobules and ducts contributes to the discomfort. The congestion causes throbbing pains in the breast; pains may extend into the axilla.

Physiology of Lactation

Several pituitary hormones, including prolactin, growth hormone (GH), thyroid-stimulating hormone (TSH), adrenocorticotropic hormone (ACTH), and oxytocin, play parts in mammary development and lactation. In addition, hPL, estrogen, progesterone, and insulin are necessary for production and maintenance of lactation.

Prolactin is essential to initiation of lactation,[3] and it has a central role in preparation of the breasts for lactation. During pregnancy levels of prolactin rise progressively; however, high levels of estrogen and progesterone inhibit the actions of prolactin on breast tissue. In combination with estrogen and progesterone, prolactin is involved in the increase in breast size and in the number and complexity of the ducts and alveoli. Estrogen and progesterone stimulate ductal and alveolar growth. Although the mechanism is as yet unknown, some studies suggest that prolactin also may play a part in induction of the mammary secretion of immune globulins.[3] In nonbreast-feeding mothers prolactin levels return to nonpregnant levels within 4 to 6 weeks post partum. In lactating women prolactin levels remain elevated, and levels markedly increase in response to suckling. This phenomenon ends approximately 3 months after delivery. Oxytocin causes contraction of myoepithelial cells sur-

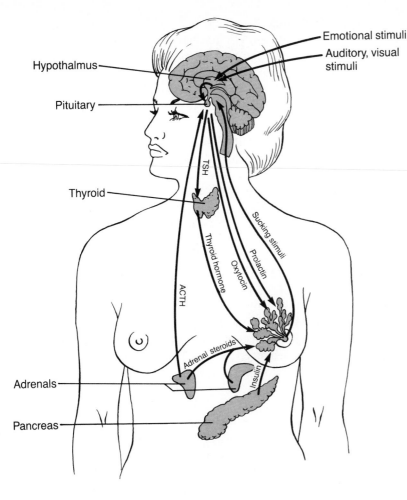

Hypothalmus

Pituitary

Thyroid

Adrenals

Pancreas

Emotional stimuli

Auditory, visual stimuli

TSH

Thyroid hormone

ACTH

Oxytocin

Prolactin

Sucking stimuli

Adrenal steroids

Insulin

FIGURE 16-4
Neurohormonal Pathways Influencing
Lactation and Milk Ejection.
Adapted from Hytten FE, Leitch I: The Physiology of
Human Pregnancy, 2nd ed. Oxford, Blackwell
Scientific Publications, 1971.

rounding each alveolus and is responsible for the milk ejection ("let-down") reflex.

Milk secretion begins at the base of the alveolar cells where small droplets are formed and migrate to the cell membrane. These droplets collect in the alveolar ducts for storage. Milk ejection is the process by which contraction of myoepithelial cells in the breasts propels milk along the ducts into the lactiferous sinuses. These sinuses are located beneath the areola, and milk is removed from them by the infant's suckling. A neurohormonal reflex controls the release of oxytocin through afferent neural pathways to the hypothalamus. Figure 16-4 illustrates the lactation and milk ejection pathways.

The importance of higher cortical centers in the brain is demonstrated by the sensitivity of the let-down reflex to various noxious stimuli. Emotional distress, i.e., anxiety, tension, pain, and severe cold inhibit the reflex and decrease milk ejection. Chronic maternal stress also may contribute to ineffective lactation.

Breast Milk

Breast size is influenced by the amount of adipose tissue and is unrelated to success in breast-feeding. Since only the secreting tissues of the mammary glands produce the breast milk, the amount of glandular tissue determines lactation. Supply of breast milk is influenced also by the mother's diet, the amount of rest and exercise she gets, and her level of contentment. Breast milk varies markedly in quality and quantity among individuals and in the same individual at different times. In general, the amount of breast milk increases as the infant's need for it increases.

Lactation is stimulated by the infant's suckling. If the infant is put to breast consistently, by the end of the first week a healthy mother usually produces 200 ml to 300 ml (6 to 10 ounces) of breast milk daily. This amount nearly doubles by the end of 4 weeks, and the mother produces approximately 600 ml (20 ounces) a day. Breast milk is produced on the basis of "demand and supply," i.e., the amount secreted gradually adjusts in relation to what the baby takes at an average feeding. In time, as the baby grows, the mother may produce 900 ml (30 ounces) daily.

Other Systemic Changes
Cardiovascular System

Within a few days of delivery, heart rate, blood pressure, oxygen consumption, and total body water have returned to nonpregnant levels. Most of the major circulatory changes caused by pregnancy disappear within 2 weeks of delivery.[3]

Cardiac Output

Immediately following placental separation, cardiac output increases suddenly as a result of uterine contractions' forcing a large volume of blood into the circulation.[6] For at least 48 hours after delivery, the pregnancy-induced increase in stroke volume and cardiac output continues because of increased venous return related to loss of the placental circulation and reduced uterine blood flow. Normal postpartum diuresis causes a transient increase in circulating blood volume as excess interstitial fluid is mobilized for excretion. Within 2 weeks after delivery a 30% decrease in cardiac output has occurred.[7] Cardiac output returns to nonpregnant levels by the third week post partum.[2]

Blood Volume

The normal pregnancy-related increase in blood volume adds 1000 ml or more to the maternal circulation; the total blood volume at term is 5 to 6 L. The average blood loss with a normal vaginal delivery is 500 ml; with cesarean delivery it may be 1000 ml or more.

Changes in blood volume occur rapidly in the postpartum period. Between 12 to 48 hours after delivery postpartum diuresis causes a transient increase of 15% to 30% in circulating blood volume. The increase in fluid component results in hemodilution. Within 72 hours of normal vaginal delivery, the total pregnancy-related blood volume has declined by 16%.[3] By the fourth postpartum week, the total blood volume has decreased to nonpregnant levels.

Blood Constituents

During pregnancy high estrogen levels affect protein and fat synthesis, resulting in an increased production of free fatty acids, cholesterol, triglycerides, lipoproteins, fibrinogen, and other clotting factors. A signif-

Hematologic Changes

Postpartum Week 1

Hematocrit level: Early postpartum—may reflect hemodilution caused by
diuresis; days 3 to 7—may reflect hemoconcentration caused by diuresis
with loss of more plasma fluid than red blood cells
Marked leukocytosis immediately post partum; WBC level up to 30,000/ml
Clotting factors I, II, VIII, IX, and X: decline to prepregnant levels; fibrinogen
level still elevated

Postpartum Week 2

WBC count within normal limits
Nonpregnant lipid level reestablished within 10 days
Total protein and serum electrolyte levels reestablished within 2 weeks

Postpartum Week 3

Sedimentation rate within normal limits by end of week 3
Fibrinogen level within normal limits by end of week 3

Postpartum Week 4

Total blood volume at nonpregnant level (4 L)

icant drop in lipid components is noted within 24 hours of delivery, and
nonpregnant levels are reestablished within 10 days. The hypercoagulability of pregnancy continues into the postpartum period. Fibrinogen
levels and sedimentation rates return to normal within 3 weeks after
delivery.[1,3]

A marked leukocytosis occurs during labor and continues into the early
puerperium. Blood values may reach as high as 30,000 white blood cells/
ml. Hemoglobin, hematocrit, and erythrocyte counts may fluctuate but
should not fall much below prelabor levels.[1] Often the red blood cell
count and hematocrit are elevated because of hemoconcentration that
accompanies the disproportionate loss of plasma volume during diuresis.[2]
The display above summarizes hematologic changes.

Pulse

Often after delivery there is a transient physiologic bradycardia, with
pulse rates as low as 40 to 50 beats per minute. Postpartum bradycardia
results from normal hemodynamic changes, e.g., increased stroke volume
and cardiac output, and a vagal response to the increased sympathetic
nervous system activity during labor.[3] Physiologic bradycardia usually
persists for 24 to 48 hours.

Blood Pressure

Under normal conditions the physiologic response to parturition produces
no significant changes in systolic or diastolic readings.

Respiratory System

During pregnancy progesterone creates a type of hyperventilation at the
alveolar level, increasing oxygen saturation. The lower CO_2 tension in
the blood encourages diffusion of fetal CO_2 to the maternal circulation.[6]
During labor the pregnancy-related respiratory alkalosis and compensated

metabolic acidosis begin to change. A rising blood lactate level, falling pH, and hypocapnia occur toward the end of the first stage. These conditions persist into the early puerperium.

Changes in abdominal pressure and thoracic cage capacity after delivery result in rapid alterations of pulmonary function. Residual volume, resting ventilation, and oxygen consumption increase. Decreases occur in inspiratory capacity, vital capacity, and maximum breathing capacity. Pulmonary functions return to nonpregnant levels within 6 months of delivery.

Urinary System

Pregnancy-related changes in urinary system function also return to nonpregnant levels in the early postpartum period. Dilation of the renal pelvis, calyces, and ureters regresses within 5 days of delivery. Renal plasma flow, glomerular filtration rate (GFR), and creatinine clearance rate return to nonpregnant levels within 6 weeks of delivery.[3]

The water metabolism of pregnancy is reversed because of the rapid drop in steroid hormone levels and uterine involutional processes. Within 12 hours of delivery marked diuresis usually begins.[4] The catabolic autolytic processes contribute to proteinuria and elevations in blood urea nitrogen. On occasion acetonuria may occur. Changes in blood volume and hormone levels affect the GFR and serum electrolytes.

The GFR remains elevated during the first week after delivery. Postpartum diuresis may reach 3000 ml/day for the first 4 to 5 days. Excretion of interstitial fluid retained during pregnancy, combined with involutional changes, contributes to a postpartum weight loss of approximately 9 pounds. Glycosuria occurs approximately 20% of the time. Lactosuria is present, especially in lactating women, and in approximately 50% of women proteinuira may be present for 1 or 2 days.

After delivery the bladder mucosa shows varying degrees of edema and hyperemia, with diminished bladder tone. The pregnancy-related increase in bladder capacity and decreased sensitivity of bladder stretch receptors to pressure contribute to a tendency to overdistention, incomplete emptying, and excessive residual urine in the early puerperium.[1] With adequate emptying, bladder tone is usually restored within 5 to 7 days.

Gastrointestinal System

Most women are thirsty for the first 2 to 3 days post partum. This thirst probably is due to fluid shifts within the body associated with postpartum diuresis. Constipation, caused by the residual effects of progesterone, is common during the early postpartum period. Pain from an episiotomy or from hemorrhoids may further deter defecation. Tone and motility of the gastrointestinal system usually return to normal within 2 weeks.

Weight Loss

The average weight loss after delivery totals 22 pounds. Table 16-3 describes sources and amount of weight loss during the postpartum period.

TABLE 16-3

*Sources and Amount of Weight Loss
During the Postpartum Period*

Source of Weight Loss	Amount of Weight Loss	
	Pounds	Kilograms
Fetus and placenta; amniotic fluid and blood loss at delivery	12-13	5.5-6.0
Perspiration and diuresis during the first postpartum week	5-8	2.5-4.0
Uterine involution and lochia	2-3	1
TOTAL WEIGHT LOSS	19-24	9-10

Integumentary System

Pigmentary Changes

Approximately 90% of pregnant women experience pigmentary changes. Increased melanin activity appears related to high levels of estrogen and progesterone.[7] Pregnancy-induced chloasma and hyperpigmentation of the nipples, areola, and linea nigra gradually diminish after delivery. Although the darker coloration of these areas regresses, the skin may not return to prepregnant character, and some women have persistent darker pigment.

Vascular Changes

Falling estrogen levels also cause regression of spider angiomas, darker nevi, palmar erythema, and other pregnancy-related phenomena related to vascular changes. Most other pregnancy-related skin lesions also regress spontaneously, e.g., granuloma gravidarum of the gums.[8]

Connective Tissue Changes

Because of the rupture of the elastic fibers underlying the skin, the striae usually remain. Over time the striae fade to a silvery appearance.

Hair Growth Cycle

Pregnancy levels of estrogen decrease the rate of growth and lengthen the amount of time required for hair growth. Estrogen withdrawal in the postpartum period may result in a diffuse, transient hair loss. Usually the degree of hair loss is not significant, and regrowth occurs gradually without treatment.[8]

Musculoskeletal System

Pelvic Muscular and Fascial Support

During pregnancy, labor, and delivery, the ligaments that support the uterus, ovaries, and tubes have been subjected to great tension and stretching. In the postpartum period they are somewhat relaxed. The broad and round ligaments require considerable time to regain normal size, tone, and position.

The muscular and fascial support structures of the uterus and vagina may be injured during childbirth. The weakening and lengthening of support structures for the uterus, vaginal wall, rectum, urethra, and/or bladder may result in later pelvic relaxation. The most common types of pelvic relaxation include rectocele, enterocele, cystocele, urethrocele, and uterine prolapse.[4] Symptoms and signs of pelvic relaxation appear around menopause when the tonic effects of estrogen diminish and atrophic changes occur in fascia. They tend to be progressive over time and often are not responsive to rest or exercise.

Abdominal Wall

The abdominal wall recovers partially from the overstretching caused by pregnancy but remains soft and flabby for some time. The process of involution in the abdominal structures requires at least 6 weeks. Provided that the abdominal walls have retained their muscle tone, they gradually return to their original condition. However, if these muscles have lost their tone, a marked separation, or diastasis, of the recti muscles with diminished support to the abdominal organs may occur. Abdominal tone may be regained with prescribed exercises, rest, and diet.

Joint Mobility

The pregnancy-related endocrine effects on fibrocartilage gradually are reversed during the postpartum period. The relative relaxation and in-

TABLE 16-4

Postpartum Physiologic Adaptations

Changes	Time Frame
Breasts	Lactation established by day 3 or 4
Uterus	Involutes at rate of one fingerbreadth daily; nonpalpable by day 9 or 10; placental site healed by 6 weeks post partum
Vagina	Reappearance of rugae by week 3
	Restoration of normal estrogen index and vaginal lubrication by weeks 6 to 10
Ovulation	Widely varied time of return, influenced by lactation; average—10 to 12 weeks in nonlactating women, 12 to 36 weeks in nursing mothers
Cardiovascular system	Increased cardiac output and stroke volume diminished after 48 hours
	Total blood volume affected by blood loss and postpartum diuresis; at nonpregnant level by week 4
Respiratory system	Increased residual volume, resting capacity, and oxygen consumption
	Decreased inspiratory capacity, vital capacity, and maximum breathing capacity
	Restoration of nonpregnant pulmonary function within 6 months
Urinary system	Beginning of diuresis within 12 hours of delivery; output to 3000 ml for 4 to 5 days
	Restoration of nonpregnant renal functions by week 6
	Restoration of bladder tone by end of week 1
Gastrointestinal system	Restoration of normal tone and motility by week 2
Musculoskeletal system	Involution of abdominal wall by minimum of 6 weeks; improvement of tone through abdominal exercise

creased mobility of pelvic articulations return to nonpregnant stability within 6 to 8 weeks of delivery. Postural changes induced by the enlarged uterus regress, improving lumbar lordosis and compensatory dorsal kyphosis. However, enlarged lactating breasts and a weakened abdominal wall may contribute to poor posture after delivery. Table 16-4 summarizes the average time frame required for anatomic and physiologic return to nonpregnant status.

REFERENCES

1. Cunningham F et al: William's Obstetrics, 18th ed. Norwalk, Conn, Appleton & Lange, 1989
2. Easterling W, Herbert W: The puerperium. In Danforth D, Scott J: Obstetrics & Gynecology, 5th ed. Philadelphia, JB Lippincott, 1986
3. Resnick R: The puerperium. In Creasey R, Resnick R: Maternal-Fetal Medicine: Principles and Practice, 2nd ed. Philadelphia, WB Saunders, 1989
4. Willson R: The puerperium. In Willson R et al (eds): Obstetrics and Gynecology, 8th ed. St. Louis, CV Mosby, 1987
5. Oppenheimer L et al: The duration of lochia. Br J Obstet Gynaecol 93(7):754-757, July 1986
6. Laros R: Physiology of normal pregnancy. In Willson R et al (eds): Obstetrics and Gynecology, 8th ed. St. Louis, CV Mosby, 1987
7. Robson S et al: Haemodynamic changes during the early puerperium. Br Med J 294:106, 1987
8. Rappini R, Jordon R: The skin and pregnancy. In Creasey R, Resnick R: Maternal-Fetal Medicine: Principles and Practice, 2nd ed. Philadelphia, WB Saunders, 1989

SUGGESTED READING

Jacobson H: A standard for assessing lochia volume. MCN 10(3):174, 1985

Biophysical Aspects of Neonatal Adaptation

IMPORTANT TERMINOLOGY

brown fat Specialized adipose tissue found in the newborn; primary source of heat production in response to cold

neonate Newborn infant from birth to 28 days of age

nonshivering thermogenesis Heat produced by metabolism of brown fat

physiologic jaundice Condition resulting from normal hemolysis of aging red blood cells' liberating amounts of bilirubin that exceed the newborn's conjugation and excretion abilities

pulmonary surfactant Phospholipid agent in lungs that acts to maintain alveolar patency; reduces surface tension

The neonatal period is a time of profound adjustment and adaptation. Successful transition from dependent intrauterine fetal life to independent extrauterine survival requires several vital physiologic and metabolic alterations. During the many weeks before birth, all fetal needs have been met by the mother's body. Oxygen and nutrients from the maternal circulation have been transported parenterally to the growing fetus, and metabolic wastes have been removed. However, after birth newborn infants must adapt physiologically to meet their own survival needs: (1) the neonate must obtain oxygen from the environment; (2) the systemic circulation must be modified, and blood flow to the lungs must increase and gas exchange occur; (3) enteral nutrition and hydration must be obtained and assimilated; (4) wastes must be excreted; and (5) metabolic mechanisms must be altered to respond to the new internal and external environment. Many adaptations must occur immediately; others take place over the next several days or weeks.

The nurse's ability to assess the **neonate's** status and intervene appropriately to support, maintain, and promote successful adaptation is dependent on an understanding of these adaptive changes, the parameters of normal adaptation, and evidence of unsuccessful adaptation. Table 17–1 summarizes clinical aspects of successful neonatal transition to ex-

TABLE 17-1

Clinical Aspects of Newborn Physiologic Responses to Extrauterine Transition

Physiologic Response	Clinical Aspect
Vital Signs	
Temperature	Elevated temperatures may indicate prolonged exposure to high environmental temperatures, infection, drug addiction, or dehydration.
Rectal: 35.6°-37.5° C (96.8°-99.5° F)	
Axillary: 36.5°-37.2° C (97.7°-98.9° F)	Subnormal temperatures are associated with prolonged exposure to low environmental temperature, respiratory distress syndrome (RDS), and prematurity. Cold stress rapidly exceeds the newborn's compensatory resources and results in jeopardy because of metabolic acidosis.
Pulse	Persistent tachycardia is associated with RDS. Persistent bradycardia may indicate congenital heart block.
Normal rate: 120 to 150 beats per minute	
Respirations	Bradypnea may indicate narcosis or birth trauma. Tachypnea is associated with RDS, atelectasis, meconium aspiration, and diaphragmatic hernia.
Normal rate: 30 to 50 per minute	
Blood pressure	Any marked difference between blood pressure in the upper and lower extremities may indicate coarctation of the aorta; hypertension may be present in infants with RDS.
Normal: 60/40 to 80/50	
Color	Within the first 24 hours of birth, jaundice may indicate premature bilirubin overload resulting from pathologic hemolysis (e.g., Rh incompatibility; cyanosis, unrelieved by O_2, may indicate persistent fetal circulation or RDS.

trauterine life. Essential components of the nursing assessment of neonatal status and the implications of assessment findings are discussed in Chapter 20.

Biologic Adaptations

Respiratory Changes

Development of the fetal respiratory system begins between the 5th and 16th weeks of gestation.[1] By 25 weeks gestation, lung alveoli are developed, and by 35 to 36 weeks gestation, adequate amounts of pulmonary surfactant are being produced.[2] By the time of birth, the respiratory system is ready to begin extrauterine gas exchange. A combination of physiologic (internal) and physical (external) stimuli associated with the birth process generate spontaneous respiration in the newborn (Fig. 17-1).

Internal Respiratory Stimuli

During labor uterine contractions interrupt placental perfusion and cause repeated, transitory fetal hypoxia. Changes in fetal blood chemistry that

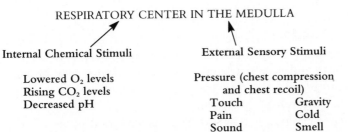

FIGURE 17-1

Initiation of Respiration in the Newborn. Spontaneous initiation of respiration in the newborn involves the interaction of chemical, mechanical, and sensory stimuli. These internal and external stimuli activate the respiratory center in the medulla, and the vigorous infant usually breathes spontaneously seconds after birth.

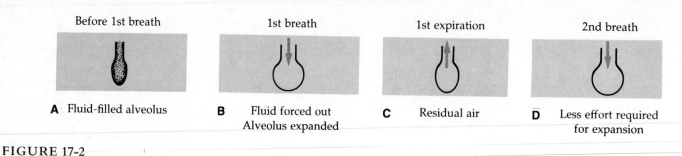

Before 1st breath   1st breath   1st expiration   2nd breath

A Fluid-filled alveolus   **B** Fluid forced out   **C** Residual air   **D** Less effort required
                                      Alveolus expanded   for expansion

FIGURE 17-2

Physiology of Initiation of Respiration in the Newborn. **A,** While in utero, the fetal lungs are filled with fluid. **B,** The first inspiration distends the alveolar spaces with air, forcing fluid out. **C,** On expiration a residual volume of nearly 20 ml of air remains. **D,** The pulmonary surfactant lessens alveolar resistance to expansion and decreases the pressure required to inflate the lung.[2] Therefore the second breath takes less effort than the first and the third breath even less; by this time most of the small airways are open. After several minutes of breathing, lung expansion is usually complete.

result from the hypoxia seem of paramount importance in stimulating spontaneous respiration. These changes include lowered oxygen tension (PO_2), elevated carbon dioxide tension (PCO_2), and lowered pH.[3] However, if fetal asphyxia continues, the respiratory center is depressed.

External Respiratory Stimuli

During fetal life the lungs are filled with fluid. In the process of the normal vaginal delivery of a vertex presentation, compression of the infant's chest expresses tracheal fluid. As the body is born, chest recoil causes shallow passive inspiration of air. **Pulmonary surfactant** lowers the surface tension and maintains alveolar patency when air enters (Fig. 17-2). The remaining alveolar fluid is absorbed through the pulmonary capillaries and lymphatics.[2]

Sensory stimuli such as cold, light, sound, gravity, touch, and pain contribute to spontaneous initiation of respirations. Cold is considered a major stimulus for initiating respiration,[4] normal room air of approximately 22° C (72° F) is more than 15° C (25° F) below the mother's normal body temperature.

Initiation of Respirations

Great effort is required to expand the newborn's lungs and to fill the collapsed alveoli. Surface tension in the respiratory tract, as well as resistance in the lung tissue itself, the thorax, the diaphragm, and the respiratory muscles, must be overcome. Any obstruction such as mucus must be cleared. The first active inspiration results from a powerful contraction of the diaphragm, creating a high negative intrathoracic pressure and causing marked retraction of the ribs.

Respiration in First and Second Periods of Reactivity

The first period of reactivity (Fig. 17-3) begins immediately after delivery. At this time the newborn's respiration is rapid and may reach as high as 80 breaths per minute. During this initial transition period the infant may experience a brief, transitory episode of respiratory distress with obvious nasal flaring, chest retraction, or grunting.

After this initial response, the newborn becomes relatively quiet and does not respond intensely to either internal or external stimuli. He or she relaxes and may fall asleep. The first sleep occurs, on average, 2 hours after birth and may last from a few minutes to several hours. While the newborn is quiet or asleep, respirations usually are 30 to 50 per minute, shallow, and relatively regular.

On awakening the newborn begins the second period of reactivity and again is overreactive to stimuli. His or her color may change rapidly (from pink to moderately cyanotic), and his or her heart rate becomes

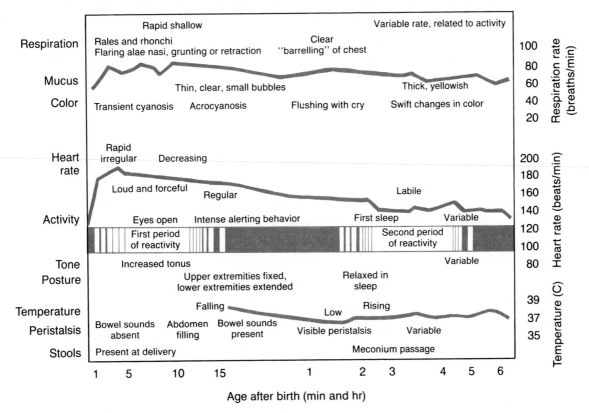

FIGURE 17-3

Reactivity in the Newborn. During the initial transition to extrauterine life, the newborn exhibits two periods of reactivity divided by a period of quiet sleep. In the first period of reactivity the newborn responds to physical and sensory stimuli with immediate vigorous activity. He or she exhibits outbursts of diffuse, purposeless movements that alternate with periods of relative immobility. Tachycardia is associated with high activity; the heart rate may reach 180 beats per minute in the first minutes of life. Thereafter, it falls to an average of 120 to 140 beats per minute. After the first sleep, the newborn awakens to the second period of reactivity.

rapid. Oral mucus may be a major problem during this period. Choking, gagging, and regurgitation may occur. Since the length of the second period of reactivity varies widely, the nurse must be particularly alert for the first 12 to 18 hours of the infant's life.

Circulatory Changes

During fetal life oxygenated blood is transported from the placenta by the umbilical vein and through the hepatic veins and ductus venosus to the inferior vena cava. The blood then passes from the right atrium through the foramen ovale into the left atrium. It then enters the left ventricle and ascending aorta to supply the head and upper extremities. Returning to the right atrium through the superior vena cava, the blood flows into the right ventricle and pulmonary artery. Much of the blood flow from the pulmonary artery flows through the ductus arteriosus and through the aorta to the lower extremities and abdomen. The blood returns to the placenta through the two umbilical arteries. Before birth only comparatively small amounts of blood enter the pulmonary circulation to nourish the lung tissue.

Several interrelated events result in closure of fetal circulatory structures: (1) the first breath inflates the lungs, creating a negative intrathoracic pressure, which contributes to (2) a sudden, marked decrease in pulmonary vascular resistance that opens the pulmonary capillary bed; (3) blood flowing from the aorta to the pulmonary artery increases the pulmonary circulation and (4) lowers pressure in the right atrium; (5) clamping the umbilical cord reduces the amount of blood entering the heart through the inferior vena cava and further lowers pressure in the right atrium; (6) increased peripheral vascular resistance raises systemic blood pressure; (7) the rise in systemic blood pressure increases pressure in the

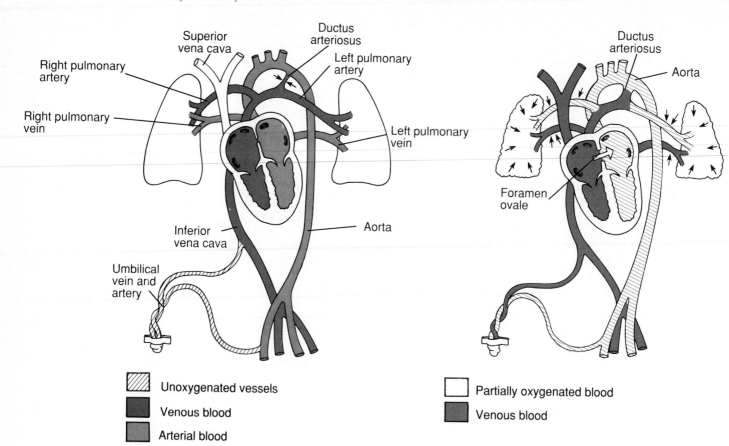

Right pulmonary artery
Right pulmonary vein

Superior vena cava

Ductus arteriosus
Left pulmonary artery
Left pulmonary vein

Ductus arteriosus
Aorta

Inferior vena cava

Aorta

Umbilical vein and artery

Foramen ovale

Unoxygenated vessels
Venous blood
Arterial blood

Partially oxygenated blood
Venous blood

FIGURE 17-4

Onset of Respiration. **A,** After expansion of the lungs and clamping of the umbilical cord, the pulmonary blood flow increases, and left atrial and systemic arterial pressures rise. Pressures in the right atrium and pulmonary artery fall. The higher pressure in the left atrium closes the foramen ovale. Blood entering the right atrium from the inferior and superior vena cava is pumped from the right ventricle through the pulmonary artery toward the lung. The rise in systemic arterial pressure and the fall in pressure in the pulmonary artery cause a left-to-right blood flow through the ductus arteriosus. The ductus constricts and closes, and normal (adult) circulation is established. **B,** With incomplete expansion of the lungs, pulmonary vascular resistance is high, and pulmonary blood flow is low. Because the pressure in the right atrium is higher than that in the left atrium, the foramen ovale opens, and vena caval blood flows through it into the left atrium. The fetal circulation pattern returns; however, the umbilical vein no longer supplies oxygenated blood to the inferior vena cava.

left atrium; (8) the difference in the two atrial pressures forces closure of the foramen ovale; and (9) diminished blood flow through the ductus arteriosus and ductus venosus, in conjunction with (10) a neuromuscular mechanism associated with the rising oxygen tension of the blood, is thought to influence closure of these fetal structures (Fig. 17-4A). Under the influence of prostaglandins interacting with the rising oxygen tension of the blood, the ductus arteriosus gradually closes. Closure of the ductus arteriosus is completed within 24 hours of birth.[2,4] However, under abnormal conditions, e.g., drop in blood oxygen tension, fetal circulation may be reestablished during the early transitional period (Fig. 17-4B).

Peripheral Circulation

Peripheral circulation in the newborn is somewhat sluggish. This accounts for the normal **acrocyanosis** of the infant's hands and feet. These areas often remain mildly cyanotic for 1 to 2 hours after birth. The general circulatory lability probably accounts for the mottled appearance of the infant's skin when it is exposed to air and for the "chilliness" of the infant's hands and feet.

Pulse Rate

Like the rate of respiration, the pulse rate also is labile and follows a pattern similar to that of respiration. When respiration is rapid, the pulse tends to be rapid; similarly, when respiration slows, so does the pulse. Like the fetal heart rate, the newborn's pulse rate is usually 120 to 150 beats per minute. During sleep the pulse rate may drop to 100 beats per minute. With crying and other intense activity, the rate may rise to 180 beats per minute.

Blood Pressure

Although normal newborn blood pressure varies with the neonate's size, weight, and activity, it usually ranges from 60/40 to 80/50; lower average pressures are found in preterm infants. The infant's blood pressure rises with crying and activity.[5]

Total Blood Volume

Several factors influence the total blood volume of the newborn: (1) gestational age; (2) type of delivery (vaginal or cesarean); and (3) time of cord clamping.

While in utero, the low oxygen tension of the maternal blood in the intervillous spaces stimulates fetal erythropoiesis. Thus the total blood volume in the term infant is comparatively greater than that in the adult. The newborn's total blood volume is approximately 300 to 370 and represents 10% to 15% of total body weight.

If the infant is held below the level of the placenta and clamping of the cord is delayed until the cord stops pulsating, 50 ml to 100 ml of additional blood may enter the infant's circulation.[6] Delayed clamping of the cord may increase the blood volume as much as 40% to 60%.[7] A question has arisen as to whether or not the additional placental transfusion is advantageous for the infant. The rapid increase in blood volume may stress the heart and pulmonary circulation; however, some reports indicate that the incidence of neonatal respiratory distress is decreased with delayed clamping.[5] Infants who receive the extra blood gain an increased storage supply of iron from the breakdown of additional hemoglobin. These iron stores may be advantageous later when iron is needed for rapid growth or when dietary intake of iron is inadequate. However, hemolysis of the extra blood can contribute to hyperbilirubinemia in the first 72 hours of life.[8]

Erythrocyte Count and Hemoglobin Concentration

To ensure adequate oxygenation for intrauterine survival, growth, and development, the fetus must have higher hemoglobin and hematocrit blood values than an adult. Table 17-2 lists hematologic values of the newborn. These values are influenced by the following:

1. Duration of gestation. The hemoglobin concentration rapidly increases during the final weeks of gestation. Preterm infants do not have this benefit and, compared with the normal term infant, have low hemoglobin values.

2. Time of cord clamping. Infants who receive additional blood as a result of delayed cord clamping demonstrate increased hemoglobin and hematocrit levels for the first 3 to 4 days after birth.

3. Hemoconcentration. Immediately after birth there is an increase in the erythrocyte count over cord blood levels because of a decrease in plasma volume. This increase reaches a maximum level 2 to 6 hours later.

Red blood cell production (erythropoiesis) is suppressed for several months after birth; when added to the increased blood volume caused by the infant's rapid growth, this suppression results in a progressive decline in the hemoglobin concentration. A low point of 9 to 13 g/dl may be reached after 2 to 3 months. This physiologic anemia does not represent any abnormality or nutritional deficiency in the infant and is unaffected by iron therapy. Active erythropoiesis resumes near this time. If the iron

TABLE 17-2

Newborn Laboratory Values

Laboratory Test	Cord blood
Hemoglobin concentration	14.0–20.0 g/dl
Hematocrit	43%–63%
Red blood cell count	4,200,000–5,800,000/mm
White blood cell count	10,000–30,000/mm
Platelet count	150,000–350,000/mm
Bilirubin	1.0–1.8 mg/dl
Prothrombin time (seconds)	14
Partial thromboplastin time (seconds)	51

Adapted from Shurin S: Hematologic problems in the fetus and neonate. In Fanaroff A, Martin R (eds): Neonatal-Perinatal Medicine, 4th ed. St. Louis, CV Mosby, 1987; and Maisel M: The epidemiology of neonatal jaundice. In Avery G: Neonatology: Pathophysiology and Management of the Newborn, 3rd ed. Philadelphia, JB Lippincott, 1987.

supply is adequate, the hemoglobin concentration gradually increases to an average level of 12.5 g/dl, where it stays during early childhood.

Physiologic Jaundice

Normal destruction of fetal red blood cells liberates bilirubin. The bilirubin is bound tightly to serum albumin and is transported to the liver for conjugation. A marked deficiency of the enzyme glucuronyl transferase reduces the ability of the newborn's liver to alter the fat-soluble bilirubin to a conjugated, water-soluble form for excretion. Figure 17-5 depicts the pathways of bilirubin synthesis, transport, and metabolism. Mean newborn total serum bilirubin levels are illustrated in Figure 17-6.

Jaundice is the visible evidence of a rise in the serum concentration of unconjugated bilirubin to 5 mg/dl or above. Approximately 40% to 60% of full-term newborns (and a higher percentage of preterm infants) develop jaundice between the second and fourth day of life. In the absence of disease this is called **physiologic jaundice**. Although its cause is as yet unclear, several physiologic characteristics of the newborn appear to contribute to the development of physiologic jaundice (see the display below). Some genetic and ethnic factors seem to influence the incidence of physiologic jaundice also (see Cultural Implications: Physiologic Jaundice). However, the following should be investigated promptly: (1) bil-

Newborn Physiologic Mechanisms Related to Development of Physiologic Jaundice

The newborn's high erythrocyte count and the shorter life span of the red blood cells (70 to 90 days) result in increased breakdown of red blood cells.

With cell breakdown the hemoglobin splits into two fragments, heme and globin. While the globin is used by the body, the heme forms unconjugated bilirubin.

Normal newborns produce 6 to 8 mg of bilirubin/kg/24 hours.

Liver uptake of bilirubin is limited by the available enzymes for conjugation.

Newborn serum albumin does not bind bilirubin as effectively as does adult albumin.

The lack of intestinal bacterial flora may result in bilirubin's being reabsorbed and recirculated.

Levels of circulating unconjugated bilirubin may exceed the conjugating ability of the liver and the binding capacity of serum albumin.

Adapted from Korones S: High-Risk Newborn Infants. St. Louis, CV Mosby, 1986.

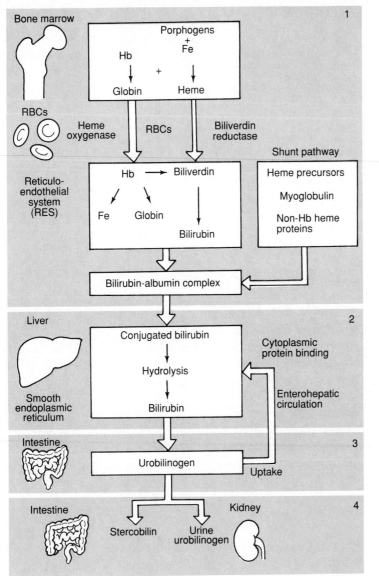

FIGURE 17-5

Physiology of Bilirubin. Bilirubin, liberated by the destruction of red blood cells is (1) bound to serum albumin, (2) transported to the newborn infant's liver, and (3) altered by the actions of liver enzymes into a water-soluble form that can be (4) excreted through the gastrointestinal and renal systems. Conjugated bilirubin is then excreted in the stool and urine. When the amount of bilirubin exceeds the capacity of the liver to convert it to a form that can be excreted, the excess remains in the circulating blood. Because of its neurotoxic effects, high circulating levels of bilirubin pose a hazard to the newborn.

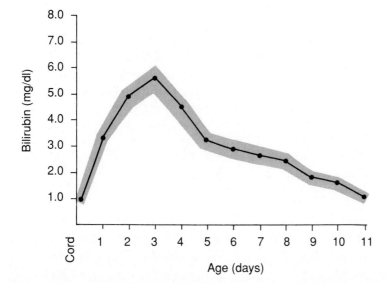

FIGURE 17-6

Unconjugated Bilirubin. Mean serum bilirubin values in normal newborn cord blood range from 1.0 to 1.8 mg/dl. Between 60 and 72 hours after birth, the unconjugated bilirubin concentration reaches a mean peak of 6 mg/dl. The concentration then declines to approximately 2 mg/dl by the fifth day of life. The rate of decline slows somewhat thereafter, and the normal adult value of approximately 1 mg/dl is reached by day 10 or 11 of life.

▲ CULTURAL
IMPLICATIONS

Physiologic Jaundice

Increased neonatal serum bilirubin levels have been noted in infants of the following ancestry: Oriental, Greek, and American Indian.

Japanese-American infants have a significantly higher incidence of hyperbilirubinemia.

Lower serum bilirubin levels have been noted in black infants in the United States and Great Britian.

A hereditary deficiency of the liver enzyme glucose 6-phosphate dehydrogenase has been linked with a higher incidence of hyperbilirubinemia. This disorder occurs more commonly in Oriental, Greek, and black infants. Because of the greater difficulty in detecting jaundice early in black infants, they should be observed carefully.

Adapted from Maisel M: The epidemiology of neonatal jaundice. In Avery G: Neonatology: Pathophysiology and Management of the Newborn, 3rd ed. Philadelphia, J B Lippincott, 1987.

irubin levels greater than 5 mg/dl or the appearance of jaundice during the first 24 hours and (2) bilirubin levels greater than 12 mg/dl at any time during the neonatal period.

Breast Milk Jaundice

A strong association has been found between breast-feeding and rising serum bilirubin levels during the first 3 to 6 days of life. The most likely reason for this phenomenon is a lack of sufficient caloric intake and subsequent weight loss.[8] Breast-fed infants who nurse every 3 hours for the first 3 days of life demonstrate lower bilirubin levels than those who nurse less frequently.[9] Infants who receive supplementary formula feedings also demonstrate lower bilirubin levels.[10] If the serum bilirubin level rises to 14 to 16 mg/dl, interrupting nursing for 48 hours and instituting formula feedings result in a rapid fall in the serum bilirubin level. Although the bilirubin level rises 1 to 3 mg/dl when nursing is resumed, it does not reach the previous level.[8]

Pathologic Jaundice

Very high circulating levels of unconjugated bilirubin pose significant threat to the newborn. Bilirubin pigment is neurotoxic and can cause irreversible damage to cells in the brain and spinal cord. An increase in total serum bilirubin of 5 mg/dl per day should be reported promptly.[8] Pathologic jaundice is discussed in Chapter 26.

Blood Coagulation

At birth the vitamin K–dependent blood clotting factors (Factors VII, IX, X, and prothrombin) are significantly low. Also the intestinal tract of the newborn does not contain the bacteria necessary to help synthesize vitamin K. Thus the infant has a transitory deficiency in blood coagulation that occurs between the second and fifth days after birth. On occasion this deficiency is severe enough to cause clinical bleeding. As a preventive measure, many pediatricians order administration of an intramuscular injection of 1 mg of vitamin K shortly after the birth.

Leukocytes

Although there is a wide range of normal for the white blood cell count at birth, the average is approximately 20,000 cells/μl; approximately 70% of the white blood cells are neutrophils. During the first few days after birth, the total white cell count decreases considerably, and lymphocytes replace the neutrophils as the predominant type of cell.

Immune System Changes

Most of the immunologic mechanisms develop early in fetal life; however, many are not yet fully developed in the newborn. Consequently, the infant's resistance to disease is limited.[11] For example, although the fetus or newborn produces phagocytes, the membranes of these cells are more rigid than those of adult cells. This rigidity impairs effective movement to a site of infection. Further, their efficiency in localizing and killing bacteria is limited.[12]

Antibody Immunity

Until 20 to 22 weeks of gestation, serum immunoglobulin levels are very low; transfer of maternal immunoglobulin G (IgG) across the placenta accelerates during the sixth month of gestation. IgG antibodies are responsible for immunity to bacteria, bacterial toxins, and viral agents. Levels reflect maternal response to present and previous infections. At birth the newborn's IgG serum level is 5% to 10% higher than that of the mother. Thus the infant has passive immunity to the infections that generated maternal antibody formation.[12] However, this is a transient immunity that declines rapidly during the first few months of life.

The infant produces only small amounts of IgM, the antibody category that protects against blood-borne infection. The low levels of IgM may explain, in part, the newborn's susceptibility to gram-negative bacterial infections.[12] Elevated levels of IgM in cord blood indicate intrauterine exposure to syphilis, rubella, cytomegalovirus, or other members of the TORCH group of infections (*T*, toxoplasmosis; *O*, other; *R*, rubella; *C*, cytomegalovirus; *H*, herpes).

The newborn also produces very small quantities of IgE antibodies; these antibodies are important in hypersensitivity allergic reactions. Further, the newborn produces little or no IgA; these antibodies are important in providing local mucosal immunity to respiratory and gastrointestinal viruses and bacteria. However, IgA is the predominant immunoglobulin in human colostrum and breast milk and may provide the breast-fed infant some passive immunity to these agents.[12]

Response to Inflammation

The newborn's response to inflammation is functionally immature; thus traditional measures for detecting inflammation such as fever and leukocytosis are not valuable signs of infection.[11]

Neurologic Changes

The nervous system of the newborn is immature; it is neither anatomically nor physiologically fully developed. Although all neurons are present, many remain immature for several months—some, for years. Thus the infant (1) is uncoordinated in his or her movements, (2) is labile in his or her temperature regulation, and (3) has poor control over his or her musculature—he or she startles easily and is subject to tremors of the extremities. However, development is rapid during the neonatal period. As the various nerve pathways controlling the muscles are used, the nerve fibers connect with one another. Gradually, more complex patterns of behavior emerge, and the higher cerebral levels begin to function.

Reflexes

The reflexes are important indices of the infant's normal development. Their presence or absence at certain times reflects the extent of normality in central nervous system functions (individual reflexes are discussed in Chapter 18).

Metabolic Changes

While the fetus is in utero, the mother's body systems maintain fetal body temperature, nutrition, hydration, and acid–base and electrolyte balances. At birth, however, newborns become dependent on their own bodies to maintain metabolic stability. The absence of necessary enzymes and the immaturity or inefficiency of the newborn's body systems increase the potential for serious metabolic compromise.

Temperature Regulation

Before birth the fetal temperature is 0.5° C (0.9° F) higher than that of the mother and is relatively stable.[3] Although some heat is transferred to the surrounding amniotic fluid, the majority of heat transfer occurs in the intervillous spaces of the placenta. At birth the newborn infant enters an environment that is considerably cooler than that of the mother's body. Because of the sudden change in environmental conditions, the newborn's temperature may drop several degrees after birth. The newborn's temperature tends to vary with environmental temperature because of the newborn's limited supply of insulating subcutaneous fat and large surface area in relation to body weight. In addition, the infant's ability to generate heat is limited.

Shivering is the most common mechanism by which adults produce heat in response to chilling. Newborns, however, rarely shiver. Their primary mechanism of heat production is **nonshivering thermogenesis**, which refers to heat that is produced by an increased metabolic rate. The heat is a by-product of a chemical reaction in **brown fat**.

Brown fat usually is not found in adults. However, this unique form of adipose tissue accounts for approximately 1.5% of total body weight in the newborn.[3] Brown fat cells contain many small fat vacuoles in contrast to the single large vacuole of white fat. Thus brown fat is metabolized easily to generate heat. It also has a richer blood supply, which helps account for its darker color and aids in the distribution of the heat produced. However, newborns have a limited amount of brown fat (Fig. 17-7), and when it is used to produce heat, the fat cells may be depleted rapidly.

Newborn Response to Cold

Nonshivering thermogenesis is activated by chilling: (1) thermoreceptors in the infant's skin transmit messages to the hypothalamus; (2) the hypothalamus triggers the release of norepinephrine from sympathetic nerve

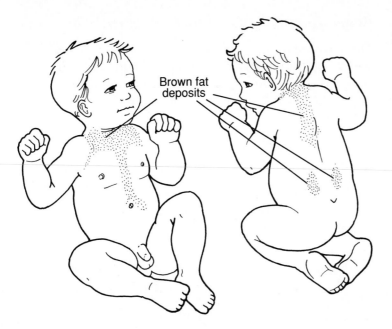

Brown fat
deposits

FIGURE 17-7

Brown Fat. Deposits of brown fat are found between the scapulae, at the nape of the neck, in the axillae, in the mediastinum, and surrounding the kidneys and adrenals. The skin overlying brown fat deposits feels slightly warmer to the touch. Brown fat reserves usually persist for several weeks after birth unless depleted for heat production required by cold stress.

endings; (3) norepinephrine stimulates brown fat metabolism; (4) intracellular fat is broken down to form triglycerides, glycerol, and fatty acids; and (5) oxidation of the fatty acids liberates heat. Mechanisms of heat loss and production are summarized in Table 17-3.

Effects of Cold Stress

The high metabolic rate associated with nonshivering thermogenesis increases both oxygen and energy consumption. To replace the heat lost during a temperature drop of 3.5° C (6.3° F), the infant must increase oxygen consumption by 100% for more than 1½ hours. The physiologic stress of responding to hypothermia contributes to rapid development of metabolic acidosis, even in vigorous full-term infants.

TABLE 17-3

Thermal Regulation in the Newborn

Heat Loss	Heat Production
Evaporation: loss of heat to the air by way of moisture from the skin or lungs; occurs when wet infant exits the mother's body at birth, during bathing, when the environmental humidity is low, and (from the lungs) when the infant has tachypnea.	Nonshivering thermogenesis: metabolic mobilization of brown fat deposits to produce heat Associated problems: limited brown fat deposits; large amounts of energy and oxygen required; impaired by hypoxia; may contribute to development of metabolic acidosis
Conduction: transfer of heat from a warm object to a cooler one by direct contact; occurs when the infant is placed on a cold surface or when cool blankets or clothing are applied.	Increased activity of voluntary muscles Associated problems: requires large amounts of energy and oxygen; may rapidly exceed energy resources

Convection: transfer of heat from the body to the surrounding air; infant's temperature is affected by the air currents in the environment	Heat conservation mechanisms
	  Peripheral vasoconstriction—maintains heat in body core
	  Assumption of fetal position—decreases exposed surfaces

Radiation: transfer of heat from a warm object to a cooler one when the objects are not in direct contact; occurs if the walls of the crib are cool or if the crib is close to a cool outside wall or window.	

Renal Changes and Urinary Excretion

The renal and respiratory systems are important in adjusting to acid-base disturbances. The fetal kidneys demonstrate function in the fourth gestational month. However, their relative immaturity at birth seriously impairs their ability to regulate effectively the infant's internal environment.

The newborn's kidneys are unable to concentrate or dilute urine efficiently. The average maximum urinary concentration is a specific gravity of 1.018 to 1.021. The average maximum urinary dilution is 1.001. The newborn's glomerular filtration rate (GFR) is approximately 30% to 50% that of the adult, and the newborn's tubular secretion and reabsorption are less efficient. The low GFR limits the newborn's ability to excrete a fluid load rapidly and may result in overhydration.[13,14] The inefficiency in tubular reabsorption may result in loss of amino acids and bicarbonate. The inability to concentrate urine efficiently may result in dehydration.

The renal threshold for glucose, amino acids, phosphate, and bicarbonate is low. Proteinuria is common in the first week of life, and the urine may contain large amounts of urates. The lower thresholds for glucose and protein increase potential for newborn hypoproteinemia and hypoglycemia. Three factors contribute to the newborn's tendency toward transient elevations in blood urea nitrogen level: (1) the ability to concentrate urine is limited; (2) urea clearance is low; and (3) production of ammonia is limited.[15]

Gastrointestinal Changes

Nutrition

By the end of the third gestational month, insulin may be detected in fetal plasma, and the small intestine is capable of actively transporting glucose. In the final weeks of gestation large carbohydrate reserves accumulate in the liver and skeletal muscle. These reserves are metabolized for energy needs during the first few days of life.

Since the infant does not have the ability to transfer food from the lips to the pharynx, food must be placed well back on the tongue to aid swallowing. Sucking is facilitated by strong sucking muscles and ridges in the anterior portion of the mouth. In addition, the sucking pads (deposits of fatty tissue in each cheek) prevent the collapse of the cheeks during nursing and make sucking more effective. This fatty tissue remains (even when fat is lost from the rest of the body) until sucking is no longer essential to obtain food. The salivary glands are immature at birth and manufacture little saliva until the infant is approximately 3 months old.

The newborn's intestinal tract is proportionately longer than that of an adult. Although the musculature of the gastrointestinal system is somewhat underdeveloped at birth, the term infant can ingest, digest, and absorb some foods in liquid form. Sufficient intestinal and pancreatic enzymes are present to digest most simple carbohydrates and proteins; however, fat digestion is poor.[16] Pancreatic amylase and lipase are not present at birth, and digestion of complex sugars, starches, and fats occurs more readily in later infancy.

Hydration

By 16 weeks gestation, fetal gastrointestinal function is sufficient to permit absorption of water ingested as amniotic fluid. At term the fetus swallows approximately 450 ml of amniotic fluid per day.[16] At birth approximately 80% of the newborn's total body weight is water, 35% to 40% of which is extracellular fluid. The 10% to 15% total weight loss that occurs in the first week of life is due largely to loss of extracellular fluid.[15] Water is lost through the lungs during respiration, by evaporation from the skin, and in urine and stool. The infant's daily requirement for water increases progressively after birth. A 30% increase in the amount of water needed to maintain hydration accompanies exposure to radiant warmers. A 10% increase in water requirements is associated with phototherapy.[17]

REFERENCES

1. Farrell P, and Perelman R: The developmental biology of the lung. In Fanaroff A, Martin R (eds): Neonatal-Perinatal Medicine, 4th ed. St. Louis, CV Mosby, 1987
2. Nelson N: The onset of respiration. In Avery G: Neonatology: Pathophysiology and Management of the Newborn, 3rd ed. Philadelphia, JB Lippincott, 1987
3. Korones S: High-Risk Newborn Infants, the Basis for Intensive Nursing Care, 4th ed. St. Louis, CV Mosby, 1986
4. James L, Adamsons K: The newborn infant. In Danforth D, Scott J: Obstetrics and Gynecology, 5th ed. Philadelphia, JB Lippincott, 1986
5. Cabal L et al: Neonatal clinical cardiopulmonary monitoring. In Fanaroff A, Martin R (eds): Neonatal-Perinatal Medicine, 4th ed. St. Louis, CV Mosby, 1987
6. Cunningham F et al: William's Obstetrics, 18th ed. Norwalk, Conn, Appleton & Lange, 1989
7. Shurin S: Hematologic problems in the fetus and neonate. In Fanaroff A., Martin R (eds): Neonatal-Perinatal Medicine, 4th ed. St. Louis, CV Mosby, 1987
8. Maisels M: The epidemiology of neonatal jaundice. In Avery G: Neonatology: Pathophysiology and Management of the Newborn, 3rd ed. Philadelphia, JB Lippincott, 1987
9. DeCarvalho M, Klaus M, Merkatz R: Frequency of breast-feeding and serum bilirubin concentration. Am J Dis Child 136:737-738, 1982
10. Osborn L, Bolus R. Breastfeeding and jaundice in the first week of Life. J Fam Pract 20:475-480, 1985
11. Bellanti J et al: Immunology of the fetus and newborn. In Avery G: Neonatology: Pathophysiology and Management of the Newborn, 3rd ed. Philadelphia, JB Lippincott, 1987
12. Palmer S, Manthel U: Immunology. In Fanaroff A, Martin R, (eds): Neonatal-Perinatal Medicine, 4th ed. St. Louis, CV Mosby, 1987
13. Jose P et al: Renal disease. In Avery G: Neonatology: Pathophysioloy and Management of the Newborn, 3rd ed. Philadelphia, JB Lippincott, 1987
14. Spitzer A et al: The kidney and urinary tract. In Fanaroff A, Martin R (eds): Neonatal-Perinatal Medicine, 4th ed. St. Louis, CV Mosby, 1987
15. Behrman R, and Vaughan V: Nelson Textbook of Pediatrics, 13 ed. Philadelphia, WB Saunders, 1987
16. Bucuvalas J, Ballistreri W: The neonatal gastrointestinal tract: Development. In Fanaroff A, Martin R (eds): Neonatal-Perinatal Medicine, 4th ed. St. Louis, CV Mosby, 1987
17. Nash M: Provision of water and electrolytes. In Fanaroff A, Martin R (eds): Neonatal-Perinatal Medicine, 4th ed. St.Louis, CV Mosby, 1987

SUGGESTED READINGS

Anderson C: Integration of the Brazelton Neonatal Behavioral Assessment Scale into routine neonatal nursing care. Issues Compr Pediatr Nurs 9:341-351, 1986

Avery G: Neonatology: Pathophysiology and Management of the Newborn, 3rd ed. Philadelphia, JB Lippincott, 1987

Banta S: Transition to extrauterine life. Neonatal Network 3:35, June 1985

Bernhardt J: Sensory capabilities of the fetus. Am J Matern Child Nurs 12(1):44, January/February 1987

Blanchette V, Zipursky A: Neonatal hematology. In Avery G: Neonatology: Pathophysiology and Management of the Newborn, 3rd ed. Philadelphia, JB Lippincott, 1987

Brazelton T: Behavioral competence of the newborn infant. In Avery G: Neonatology: Pathophysiology and Management of the Newborn, 3rd ed. Philadelphia, JB Lippincott, 1987

Brazelton T: Neonatal Behavioral Assessment Scale. London, Spastics International Medical Publications, 1973

Brazelton T: Neonatal Behavioral Assessment Scale, 2nd ed. Philadelphia, JB Lippincott, 1984

Buckner E: Use of Brazelton Neonatal Behavioral Assessment in planning care for parents and newborns. JOGN, 12:26–30, 1983

Crelin E: Functional anatomy of the newborn. New Haven, Conn, Yale University Press, 1973

Daze A, Scanlon J: Neonatal Nursing. Baltimore, University Park Press, 1985

Hey E, Scopes J: Thermoregulation in the newborn. In Avery G: Neonatology: Pathophysiology and Management of the Newborn, 3rd ed. Philadelphia, JB Lippincott, 1987

Judd J: Assessing the newborn from head to toe. Nurs '85 15(12):34, 1985

Korones S: The normal neonate: Assessment of early physical findings. In Sciarra J et al (eds): Gynecology and Obstetrics, Vol 2. Hagerstown, Md, Harper & Row, 1985

Lochlin M: Assessing jaundice in full-term newborns. Pediatr Nurs 13(1):15, 1987

Lubchenco L, Koops B: Assessment of weight and gestational age. In Avery G: Neonatology: Pathophysiology and Management of the Newborn, 3rd ed. Philadelphia, JB Lippincott, 1987

Ouimette J: Perinatal Nursing. Boston, Jones & Bartlett Publishers, 1986

Ruchala P: The effect of wearing head coverings on the axillary temperature of infants. Am J Matern Child Nurs 10:240, July/August 1985

Tan K: Blood pressure in full term healthy neonates. Clin Pediatr 26:21, January 1987

CHAPTER 18

Psychosocial Aspects of the Postpartum Family

IMPORTANT TERMINOLOGY

attachment Ongoing development of a mutually satisfying relationship between parent and infant

bonding Development of parental feelings of affection and concern for the newborn

en face Face-to-face position in which there is eye contact between parent and newborn

engrossment State of being focused on interacting with the newborn

letting-go phase Mother recognizes and accepts infant as a separate person; adapts her personal life-style to meet the infant's needs

postpartum blues Transitory period of mild depression; related to effects of puerperal hormonal changes and alterations in self-concept and life-style

taking-hold phase Beginning of active entry into maternal role

taking-in phase Initial discovery of maternal role transition

Pregnancy and parenthood may be viewed as common developmental tasks of the normal family life cycle.[1] Childbearing generates changes in self-image, life-style, and social role. Pregnancy is the anticipatory phase of the role transition to parenthood. The postpartum period marks the honeymoon phase of the transition. Prenatal parent education and family-centered care appear to expedite the processes of bonding, attachment, and coping with role transition.[2] This chapter discusses common responses of family members that occur during the postpartum period.

Transition to Parenthood

Anticipatory Phase

During pregnancy couples are in the anticipatory phase of role transition. The total life experiences of both parents influence their perceptions of pregnancy, parenthood, and family.[3,4] Expectant parents often experience intense feelings, challenges, and responsibilities.

Feeling some ambivalence toward parenthood is not unusual. Expectant couples experience varying degrees of psychologic stress caused by the developmental tasks of pregnancy. Family decision-making patterns, individual and joint responsibilities, allocation of time, space, and resources, and many other aspects of their lives are affected. Either or both partners may be concerned about the effect of children on their careers. Each may worry about the personal, interpersonal, and economic impact of the impending changes in roles, responsibilities, and relationships. Incorporating children into the family challenges the parents' ability to give of themselves.[5]

Males and females undergo different processes of gender-identity maturation.[5] As young children, both boys and girls identify with their mother. However, as they grow older, boys are encouraged to separate themselves from the female role, whereas the mother remains a role model for girls. Pregnancy and anticipation of parenthood require both partners to expand their individual self-concepts to include the new role of "mother" or "father." For the pregnant woman the unconscious continuing connection to her mother often reactivates unresolved old conflicts. The expectant father may experience similar feelings as he remembers his relationship with his own father.[6] The woman's perception and expectations of the man's role as father may induce additional stress.[7] The manner in which couples resolve their individual and mutual developmental tasks influences the later structure and function of their families.[8]

Generally, expectant parents are pleased and excited about having a baby. They are open and responsive to experiences that help them anticipate, understand, and prepare for the changes of pregnancy, labor and delivery, and parenting. Many actively seek out knowledge and aid in planning for the future.

Honeymoon Phase

The honeymoon phase refers to the postchildbirth period. Through prolonged contact and intimacy, a bond between the parents and their newborn is established. It is a period of intense activity when both parents are focused on exploring the newborn and their new roles. The couple's personal relationship is no less important; however, each is engaged in trying to adjust the "fit" of his or her personality to the demands of the new role. With the extensive demands on their limited energy, emphasis often is placed on development of the new relationship with the infant. Although they may not as yet acknowledge the need, new parents require some time alone together to mutually discover, explore, and reinforce their relationship with one another.

Bonding and Attachment

Authorities agree that **bonding** is the tie from parent to infant; **attachment** refers to the tie from infant to parent.[9,10] The parent-to-infant bond es-

Infant Influences on Bonding

Physical Characteristics

Appearance: tiny, cute, defenseless
Resemblance to parent(s)

Behavioral Characteristics

Responsive
    Maintains direct eye contact
    Is quiet, alert
    Exhibits interest in parent(s)
    Listens when parent talks; turns head in direction of parent's voice
    Mimics parent's facial expression, e.g., smiles
    Grasps parent's finger
Signals need for attention (i.e., cries) and is soothed by attention from mother
    or father (i.e., quiets promptly)
    Talking to infant
    Touching infant
    Holding, carrying, cuddling, rocking infant
    Providing direct care (e.g., feeding, diaper change)
Temperament ("happy" baby)
    Predictable; regular sleep-awake pattern
    Adaptable

Adapted from Sameroff A: Psychologic needs of the parent in infant development. In Avery G: Neonatology: Pathophysiology and Management of the Newborn, 3rd ed. Philadelphia, JB Lippincott, 1987.

tablished in the early postpartum period provides the foundation for the infant's later attachments to his or her parents and others. The quality of the early parent-infant relationship thus influences the quality of all future ties.[11]

Bonding involves parent-infant interaction. Prolonged, early contact is important to the psychologic process of bonding.[11] The honeymoon phase begins during the fourth stage of labor; the opportunity to touch, hold, and interact with the newborn facilitates parental bonding, which is enhanced by the infant's response to the parents' faces, touch, and voices (see above). However, an estimated 40% of "normal" new parents take 1 week or more to feel the infant is truly theirs.[12]

Behavioral studies of the bonding process have identified the following important aspects:

- There may be a sensitive period in the first hours and days after birth when close parent-infant contact is especially beneficial in promoting optimum bonding. However, the process occurs at different times for different people.[12]
- Species-specific parental responses occur when the infant is first given to the mother or father.[9]
- The process seems structured so that parents become attached to only one infant at a time. This phenomenon is known as *monotropy*.[13]
- Bonding may be impaired if the infant fails to interact with the parent(s). This principle has been called the "You can't love a dishrag" phenomenon.[9]
- It is difficult (but not impossible) to go through the attachment and detachment processes simultaneously. Thus it is difficult (but not impossible) for parents to attach to an infant while mourning the loss or threatened loss of another person.[9]
- Affectional ties can be disturbed (and may be altered permanently) by temporary newborn disorders that occur during the transitional period.[14]

- Emotional support, guidance, appropriate reassurance, and encouragement of parents by health care providers (e.g., nurses) can reduce the impact of temporary newborn disorders and facilitate effective parent-infant bonding.[11,14,15]

Assumption of Parental Role

As parents continue in their role transition, certain behaviors become apparent. Most research into assumption of parental role has focused on maternal behaviors. However, recent studies reveal that the father's responses are markedly similar.[3]

Influences on Parental Behavior

A schematic diagram of major influences on parental behavior and their potential outcomes is presented in Figure 18-1. Parental background and experiences in the immediate postpartum period apparently are important variables. The health status and ability of the newborn to interact with the parents also are important. The influence of parental variables can be altered by (1) the psychologic crisis of birth and (2) the nurturing, support, and guidance provided by the health caregiver.[11,14]

Cognitive Level

Cognitive level refers to the sequential development of the intellectual ability to deal with the abstract and plan for the future. Concrete thinking is typical of childhood when judgments are based on the outward appearance of things. Parents who are concrete thinkers may experience greater difficulty in attaching to infants (1) who look different (do not resemble the fantasy child), (2) who are premature, or (3) who are ill.[15]

Newborn Behavior

Bonding is facilitated by the infant's behavioral responses. After the initial response to birth, healthy newborns who are warm and comfortable enter a quiet, alert state. Their eyes are open, and they display interest in the human face. Held **en face,** they will gaze into the parent's eyes and turn their heads toward the sound of a human voice. Often, they may mimic the parent's facial expression. Usually, parents are enchanted and delighted; the positive response of infant to parent supports and reinforces attachment.[9,12] Conversely, poor newborn-parent interaction discourages bonding. For example, infants who are hyperreactive to sensory stimuli, cannot maintain eye contact, and fail to respond to usual comforting measures do not reinforce positive parenting behaviors.[16]

Maternal Behavior

Reva Rubin[17] pioneered nursing research into parental behavior. Her early studies identified three phases of orderly progression in maternal behavior (Table 18-1 p. 432). Rubin described the tasks of mothering as (1) identifying the new child, (2) determining one's relationship to the child, and (3) guiding and reconstructing the family constellation to include the new

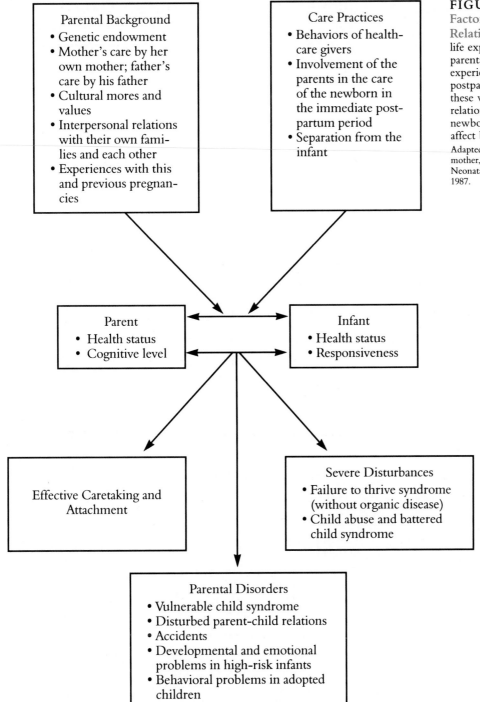

FIGURE 18-1
Factors Affecting Parent–Infant Relationship. The interplay of previous life experiences and care variables influences parental behavior. Positive parental experiences during the immediate postpartum period may alter the effects of these variables on the parent-infant relationship. The health and ability of the newborn to interact with the parents also affect bonding and attachment.

Adapted from Klaus M, Kennell J: Care of the mother, father and infant. In Fanaroff A, Martin R: Neonatal-Perinatal Medicine. St. Louis, CV Mosby, 1987.

member. Rubin maintained that certain behaviors accompany these various tasks and the assumption of the maternal role. Current research suggests that contemporary mothers progress through similar phases. However, maternity-nursing practices that involve parents immediately in the infant's care appear to expedite achievement of developmental tasks and attainment of maternal role.[18,19] Table 18-2 describes clinical aspects of maternal role transition.

TABLE 18-1

Rubin's Phases of Maternal Behavior

Phase	Behavior
Taking-In Present: First 2-3 days after delivery	Relives birth experiences Focuses on her own needs, e.g., sleep, food Passive and dependent
Taking-Hold Present: Day 3 or 4 to day 14	Expresses concern over her own body functions and ability to care for infant Seeks reassurance and assistance Actively participates in care of self and infant
Letting-Go Begins during week 3	Acknowledges infant as separate individual Demonstrates increased independence in care of self and infant

TABLE 18-2

Clinical Aspects of Maternal Psychologic Adaptations to Parturition: Rubin's Phase of Maternal Role Transition

Assessment	Rationale
Verbalization and discussion of labor and delivery experiences *Taking-in*: Verbally relives labor and delivery experiences	Reinforces reality of end of pregnancy; enables beginning realization of infant as a separate being
Maternal touch behaviors *Taking-in*: Tentative fingertip touch; progresses to palmar touch and enfoldment	Reflects psychosocial progress from acquaintance to acceptance, ownership, comfort, and protectiveness
Involvement with self-care *Taking-in*: Passive dependence; accepts nursing aid in meeting her needs for care; comfort, sleep, and food are major concerns	Reflects depleted energy reserves, focus on self, and need for nurturing
Taking-hold: Active participation in own health maintenance; concern with control over own body function	Reflects increasing focus on return to independence
Involvement with infant care *Taking-in*: Passive dependence; accepts nursing responsibility for infant care	Reflects inward focus on integrating reality of end of pregnancy, depleted energy stores, and focus on self
Taking-hold: Actively seeks practice, aid, and reassurance in developing infant care skills; assumes increasing responsibility for infant care	Reflects acceptance and assumption of maternal role and responsibilities

Taking-In Phase

In the **taking-in phase** the mother is concerned primarily with her own needs. She may be quite passive and dependent. Some mothers may not initiate contact with their infants—not out of disinterest but because of their own immediate dependency. Although the mother may not indicate much interest in assuming responsibility for the infant's care, she is taking in information that helps her identify the infant as her own.

Taking-in involves discovery. Three processes assist the mother in discovery as she becomes acquainted with her infant: identification, relating, and interpreting with the infant. In *identification* the mother points out physical aspects or features of the infant that provide a frame of

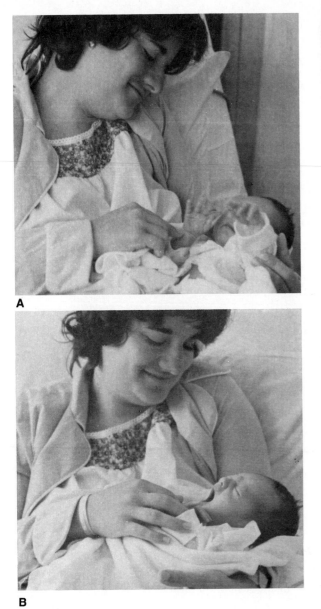

A

B

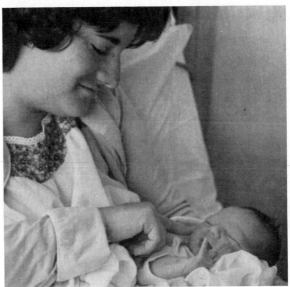

C

FIGURE 18-2

Aspects of Taking-In Phase. **A,B,** The mother may lay the infant on her lap and gently explore him or her with her fingertips. Palmar contact with larger surfaces of the infant's body (not shown) is followed by, **C,** enfoldment of the arms. Engrossment is typical of the first steps in the idenfication process and is evidence of an awakening interest in the newborn.

reference (e.g., "He has his father's eyes/nose/chin"). From there she *relates* actions and characteristics to some familiar person, object, or fantasy (e.g., "She has hiccoughs just like her sister did"). Finally, in *interpreting* she gives meaning to the infant's actions and perceived needs. For instance, if the infant is crying and difficult to quiet, she may say, "He's going to be a holy terror; I just know it." All these behaviors help the mother realize the infant is a separate person.

MATERNAL TOUCH. Initial interactions with the infant may be somewhat tentative. *Fingertip touch* with the infant (Fig. 18-2, *A*) is the first stage in maternal touch. As the mother becomes more comfortable with her infant, she moves to the second stage, *palmar contact* (Fig. 18-2, *A-C*). The third stage of maternal touch is *enfoldment* (Fig. 18-2, *C*).

INTEGRATING THE EXPERIENCE. During the taking-in phase the mother relives the birth experience to integrate it fully into reality. She is apt to

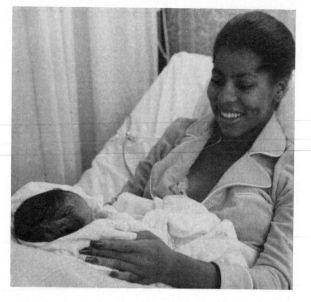

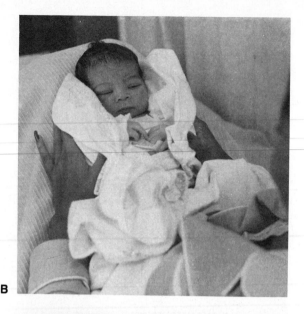

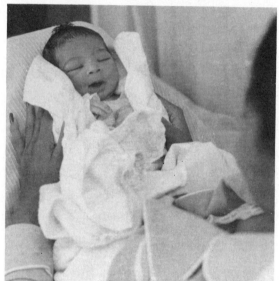

FIGURE 18-3

Mother-Infant Interactions. A,B, The mother positions herself or the infant so they can have eye contact (en face) and mutually explore each other's face. **B,** The infant establishes eye contact with the mother. **C,** The infant responds to an animated smiling face and begins to move his or her mouth as the mother smiles and talks.

be very talkative at this time. She may want to know specifics and details of the delivery so that she can form a total picture of what "really" happened. This information reinforces the realization that pregnancy and delivery are truly over and that her infant is now an individual separate from herself. Figure 18-3 shows mother-infant interactions. This task involves profound changes in attitudes and feelings.

NEED FOR SLEEP AND FOOD. Sleep and food play an important part during this phase. The mother is more able to begin the activities required for her if she is allowed to rest and sleep after the energy expenditures of labor and delivery. If this necessary rest is disrupted, the mother may experience "sleep hunger" that may last for several days. Irritability and complaints of fatigue reflect sleep hunger.

Food has tremendous psychologic significance. A concern about food is part of the mother's general need for nurturing. The mother may talk a great deal about the adequacy or inadequacy of her meals or request between-meal nourishments.

Taking-Hold Phase

In the **taking-hold phase** the mother actively seeks independence. One of her main concerns is her ability to control her body functions. She takes an active part in her own care. She wants to walk, to sit, and to move as she did before the delivery. It is as if she is thinking, "How can I possibly assume responsibility for others if I cannot control my own body?" If she is nursing her infant, she is concerned about producing an acceptable quantity and quality of milk. She cannot have enough reassurance that she is "performing" well.

As the woman develops a relationship with her newborn, she integrates the new concept of "mother" into her self-image, i.e., she attains the maternal role.[20] Her first mothering tasks are vitally important to her. If she feels awkward at handling her child or when the infant sleeps rather than nurses, she perceives she has failed as a mother and may show signs of despair. When she succeeds at a task, her relief and delight also are clearly evident.

Letting-Go Phase

As her mothering functions become more established, the mother enters the **letting-go phase.** Generally, this occurs after the mother returns home. In this phase the mother must accomplish two psychologic separations: (1) she must realize and accept the physical separation from her infant, and (2) she must relinquish her former role of childless person. The implications are enormous. She must adjust her life-style to the dependency and helplessness of her child. If she stops working, she must adapt to less freedom, autonomy, and social stimulation. If she continues to work, the complex task of finding mother substitutes and other household caretakers must be resolved (Fig. 18-4).

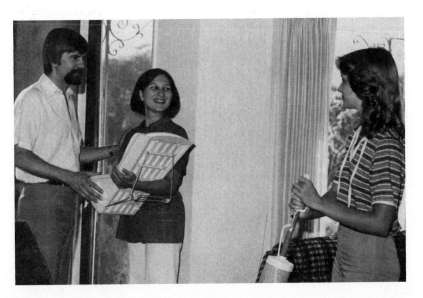

FIGURE 18-4
Adjusting to Shifts and Changes in Household Responsibilities. "Mother's helpers" allow parents more time to enjoy an outing with their infant.

Postpartum Blues

A brief, transient period of mild depression commonly occurs during the first postpartum week.[2,21] This condition is known as **postpartum blues,** or the baby blues (see above). It is thought related both to dropping hormone levels and to the ego stress associated with role transition and altered life-style. Discomfort, fatigue, and exhaustion certainly contribute to this condition. Baby blues is self-limiting and usually ends within 2 to 3 days.

Postpartum Depression

Serious depressive disorders of the puerperium are rare.[2] Most commonly, they reflect situational aspects of other long-standing problems.[22] However, if the depression (1) persists longer than 10 days, (2) deepens, or (3) interferes with the mother's ability to cope with the activities of daily living, psychiatric consultation may be needed. Severe maternal postpartum depression affects the mental and emotional health of the entire family. Marital discord, inadequate parenting, and child behavior problems may result.[23]

Paternal Behavior

Most researchers agree that more studies need to be done about paternal role adaptation and behaviors. Parke,[24] a pioneer in this area, has concluded that there are no significant behavioral differences between maternal and paternal role adaptation. Alone with their infants, fathers exhibit the same behaviors as mothers (Fig. 18-5). Parke found that if the trio is together, the father tends (1) to hold the infant twice as much as the mother, (2) to vocalize more, and (3) to touch the infant slightly more; however, he smiles significantly less. A recent study also found that fathers who had extended contact with their infants during the early postpartum period demonstrated intense **engrossment** and interaction with their newborns, were more involved in caretaking, and exhibited greater self-esteem.[25]

The father's presence at the birth and early contact with the infant do not appear as important in bonding as once was believed.[3] However, fathers who have been actively involved in the birth process seem to display significantly more bonding behaviors. In addition, the amount of time spent with the newborn in the early postpartum period appears important to paternal bonding. The more time a father can spend with his newborn in the first few days after birth, the greater is his engrossment and pleasure in interacting with the infant.[12,15]

After the early honeymoon phase (in the hospital and perhaps the first few days after discharge), work and other normal pursuits also occupy the father's attention. He, too, experiences role change. If this is their

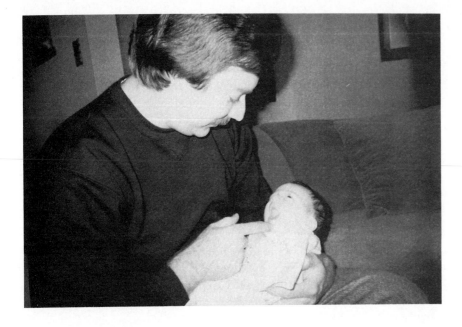

FIGURE 18-5
Father-Infant Interaction. The father positions himself to gain eye contact with the infant. Engrossment and exploratory touch also are evident.

first child, because of the mother's seeming preoccupation with the infant's needs, he may feel neglected or in competition with it. When there are older siblings in the family, the father may assume a more active role as caregiver for them.

Sibling Behavior

Several variables influence the response of a sibling to the new baby. Influential factors include the child's (1) age; (2) participation in the pregnancy experience, e.g., accompanying mother on prenatal visits, hearing the fetal heart tones, helping prepare the home for a new baby; (3) preparation for the event, e.g., attending sibling programs that teach what infants are like; (4) feelings of security and parental love and the quality of the family life; (5) opportunities to discuss his or her feelings about the new infant before it comes; (6) attendance at the birth; and (7) opportunity for immediate bonding interactions, e.g., touching, holding.

The newborn's response to the sibling, e.g., eye contact, often elicits feelings similar to those of the parents. Some siblings may speak of "our baby" or "my baby sister/brother." They may display pride, excitement, curiosity, and ownership; they may seek involvement with the care and avidly accept the new expectations of them as "big brother" or "big sister." They may see helping out with the infant or watching over the newborn as a positive alteration in status. For others, the sudden reality of the new infant and the personal loss of parental time and attention may cause transient feelings of insecurity, frustration, and anger. These children may feel they have been replaced in their parents' affections and demand attention and reassurance; some may withdraw into themselves. Young children may view the closeness of the breast-feeding mother and new infant with jealousy and rage and want to suckle also. Some siblings may exhibit open hostility toward the infant; others may regress to an earlier developmental stage, exhibiting thumb sucking, bedwetting, or baby talk.

Adjustment of Grandparents

Grandparents also are faced with psychosocial adjustments to their new roles and, perhaps, alterations in self-image. Some may perceive the newborn as undesired, irrefutable evidence of their own aging. However, most grandparents are thrilled and delighted with the arrival of a new infant. For many the event revives warm and happy memories. The earlier days of their own relationship, the birth of the child who now has become a father or mother, and the events of that early childhood are recalled. Further, grandchildren assure the continuance of the family throughout time.

Bonding Behaviors

Grandparents often display the same bonding behaviors as do the parents and siblings. They, too, seek eye contact with the infant and talk to it. Their touch may be tentative as they explore the newborn and discover his or her unique (and family) features and personality, but enfoldment usually occurs with the first opportunity.

Grandparents often are a stabilizing influence on the entire family. For most new parents their own parents are invaluable resources. They provide emotional support, share their experiences and knowledge, and offer needed comfort during the minor (and major) crises that usually occur in any new family. They can offer older siblings needed attention, love, and reassurance of their importance in the family. Some are delighted to care for the infant so that the new parents will have opportunities for recreation and time together. However, many contemporary American families lack easy access to the help and support provided by grandparents because of geographic separation. Legal or psychologic separation (e.g., related to a previous divorce) also may deprive the new family of this important support system.

Cultural Influences

Often parental role behavior is prescribed by cultural mores and values. For example, the type and amount of paternal involvement with childbirth and infant care may be influenced or dictated by the culturally defined male social role.[26] In some cultures even maternal involvement with the newborn may be limited. The responsibility for infant care during the first month post partum may be assumed by female members of the extended family.[27] Grandmothers may exert major influences on the behaviors of new parents.[28]

Culturally related health beliefs and practices also influence maternal behaviors during the postpartum period. Some cultures impose specific bathing, dietary, and activity restrictions on the new mother.[29,30]

Clients With Special Needs
Adolescent Parents

Data from the National Research Council[31] reveal that adolescent parents are less likely to complete their own education, to be able to meet their economic needs, or to establish stable marriages and families. Adolescent mothers are more likely (1) to have another baby within 2 years and more children within 3 to 5 years; (2) to be single parents (unwed or become divorced); (3) to become welfare recipients; and (4) to experience serious family problems. Adolescent fathers often fail to complete their basic schooling, have fewer opportunities for employment and career advancement, and have limited earning potential.

Adolescent mothers (and fathers) often fail to achieve the rapid, smooth transition to parenthood they (and others) may expect. Coping with the developmental tasks of parenthood often is complicated by the unmet developmental needs and tasks of adolescence. They may experience difficulty accepting a changing self-image, altering life-style, and adjusting to new roles required by the responsibilities of infant care. They may feel "different" from their peers, excluded from normal adolescent activities, i.e., "fun," and forced into undesired aspects of an adult social role. The conflict between their own desires and the demands of the infant and the low tolerance to frustration typical of adolescence further contribute to the normal psychosocial stress of the postpartum period.

Factors that influence their successful transition to responsible parenthood include (1) their previous life experiences, (2) their current level of developmental maturity, (3) their perception of and response to the impact of their responsibilities as parents on their own lives and plans; (4) their ability to seek and accept help; and (5) the amount, type, and quality of support available.[32]

Antepartum Aspects of Care

Effective anticipatory guidance and client teaching help prepare adolescents for the psychosocial challenges of pregnancy and parenting. Guided antepartum discussions can assist them in examining the present and potential impact of childbearing on their lives. Determining their individual knowledge deficits and meeting their needs for information and counseling facilitates informed decision making and planning for the future (see below).

Postpartum Aspects of Care

During the hospital stay prenatal teaching and counseling are reviewed, reinforced, and, when necessary, augmented. Additional nursing emphasis is placed on assessment of (1) the adolescents' responses to the infant, (2) the adequacy of their current support system, (3) their individual psychosocial and economic needs, (4) their plans for the future, and (5) their knowledge of community resources.

Adolescent Adaptation to Childbearing: Common Areas for Counseling

Parenting and childrearing
   Family role and responsibilities
   Normal infant growth and development
   Parenting skills
Decision making
   Continuing education or vocational training
   Contraception
Opportunities for socialization
   Provision for child care in the parent's absence

Anticipatory guidance includes preparing them (1) to understand their own postpartum needs and responses; (2) to identify the changing needs of the infant as it grows and develops; (3) to recognize the implications for the future; and (4) to use appropriate resources. Client teaching includes self-care, infant care, and information specific to their individual needs, e.g., contraception. When given adequate support, guidance, instruction, and encouragement in the postpartum period, adolescent parents can (1) cope effectively with the common stresses of the postpartum period; (2) achieve their developmental tasks; (3) make informed decisions; and (4) succeed at parenthood.[32]

Older Parents

Increasing numbers of women and couples are experiencing childbearing beyond the age of 30. The emergence of this contemporary phenomenon may have been influenced both by biomedical advances, i.e., the advent of effective methods of contraception that allow individual family planning choices, and social changes. Social changes include (1) the women's liberation movement and emphasis on a woman's right to control her own destiny; (2) expanded educational and career opportunities for women; (3) women's desire to postpone childbearing until personal goals and financial security have been achieved; (4) elective single parenting; (5) later marriage, e.g., in young adulthood; and (6) greater numbers of early divorce with later remarriage.

Many of these mothers are successful career women who are secure in their job-related self-image and skills. Others have been successful in previous parenting experiences. However, this pregnancy and its outcome may generate stresses similar to those confronting clients in other age groups. Anticipatory guidance and client teaching in the antepartum period assist older women in planning for the new parenting experience. Postpartum psychosocial adaptation varies among all clients, and nursing assistance must be tailored to the individual client's needs.

Family Adaptation

The entire family is affected by the arrival of a new baby. Each member experiences psychologic stress related to the challenges of new developmental tasks and alterations in self-concept. Roles, responsibilities, and relationships must be redefined and life-styles adjusted to meet the new demands. Family adaptation and functioning are influenced by intrafamily and external forces.[33] These forces include (1) the degree to which each member has achieved previous developmental tasks; (2) social, cultural, and religious values; and (3) the availability and use of support systems.

The birth of the first child requires the couple to expand their individual self-concepts to include the new dimensions of "mother" and "father." Further, together they must achieve the joint developmental tasks of the "family" (see display on p. 441). They must align their personal expectations for their new roles, responsibilities, and relationships and develop a shared concept of family.

Sporadic ambivalence, anger, and hostility toward the infant commonly arise during its first weeks at home. New parents may be over-

Developmental Tasks of the Childbearing Family

Adapting housing arrangements to meet infant's needs
Meeting financial expenses of the new infant
Realigning individual and shared responsibilities
Reestablishing mutually satisfying sexual relationships
Refining patterns of communication
Redefining relationships with extended family
Developing a shared concept of family
Entering new roles in the community
Deciding whether or not to have more children

Adapted from Duvall E: Marriage and Family Development, 5th ed. Philadelphia, JB Lippincott, 1977.

whelmed by these (normal) feelings, which usually are related to unrealistic self-expectations and to sleep deprivation. Their (self-perceived) inability to meet the total needs of infant, self, and family engenders feelings of inadequacy in the parental role. These feelings erode self-confidence and, consequently, self-image. Effective anticipatory guidance during the antepartum and postpartum periods facilitates successful achievement of parental developmental tasks and smooths transition into the parental role.

REFERENCES

1. Rossi A: Transition to parenthood. J Marr Fam 30:26-39, February 1968
2. Easterling W, Herbert W: The puerperium. In Danforth D, Scott J: Obstetrics and Gynecology, 5th ed. Philadelphia, JB Lippincott, 1986
3. May K, Perrin S: Prelude: Pregnancy and birth. In Hanson S, Bozett F (eds): Dimensions of Fatherhood. Beverly Hills, Calif, Sage Publishing, 1985
4. Curry M: Variables related to adaptation to motherhood in "normal" primiparous women. JOGN 12(2):115-121, December 1983
5. Daly M, Hotelling K: Psychology and the life stages of women. In Willson R et al (eds): Obstetrics and Gynecology, 8th ed. St. Louis, CV Mosby, 1987
6. Lederman R: Psychosocial Adaptation in Pregnancy. Englewood Cliffs, NJ, Prentice-Hall, 1984
7. Fishbein E: Expectant father's stress—Due to mother's expectations? JOGN 13:325, September/October 1984
8. Broom B: Consensus about the marital relationship during transition to parenthood. Nurs Res 33(4):223-228, July/August 1984
9. Klaus M, Kennell J: Parent-Infant Bonding. St. Louis, CV Mosby, 1982
10. Brazelton T: Comments. In Klaus M, Klaus P: Parent-Infant Bonding, 2nd ed. St. Louis, CV Mosby, 1982
11. Brown J, Bernstein D: Family-centered nursing care. In Avery G (ed): Neonatology: Pathophysiology and Management of the Newborn. Phildadelphia, JB Lippincott, 1987
12. Klaus M, Klaus P: The Amazing Newborn. Menlo Park, Calif, Addison-Wesley, 1985
13. Bowlby J: Attachment and Loss. New York, Basic Books, 1969. Quoted in Sameroff A: Psychologic needs of the parent in infant development. In Avery G (ed): Neonatology: Pathophysiology and Management of the Newborn. Philadelphia, JB Lippincott, 1987
14. Klaus M, Kennell J: Care of the mother, father, and infant. In Fanaroff A, Martin R: Neonatal-Perinatal Medicine. St. Louis, CV Mosby, 1987
15. Sameroff A: Psychologic needs of the parent in infant development. In Avery G (ed): Neonatology: Pathophysiology and Management of the Newborn. Philadelphia, JB Lippincott, 1987
16. Poulsen M: Children exposed to drugs: Challenge of the nineties. Paper presented at the Third Annual Conference on Substance Abuse and Pregnancy, St. Petersburg, Fla, February 7, 1990
17. Rubin R: Puerperal change. Nurs Outlook 9:753, 1961a
18. Gay JT, Edgil AE, Douglas AB: Reva Rubin revisited. JOGN 11:394-399, November/December 1988
19. Martell L, Mitchell SK: Rubin's "puerperal change" reconsidered. JOGN 13:145, May/June 1984
20. Rubin R: Maternal Identity and the Maternal Experience. New York, Springer Publishing, 1984
21. Cunningham F et al: Williams Obstetrics, 18th ed. Norwalk, Conn, Appleton & Lange, 1989
22. Watson J et al: Psychiatric disorders in pregnancy and the first postnatal year. Br J Psychol, pp 144-453. Quoted in Cunningham et al, 1989, p 253
23. Martell L: Postpartum depression as a family problem. MCN 15:90-93, March/April 1990

24. Parke R: The father's role in infancy: a reevaluation. Birth Fam J 5:211-213, Winter 1978
25. Keller W, Hildebrandt K, Richards M: Effects of extended father-infant contact during the newborn period. Infant Behav Dev 9:337, 1985
26. Kay M: Anthropology of Human Birth. Philadelphia, FA Davis, 1982
27. Pillsbury B: Doing the month: Confinement and convalescence of Chinese women after childbirth. In Kay M: Anthropology of Human Birth. Philadelphia, FA Davis, 1982
28. Grosso C et al: The Vietnamese American family: And grandma makes three. MCN 6:177, 1981
29. Engel N: An American experience of pregnancy and childbirth in Japan. Birth 16(2):81-86, June 1989
30. Anderson S, Bauwens E: An ethnography of home birth. In Kay M: Anthropology of Human Birth. Philadelphia, FA Davis, 1982
31. National Research Council: Risking the future: Adolescent sexuality, pregnancy and childbearing. Washington, DC, National Academy Press, 1987
32. Hofman A: Adolescent Medicine. Menlo Park, Calif, Addison-Wesley, 1983
33. Belsky J: Experimenting with the family in the newborn period. Child Dev 56:407-414, 1985

SUGGESTED READINGS

Affonso D: Assessment of maternal postpartum adaptation. Pub Health Nurs 4(1):9-20, April 1987
Choi E, Hamilton R: The effects of culture on mother-infant interaction. JOGN 15:256, May/June 1986
Fishman SH et al: Changes in sexual relationships in postpartum couples. JOGN, 15:58, January/February 1986
Hampson S: Nursing interventions for the first 3 postpartum months. JOGN, 18(2):116-121, March/April 1989
Humenick S, Bugen L: Parenting roles: Expectation versus reality. MCN 12:36-39, December 1987
Konrad CJ: Helping mothers integrate the birth experience. MCN 12:4:268, December 1987
Mansell KA: Mother-baby units. The concept works. MCN 9:132, 1984
Meleis A, Sorrell L: Arab American women and their birth experiences. MCN 6:171, 1981
Orque MS, Bloch B, Monrroy LA: Ethnic Nursing Care, A Multicultural Approach. St. Louis, CV Mosby, 1983
Pridham K: The meaning for mothers of a new infant: Relationship to maternal experience. Matern Child Nurs J 16(2):103-122, Summer 1987
Rubin R: Basic maternal behavior. Nurs Outlook 11:683-686, 1961b
Tomlinson P: Father involvement with first-born infants: Interpersonal and situational factors. Pediatr Nurs 13:101, March/April 1987
Tulman L, Fawcett J: Return of functional ability after childbirth. Nurs Res 37(2):77-81, 1988
Tribotti S et al: Nursing diagnoses for the postpartum woman. JOGN 11:410-416, November/December 1988

CHAPTER 19

Maternal Nursing Care in the Postpartum Period

IMPORTANT TERMINOLOGY

anticipatory guidance Nursing interventions designed to assist the mother in coping with predictable future needs

atony Lack of normal muscle tone

coitus Vaginal intercourse

colostrum Thin, yellowish breast fluid; precursor to breast milk

fundal height Relationship of the position of the uterine fundus to the umbilicus; identified as U/1 (one fingerbreadth below the umbilicus) or 1/U (one fingerbreadth above the umbilicus)

fundus Rounded "crown" area of the uterus between the fallopian tubes

Homans' sign With the leg extended, forced dorsiflexion of the foot causes calf pain; a sign of lower-extremity thrombophlebitis

involution Return of the uterus to normal nonpregnant size, shape, and consistency; accomplished by contractions and autolysis

lochia Postpartum vaginal discharge that lasts 1 to 3 weeks after delivery

puerperium The 6-week period following childbirth; begins with the fourth stage of labor

Q.S. Abbreviation for "quantity sufficient"; describes voiding in adequate amounts

This chapter continues discussions of the postpartum period. Content focuses on nursing care of the new mother and supportive actions that assist families in successfully adapting to the new demands of parenthood. Emphasis is placed on nursing assessment of factors that influence the mother's recovery, her caregiving abilities, and her successful role transition. Also included are **anticipatory guidance** and the teaching role of the nurse, which are important components of effective postpartum care.

Nursing Assessment

Following delivery, nursing assessments monitor maternal status and progress through the stages of the **puerperium**. Postpartum assessments focus on signs and symptoms that indicate maternal response to labor and delivery events, the biophysical changes affecting her body systems, and the psychologic adjustments to parenthood. Assessment findings can also identify early signs of postpartum complications and enable prompt medical and nursing management. Although the greatest risk for postpartum complications is during the first 24 hours, the potential for problems associated with childbirth persists throughout the puerperium. Because of the greater risk for complications immediately post partum, more frequent nursing assessments are required to monitor the mother's physical status during the first 24 hours.

Admission to the Postpartum Unit

Once the newly delivered mother's body systems are determined stable and there has been opportunity for initial bonding with the newborn, the mother is transferred from the labor / delivery / recovery area to the postpartum unit. The recovery room nurse who transports the mother to her new room is responsible for providing detailed information about the mother's history and labor and delivery events to the staff of the postpartum unit (see Assessment Tool: Admission to Postpartum Unit Checklist). This information provides the initial data base for implementing the nursing process.

Initial Nursing Assessment

For the first 1 to 2 hours after admission to the postpartum unit, status checks are usually conducted every 30 minutes (see Assessment Tool: Initial Postpartum Assessment Checklist). If findings are within normal

---

ASSESSMENT
TOOL

Admission to Postpartum Unit Checklist

The initial data base provided by recovery personnel includes the following information:
  Gravida and parity
  Term or preterm gestation
  Any pertinent prenatal and intrapartum information
  Date, time, and type of delivery
  Sex, weight, and status of newborn
  Estimated blood loss
  Intravenous fluids or medications
  Bonding behaviors
  Breast or bottle feeding
  Recovery room discharge status
    Vital signs
    Fundal height and character
    Lochial amount and character
    Condition of bladder, rectum, perineum
  Any special orders

Initial Postpartum Assessment Checklist

Vital signs
   Temperature: every 4 hr in the absence of elevation
   Pulse and blood pressure with each status check for first 2 hr, then
      every 4 hr
Complaints of discomfort
Intake and output
   Hydration and nutrition
   Time and amount of first one to three voidings
Fundal height and character
Lochial amount and character
Bladder status (nonpalpable or palpable, distended)
Condition of perineum and rectum
   Episiotomy
   Lacerations
   Hemorrhoids
Status on initial ambulation (stable; weak, dizzy)

limits, the intervals for subsequent assessments are lengthened gradually throughout the first 24 hours following delivery, e.g., hourly, every 2 hours.

Ongoing Nursing Assessment

For the remainder of the hospital stay, the nursing assessments of the postpartum mother's physical status are done once each shift. Nursing assessments of the biophysical changes that occur in the puerperium usually include vital signs, breast changes, condition of the abdomen, signs of uterine **involution**, condition of the perineum and episiotomy, urinary and intestinal elimination, and **Homans' sign**. In addition, the nurse is concerned with the mother's general comfort and well-being. Assessment areas also include appetite, rest and sleep patterns, activity, emotional status, how she is adjusting to her role as a new mother, and her individual needs for health teaching (see Assessment Tool: Ongoing Postpartum Nursing Assessment Checklist). Each component of the postpartum checklist is carefully charted. Some hospitals require narrative nurse's notes or checklists of postpartum status and activities of daily living, i.e., voiding, bathing, or both.

Vital Signs

Vital sign assessment data also suggest and support nursing diagnoses of the client's current state of health. Changes in maternal vital signs may reflect complications that affect the mother's recovery. During the first 24 hours after delivery, the mother's temperature, pulse, respirations, and blood pressure are usually assessed every 4 hours.

TEMPERATURE. In the immediate postpartum period temperatures up to 30°C (100.4°F) can be caused by dehydration or excessive intrapartum blood loss. If there is no temperature elevation after the first 24 hours, the temperature, pulse, and respiration are monitored every 8 hours. Temperature elevations suggest possible infection and, when correlated

Ongoing Postpartum Nursing Assessment Checklist

Physical Status
A. Vital signs
B. Breasts
   1. Skin integrity (nipples supple; intact, reddened, fissures)
   2. Consistency (soft, firm, engorged)
   3. Lactation status (suppressed; colostrum, milk)
C. Abdomen (soft, distended, bowel sounds)
D. Involution
   1. Uterus (fundal height and consistency)
   2. Lochia (amount, character, type)
E. Perineum and perianal area (suture line, edema, pain; hemorrhoids)
F. Elimination
   1. Urinary (first three voidings, amount, color, character)
   2. Bowel (flatulence; stool)
G. Homans' sign (absent; present, right, left)
H. Other: complaint of pain or discomfort
   1. Characteristics (sharp, dull, aching)
   2. Degree of discomfort (mild, moderate, severe)
   3. Location (localized, incisional, general)
   4. Cause (precipitated by, associated with, relieved by)
I. Laboratory values
   1. Hematocrit
   2. Hemoglobin
   3. White blood count

Sample Narrative Charting
Routine Postpartum Assessment: Alert and responsive. No complaint of pain. Breasts soft. Nipples supple and intact, no evidence of redness or cracking. Fundus firm and in midline, U/1; moderate lochia rubra. Active bowel sounds present. Episiotomy clean and healing, suture line intact. Voiding Q.S. Homans' sign absent. Ambulates easily without assistance. Bonding evidenced by eye contact, stroking, snuggling; calls newborn by name.

with other assessment data, may identify the underlying health problem, e.g., the nursing history may disclose a preadmission upper respiratory or urinary tract infection; the intrapartum history may reveal an increased risk of uterine infection secondary to prolonged rupture of the membranes.

PULSE. Normal postpartum physiologic bradycardia persists for the first 6 to 10 days and is reflected in pulse rates of 50 to 70. Tachycardia (rate >100) may indicate anxiety or pain. A rapid, thready pulse and hypotension suggest possible hemorrhage, shock, or embolism.

BLOOD PRESSURE. Postpartum blood pressure readings should remain stable. Elevated blood pressure may indicate pregnancy-induced hypertension (PIH), which can develop as late as 72 hours after delivery.

Breast Assessment

During pregnancy progressive changes occur that prepare the breasts for lactation. Postpartum nursing assessment includes inspection and palpation of the mother's breasts to determine lactation status. Normal post-

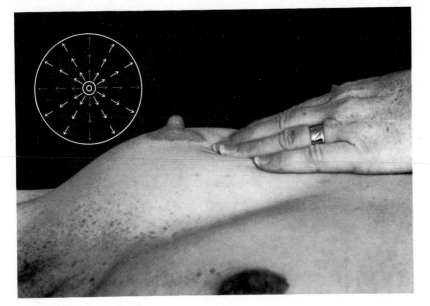

FIGURE 19-1
Palpation for Breast Engorgement.
With the woman supine, the nurse inspects
the breast and axilla. Occasionally accessory
breast tissue and supernumerary nipples may
be found in the axilla. The nurse applies
light pressure with the palmar surface of the
fingers and, using a circular, rotary motion,
palpates both breasts and axillae. One
systematic approach to breast palpation is to
visualize the breast as a clockface and
mentally divide it at 12, 3, 6, and 9 o'clock
into four quadrants. The nurse palpates each
quadrant until the entire breast has been
examined and repeats the procedure to
examine the other breast.

partum hormonal changes establish lactation within 2 to 4 days (average—
3 days) after delivery. Characteristic assessment findings accompany
breast engorgement.

INSPECTION. Age, nutrition, and genetic inheritance influence breast
structure. Considerable variation in size and amount of fatty and glandular
tissue occurs. Breasts may be small, large, or pendulous. Often one breast
is somewhat larger than the other, but the contour is essentially symmetric. The skin is smooth; striae may be noted. Dark areolae surround
the circular nipples. Nipples may protrude, lie flush with the areolae, or
be inverted.

In the first few days after delivery, breast appearance changes little.
Initial postpartum nursing assessments include size, contour, and symmetry of the mother's breasts. In addition, general skin color, texture,
vascular patterning, and the appearance of the areolae (pigmented areas
surrounding the nipples) and nipples are recorded; trauma caused by the
baby's latching on incorrectly may be identified.

For the first 1 to 3 days the breasts secrete **colostrum**, a thin, yellowish
fluid. The breast milk "comes in" 2 to 4 days post partum. Breast engorgement can occur and is due primarily to milk retention in breast
alveoli, compression of the milk ducts, and vascular and lymphatic stasis.
When engorged, the breasts appear larger, tense, and shiny, with distended blue veins, and are a source of discomfort to the mother.

PALPATION. Palpating for signs of impending breast engorgement (Fig.
19-1) is similar to self-examination. During the first few days after delivery the breast tissue feels soft. A generalized, uniform nodularity, which
is caused by the normal hypertrophy of breast alveoli during pregnancy,
can be felt. The nipples are intact and supple and become erect with
stimulation. Colostrum can be expressed by gently grasping the breast
approximately 1/2 inch behind the areola with the thumb and forefinger
so the two fingers form a **C** position. Pressing toward the chest wall and
gently squeezing the fingers together will open the duct so colostrum can

be visualized. When they become engorged, breasts feel uniformly firm, taut, and warm to the touch. Tenderness is common, and palpation is often painful for the mother.

Involution

The potential for hemorrhage or infection through the placental separation site is an element of risk that accompanies normal childbirth. Normal involutional progress reduces the risk of major postpartum complications and is essential to an uneventful recovery after childbirth. The purpose of assessing uterine involution is to identify early signs of deviation from the normal process that indicate a potential threat to the mother's well-being.

The progress of involution is monitored by assessing the height and consistency of the uterine **fundus** and the amount and character of **lochia** (see Nursing Procedure: Fundal Check). Characteristic assessment find-

---

NURSING
PROCEDURE   *Fundal Check*

Intervention

1. Explain procedure and rationale.

2. Have woman empty her bladder.
3. Position client supine in bed, knees bent and apart.
4. Put on gloves.
5. Disengage perineal pad.
   a. Note amount of saturation.
   b. Ask about the time elapsed and amount of time since last pad change.
   c. Explain importance of frequent perineal pad changes.
6. With one hand supporting the lower fundus just above the symphysis pubis, rest other hand on abdomen with middle finger across the umbilicus. Keeping fingers flat, press down; note position of fundus in relation to umbilical landmark.
7. Repeat actions, moving hand down by one fingerbreadth until the fundus is located. Note its position.
8. Discard soiled perineal pad and underpad; provide perineal care and apply fresh perineal pad.
9. Fold discarded perineal pad with soiled surfaces inside; place in paper bag. Dispose of perineal pad and bed pad per agency protocol.
10. Remove gloves and discard; wash hands.
11. Record pad count for first 24 hours after delivery.
12. Record assessment findings related to the following:
    a. Fundal height and consistency
    b. Amount and character of lochia
    c. Status of perineum

Rationale

1. Decreases anxiety; an informed client is more cooperative
2. Distended bladder displaces uterus
3. Relaxes abdominal muscles

4. Observe universal precautions
5.
   a. Estimates blood loss
   b. Provides index of lochial flow in relation to time and activity
   c. Infrequent pad changes increase odor and risk of infection
6. Locates fundal height

7. Identifies rate of descent

8. Promotes comfort and hygiene; reduces potential for infection
9. Minimizes risk of contamination of housekeeping personnel

10. Observe universal precautions
11. Estimates blood loss in the immediate postpartum period
12. Provides data for later assessment comparison

Sample Narrative Charting: Fundus firm and in midline, U/1. Moderate lochia rubra. Episiotomy clean and healing, suture line intact.

Deviations From Expected Patterns

The following uterine assessment findings indicate involution is **not** progressing normally and should be reported to the primary health care provider:

The uterus fails to become progressively smaller in size; fundal height in relation to the umbilicus remains unchanged.

A lack of uterine firmness is noted, i.e., boggy (spongy).

Pelvic discomfort, pressure, or backache persist.

Lochia remains heavy.

Foul lochial odor is present.

ings during the average 2- to 3-day hospital stay are (1) the fundus is firm, (2) fundal position recedes daily, and (3) a moderate amount of lochia rubra is present. The display above shows assessment findings that indicate involution is not progressing as expected.

FUNDAL HEIGHT. **Fundal height** in relation to the umbilicus decreases by approximately one fingerbreadth per day (Fig. 19-2). To assess fundal height accurately, the woman should empty her bladder shortly before palpation; a full bladder pushes against and raises the height of the uterus.

FUNDAL CONSISTENCY. The fundus of the normal involuting uterus feels similar to a round, firm, grapefruit.

LOCHIA. Inspecting the mother's lochia provides an indirect assessment of the progress of endometrial healing. During the normal healing process the amount of lochia gradually diminishes, and the characteristic color changes reflect a decrease in the blood component of the lochial flow.

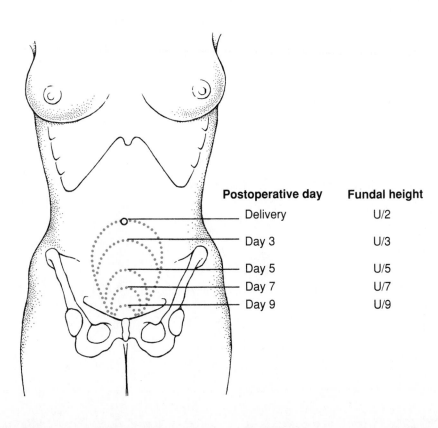

Postoperative day	Fundal height
Delivery	U/2
Day 3	U/3
Day 5	U/5
Day 7	U/7
Day 9	U/9

FIGURE 19-2

Rate of Uterine Involution. After rising to the height of the umbilicus in the immediate postpartum period, the uterus descends into the pelvis at the approximate rate of one fingerbreadth each day. Fundal height in relation to the umbilicus is noted as, for example, U/1, U/2, U/3. By the 10th postpartum day, it cannot be palpated abdominally. Any marked deviation from this rate of descent should be reported to the physician or nurse midwife.

TABLE 19-1

Characteristics of Normal Lochia★

Characteristic	Normal Lochial Progression				
	Rubra	*to*	Serosa	*to*	Alba
Color	Dark red; may have small clots		Pinkish; thin, watery, no clots		Cream to yellowish
Odor	Similar to menstrual flow		No odor		No odor
Occurrence	Days 1 to 3		Days 4 to 10		Days 11 to 21
Amount	Moderate		Moderate to small		Scant

★The lochial pattern is characteristic of the stage of endometrial healing. Immediately following the tissue trauma of placental separation, lochia is red to dark red; as venous sinuses are constricted and healing begins, the amount of blood diminishes. Marked alterations from this pattern suggest possible inflammatory interference with normal healing processes.

Quantity. The quantity of lochia varies somewhat among women but may be more profuse in multiparas. A moderate amount of discharge is the usual finding. The amount of lochia may appear to increase on first ambulation because of prior vaginal pooling. The amount and character of the lochia are observed and recorded daily. These observations indicate the healing progress of the uterine endometrial surface. To assess the amount of lochial volume, the nurse compares it against established standards.[1] Table 19-1 and Figure 19-3 describe characteristic findings.

Character. In the first 1 to 3 days following delivery lochia rubra (dark red) is characteristic of the initial stage of uterine healing. After the third day the character of the lochia becomes thin and more serous (serosa—pinkish), and lochia serosa persists from the fourth to the 10th day. From the 11th through the 21st day, lochia alba (white or yellowish) signifies normal healing progression.[2]

Odor. Lochia smells similar to normal menstrual flow. It should not have a disagreeable or offensive odor. If unusual odor is noted, the nurse should investigate the amount of time elapsed since the perineal pad was changed and the client's use and pattern of perineal care. Often the cost of perineal pads may prompt the woman to replace a soiled pad only when it is completely saturated. Odor results from lochial hemolysis,

FIGURE 19-3

Assessment of Lochial Volume. The degree of saturation of the perineal pad in relation to the amount of time that has elapsed since it was applied provides an estimation of the lochial volume. A moderate amount of lochia rubra is most common during the first 3 days post partum. A large amount of lochia (heavy) indicates potential excessive blood loss and should be reported to the physician or nurse midwife. Bright red vaginal bleeding in the presence of a firm, contracted uterus is indicative of lacerations and also should be reported promptly.

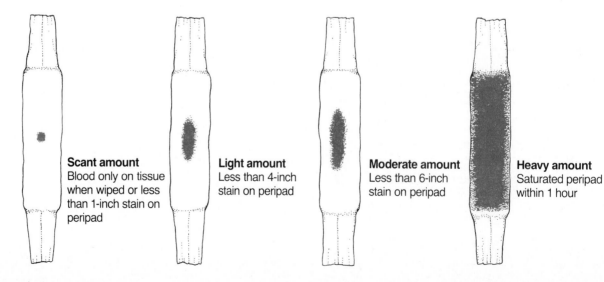

Scant amount
Blood only on tissue when wiped or less than 1-inch stain on peripad

Light amount
Less than 4-inch stain on peripad

Moderate amount
Less than 6-inch stain on peripad

Heavy amount
Saturated peripad within 1 hour

Deviations From Expected Patterns

The following assessment findings should be reported to the primary health care provider:

   Persistent bright red bleeding
   Suppression of lochial discharge
   Fresh bleeding after the lochia has become pinkish and diminished in
      amount
   Persistence of lochia rubra, serosa, or alba beyond the normal time range
   Foul lochial odor with or without fever

urine, stool, and body oils. Malodorous lochia, particularly if accompanied by fever, suggests possible infection (see above).

Hematologic Laboratory Values

Reviewing laboratory findings to gather additional data enables the nurse to plan client care and teaching to meet the individual woman's needs. The estimated blood loss associated with normal childbirth is 400 to 800 ml, with an average of 500 ml.[3] Because there is a 30% to 60% increase in circulating blood volume during pregnancy, the normal, healthy mother experiences few problems associated with this blood loss. However, anemia during pregnancy or excessive blood loss during labor and delivery affect the management of postpartum nursing care.

The extent of changes in postpartum blood values is assessed by comparing results of samples drawn during the month preceding labor with those drawn on the second postpartum day. Average findings are presented in Laboratory Values: Hematologic Changes in Blood Values. Samples drawn at other times cannot be used for comparison because of the following: (1) although findings of the initial blood work may be within normal limits for a healthy adult female, the mother may develop anemia during the months of gestation; (2) hematocrit values determined during labor may reflect hemoconcentration resulting from dehydration—when used as a baseline measure, they convey an erroneous impression of excessive blood loss; (3) hemodilution resulting from postpartum diuresis requires 12 to 24 hours to occur; and (4) even acute hemorrhage may not cause a significant drop in hemoglobin concentration. A drop of 1 g in the hemoglobin level or 3% in the hematocrit value reflects a blood loss of approximately 500 ml[4] (see below).

Urinary Elimination

The most common cause of excessive uterine bleeding during the immediate postpartum period is uterine **atony**. Uterine atony may be related

|||| LABORATORY
VALUES

Hematologic Changes in Blood Values

Blood Value	Late Pregnancy (37–40 weeks)	Post Partum (second day)
Hemoglobin	12.1-12.7 g/dl	10.0-11.4 g/dl
Hematocrit	35%-42%	32%-38%
Leukocytes	5000-12,000/mm	14,000-16,000/mm

Deviations From Expected Patterns

The following laboratory values indicate the presence of maternal anemia and should be discussed with the physician or nurse midwife:

   Preadmission: Hemoglobin concentrations <11 g/dl at 37 to 40 weeks
      gestation (most probable cause is nutritional iron deficiency anemia)
   Postpartum: Hemoglobin concentrations <10 g/dl or hematocrit values
      <30%

to bladder distention or secondary to ineffective uterine contractibility. Maternal postpartum urinary elimination assessments can identify early signs of bladder distention or bladder trauma. Early identification of bladder distention can minimize potential hazards to the mother's health and recovery. Measuring intake and ouput and determining bladder status are two important components of the nursing assessment of urinary elimination.

The newly delivered mother may not experience an urge to void even though her bladder is full. Several factors contribute to her inability to identify the physical sensation of bladder fullness: (1) the bladder capacity increases as a result of the reduced intraabdominal pressure; (2) some edema of the trigone area at the base of the bladder may be present as a result of trauma during labor and delivery; and (3) if she had regional anesthesia during labor, neural transmission of afferent impulses may be impaired. Mothers who receive intravenous fluids during labor are at increased risk to develop a full bladder rapidly. In addition, normal biophysical adaptations contribute to an increased urinary output in the early puerperium, increasing the tendency for bladder distention. To minimize the risk of bladder distention, the mother should be encouraged to void within the first 6 to 8 hours after delivery. The time and amount of the first one to three voidings are measured and recorded.

BLADDER DISTENTION. Assessments that enable the nurse to identify signs of bladder distention include observations of abdominal contour, palpation of fundal height, consistency, and position, observation of lochial volume, and percussion of the suprapubic area (see Assessment Tool: Signs of Bladder Distention). Figure 19-4 illustrates the abdominal contour seen with bladder distention.

Intestinal Elimination

Constipation is common early post partum. The relaxed condition of the intestinal and abdominal muscles and the continued effect of progesterone on smooth muscle contribute to diminished bowel motility. Often the mother's fear of pain inhibits spontaneous defecation. Hearing bowel sounds indicates returning intestinal activity, and passage of the first stool identifies return to normal bowel function.

Perineum

Inspection of the perineum and perianal area are included in postpartum nursing assessments to identify healing progress or signs of complications such as tenderness, swelling, bruising, and hematoma. If the client had

---

ASSESSMENT
TOOL

Signs of Bladder Distention

Initial voidings of <300 ml
Altered abdominal contour; elevated appearance of suprapubic area
Fundus U/U or above; not in abdominal midline; may be boggy
Increase in lochia rubra
Dull sound heard on percussion of suprapubic area

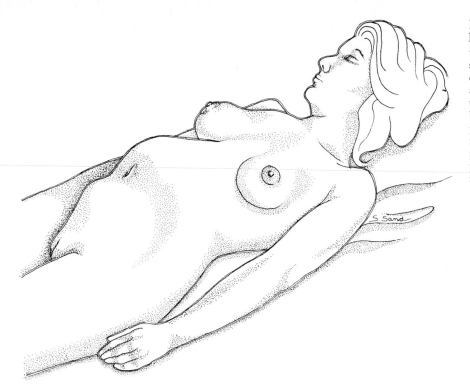

FIGURE 19-4
Bladder Distention. As the bladder fills with urine, it gradually protrudes above the symphysis pubis. If the bladder is markedly distended, the uterus may be pushed upward and to the side. When a hand is cupped over the uterine fundus to massage and bring it back to the midline position, the bladder protrudes even farther. When the hand is removed, the uterus returns to its displaced position. Palpation just above the symphysis pubis reveals a soft spongy consistency instead of firmness.

Perineal Assessment: R.E.E.D.A.   ASSESSMENT
                                                            TOOL

Redness
Edema
Ecchymosis
Discharge
Approximation

---

an episiotomy, the suture line is assessed for signs of separation, infection, and hematoma (see Assessment Tool: Perineal Assessment). The perianal area is inspected for hemorrhoids and fissures.

Perineal pain is rare after spontaneous vaginal delivery without lacerations. Pain is more common when an episiotomy has been performed or lacerations repaired and may be intensified by local edema's causing tension on the perineal sutures.

Lower Extremities

The purpose of assessing the mother's lower extremities is to identify signs of thrombophlebitis. The increased tendency for coagulation (hypercoagulability) and for decreased venous return of blood from the legs during pregnancy predisposes the woman to thrombosis. Prolonged compression of the vessels in the legs while pushing in second stage labor is another factor that also may contribute to clot formation. During routine postpartum nursing assessments the lower extremities are inspected for size, shape, symmetry, varicosities, edema, and color. A positive Homans' sign (Fig. 19-5) indicates thrombophlebitis.

FIGURE 19-5

Homans' Sign. Homans' sign is complaint of pain in the calf when the foot is dorsiflexed with the leg extended. A positive Homans' sign may be the first indication of thrombophlebitis in the leg. Other signs of thrombophlebitis in the lower extremities include unilateral swelling, erythema, and tenderness. Pedal and popliteal pulses may be absent.

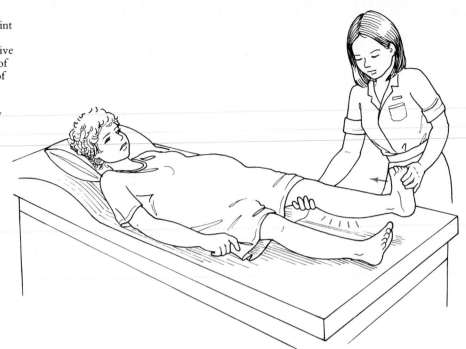

Client teaching focuses on the need to increase circulation and minimize potential for thrombophlebitis. Discussions with the mother include explaining the purpose and value of early ambulation and the importance of not elevating the knee area of the bed.

Risk Factors

Potential for infection is a primary postpartum concern (Table 19-2). The dark, warm, moist environment of the milk ducts and lactiferous sinuses and the presence of breast milk are hospitable to invading bacteria. Placental separation traumatizes the uterine endometrium and provides a portal of entry for bacteria. Lochia is a potential medium for bacterial growth. Normal postpartum diuresis increases potential for bladder distention, urinary stasis, and urinary tract infection.

Data in the client's chart describing events that occurred during labor, delivery, and recovery may suggest additional potential risks to the normal, healthy postpartum mother. Prolonged labor may result in maternal exhaustion and dehydration. Preexisting and coexisting disorders such as PIH, diabetes, and cardiac disease also pose potential risks during the postpartum period. Nursing assessment findings enable the nurse to identify early signs of deviations from expected postpartum patterns.

Psychosocial Assessment

Psychosocial or behavioral assessments enable the nurse to identify (1) maternal and family strengths and needs for emotional support, client teaching, and anticipatory guidance; (2) factors that influence client or

TABLE 19-2

Postpartum Risk Factors

Risk Factor	At Risk For	Assessment Findings
Breast-feeding	Infection (mastitis)	Nipples red, appear irritated; nipple fissures; pain on palpation or breast-feeding
Uterine over-distention (hydramnios, large fetus, multiple pregnancy)	Uterine atony, immediate postpartum hemorrhage (within first 24 hr)	Fundus boggy; heavy lochia rubra; hypotension, tachycardia
Prolonged labor		
Operative (forceps) delivery	Lacerations	Bright red vaginal bleeding
	Uterine atony, hemorrhage	Fundus boggy; heavy lochia rubra
	Hematoma	Distended, firm, often bluish mass (labial, perineal); perineal pain
	Edema of trigone area of bladder; impaired urinary elimination	Unable to void; inadequate urinary output
Premature rupture of membranes	Infection (endometritis)	Temperature elevation, tachycardia, malaise; fundus tender to palpation; lochial change
Prolonged second stage of labor	Thrombus formation; thrombophlebitis	Presence of Homans' sign
Retained placental fragments	Delayed postpartum hemorrhage (after first 24 hr)	Bright red vaginal bleeding

family response to the childbearing experience or the present approach to nursing care; and (3) progress in parenting.

Childbearing is an intensely personal experience that occurs within the social context of the individual family. All members of the family are affected by the birth. For each there is potential stress associated with a changing perception of self, altered intrafamily relationships and life-style, and accepting and integrating the newborn into the family unit. Effective anticipatory guidance is based on accurate assessments of the strengths and needs of the individual family.

Nursing assessments of parenting behaviors focus on identifying response to the newborn, phases of postpartum adjustment, progress toward developmental tasks, and factors that influence merging of the new family unit. Additional assessments focus on identifying the mother's current knowledge about self-care, infant care, and health maintenance (see Assessment Tool: Postpartum Nursing Assessment Checklist: Psychosocial Status). The contemporary trend of visiting by the siblings and grandparents enables the nurse (1) to observe interactions between family members and with the newborn; (2) to assess family adaptation and progress toward merging the new family unit; (3) to identify cultural factors that influence health-related behaviors, postpartum adjustments, and development of the family unit; and (4) to identify needs for emotional support, anticipatory guidance, and client teaching.

Postpartum Psychologic Adjustment Phases

Maternal psychologic responses to the childbearing experience appear to follow a predictable sequence, i.e., "taking-in," "taking-hold," and "letting-go."[5] Characteristic maternal behaviors that reflect underlying changes in self-concept and role perception are associated with each phase (see Assessment Tool: Characteristic Phases of Maternal Postpartum Ad-

Postpartum Nursing Assessment Checklist: Psychosocial Status

Mother

Attachment (bonding) behaviors
  Eye contact; in-face position
  Touching, stroking
  Cuddling
  Calls by name; talks to infant
Adjustment phase
  Taking-in
  Taking-hold
  Letting-go
Cultural variables
  Role definition and responsibilities
  Expectations of caregivers
  Limitations on activities (self-care, infant care)
  Dietary restrictions (food, fluids)
Knowledge level and learning needs
  Self-care
  Infant care
  Family planning

Family

  Nuclear
  Extended
  Communal
  Single parent
  Adolescent
Development and adaptation of family unit
  Attachment (bonding) behaviors of father, siblings, grandparents
  Relationships between family members (roles played, type and quality of
    interactions)
  Evidence of interactive role changes (to father, brother, sister)
Cultural variables
  Role, influence of extended family
  Expectations of caregivers

justment). The mother's psychologic adaptation to parenthood can be assessed based on evidence of these expected behaviors. The amount of time an individual mother requires to complete each phase varies.[6] Today's prenatal care and preparation for childbirth may expedite postpartum adjustment; routine ultrasonography often identifies fetal sex, allowing parents to select and use the child's name before birth, encouraging prenatal bonding, and expediting taking-in.[7] Because of the shortened hospital stay, the nurse may see only the beginning of maternal progress in taking-hold.

Cultural Variations

Psychosocial nursing assessments of the client and family focus also on identifying any ethnic or culturally related health beliefs and practices that influence behaviors expected of the new mother during the puerperium (see Assessment Tool: Cultural Health Beliefs and Health Practices in the Postpartum Period). The greatest difference between American and non-Western health management during pregnancy and childbearing apparently is in perceptions of the postpartum period. Many non-Western

Characteristic Phases of Maternal Postpartum Adjustment

Taking-In Phase

Passive, dependent, concerned with own needs
Talkative; repeatedly relives the delivery experience verbally
Explores the reality of the infant, demonstrates bonding
   Touches with fingertips
   Seeks eye contact; frequently holds infant in facing position
   Identifies infant's image and behavior as similar to that of self, husband,
     other children, members of extended family
   Predicts future talents and behaviors

Taking-Hold Phase

Verbalizes concern about exerting control over her own body functions
Expresses worry about her ability to "be a good mother"
Actively seeks information and assistance needed to meet her perceived needs;
  responsive to teaching
Demonstrates increasing comfort with infant; exhibits total hand contact and
  enfolding

Letting-Go Phase

Early stage
Expresses feelings of insecurity and inadequacy
Hesitant in approaching infant care task without support and guidance
Identifies infant as separate individual
Relinquishes role of childless individual; integrates concept of self as "mother"

Later stage
Developing confidence in own abilities as "mother"
Actively assumes independent responsibility for self and infant
Establishes new interdependent roles with significant others
Integrating infant into family

Postpartum let-down
Irritable
Cries without reason
Loss of appetite
Altered sleep patterns

Cultural Health Beliefs and Health Practices in the Postpartum Period

Ask client to describe the following:

Personal meaning of this birth
   Impact on health and balance of body systems (e.g., yin/yang)
   Self-image, role change, and responsibilities
Expectations regarding recovery
   Length of time required
   Factors affecting recovery
Accepted behaviors and health practices (cultural prescriptions)
   Amount of rest required
   Beginning activities (what? when?)
   Hygienic practices needed or avoided
   Dietary needs or restrictions

cultures hold strong folk beliefs about the new mother's state of health and prescribe specific "do's and don'ts" during the puerperium. Common cultural beliefs and associated postpartum behaviors identified by contemporary researchers are summarized in the Cultural Implications box below.

Insight into the influence of cultural factors on maternal and family expectations and behaviors enables the nurse (1) to establish a therapeutic nurse/client relationship; (2) to plan and implement effective, individualized, client-centered, goal-directed postpartum care and client teaching; (3) to project and encourage compliance with medical and nursing recommendations; and (4) to evaluate client responses accurately.

Learning Needs

An important component of the nursing assessment is identification of the mother's knowledge deficits and learning needs. Effective anticipatory guidance, e.g., client teaching and referral to community resources, is planned and implemented on the basis of the client's present and projected future needs. Each client's level of knowledge and ability to assume responsibility for self-care, infant care, and health maintenance activities varies. The mother's background and previous life experiences provide a foundation for learning. Some mothers need guided learning in self-care and infant care activities; others are comfortable with those skills but may need help in understanding and dealing with sibling rivalry. Mothers who have no experience with childbirth or in caring for infants may require more teaching and emotional support.

CULTURAL IMPLICATIONS

Beliefs: Body imbalance (hot/cold; yin/yang)
The postpartum woman is believed polluted with fetal blood or in a "cold" state of health. She is vulnerable to illness unless she follows specific cultural prescriptions.

Culturally prescribed postpartum behaviors
1. Observe a long period of seclusion, rest, and avoidance of physical activity and sexual intercourse. Often household responsibilities and infant care are provided by another female family member during this time.
   Two weeks: Filipino
   One month: Chinese, Japanese
   Forty days: Mexican Americans, Southeast Asians (Vietnamese, Cambodians, Laotians)
2. Avoid cold and maintain and increase body warmth.
   Avoid bathing: Chinese, Mexican Americans, Southeast Asians, Japanese, Shinto (may shower; ritual bath at end of seclusion period)
   May not wash hair: Chinese, Raza/Latina
   Add external heat (remain covered at all times, extra blankets, slippers): Hispanics, Filipinos, Asians
   Avoid exposure to any breeze or wind: Chinese, Southern blacks, Mexican-Americans, Filipinos, Southeast Asians
3. Follow dietary prescriptions and restrictions (hot/cold)
   Chinese: Eat five or six meals daily; rice, eggs, organ meats, chicken are considered "hot" foods; hot herbal teas are encouraged; water, cold, and raw foods are avoided
   Hispanics: Fresh fruit and vegetables and cold and sour (acidic) foods are avoided

---

Compiled from discussions in references 8 through 13.

Nursing Diagnosis

Nursing diagnoses are used to define the focus for individualized post-partum care. They are derived from the individual client's total data base (see Potential Nursing Diagnoses, p. 460.) Integrating knowledge of normal postpartum biophysical and psychosocial aspects with analyses of assessment findings enables the nurse (1) to identify actual present nursing diagnoses; (2) to project potential nursing diagnoses; (3) to establish client-centered goals; (4) to plan appropriate, goal-directed nursing care; and (5) to evaluate the effects of nursing interventions and goal attainment.

Planning and Intervention

Nursing interventions during the postpartum period are designed to maximize potential for an uneventful recovery and to facilitate development of a stable family unit. Current trends in maternity care such as a shortened hospital stay have caused the nursing profession to realign priorities for care. The amount of time that physical care is provided by the nurse has diminished, and the emphasis on client teaching for self-care and health maintenance has increased.

In the early postpartum period, i.e., the first 24 to 48 hours after delivery, the mother's dependency needs must be met. Providing or assisting the mother with basic bedside activities allows her to rest, relax, and focus on taking-in. Interventions that increase her sense of psychologic security and encourage a positive self-concept include facilitating adequate comfort, rest, and nutrition and providing guidance and emotional support as the woman begins to examine her new identity of

---

Focus Assessment

Physiologic Aspects

Identify presence of contribution factors.
    Review admission bloodwork for signs of antepartum anemia or infection.
    Identify estimated blood loss during labor and delivery.
    Determine use and amount of intravenous fluids during labor and delivery.
    Determine use of regional anesthesia for delivery.
    Estimate time elapsed since delivery.
    Evaluate postpartum laboratory studies, i.e., complete blood count, hemoglobin and hematocrit values.
    Monitor intake and output and bladder status.
    Monitor bowel sounds, passage of gas, stool.

Psychosocial Aspects

Identify client's perception of personal knowledge and skills needed for self-care and infant care.
Identify anticipated demands on parental time.
Elicit description of client's plans for organizing time/activities to meet anticipated needs.
Estimate effectiveness of available client support system.
Identify individual learning needs.
Estimate readiness to learn.
Determine past/present coping behaviors.
Evaluate ability to problem solve.

POTENTIAL NURSING DIAGNOSES

Postpartum Care

Biophysical Aspects

Fluid Volume Deficit (2): Immediate—related to excessive blood loss secondary to uterine atony, cervical, or vaginal lacerations

Fluid Volume Deficit (2): Delayed—related to excessive blood loss secondary to retained placental fragments

Potential for Infection: Mastitis, Endometritis, Wound Infection—related to bacterial invasion of body structures secondary to impaired tissue integrity, lactation, open placental site; indwelling catheter secondary to inability to void or bladder distention, surgery

Impaired Skin Integrity—related to surgical incision or episiotomy/laceration

Urinary Retention—related to regional edema secondary to delivery trauma, increased capacity; overdistention secondary to postpartal diuresis

Pain—related to breast engorgement, uterine contractions or afterpains, surgical incision or episiotomy, hemorrhoids

Altered Nutrition: Less than Body Requirements for Lactation and Successful Breast-feeding

Constipation—related to reduced bowel motility and decreased abdominal muscle tone or pain medication

Psychosocial Aspects

Knowledge Deficit (Learning Need)—regarding self-care, infant care, health maintenance activities (nutrition, family planning, adaptation to parenting)

Ineffective Individual Coping—related to personal perception of inability to parent effectively, response to normal postpartum physiologic changes ("baby blues")

Family Coping: Potential for Growth—related to bonding and integration of newborn into the developing family unit

Potential Altered Parenting—related to feelings of inadequacy, incompetence, disappointment regarding newborn

Situational Low Self-Esteem—related to altered body image, role transition, personal identity, "baby blues"

Family Process, Altered—related to stress of demands of developmental tasks, change in role, and life-style

Sleep Pattern Disturbance—related to life-style changes associated with breast-feeding, infant care

Diagnoses abstracted and expanded from the approved NANDA list of Approved Nursing Diagnoses, June 1988.

"mother." The mother needs attention, guidance, encouragement, and positive reinforcement to begin exploring her new role and responsibilities.

Anticipatory Guidance

Planning for discharge begins with the client's admission to the hospital. Contemporary trends in maternal-newborn care have increased the importance of anticipating common problems experienced by clients after discharge and integrating guidance toward preventing or resolving future problems into in-hospital nursing care. Most new mothers are eager to go home. However, after they and their infants have been discharged from the hospital, many women find they are overwhelmed by the multiple demands of parenthood; they report feelings of insecurity about their own abilities to care for themselves and their infants, concern about their own worth as mothers, and disturbances in self-concept.[14,15] Effective anticipatory guidance is designed to assist mothers in coping with predictable future stresses and to minimize the impact on postpartum mental health. Client teaching during in-hospital postpartum care and providing reference materials such as pamphlets on breast-feeding, infant care and development, when to call the doctor, and referral information for future use are important components of postpartum nursing care.

Client Teaching

Postpartum client teaching is directed toward meeting the client's individual needs for knowledge of self-care, infant care, and health maintenance actions (see Client Self-Care Education: Checklist). The purpose of client teaching is to enable mothers to gain knowledge and skills needed for safe, effective health maintenance care of self and infant; to develop confidence and competence in applying knowledge and skills in providing care; to make informed judgments about health options; and to take appropriate health maintenance actions (see Client Self-Care Education: General Outline, p. 462).

Specific client-centered nursing goals are set for each identified knowledge deficit. Mothers who have had no previous childbirth or infant care experience may require extensive teaching for self-care and infant care.

Checklist

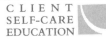

CLIENT
SELF-CARE
EDUCATION

I. Physical aspects of self-care
  A. Bathing and breast care, support, and comfort
    1. Breast-feeding (bra, milk expression, ice packs)
    2. Bottle-feeding (bra, ice packs)
  B. Involution: fundus and characteristic lochia; afterpains
  C. Perineal care (solutions, witch hazel pads)
    1. Sitz bath
    2. Perineal heat lamp
  D. Nutrition and hydration (breast-feeding, bottle-feeding)
  E. Rest and sleep
  F. Exercise (ambulation, postpartum and Kegel's exercises)
  G. Bowel elimination
  H. Signs to report promptly
  I. Available assistance with household tasks
II. Psychosocial aspects of self-care
  A. Emotional adjustment (bonding, taking-in, taking-hold, letting-go)
    1. Self-image
    2. Baby blues
  B. Family relations
    1. Family adjustments to the new baby (parental, sibling, extended family)
    2. Role change
    3. Alterations in life-style
  C. Sexuality and family planning
  D. Visitors
III. Infant care
  A. Feeding (breast, formula)
  B. Positioning and handling
  C. Bathing
  D. Cord and circumcision care
  E. Clothing and diapering
  F. Temperature and thermometer use
  G. Suctioning with bulb syringe
  H. Infant behavior patterns (sleeping, crying, fussing, neuromuscular control, eye movements, developmental patterns, elimination patterns)
  I. Safety (car seat use, never leaving baby alone on bed or table, non-flammable clothing)
  J. Recognizing signs of illness; signs to report promptly to physician
IV. Community resources (La Leche International, family service agencies, local mother's support groups, parenting education sources)

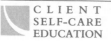

CLIENT
SELF-CARE
EDUCATION

General Outline

Intervention	Rationale
1. Discuss and demonstrate care activities.	1. Introduces learning task
2. Guide the mother through each new experience, explaining underlying rationale for actions.	2. Increases security; associates words and actions

3. Include concepts and principles of the following:
  a. Health maintenance
  b. Signs and symptoms of normal postpartum progress
  c. Signs of common potential postpartum health problems
	3. Provides learning content; enables woman to participate actively in her own health care; facilitates early diagnosis and treatment of complications

4. Guide and supervise hands-on learning experiences for care of self and baby, i.e., return demonstrations.	4. Reduces anxiety, increases security; optimizes learning
5. Ask mother to explain reasons for actions in her own words.	5. Enables her to identify and understand the relationship between words and actions; crystallizes learning; increases compliance with recommendations
6. Correct errors in understanding and performance.	6. Minimizes integration of misconceptions
7. Make positive comments regarding skills and "mothering" behaviors; identify infant response to comfort measures.	7. Generates and reinforces growing confidence in own abilities

At first they may be timid because they do not know what to expect of their infants. Some feel inadequate and are afraid of harming their infants. Many are hesitant to ask for help in changing diapers or handling the baby. Some multiparas may need guidance and assistance in planning approaches to sibling rivalry. Various approaches to both nursing care and the teaching/learning process may be required to meet the identified individual needs, desires, and abilities of the woman and family. Care and teaching must be based on the woman's present knowledge level, cultural values and traditions, and resources available.

As soon as her physical status is stable, the nurse should encourage, prompt, and assist the new mother to take an active part in her own care and in caring for her infant. Nursing interventions should incorporate anticipatory guidance toward meeting the discharge goals. Although anticipatory guidance and health teaching are most effective when they correlate with the mother's readiness to learn, today's typical short (2 to 3 day) hospital stay severely limits opportunities for nurse/client interactions. Nurses must make every effort to maximize any and all contact time with mothers to expedite progress through the "taking-in" phase and entry into "taking-hold." Client teaching should be integrated into all care activities.

Effective teaching/learning techniques include discussing and demonstrating care activities, guiding the mother through each new experience, and explaining the underlying rationale. Sharing information on basic concepts and principles of health maintenance, signs and symptoms of normal postpartal progress, and common potential health problems in the puerperium enables the woman to be an active participant in her own health care. For many mothers, nurse-guided, supervised "hands-on" experiences increase security and optimize learning. Many nurses use positive comments regarding the infant's response to mothering behaviors to reinforce maternal confidence in her own abilities. Asking the mother to return-demonstrate care and to explain the reasons for procedures in her own words often enables her to understand the relationship between words and actions and crystalizes learning. In addition the nurse is able to correct errors in understanding or performance and to reinforce the mother's growing confidence and skills.

DIRECT CARE AND CLIENT TEACHING. Current trends in maternal-newborn nursing encourage client self-care as soon as the new mother's physical status is stable. Direct nursing care of normal, healthy postpartum women is limited to the first 24 hours after delivery. Health maintenance information should be included in nurse-client contacts throughout the hospital stay.

Prevention of Infection

Client teaching enables the woman to minimize the potential for postpartum infections of the breast, uterus, and surgical wounds during and after hospitalization. Self-assessment is emphasized to enable early identification and prompt treatment of any infection-related complications that may arise in the postpartum period.

BATHING. Biophysical adaptations in the early postpartum period result in excretion of interstitial fluids retained during pregnancy. Marked diaphoresis and night sweats are common during this period. A shower is refreshing and a source of comfort. If they desire, most mothers who experienced an uncomplicated normal delivery are permitted to shower within a few hours of the delivery or on the following morning. When the mother is ready for her first postpartum shower, the nurse provides health teaching about bathing aspects of self-care. Breast care and perineal care are reviewed. For safety the nurse should remain nearby while the mother showers.

BREAST CARE. Routine breast care maintains cleanliness and comfort and minimizes potential for infection (mastitis). Client teaching includes hygiene, comfort, self-examination, and signs to report promptly (see Client Self-Care Education: Breast Care for the Breast-Feeding Mother, p. 464). Formula-feeding mothers may receive lactation-suppressant medications (see Drug Guide: Bromocriptine Mesylate, p. 465). These mothers may bathe with soap and water but should be cautioned to rinse the breasts and nipple areas well. Occasionally they may experience engorgement discomfort. If this occurs, they should follow directions for discontinuing breast-feeding in the client self-care education about breast care.

Involution

If on assessment the fundus is atonic (boggy), the nurse should perform intermittent fundal massage until the uterus is firm and maintains adequate

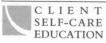

Breast Care for the Breast-Feeding Mother

Action	**Rationale**
1. Wear bra 24 hr/day.	1. Maintains support; reduces discomfort from normal movement.
a. May use breast pads or clean handkerchief	a. Absorbs milk leakage; protects clothing
b. Avoid plastic liners or pads	b. Plastic retains body heat and moisture
c. Air dry nipples after each feeding	c. Reduces nipple irritation
2. Bathe breasts and nipples with clear water daily.	2. Soap removes natural nipple secretions, is drying, and can lead to cracking
3. Gently pat dry.	3. Friction is irritating to nipples, may traumatize tissue
4. Inspect nipples for signs of redness, cracking.	4. Facilitates early detection and prompt management of irritation; minimizes potential for infection
Sore nipples care	
a. Expose to air for 15 to 30 min several times daily	a. Reduces nipple irritation; promotes healing
b. Express colostrum and rub over nipple area	b. Colostrum is very healing
c. If ordered, may use hydrous lanolin	c. Soothing
d. Alternate breast for start of each feeding	d. Vigorous sucking is most pronounced at beginning of feeding
e. Check that most of areola is in infant's mouth	e. Distributes sucking pressures; protects nipple
f. Change nursing positions with each feeding	f. Subjects different nipple areas to stress of sucking
5. Examine breasts after each feeding.	5. Reveals signs of infection
Signs to report promptly NOTIFY PRIMARY HEALTH CARE PROVIDER IF THE FOLLOWING OCCUR:	
a. Acute tenderness or pain	Usually involves only one breast; may occur in either breast or both breasts may be involved
b. Local or general redness, heat, swelling	
c. General feeling of malaise	
d. Marked rise in body temperature	
e. Chills	
6. Engorgement.	
a. Massage breasts with gentle, downward milking motion; may be done during shower	a. Increases circulation, opens lacteal ducts; expresses milk
b. May apply ice packs for 15 to 20 min between nursing periods	b. Reduces discomfort by decreasing circulation to breast(s)
7. Discontinuing breast-feeding	
a. Do not massage breasts or express milk to relieve discomfort	a. Stimulates further milk production; prolongs lactation
b. May apply ice packs for 15 to 20 min several times daily	b. Relieves discomfort
c. Wear well-fitting bra 24 hours each day until discomfort subsides	c. Minimizes pain from movement; provides support to breasts that have become larger and heavier during pregnancy and engorgement
d. May take aspirin or acetaminophen for pain as directed by primary health care provider	d. Analgesia; discomfort usually lasts 1 to 2 days
e. May drink to satisfy thirst but avoid excessive amounts of fluids	e. Excessive fluid may increase engorgement

Bromocriptine mesylate (Parlodel): Ergot derivative; stimulates dopamine receptors; commonly used in treatment of Parkinson's disease

Obstetric Action: Inhibits prolactin secretion, postpartum physiologic lactation, and breast engorgement

Postpartum Administration:
Average dosage: 2.5 mg b.i.d. for 14 to 21 days
Special note:
It must *not* be administered until vital signs are stable.
Therapy must begin a minimum of 4 hr after delivery.
Administer orally with food.

Maternal Contraindications: Uncontrolled hypertension, pregnancy-induced hypertension, allergy to ergot alkaloids

Potential Side Effects and Complications: Symptomatic transient hypotension, dizziness, nausea, severe headaches, blurred vision, seizures, stroke, hypertension during second week of therapy

Nursing Implications:
1. Assess client's medical and prenatal history to identify contraindications to administration.
2. Monitor status closely after administering initial dose (most common time of negative reaction to drug is 15 to 20 min after first dose).
3. Assess client's blood pressure and general status before each administration and/or every 4 hr while awake.
4. Hold medication and notify physician if client becomes hypotensive or hypertensive or complains of other above-listed signs or symptoms of side effects.
5. Ambulate client with assistance if necessary.

Client Teaching:
Advise client to continue taking drug, as ordered, with meals or milk; avoid alcohol.
Advise her to store drug in tightly closed container.
Stress importance of return visit to physician as instructed.
Discuss possibility of pregnancy's occurring before reinitiation of menses.
Recommend use of barrier contraceptives during postpartum period; use of oral contraceptives is contraindicated.
Inform about possible transient mild-to-moderate rebound engorgement when discontinuing drug.
Emphasize need to notify physician promptly if she experiences one or more episodes of severe headaches, blurred vision, dizziness, nausea, chest pain.

tone (see Emergency Nursing Intervention: Fundal Massage and Fig. 19-6, p. 466). Should fundal massage be ineffective in stimulating the uterus to maintain tone, the primary health care provider should be contacted promptly. An oxytocic medication may be ordered to stimulate uterine contractions.

Because most mothers are discharged within 72 hours of delivery, client teaching should include self-assessment of the progress of involution and signs of deviation from expected patterns. Instructing the mother in self-examination of fundal height and lochial characteristics should be integrated into the daily nursing assessment activities. Clients are taught to follow the same assessment pattern at home (see Client Self-Care Education: Involution, p. 467). Figure 19-2 and Table 19-1 describe characteristic postdischarge findings.

AFTERPAINS. Uterine contractions continue after delivery as part of the involution process. Afterpains, a discomfort similar to menstrual cramps, are not experienced by all new mothers. Because the primiparous uterus remains tonically contracted, afterpains occur more frequently in multiparas. Afterpains are more common or severe when the uterus has been overdistended by a large baby, hydramnios, or multiple pregnancy. Nursing mothers may notice afterpains during breast-feeding since suckling stimulates release of oxytocin, which increases uterine contractions. The

>> EMERGENCY NURSING
INTERVENTION

Immediate Postpartum Hemorrhage:
Fundal Massage

If on assessment the fundus is not well contracted and it feels soft and boggy, the nurse should immediately begin fundal massage.
1. Explain procedure and rationale; inform client procedure may be somewhat uncomfortable; reassure her.
2. To relax her abdominal muscles, position client supine in bed with knees bent and apart.
3. To avoid inversion of the atonic uterus, support her lower fundus with one hand just above the symphysis pubis; cup the other hand around the fundus and rotate and massage *gently* until fundus is firm (see Fig. 19-6).
4. To avoid the hazard of uterine inversion, express blood that has collected in the uterine cavity with gentle pressure *only after the fundus is firm.*
5. Maintaining hands in position, observe client's vulva for passage of blood clots; if the fundus begins to relax, reinstitute massage until it is firm.
6. Provide perineal care; apply fresh perineal pad and fresh bed pad.
7. Palpate fundus for height and consistency.

Sample Narrative Charting: Boggy fundus, 1/U. One large clot size of ¾ cup and several dime-sized clots expressed with fundal massage. Fundus firm after massage, U/1; scant lochia rubra.

FIGURE 19-6

Fundal Massage. Effective fundal massage stimulates contraction of the uterine muscles and helps to restore normal tonicity and reduce bleeding.

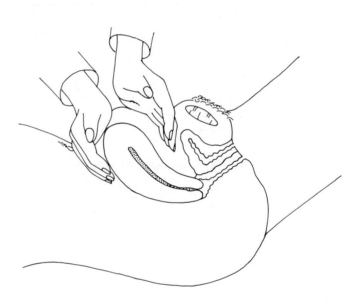

cramps gradually diminish and usually become quite mild within 48 hours after delivery. If they are severe, analgesics may be ordered to relieve the discomfort.

Client teaching emphasizes the origin and purpose of the uterine contractions. The mother should be reassured that they are not harmful and will soon end. Simple self-care measures, e.g., fundal massage and applying external heat, may alleviate discomfort (see Client Self-Care Education: Afterpains).

Bladder Distention

Most mothers void spontaneously and in adequate amounts within 6 to 8 hours after delivery. The time and amount of the first three voidings are recorded; failure to void spontaneously in adequate amounts (>300 ml) may indicate bladder distention and urinary retention. Voiding frequently in small amounts in the postpartum period often represents the overflow from a distended bladder and requires careful nursing assessment and intervention. In the early postpartum period diminished bladder tone

Involution

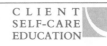

Intervention

1. Explain assessment process, pattern, and rationale.

2. Demonstrate assessment of location of fundal height.

3. *Signs to report promptly.*
NOTIFY DOCTOR OR MIDWIFE IF THE FOLLOWING OCCUR:
   a. Fundal height and character
      (1) Fundal height unchanged
      (2) Uterus spongy to touch
      (3) Increased uterine tenderness to touch
      (4) Pelvic pain or backache
   b. Alterations in lochia
      (1) Persistent bright red bleeding
      (2) Lochial characteristics vary from normal pattern
         (a) Stops suddenly
         (b) Fresh bleeding occurs
         (c) Lochia rubra, serosa, alba persist longer than usual (rubra to day 3; serosa to day 10; alba to day 20)
      (3) Foul lochial odor with or without fever

Rationale

1. Increases mother's understanding; encourages compliance with recommendations

2. Return-demonstration enables nurse to evaluate performance and correct errors

3. Requires professional evaluation

Afterpains

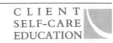

Action

1. Empty bladder.

2. If necessary, massage fundus until firm.
3. Lie on stomach for 5 to 10 min.

4. Perform 10 repetitions of leg lifts (postpartum exercises).
5. Use heating pad intermittently.

6. If breast-feeding, take analgesic 15 to 30 min before nursing.

Rationale

1. Distended bladder increases discomfort

2. Expresses clots, increases uterine tone, stimulates circulation
3. Body heat causes mild local vasodilation; increases circulation
4. Contraction of abdominal muscles stimulates circulation
5. Causes local vasodilation, increases circulation
6. Nursing stimulates release of oxytocin and uterine contractions; promotes comfort

or edema of the area at the base of the bladder and surrounding the urethra may cause difficulty in voiding. If a mother is unable to void spontaneously, assistive nursing measures are necessary (see Nursing Procedure: Bladder Distention). Some mothers void spontaneously, but the first voiding may not empty the bladder (<300 ml). If her bladder is not distended, instruct the mother to wait approximately 1 hour before attempting to void. During the time between voiding attempts, nursing interventions are directed toward encouraging her to relax. Emphasizing the importance of voiding may increase her anxiety and tension. Administering the prescribed analgesic to relieve perineal discomfort and offering warm beverages also may aid the mother in relaxing. Unless the bladder appears markedly distended, three attempts to void spontaneously in an adequate amount are permitted. Catheterization may be necessary if the mother is unable to empty her bladder within 8 hours of delivery and nursing assessments reveal bladder distention.

If the mother does not void in sufficient quantity after catheterization and the bladder is again distended, many physicians and nurse midwives will order insertion of an indwelling catheter because repeated intermittent catheterization increases the potential for trauma to the bladder sphincter and for infection. If an indwelling catheter is used, it should be used for the shortest time possible, and it is usually removed in 48 hours. Before

---

NURSING PROCEDURE   *Bladder Distention*

Intervention

1. Explain procedure and rationale.

2. If mother complains of perineal discomfort, administer analgesic as ordered by the physician or nurse midwife; offer warm beverages.
3. After 15 to 30 min assist woman either to:
   a. Ambulate to bathroom *or*
   b. transfer to bedside commode
4. If bed rest has been prescribed for the mother, provide privacy and position her comfortably on bedpan; elevate head of bed to sitting position.
5. Institute the following measures:
   a. Run water in sink.
   b. Have mother dip fingers in warm water.
   c. Pour warm water over perineum.
   d. If she is ambulatory, use continuous-flow sitz bath.
6. If mother is stable, allow her privacy; remain in close proximity to provide help if needed.
7. Provide perineal care.
8. Assist with application of fresh perineal pad and return to bed.
9. Measure voiding; subtract amount of fluid used for perineal care.
10. Assess bladder by palpation on her return to bed.
11. Assess height of fundus.

12. Record time and amount voided.

Rationale

1. Decreases anxiety; an informed client is more cooperative
2. Encourages relaxation

3. Allows time for effects of analgesic
   a.-b. Normal anatomic position may facilitate voiding
4. Reduces tension related to embarrassment

5. Provides sensory input that often stimulates voiding

6. Reduces embarrassment

7. Cleanses; promotes comfort

9. Accurate measurement of amount voided required
10. Identifies emptying vs. retention

11. Bladder displaces fundus; after emptying, bladder fundus returns to expected position
12. Component of intake and output evaluation

Sample Narrative Charting: Fundus slightly boggy, 2/U, laterally displaced to the right. Moderate to heavy lochia rubra. Fundal palpation elicits c/o suprapubic pressure and urge to void. Bladder markedly distended. Up to bathroom with assistance. Voided 600 ml. Demonstrated appropriate perineal self-care without error. Returned to bed without incident. Fundus firm, in midline, U/1. Moderate lochia rubra.

catheter removal, a urine specimen is sent for culturing and sensitivity testing. An antibiotic may be ordered to be taken for 7 to 10 days.

CATHETERIZATION. Vulvar and perineal edema is a common tissue response to pushing during second-stage labor and delivery. Tenderness and distortion of vestibular landmarks may result. The use of variations in the nursing approach to catheterizing the postpartum woman is necessary to reduce maternal anxiety, enable smooth, accurate catheterization, and minimize potential for infection (see Nursing Procedures: Postpartum Catheterization).

Postpartum Catheterization

Intervention

1. Explain procedure step by step; provide rationale.
2. Convey awareness of her soreness; assure her that, although she may be uncomfortable, catheterization is not painful.
3. Provide perineal care before beginning procedure.
4. Gently separate vulva.
5. After cleansing the vestibule, place a sterile cotton ball at introitus.
6. Inform woman that catheter will be introduced shortly; request that she take a deep breath and slowly exhale while visualizing perineal relaxation.
7. Follow standard procedure for introducing catheter.
8. If bladder is markedly distended, do the following:
   a. Clamp catheter with fingers after drainage of every 300 ml, count slowly to 10, and allow flow to resume
   b. Continue pattern until
      (1) Flow of urine has diminished
      (2) Abdominal contour is restored
      (3) Fundus is firm in abdominal midline
9. Withdraw catheter or inflate balloon if it is indwelling; set equipment aside, apply fresh perineal pad, and ensure client comfort.
10. Measure and record amount, color, and character of urine; label it and send specimen(s) to laboratory if ordered.

Rationale

1. Reduces anxiety; enables cooperation
2. Fear results in increased muscle tension, resistance to passage of catheter, and pain

3. Increases comfort; cleanses area, reduces potential for infection
4. Minimizes strain on perineal sutures
5. Absorbs lochia during catheterization; reduces risk of introducing contaminants
6. Reduces maternal tendency to tense involuntarily; encourages relaxation of tissues surrounding urethra

7. —

8. Bladder capacity may exceed 1500 ml
   a. Allows slow bladder deflation; minimizes risk of "bladder shock"
   b. Encourages return of bladder tone

Perineal Care

Gentle perineal cleansing is a postpartum comfort measure that also reduces potential for infection. The most common method of perineal care is pouring a cleansing cascade of warm water or antiseptic solution over the vulva and perineum after voiding and defecation (see Client Self-Care Education: Perineal Care). Universal precautions (gloving) are observed whenever the nurse may come in contact with lochial flow. Client teaching starts with the first perineal care procedure in the immediate postpartum period, and it is reinforced during each following procedure. Instructing and demonstrating the appropriate technique for changing and disposing of soiled perineal pads is included.

COLD AND HEAT THERAPY. Cold therapy may be used immediately after delivery when there has been significant perineal trauma or an extensive episiotomy. A perineal ice pack is applied to reduce edema and provide local anesthesia. Its frequent replacement may be required to maintain the cold temperature over several hours. Moist heat therapy is used to reduce edema and promote comfort and healing by increasing perineal circulation. Procedures and equipment for application of perineal heat are agency-specific. In some agencies a special continuous-flow sitz bathtub is used; in others, personal portable sitz basins are provided. The mother submerges the perineal area in water maintained at 38°C to 41°C (100° to 105° F) for 20 minutes two or more times daily. She should be instructed in the use of the portable sitz bath for self-care and may continue this procedure after discharge. Dry heat therapy is another method used to provide comfort and healing. Perineal lamps are used to generate heat; dry heat treatments usually are ordered for 20 minutes three times daily (see Nursing Procedure: Perineal Lamp).

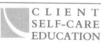

CLIENT
SELF-CARE
EDUCATION

Perineal Care

Action

1. Wash hands.
2. Remove soiled perineal pad from front to back; discard.

3. With labia closed, flush vulva and perineum with a gentle cascade of warm water or antiseptic solution; may use squeeze bottle, pitcher, or other clean container.
4. Use tissue to pat dry from front to back.

5. Use witch hazel pads, ointments, or sprays as directed.
6. Apply a fresh perineal pad from front to back; avoid touching surface of pad that will touch perineum; secure pad with sanitary belt or perineal panty.
7. Wash hands.

Rationale

1. Removes microorganisms
2. Minimizes potential for transfer of microorganisms from rectum to vagina
3. Minimizes potential for fluid entry and transmission of microbes from vulva to the vagina; rinses away lochia

4. Reduces friction; promotes comfort; minimizes potential for fecal contamination of vagina or urethra

5. Maximizes comfort but should be used as directed
6. Prevents sliding movement between rectum and vagina; promotes comfort

7. Removes microorganisms

Perineal Lamp

Intervention

1. Explain procedure and rationale.

2. Position the woman supine with knees bent and apart.
3. If equipment used provides knee rest, pad with towels.
4. Position lamp approximately 18 in from perineum (approximately the length of the woman's thigh); disengage perineal pad.
5. Cover lower body with sheet or spread.
6. Leave lamp in place for 20 min.
7. Apply fresh perineal pad; remove lamp.
8. Client self-care teaching.
   a. May continue treatments after discharge; may use a goose necked desk lamp as perineal lamp substitute
   b. *Safety precautions*
      (1) Place lamp a mimimum distance of length of thigh from self.
      (2) Avoid contact with hot light bulb.
      (3) Limit treatments to 20 min; may wish to use cooking timer for timing treatment at home.
      (4) Wash off ointment or spray before use of lamp to avoid burning or other irritation.
9. Record treatment.

Rationale

1. Dry heat increases circulation, promotes comfort and healing
2. Exposes perineum to heat generated by lamp

3. Reduces compression of popliteal space; promotes comfort
4. Provides effective heat source; safety precaution reduces potential for contact burn

5. Reduces embarassment; promotes warmth
6. Optimum length of time for effective dry heat
7. —
8. Enables safe self-care

Sample Narrative Charting: Perineal lamp × 20 min. Episiotomy clean and healing. Instructed in procedure for self-care at home. Verbalizes understanding. Demonstrated positioning of self and lamp accurately.

MEDICATION. To relieve episiotomy or laceration discomfort, anesthetic sprays, ointments, or witch hazel pads (Tucks) are applied directly to the sutured area. The physician or nurse midwife also may prescribe analgesics for relief of perineal pain. Women with extensive perineal repair may need medication every few hours for the first 1 or 2 postpartum days. To enable the mother to relax and concentrate on her infant, analgesics should be given 30 to 40 minutes before the infant's feeding period.

Early Ambulation

Unless contraindicated, mothers are encouraged to be out of bed within 4 to 8 hours of delivery. Early ambulation stimulates circulation and reduces the risk of thrombophlebitis. Bladder function is improved, reducing the risk of complications requiring catheterization. Bowel function is stimulated, and constipation and abdominal distention occur less frequently.

Before the mother ambulates for the first time, she should dangle her legs over the side of the bed for a few minutes. If the mother does not complain of being dizzy or weak, she may be assisted to the standing position. The nurse should assess the mother's status before allowing her to walk and should accompany her to the bathroom or chair. The nurse should remain close at hand so that immediate assistance is available should the mother become weak or faint. Initial ambulating and sitting in a chair usually is limited to 5 to 15 minutes. Client teaching should include discussing the importance and purposes of early ambulation. The need to increase activity gradually should be emphasized.

Sitting

Mothers who have discomfort from perineal sutures usually find sitting uncomfortable for the first few days. Client teaching includes instructing the woman to splint the perineal area by tensing her buttocks together as she sits and rises. She should maintain the tension briefly after sitting down, then relax. This action minimizes pressure on the perineum and promotes comfort. If the mother is unable to splint the perineal area, the nurse can assist by manually squeezing the buttocks together as the mother sits.

Exercise

As a result of diminished muscle tone, the vagina may be flaccid and distended after delivery. Exercise can hasten recovery, prevent complications, and strengthen the muscles of the back, pelvic floor, and abdomen. Kegel's exercise, an isometric activity, facilitates perineal healing, helps restore muscle tone, and increases circulation. It also helps prevent urinary stress incontinence and pelvic relaxation and enhances orgasmic capacity (see Client Self-Care Education: Kegel's Exercise).

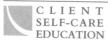

CLIENT
SELF-CARE
EDUCATION

Kegel's Exercise

Action

1. Institute exercise whenever urinating and at intervals throughout the day.
   a. Contract the perineal muscles with sufficient force to stop a stream of urine.
   b. Hold contraction for 5 seconds and release.
   c. Repeat 50 to 100 times.

Rationale

1. Strengthens the pubococcygeal and levator ani muscles; increases tone and circulation

---

Muscle toning exercises also assist the mother to regain her figure and can be beneficial psychologically. Client teaching emphasizes beginning with a few repetitions of one exercise and gradually increasing the number of exercises and repetitions (see Client Self-Care Education: Abdominal Exercise and Figs. 19-7 to 19-12). Mild exercise such as abdominal breathing can be started on the first postpartum day.

Abdominal Exercise: General Principles

Action

1. Avoid overexercising.
   a. Begin with five repetitions.

   b. Add one to two repetitions each day.
   c. Set goal of 30 repetitions each day.
   d. Perform in sets of 10 repetitions; rest between sets.

2. Progress slowly in adding to routine.
   a. Add one exercise each day.

   b. Begin each new exercise with five repetitions.

   c. Add one to two repetitions each day.
   d. Set goal of 30 repetitions of each exercise.

Rationale

1. a. Overexercising causes fatigue and muscle soreness, discourages consistent exercising.
   b. Gradually adding repetitions increases tone and stamina
   c. Sufficient to maintain good muscle tone
   d. Resting between sets allows muscle relaxation, restores energy, and enables more repetitions

2. Avoids fatigue and soreness

   a. Varies active muscle groups; enhances effects of other exercises
   b. Gradual increase in active exercise time achieves effects without fatigue or soreness
   c. Facilitates goal achievement

   d. Maintains good muscle tone; increases energy level

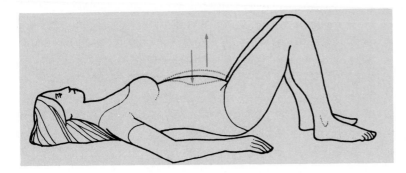

FIGURE 19-7

Firming the Abdomen. Phase I. Abdominal Breathing.

1. Lie on back with knees bent.
2. Inhale deeply through the nose, keeping ribs as stationary as possible and allowing the abdomen to expand up.
3. Exhale slowly but forcefully while contracting the abdominal muscles.
4. Hold for about 3 to 5 seconds while exhaling. Relax.
5. Begin with 2 repetitions, gradually progressing to 10.

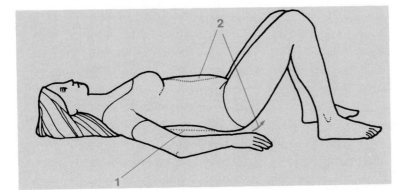

FIGURE 19-8

Phase II. Combined Abdominal Breathing and Supine Pelvic Tilt.

1. Lie on back with knees bent.
2. While inhaling deeply, roll pelvis back by flattening the lower back on the floor or bed
3. While exhaling slowly but forcefully, contract the abdominal muscles and tighten the buttocks.
4. Hold for about 3 to 5 seconds while exhaling. Relax.
5. Begin with two repetitions, gradually progressing to 10.

FIGURE 19-9
Phase III. Reach for the Knees.

1. Lie on back with knees bent.
2. While inhaling deeply, bring the chin onto the chest.
3. While exhaling, raise the head and shoulders slowly and smoothly, reaching for the knees with outstretched arms. The body should only rise as far as the back will naturally bend while the waist remains on the floor or bed (about 6 to 8 inches).
4. Slowly and smoothly lower head and shoulders to the starting position. Relax.
5. Begin with 2 repetitions, gradually progressing to 10.

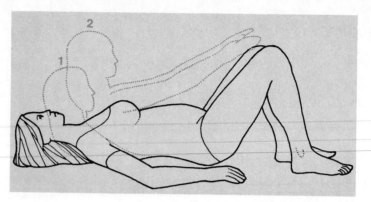

FIGURE 19-10
Firming the Waist. Phase I. Double Knee Roll.

1. Lie on back with knees bent.
2. Keeping shoulders flat and the feet stationary, slowly and smoothly roll the knees over to touch the right side of the bed.
3. Maintaining a smooth motion, roll the knees back over to touch the left side of the bed.
4. Return to starting position. Relax.
5. Begin with 2 repetitions, gradually progressing to 10.

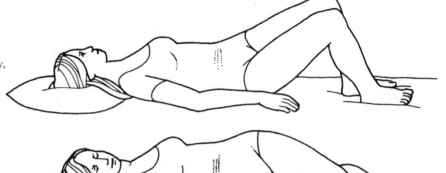

FIGURE 19-11
Phase II. Single Knee Roll.

1. Lie on back, right leg straight, left leg bent at the knee.
2. Keeping the shoulders flat, slowly and smoothly roll the left knee over to touch the right side of the bed and back to starting position.
3. Reverse position of legs, touch left side of the bed with the right knee, and return to starting position. Relax.
4. Begin with 2 repetitions, gradually progressing to 10.

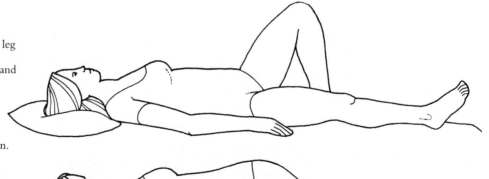

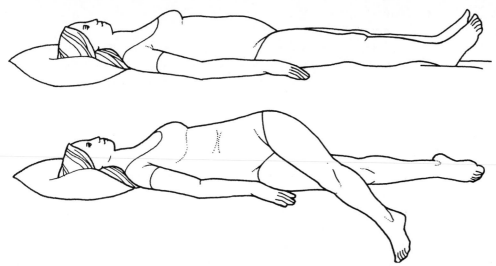

FIGURE 19-12
Phase III. Leg Role.

1. Lie on back with legs straight.
2. Keeping shoulders flat, slowly and smoothly lift the leg and, keeping it straight, roll it over to touch the right side of the bed and return to starting position.
3. Repeat, using the right leg to touch the left side of the bed. Relax.
4. Begin with 2 repetitions, gradually progressing to 10.

Nutrition and Hydration

Because energy reserves may have been depleted during the course of a long labor, nutrition and hydration are important aspects in care of the postpartum mother. For women who have experienced uncomplicated vaginal deliveries, encouraging oral fluids and light nourishment during the immediate postpartum period enhances their feelings of well-being. Later mothers usually enjoy a regular diet. Partaking of nourishing snacks and beverages should be encouraged if the mother is hungry between meals. Client teaching should include discussing the need for sufficient oral fluids and an adequate diet. Breast-feeding mothers should be counseled about the additional calories and nutrients required during lactation.

Rest and Sleep

After the physical and emotional stress of labor and delivery, many mothers complain they feel exhausted. Obtaining adequate rest is important to recovery from the energy expenditure of childbirth. Mothers should be encouraged to rest, relax, and sleep whenever possible. Necessary nursing procedures should be organized to provide the mother with uninterrupted rest periods. Client teaching emphasizes the need for adequate rest after discharge (see Client Self-Care Education: Rest and Sleep).

Rest and Sleep

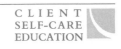

CLIENT
SELF-CARE
EDUCATION

Action

1. Suggest that family and friends call or visit at specific times during the day.
2. Nap during the day when baby sleeps.

3. Allow some time during the day for own self; do something enjoyable, e.g., read, soak in tub.

Rationale

1. Allows time for rest, relaxation, naps

2. Insufficient rest contributes to irritability, decreases tolerance to stress; may inhibit effective nursing
3. Relaxing; increases tolerance to stress; supports positive self-concept

Intestinal Elimination

CONSTIPATION. In the early postpartum period reduced intestinal motility and relaxed abdominal muscles contribute to constipation. Also, fear of pain on defecation may be an inhibiting factor. The primary health care provider may order a stool softener for the first few days. The nurse should explain the purpose of the medication and reassure the mother that her first stools should not be painful. Client teaching should emphasize that early ambulation assists return of normal bowel function and that increasing dietary roughage and maintaining adequate fluid intake is helpful. The presence or absence of bowel sounds before the first post-delivery bowel movement and the passage of the first stool after delivery are noted and recorded in the client's chart.

If the mother has not responded to dietary management and medication by the second or third postpartum day, the primary health care provider may order a rectal suppository or a cleansing enema. Should these measures also fail, an oil retention enema, followed some hours later by a cleansing enema, may be ordered.

Client teaching for self-care emphasizes dietary management and fluid intake. Breast-feeding mothers should be instructed to take only the specific medication recommended by the primary health care provider because certain laxatives are excreted in breast milk and therefore affect her infant.

HEMORRHOIDS. Hemorrhoids are a common problem during the postpartum period. The pressure exerted by the presenting part on the pelvic floor during labor and the straining of the expulsive phase are contributing factors. Although they gradually shrink and regress, hemorrhoids may be most painful during the first 2 to 3 days after delivery. Sitz baths, topical ointments, or anesthetic sprays and cool, astringent compresses (witch hazel pads) provide relief. Some physicians prescribe hydrocortisone suppositories. Comfort measures include loosening perineal pads and lying in the Sims' position while in bed. Client teaching emphasizes preventing constipation through dietary measures and avoiding straining at stool.

Psychosocial Aspects of Postpartum Care
Cultural Considerations

Nursing care may require modification to accommodate culturally prescribed postpartum behaviors and to demonstrate respect for client health beliefs (see Cultural Implications: Postpartum Care). In many cultures males or family matriarchs, the maternal and paternal grandmothers, are the decision makers.[10] Performing extensive, creative, and persuasive client teaching for both parents and the extended family may be necessary to encourage client ambulation, bathing, nutrition, hydration, and infant care. Special care should be taken in determining the client's desire for counseling or teaching about psychosocial aspects of the postpartum period. Non-Western clients, in particular, may be offended by unsolicited discussions about psychologic adjustments to childbearing, postpartum sexuality, or contraception.

Implication	Suggested Interventions
Avoidance of	
Physical activity	Organize care to maximize uninterrupted rest. Assist with ambulation. Provide health teaching about the importance of graduated activity as accepted by client.
Bathing	If sitz baths are unacceptable, discuss use of perineal lamp as alternative therapy with physician or nurse midwife and client. Provide health teaching about breast and perineal care and handwashing.
Cold foods and fluids	Offer hot beverages.
	Encourage client selection of menu items.
	Request consultation with dietician.
Cold and drafts	If client desires, provide extra blankets.
	Offer robe and slippers before she ambulates.
	If client desires, cover her with blanket when sitting in chair.

CULTURAL
IMPLICATIONS

Postpartum Care

Sexuality

Sexual adjustment after the birth of a baby is a major concern of new parents. Often it becomes a source of conflict and confusion. When possible, discussions of postpartum sexuality should include both the mother and her sexual partner. Client teaching emphasizes the value and importance of open communication between partners and of mutual emotional support. Discussion content should include (1) normal postpartum biophysical changes, (2) psychosocial factors that influence the sexual relationship during the puerperium, and, if the couple desires, (3) comparisons of contraceptive options (see Client Self-Care Education: Psychosocial Aspects of the Postpartum Period and Client Self-Care Education: Sexuality, pp. 478 and 479).

One common source of confusion and stress concerns when to resume sexual activity. Many couples believe that intercourse should be avoided until after the 6-week postpartum checkup; this belief is common among non-Western cultures. However, **coitus** may be resumed as soon as mutually desired if sexual activity does not cause the woman discomfort. For clients with an episiotomy, by the third week post partum the lochial flow usually has subsided, and the perineum has healed sufficiently to allow intercourse without discomfort.[2]

Some couples also are concerned about when menstruation will return. Nonlactating women usually resume menses by 9 weeks and breast-feeding mothers by 30 to 36 weeks post partum.

Contraception

Counseling about contraceptive options should begin during the prenatal period.[16] One question the couple should discuss is whether they desire future pregnancies. Contemporary contraceptive techniques enable clients to avoid unwanted pregnancy and plan their families, and a wide variety of choices are available. If during the antepartum period the couple decides to terminate their ability to conceive, a tubal ligation can be performed immediately after the delivery or on the following day.

More commonly, couples elect to interrupt fertility temporarily. For those who prefer to use oral contraceptives, the physician or nurse midwife may prescribe the mini-pill (progestin-only pill) immediately post

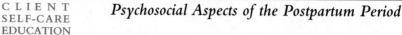

CLIENT SELF-CARE EDUCATION

Psychosocial Aspects of the Postpartum Period

Intervention	Rationale

1. Discuss sequential phases of maternal postpartum psychologic adjustment (taking-in, taking-hold, letting-go).
   a. Describe feelings characteristic of each phase.
   b. Explain their origins.
	1. Enables client(s) to understand and accept feelings and behaviors as they arise.

2. Identify common sources of emotional distress; emphasize normalcy.
   a. Changing self-concept
     (1) Altered body image, need to lose weight and tighten muscles
     (2) Assuming new role as mother or father
     (3) Transient feelings of jealousy toward infant
   b. Unrealistic self-expectations (fantasy image of what is a "good" or "perfect" mother or father)
     (1) Frustration when infant cries and fails to respond immediately to "parenting" actions (feeding, comfort measures)
     (2) Fear of overlooking serious potential problem, injuring infant or self
   c. Loss of energy, altered appetite, fatigue
   d. Discomforts related to breast-feeding and childbirth (afterpains, sore nipples, episiotomy healing, sexual activity)
   e. Hormonal changes
	2. Emphasis on normalcy and transitory nature reduces potential negative impact on self-concept

3. Discuss postpartum letdown.
   a. Describe common feelings of inadequacy, incompetence, depression.
   b. Emphasize normalcy of this occurrence.
   c. Reassure regarding transitory nature.
   d. Discuss self-care activities that help prevent or minimize letdown.
     (1) Adequate rest (naps while the baby sleeps help)
     (2) Adequate nutrition
     (3) Assistance with household responsibilities
     (4) Taking time for relaxation and diversion
	3. Supports positive self-image and coping abilities; minimizes symptoms

partum; its use does not interfere with lactation, and it is the hormonal contraceptive of choice for breast-feeding mothers.[17]

The choice of a specific method of birth control often is deferred until the 6-week postpartum checkup. Because of the increasing risk of ovulation, contraceptive use should not be delayed longer. Most couples resume sexual activities before the 6-week postpartum checkup, most commonly by the third postpartum week. Although it is unlikely that clients will conceive during the time between discharge and the follow-up examination, the nurse should suggest they use some method of protection against unexpected pregnancy.[17] Spermicides and condoms do not interfere with lactation and breast-feeding and can be used safely during the postpartum period by both breast-feeding and bottle-feeding mothers.

If a choice has not been made and the couple so desires, family planning

Sexuality

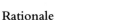

CLIENT
SELF-CARE
EDUCATION

Intervention	Rationale
1. Describe normal physical factors that affect postpartum sexuality.	1. Facilitates effective coping with or management of contributing factors
a. Low maternal hormone levels *Suggest:* Use of contraceptive cream or water-soluble lubricant	a. Diminished or absent normal vaginal lubrication may result in reduced libido; lubrication minimizes friction discomfort.

b. Healing episiotomy
    (1) Fear of injury or pain
    (2) Discomfort, tender to touch
      (a) Explore alternative methods of sexual expression.
      (b) Use preparatory lubrication (as suggested above).
      (c) Experiment with coital positions that avoid pressure from penile shaft against perineum.
	b. Anxiety or fear of pain increases tension, interferes with sexual response. If acceptable to the couple, using alternative methods of sexual expression or coital position can enable satisfaction of sexual desires.

2. Discuss normal psychosocial factors that influence sexuality.	2.
a. Fatigue associated with sleep deprivation	a. Fatigue increases irritability and inhibits sexual arousal.
b. Presence of lochia	b. Presence of lochia may affect perception of desirability.
c. Psychologic stress of role change	c. Demands of role change may affect self-concept and ability to respond.
d. Fear of pregnancy	d. Fear of pregnancy may inhibit sexual arousal.
3. Emphasize the importance of open communication between partners.	3. Enables couple to share feelings, increase mutual understanding, and develop effective problem-solving skills

4. List common criteria for resumption of coitus
  a. Mutual desire
  b. Lack of perineal discomfort to touch
  c. Lochia diminished, alba
	4. Enables couples to make informed choices about postpartum sexual activity

5. Explain potential events associated with breast-feeding.
  a. Sexual arousal
  b. Release of breast milk with orgasm
	5. Increases understanding and acceptance of natural events, minimizes fear and embarrassment

6. Explore interest in and desire for family planning information.	6.
a. Remind couple that breast-feeding inhibits but does not prevent ovulation	a. Number of weeks before ovulation occurs varies widely.

b. Important questions
    (1) Was this pregnancy planned?
    (2) What, if any, method was used to prevent pregnancy?
    (3) What was their level of satisfaction with previous method?
    (4) What do they know about other contraceptive options?
	b. Responses identify current level of knowledge and need and desire for information.

7. Provide information about the comparative advantages and benefits and disadvantages and risks of methods available to control fertility.	7. Enables couple to avoid pregnancy, make informed choices about contraception, and select the method(s) most appropriate to their individual needs and desires

options are discussed during discharge counseling. The nursing objectives are to enable couples to avoid unexpected pregnancy; to make informed decisions regarding contraception; and to select the contraceptive method best suited to their individual needs and desires. Table 19-3 presents information needed for decision making.

TABLE 19-3

Comparison of Contraceptive Methods[17]

Method*	Action/Contraindications	Disadvantages/Risks	Advantages/Effectiveness
Oral Contraceptives			
Combined estrogen and progesterone	Inhibits ovulation by suppressing follicle-stimulating hormone (FSH) and luteinizing hormone (LH)	May experience cyclic weight gain, breast tenderness, break-through bleeding, nausea	Easy administration: disassociated with sex act; predictable menses; may protect against endometrial and ovarian cancer, pelvic inflammatory disease; may diminish dysmenorrhea, acne *Lowest failure rate:* Most effective method of interrupting fertility Combined: 0.1% Progestin only: 0.5%
Progestin-only mini-pill	Causes thick cervical mucus; hostile to sperm penetration *Contraindications:* History of thromboembolic disorder, cerebral accident, coronary artery disease, breast cancer, estrogen-dependent malignancy; diabetes, sickle cell disease, active gallbladder disease, impaired liver function, migraine headaches, obesity, smoking, more than 35 years old *Early danger signs: ACHES* A Severe abdominal pain C Chest pain, cough, shortness of breath H Severe headaches, dizziness, weakness, numbness E Eye problems, vision loss S Severe calf or thigh pain	Increased incidence of spotting, irregular menses, amenorrhea *Risks:* Clot formation, stroke, heart attack, hypertension, hepatic adenoma	
Intrauterine Devices			
Intrauterine progesterone contraceptive (Progestasert) Intrauterine copper contraceptive (ParaGard T380A)	Theorized: Cause local inflammation, preventing implantation; increase fallopian tube motility; prevention of endometrial maturation and formation of thick cervical mucus by progestin-medicated devices *Contraindications:* Active pelvic infection, bleeding disorders, uterine fibroids, anemia, allergy to copper, history of ectopic pregnancy, impaired response to infection (diabetes, immunotherapy)	Possibility of spontaneous expulsion; spotting, bleeding, cramping; may need oral iron; must check for string *Risks:* Infection, hemorrhage, uterine embedding, perforation; pregnancy	Disassociated from sex act; does not affect hormonal cycle *Lowest failure rate:* Intrauterine devices 2% Progestin-medicated devices 1%

*A wide variety of contraceptive methods are available for family planning. Considering their contraindications and comparing the benefits, advantages, disadvantages, risks, and effectiveness enables clients to make informed decisions in selecting between options.

TABLE 19-3

Comparison of Contraceptive Methods[17]—*continued*

Method*	Action/Contraindications	Disadvantages/Risks	Advantages/Effectiveness
Mechanical Barrier Methods			
Diaphragm with spermicide	All methods: Prevent sperm entry to cervix *Contraindications:* History of toxic shock syndrome; anatomic abnormalities; weight gain or loss of 10 pounds; full-term delivery within past 6 wk; allergy to rubber or spermicides	Must be inserted before coitus and left in place for 6 hours after intercourse; must use contraceptive jelly or cream in dome and around rim; must wash, dry, inspect each time. *Risks:* Toxic shock syndrome; allergic reactions	May protect against sexually transmitted diseases (STD); reduces risk of pelvic inflammatory disease, cervical dysplasia *Lowest failure rate:* Diaphragm 2%-3%
Contraceptive sponge	*Contraindications:* History of toxic shock syndrome, allergy to polyurethane; anatomic abnormalities	Must check for placement; must follow directions precisely; increased risk of vaginal yeast infections	Absorbs vaginal secretions, ejaculate *Lowest failure rate:* 5%-8%
Cervical cap	*Contraindications:* History of toxic shock syndrome; allergy to rubber or spermicide; acute pelvic or vaginal infection; abnormal Papanicolaou smear; cervical lesions; full-term delivery within past 6 weeks	Difficulty removing; allergic reaction *Risks:* Chronic cervical irritation, lacerations, cervicitis, acute pelvic infection; abnormal Papanicolaou smear	Similar to diaphragm *Lowest failure rate:* 5%
Condom	*Contraindication:* Allergy to rubber	May be dislodged or break; may reduce sensation	Readily available, inexpensive; does not require prescription; may protect against STD, pelvic inflammatory disease *Lowest failure rate:* 3%-5%
Chemical Barrier Methods			
Spermicidal jelly, cream, foam; vaginal suppositories	Kill sperm	Liquify in body heat, messy; protective for approximately 30 minutes. *Risk:* Allergic reaction	Similar to condoms *Lowest failure rate:* 21%
Fertility Awareness Methods			
Calendar method	All methods: Calculation and avoidance of coitus during fertile period of menstrual cycle reduces potential for conception *Contraindications:* History of anovulatory cycles, inability to maintain accurate records	All methods: Must maintain accurate menstrual records and calculate fertile period; must abstain for 5 days during fertile time *Risks* (All methods): Sperm viable to 72 hours; intercourse 2 to 3 days before, during, and 1 day after ovulation may result in pregnancy	All methods: Safe, free or inexpensive; acceptable to most religions Calendar method: *Lowest failure rate:* 10%
Cervical mucus (Billings) method Basal body temperature	*Contraindications:* Unwilling to examine own mucus; unwilling to comply with required actions; must use special thermometer to take temperature every morning immediately on awakening	Cervical mucus method: Must consider fertile if any mucus present; must be able to identify characteristics accurately; normal sexual lubrication may interfere with ability to identify mucus pattern; may not give sufficient warning time	Cervical mucus methods: stretchable mucus indicates ovulation (spinnbarkheit) *Lowest failure rate:* 8%

Continued

Comparison of Contraceptive Methods[17]*—continued*

Method*	Action/Contraindications	Disadvantages/Risks	Advantages/Effectiveness
Fertility Awareness Methods—continued			
Symptothermal			Symptothermal: Combines cervical mucus and basal body temperature, increases accuracy *Lowest failure rate:* 6%
Surgical Termination of Fertility			
Tubal ligation	Occludes fallopian tubes; prevents transport of ovum, union of gametes *Contraindications:* Desire for future pregnancy; any factors influencing abdominal surgery	Permanent, not readily reversible; requires surgery *Risks:* Similar to major surgery, reactions to anesthetic, trauma to other organs, hemorrhage	Disassociated from sex act; if done at time of delivery, requires only one anesthetic and hospitalization *Lowest failure rate:* 0.2%
Vasectomy	Occludes vas deferens; prevents sperm exit *Contraindications:* Desire for future surgery; not acceptable to male partner	Permanent, not readily reversible; requires surgery *Risks:* Impotence related to psychologic response	Disassociated from sex act; not major surgery *Lowest failure rate:* 0.1%

Legal and Ethical Issues

Nurses are accountable for protecting client confidentiality, confirming informed consent, and planning, providing, and documenting adequate, appropriate care and teaching for postpartum clients (see Legal and Ethical Considerations). Care provided must be consistent with standards of care established by professional nursing organizations, i.e., American Nurses' Association (ANA), Nurses Association of the American College of Obstetricians and Gynecologists (NAACOG). The legal significance of clear, accurate, comprehensive documentation of nursing assessments, interventions, and evaluation of client response to care and treatment is undeniable.

Evaluation

Throughout the client's hospital stay the nurse evaluates the mother's postpartum health status, understanding and performance of self-care and infant care activities, adaptation to maternal role, and progress toward the established goals. Client teaching should provide the mother with basic knowledge and skills needed for self-assessment, self-care, and informed decision making for health maintenance. The mother should be able to (1) verbalize what physical and emotional changes to expect during the postpartum period, signs of common problems, and when to seek consultation with her physician; (2) return-demonstrate appropriate hand-washing, breast care, perineal care, and treatments (sitz bath, perineal

Accountability

Nurses are answerable legally for the quality of nursing care and for protecting client health and safety. Nurses are also held accountable for reporting through appropriate channels the substandard care provided by any other health professionals.

Confidentiality

In the course of their practice nurses have access to personal information concerning their clients. Observations, conversations with clients, families, and other health personnel, and medical records may reveal facts and feelings the client wishes kept confidential. Nurses are accountable for protecting the client's right to privacy of information.

Informed Consent

Primary health care providers are responsible for discussing and explaining the indications for and implications of medical and surgical procedures and treatments. Nurses are responsible for confirming and documenting that the provider has discussed the procedure or test with the client. The nurse also is responsible for conveying any ensuing client questions to the primary care provider. These activities and responses are to be documented thoroughly in the client's record.

If the client withdraws consent, the nurse is responsible for making this known to the primary care provider and for recording actions and activities in the chart.

Voluntary Sterilization

Because surgical sterilization is not readily reversible, the decision to terminate fertility should involve both partners. Many states acknowledge a woman's independent legal right to authorize sterilization; others require written consent of both partners. Nurses are accountable for confirming informed consent for sterilization by evaluating the client's knowledge and understanding of (1) the scheduled procedure, (2) the permanent impact of this contraceptive method on future childbearing, and (3) the option to alter the decision before surgery.

Sample Documentation

Client and husband confirm desire for postpartum tubal ligation. State they understand procedure may result in irreversible loss of ability to achieve pregnancy. State also they have discussed advantages/disadvantages of other contraceptive options with their primary health care provider; appear comfortable with their decision.

---

lamp); (3) assess the health and behaviors of her newborn, provide basic infant care, and identify signs that should be reported to the physician or nurse midwife; (4) describe the comparative benefits and risks of available family planning options; and (5) identify resources for needed future consultation, i.e., physician or nurse midwife, hospital maternity unit, social service, pastoral care, referral service, and community organizations that offer services to meet her special needs, e.g., LaLeche International, Parents Without Partners.

Evaluation findings may indicate that new nursing diagnoses are needed and previous ones are no longer applicable. Effective, ineffective, or alternative approaches to nursing care for the individual client or family may be identified. For example, initial nursing care plans may have focused on removing knowledge deficits. Evaluation may reveal that the client does understand teaching for self-care but is noncompliant because of cultural implications. Providing extra protection against drafts and chills and involving family support and encouragement may prove more effective than discussing the hazards of immobility. Final evaluation of expected outcomes of care and client teaching is made on the day of discharge (see Discharge Assessment Tool: Discharge Evaluation Checklist: Sample Form).

Discharge Evaluation Checklist: Sample Form

1. Health status: All assessments should be within normal limits
   a. Vital signs
   b. Lactation status
   c. Involutional progress (fundus and lochia)
   d. Elimination (voiding, stool)
   e. Healing (perineal, other)
   f. Homans' sign (absent)
   g. Ambulation
   h. Laboratory data (e.g., hemoglobin, hematocrit)
2. Immunizations (rubella, RhoGam)
3. Knowledge base: Self-care
   a. Self-assessment techniques
      (1) Normal physical findings
      (2) Psychologic adjustments, feelings
      (3) Signs to report promptly
   b. Self-care activities
      (1) Bathing, breast care
      (2) Perineal care, Sitz bath
   c. Nutrition, hydration
   d. Exercise, rest, sleep
   e. Bowel elimination
   f. Sexuality
      (1) Return of ovulation, menstruation
      (2) Management of fertility (contraception)
4. Knowledge base: Infant care
   a. Assessment and normal findings
      (1) Temperature
      (2) Skin (color/jaundice, newborn rash)
      (3) Behaviors (sleeping, crying)
   b. Feeding (breast, formula, burping)
   c. Bathing, cord and circumcision care
   d. Clothing, diapering
   e. Follow-up test (phenylketonuria [PKU])
   f. Signs to report promptly
5. Knowledge base: Medications, if any
   a. Drug, dose, time, route, reason
   b. Potential side effects, signs to report promptly
6. Knowledge base: Follow-up care
   a. Appointment with primary health care providers (physician, nurse midwife, pediatrician)
   b. Important phone numbers
      (1) Obstetrician or nurse midwife
      (2) Pediatrician
      (3) Hospital (maternity unit, emergency room, social service)
      (4) Emergency medical services
      (5) Other: Community resource agencies as appropriate (La Leche International, Parents Without Partners, Family Service)

Sample Narrative Charting: Ready for discharge. Status satisfactory, all assessment findings within established normal parameters. Afebrile. Breasts filling. Fundus firm, in midline, U/2. Moderate lochia rubra. Voiding q.s. Episiotomy clean, intact, and healing by primary intention. Homans' sign absent bilaterally. Reports one normal stool this A.M. Ambulates freely without discomfort. Accurately and appropriately demonstrates self-care and infant care activities. Verbalizes understanding of anticipated physiologic and psychologic changes, priciples of self-care/infant care activities, signs to be reported promptly, and need to avoid pregnancy for 3 months related to rubella immunization. Has appointment to see physician on (date). Provided with emergency phone numbers and encouraged to call unit if necessary. Will return with infant on (date) for PKU test.

Criteria for Early Discharge

Rising consumer interest in out-of-hospital birth, i.e., alternative birth centers, and early discharge from the delivery setting are further changing contemporary maternal-newborn care. Low-risk mothers and infants may be discharged from the hospital as early as 2 to 6 hours after delivery.[18] After the delivery both mother and infant are evaluated carefully; all assessment findings must remain within predetermined limits throughout the recovery period until the time of discharge (see Discharge Assessment Tool: Early Discharge: Sample Checklist).

Early Discharge: Sample Checklist

1. The client had a normal, uncomplicated term pregnancy (38 to 42 weeks gestation).
2. On admission hemoglobin and hematocrit levels were within normal limits.
3. The client had normal, uncomplicated labor and vaginal delivery; no excessive blood loss.
4. All assessment findings were within normal limits.
   a. Mother
      (1) Vital signs stable
      (2) Firm fundus
      (3) Moderate lochia rubra
      (4) Perineum intact, no evidence of hematoma
      (5) Homans' sign absent
      (6) Voiding spontaneously in adequate amounts
      (7) Tolerating fluids without nausea or vomiting
      (8) Ambulating without assistance; not weak or dizzy
   b. Infant
      (1) Appropriate for gestational age (>2500 g)
      (2) Vital signs stable; no excessive mucus
      (3) Normal cry and reflexes
      (4) Sucking well during initial feeding(s)
      (5) Initial voiding and stool observed
      (6) Coombs' test negative (if mother Rh negative and infant Rh positive)
      (7) Normal cord blood bilirubin level (if ordered)
   c. Signs of positive parental attachment
5. Appointment made for office visit within 48-72 hr (or scheduled home visit by nurse within 48-72 hr of discharge).
6. Client teaching has been completed.
   a. Accurate return-demonstrations of the following:
      (1) Self fundal check
      (2) Perineal care
      (3) Basic infant care (diapering, cord care)
   b. Verbal and written postpartum instructions provided
      (1) Self-care, infant care procedures
      (2) Limitations on activities
      (3) Signs to be reported promptly to primary health care provider
   c. Provided with important telephone numbers
      (1) Obstetrician or nurse midwife, pediatrician
      (2) Hospital maternity unit
      (3) Emergency medical service agency

Within 48 to 72 hours of discharge, mother and infant are seen in the physician's office, or a home visit is made by a nurse. Traditional aspects of postpartum care, i.e., ongoing evaluation of maternal response to physical and psychosocial stresses of childbearing, self-care and infant care skills, client teaching, and referral counseling, are incorporated into follow-up home visits.[18-20]

Research indicates that for normal, healthy middle and upper socioeconomic class mothers and infants, few unfavorable outcomes occur.[2,14,15]

NURSING
CARE
PLAN

Immediate Postpartum Period (First 24 Hours)

Goals (Expected Outcomes)	Interventions	Rationale	Evaluation
Potential Fluid Volume Deficit (2)—Related to Excessive Bleeding			
Client will adapt successfully to anatomic and physiologic changes of immediate postpartum period without incident.	Perform gentle fundal massage if necessary to firm boggy uterus.	Stimulates uterine muscle to contract; minimizes blood loss (see also Nursing Procedure: Fundus Check; Emergency Nursing Intervention: Immediate Postpartum Hemorrhage: Fundal Massage).	Condition is stable on all status: Vital signs Fundus firm, U/U, in abdominal midline Moderate lochia rubra
	Express clots from uterus.	Empties uterus, allows effective contractions; enables estimate of blood loss.	
	Report and record any deviations from normal patterns.	Enables prompt medical or nursing intervention.	
	Encourage voiding.	Distended bladder interferes with effective uterine contractions that close endometrial vessels at placental site.	Client voids spontaneously.
Altered Patterns of Urinary Elimination—Related to Postpartum Diuresis			
Client will void spontaneously to empty bladder within 6-8 hr after delivery.	Encourage client to drink warm fluids as tolerated.	Re-establishes hydration; encourages relaxation.	Client voids 300 ml spontaneously on first three occasions.
	Promote relaxation.	Promotes comfort and relaxation.	
	Administer analgesics if indicated.	"Normal" surroundings and anatomic position encourage voiding.	
	Position client for comfort.		
	Assist to bathroom or bedside commode.		

These families are perceived as having adequate economic resources, stable home environments, and immediate access to health care. Early discharge of clients appears safe and effective if specified evaluation criteria for low-risk prenatal, intrapartum, postpartum, and newborn status are met; the family is well prepared; both mother and infant are observed during the immediate postdelivery period; skilled nurses provide home visits for assessment and teaching; and physician backup is available.

NURSING
CARE
PLAN

Immediate Postpartum Period (First 24 Hours)—continued

Goals (Expected Outcomes)	Interventions	Rationale	Evaluation
Urinary Retention (Acute)—Related to Bladder Edema Secondary to Trauma During Delivery			
	Provide perineal care with warm solution.	Stimulates voiding, promotes comfort and healing; minimizes potential for autoinfection.	Fundus is firm, in abdominal midline, U/U; moderate lochia rubra.
	Measure first three voidings.	Provides estimate of adequacy of emptying bladder.	
	Perform fundal check.	Reduces potential for excessive bleeding.	
	Catheterize for bladder distention, inability to void or empty.	Empties bladder, prevents distention; allows return of normal bladder tone.	
Altered Family Processes—Related to Role Change, Taking-In, and Taking-Hold			
Client will demonstrate attachment behaviors, e.g., bonding with newborn.	Place stable infant in mother's arms. Provide privacy for new family.	Encourages attachment and bonding.	Client demonstrates bonding behaviors: Eye contact Stroking Cuddling Calls by name
Client will begin integration of newborn into family unit.	Encourage both parents to interact with infant. Reduce light in room. Assist with initial breast-feeding if necessary.	Encourages infant to open eyes and interact with parents. Encourages bonding, later success in breast-feeding; stimulates uterine contractions.	Client appears happy and comfortable with newborn.
	Encourage active participation in and assumption of responsibility for infant care; meet needs for guidance and assistance.	Introduces basic infant care concepts and skills in supportive environment; facilitates development of parental confidence and competence in infant care skills.	Client demonstrates growing confidence in own abilities to provide care.

NURSING
CARE
PLAN

Normal Post Partum

Goals
(Expected Outcomes)

Goals (Expected Outcomes)	Interventions	Rationale	Evaluation
Pain—Related to			
Breast Engorgement Secondary to Impending Lactation			
Client will demonstrate understanding and applications of client teaching. Client will experience relief of discomfort.	Perform client teaching. Explain causes. Discuss comfort measures.	Establishes shared knowledge base; encourages active participation in pain management (see also Client Self-Care Education: Breast Care for the Breast-Feeding Mother).	On request, client accurately explains comfort measures and rationale in own words. Client return-demonstrates procedures. Client complies with nursing recommendations. Client verbalizes relief of discomfort. Client displays no nonverbal evidence of pain.
	Recommend mother wear bra at all times. Explain benefit of warm packs or shower before feeding.	Provides support, minimizes movement and discomfort of engorged breasts. Heat increases circulation, facilitates expression of milk.	
	Demonstrate how to express milk.	Reduces pressure and discomfort from engorgement.	
	Discuss feeding techniques (frequency, length, infant position).	Encourages successful breast-feeding; minimizes potential for problems related to nursing.	
Afterpains Secondary to Uterine Contractions Associated With Breast-Feeding			
	Explain prevention (analgesic 15 to 30 min before feeding; empty bladder).	Promotes comfort (see also Client Self-Care Education: Afterpains).	
	Discuss fundal massage, prone position, leg lifts after feeding.	Promotes comfort and healing (see also Client Self-Care Education: Perineal Care; Nursing Procedure: Perineal Lamp).	
Perineal Tenderness Secondary to Episiotomy			
	Discuss and demonstrate perineal care, use of sitz bath/perineal lamp. Describe tensing gluteal muscles on sitting.	Enables mother to participate actively in own care, minimize potential for infection.	

NURSING
CARE
PLAN

Normal Post Partum—continued

Goals (Expected Outcomes)	Interventions	Rationale	Evaluation
Potential for Infection—Related to			
Impaired Skin Integrity, Breast (Mastitis), Secondary to Nipple Fissures Associated With Breast-Feeding			
Client will demonstrate understanding and application of client teaching. Client will minimize potential for infection. Client will experience uneventful recovery.	Perform client teaching. Explain causes. Discuss prevention. Describe early signs of infection. Advise client to: Avoid soap; bathe breasts with clear water only. Air dry nipples after nursing. Avoid use of plastic bra liners, nipple shields. Apply lanolin after feeding as directed.	Enables mother to participate actively in own care, minimize potential for infection; facilitates early identification and treatment of infection. Minimizes potential for dry skin, nipple fissures (see also Client Self-Care Education: Breast Care for the Breast-Feeding Mother).	On request, client accurately explains preventive measures in own words. Client return-demonstrates procedures. Client complies with nursing recommendations. Client exhibits no signs or symptoms of infection (e.g., afebrile).
Trauma to Uterine Endometrium (Endometritis) Secondary to Placental Separation			
	Discuss and demonstrate perineal care, pad change, handwashing.	Minimizes potential for autoinfection (see also Client Self-Care Education: Perineal Care).	
Impaired Skin Integrity, Perineal (Wound Infection), Secondary to Episiotomy			
	Discuss perineal care, pad change, handwashing.	Promotes comfort and healing; minimizes potential for autoinfection.	
Constipation—Related to Reduced Intestinal Motility			
Client will re-establish normal bowel elimination pattern.	Perform client teaching: Encourage early ambulation. Encourage free intake of fluids (water 6-8 glasses daily). Encourage intake of fresh fruits, bran, vegetables. Reassure client about lack of discomfort accompanying stool expulsion. Administer stool softener as ordered.	Encourages peristalsis; reduces potential for constipation; minimizes risk of discomfort related to hard, packed stool.	Client complies with nursing recommendations. Client has spontaneous expulsion of normal stool.

Continued

NURSING
CARE
PLAN

Normal Post Partum—continued

Goals (Expected Outcomes)	Interventions	Rationale	Evaluation
Sleep Pattern Disturbance—Related to Interrupted Rest Secondary to Breast-Feeding			
Client will maximize time for rest and sleep.	Perform client teaching: Limit visitors and calls to specific times during day. Nap while baby sleeps. Rest frequently during day. Retire early. Organize nursing care to facilitate adequate rest.	Engenders rest and reduces energy expenditures resulting from "hostessing" (see also Client Self-Care Education: Rest and Sleep). Encourages rest and relaxation; reduces potential for sleep deficit.	Client complies with nursing recommendations. Client rests and sleeps during day. Client verbalizes feeling refreshed.
Altered Family Processes—Related to Role Change, Taking-In, and Taking-Hold			
Client will demonstrate attachment behaviors, e.g., bonding with newborn.	Place stable infant in mother's arms. Provide privacy for new family.	Encourages attachment and bonding.	Client demonstrates bonding behaviors: Eye contact Stroking Cuddling Calling infant by name
Client will begin integration of newborn into family unit.	Encourage both parents to interact with infant. Reduce light in room. Assist with initial breast-feeding if necessary.	Encourages infant to open eyes and interact with parents. Encourages bonding, later success in breast-feeding; stimulates uterine contractions.	Client appears happy and comfortable with newborn.
	Encourage active participation in and assumption of responsibility for infant care. Meet needs for guidance and assistance.	Introduces basic infant care concepts and skills in supportive environment; facilitates development of parental confidence and competence in infant care skills.	Client demonstrates growing confidence in own abilities to provide care.
Knowledge Deficit (Learning Need)—Regarding **Health Maintenance, Self-Assessment of Breasts, Nipples, Involution, Episiotomy, Signs of Postpartum Complications**			
Client will demonstrate understanding and application of client teaching. Client will actively participate in her own health maintenance. Client will identify early signs of postpartum complications.	Perform client teaching: Explain reasons for self-assessment. Discuss and demonstrate each component of postpartum assessment. Breasts and nipples Fundal check (height and consistency) Lochia (amount and color) Signs of healing surgical wound	Enables active client participation in own health maintenance.	On request, client explains assessment and rationale. Client accurately return-demonstrates assessment of: Breasts and nipples Involution progress Lochial volume and character Healing progress of surgical wound
	Describe and discuss signs to report to primary health care provider.	Encourages early diagnosis of emerging health problems (see also Client Self-Care Education: Breast Care for the Breast-Feeding Mother; Client Self-Care Education: Involution).	Client describes signs and symptoms to report promptly to primary health care provider. Client experiences an uneventful recovery.

NURSING
■ CARE
PLAN

Normal Post Partum—continued

Goals (Expected Outcomes)	Interventions	Rationale	Evaluation
Self-Care Activities			
Client will gain knowledge and skills needed for implementing effective postpartum self-care. Client will develop competence and comfort in performing self-care procedures. Client will develop confidence in own abilities. Client will assume responsibility for self-care.	Perform client teaching: Breast care Perineal care Heat therapy Nutrition, hydration Elimination Exercise, rest, sleep Prevention of infection	Enables active client participation in own health maintenance; minimizes potential for postpartum complications. Encourages and supports positive self-concept.	Client verbalizes understanding of principles and self-care procedures. Client performs self-care actions appropriately; displays no evidence of anxiety. Client verbalizes and demonstrates confidence in own ability.
Infant Care			
Client will gain knowledge and skills necessary for safe, effective infant care. Client will develop competence in performing basic infant care procedures. Client will develop confidence in own abilities to provide safe, effective infant care. Client will assume responsibility for basic infant care.	Perform client teaching: Feeding Burping Suctioning with bulb syringe Bathing Cord care Circumcision care Diapering	Enables client to perform basic infant care procedures effectively. Reduces anxiety; engenders confidence in own abilities. Encourages and supports positive self-concept.	Client verbalizes understanding of principles and procedures. Client performs procedures accurately. Client appears relaxed and comfortable in providing basic infant care.
Contraception			
Client will gain knowledge and understanding of selected aspects of current methods of contraception. Client will make an informed choice among available methods for family planning.	Perform client teaching: methods available Action Contraindications Advantages Disadvantages Effectiveness Risks	Enables client(s) to make an informed choice among options available for effective family planning.	Client selects method appropriate to individual needs and desires. Client experiences success in avoiding or achieving future pregnancy.
Sexuality Patterns—Related to			
Dyspareunia Secondary Episiotomy			
Client will minimize potential for sexual dysfunction.	Provide anticipatory guidance: Suggest couple defer coitus until episiotomy is less sensitive to pressure (approximately 3 wk).	Enables client(s) to understand and minimize maternal discomfort (see also Client Self-Care Education: Sexuality).	Client verbalizes understanding of factors that may cause discomfort.
Decreased Vaginal Lubrication Secondary to Low Estrogen Level			
Client will resume mutually satisfying sexual relationship with significant other.	Recommend use of spermicidal cream for lubrication.	Reduces friction discomfort; allows satisfaction of sexual drive.	

Continued

NURSING
CARE
PLAN

Normal Post Partum—*continued*

Goals (Expected Outcomes)	Interventions	Rationale	Evaluation
Fear of Pregnancy			
Client will make an informed choice regarding method of contraception.	Suggest use of spermicidal cream during interim between discharge and postpartum check-up. Client teaching: If desired, discuss options for family planning.	Promotes comfort; minimizes risk of unexpected pregnancy. Facilitates informed decision making; encourages selection of method of contraception appropriate to individual needs and desires.	Client identifies ways to minimize discomfort and potential for unexpected pregnancy.
Self-Esteem Disturbance—Related to			
Feelings of Inadequacy and Insecurity Regarding Self-Care, Infant Care			
Client will recognize the influence of physiologic changes on emotional status.	Provide anticipatory guidance: Discuss normal psychologic changes in the postpartum period; explain transitory nature; emphasize normalcy.	Enables client(s) to understand and accept emerging feelings; minimizes fear "something is wrong." (see also Client Self-Care Education: Psychosocial Aspects of the Postpartum Period).	Client copes effectively with postpartum let-down.
Altered Hormone Levels			
	Explain physiologic changes; emphasize transitory nature and normalcy.		
Fatigue Secondary to Altered Life-Style			
Client will organize activities to allow time for rest and relaxation.	Enable future coping by aiding client to develop confidence in self-care, infant care.	Enables effective coping; supports positive self-concept; minimizes symptoms.	Client experiences uneventful transition to parenthood.

REFERENCES

1. Jacobson H: A standard for assessing lochia volume. MCN 10:174-175, May/June 1985
2. Cunningham F, MacDonald P, Gant N: Williams Obstetrics, 18th ed. Norwalk, Conn, Appleton & Lange, 1989
3. Resnick R: The puerperium. In Creasey R, Resnick R: Maternal-Fetal Medicine: Principles and Practice, 2nd ed. Philadelphia, WB Saunders, 1989
4. Whitley N: A Manual of Clinical Obstetrics. Philadelphia, JB Lippincott, 1985, pp 565, 619-627
5. Rubin R: Maternal identity and the maternal experience. New York, Springer Publishing, 1984
6. Martel LK, Mitchell SK: Rubin's "puerperal change" reconsidered. JOGN 13:145, May/June 1984
7. Gay JT, Edgil AE, Douglas AB: Reva Rubin revisited. JOGN 11:394-399, November/December 1988
8. Pillsbury B: Doing the month; Confinement and convalescence of Chinese women after childbirth. In Kay MA: Anthropology of Human Birth. Philadelphia, FA Davis, 1982, pp 119-146
9. Bernstein GL, Kidd YA: Childbearing in Japan. In Kay M: Anthropology of Human Birth. Philadelphia, FA Davis, 1982, pp 101-146
10. Horn B: Cultural concepts and postpartal care. Nurs Health Care 11:516-517, 526-527, 1981
11. Wadd L: Vietnamese postpartum practices: Implications for nursing in the hospital setting. JOGN 12:252, July/August 1983
12. Orque M: Nursing care of Filipino American patients. In Orque M, Bloch B, Monrroy L: Ethnic Nursing Care. St. Louis, CV Mosby, 1983

13. Monrroy L: Nursing care of Raza/Latina patients. In Orque et al: Ethnic Nursing Care. St. Louis, CV Mosby, 1983, pp 115-148

14. Davis J, Brucker M, MacMullen N: A study of mother's postpartum teaching priorities. Matern Child Nurs 15:41-51,1986

15. Rutledge DL, Pridham KFK: Postpartum mother's perceptions of competence for infant care. JOGN 16:3:185, 1987

16. Hatcher R et al: Contraceptive Technology 1986-1987, 13th ed. New York, Irvington Publishers, 1986

17. Hatcher R et al: Contraceptive Technology 1988-1989, 14th ed. New York, Irvington Publishers, 1988

18. Norr K, Nacion K: Outcomes of postpartum early discharge, 1960-1986, a comparative review. Birth 14(3):135-141, September 1987

19. Jansson P: Early postpartum discharge. Am J Nurs 85(5):547-550, May 1985

20. Regan K: Early obstetrical discharge: A program that works. Can Nurse 80:32-35, October 1984

SUGGESTED READINGS

Fishman SH et al: Changes in sexual relationships in postpartum couples, JOGN 15:58, January/February 1986

Grosso C et al: The Vietnamese American family: And grandma makes three. MCN 6:177, 1981

Konrad CJ: Helping mothers integrate the birth experience. MCN 12(4):268, December 1987

Mansell KA: Mother-baby units. The concept works. MCN 9:132, 1984

Meleis A, Sorrell L: Arab American women and their birth experiences. MCN 6:171, 1981

Orque MS, Bloch B, Monrroy LA: Ethnic Nursing Care, A Multicultural Approach. St. Louis, CV Mosby, 1983

Pridham K: The meaning for mothers of a new infant: Relationship to maternal experience. Matern Child Nurs J 16(2):103-122, Summer 1987

Tribotti S et al: Nursing diagnoses for the postpartum woman. JOGN 11:410-416, November/December 1988

Zepeda M: Selected maternal infant care practices of Spanish speaking women. JOGN 11:16, 371, 1982

Nursing Assessment and Care of the Newborn

IMPORTANT TERMINOLOGY

acrocyanosis Blueness of newborn's extremities seen in first hours after birth

abduction Away from body's midline

adduction Toward body's midline

bradycardia Heart rate less than 120 beats per minute

bradypnea Respiratory rate of 25 per minute or less

caput succedaneum Soft-tissue edema of scalp caused by pressure on head during labor and delivery

cephalohematoma Mass formed by collection of blood between skull and periosteum; swelling does not cross suture lines

ecchymosis Purplish discoloration caused by bruising

Epstein's pearls Small, white inclusion cysts sometimes seen on gums or hard palate or both

erythema toxicum Common nonpathologic newborn rash of unknown etiology

gestational age Number of weeks elapsed since first day of mother's last menstrual period

harlequin sign Dilatation of vessels on one side of body and constriction of vessels on other side of body caused by vasomotor disturbance, resulting in two-tone body color that resembles a clown's suit

milia Tiny pearly-white spots on forehead, nose, and chin caused by retention of sebaceous material within sebaceous glands

mongolian spots Gray-blue pigmented areas usually found on lower back and buttocks of dark-skinned and Oriental infants

mottling Lacy pattern of dark and light areas on skin caused by vasomotor response to cold

nevus flammeus Flat, purple-red, sharply defined "port-wine stain" birthmark

nevus vasculosus Dark red, rough-textured, elevated "strawberry mark" birthmark

pseudomenstruation Transient, scant, blood-tinged mucoid vaginal discharge caused by withdrawal of maternal hormones

tachycardia Heart rate greater than 160 beats per minute

tachypnea Respiratory rate of 60 per minute or more

telangiectatic nevi Tiny pink or red spots that blanch on pressure; "stork bites"

This chapter continues discussions of the neonatal period. Content focuses on nursing care of the newborn and supportive actions that assist the infant to adapt successfully to independent extrauterine life. Emphasis is placed on nursing assessment of factors that influence successful transition and later growth and development.

Assessment

Newborn Transitional Status

Successful transition to independent extrauterine life requires that all adaptive physiologic mechanisms be effective. The first 24 hours after birth comprise the period of highest risk to the newborn. Performing continuous assessments is important to assure prompt management of any emerging physiologic problems during transition. Early identification and prompt management of any interferences with newborn adaptation are vital to the infant's survival.

In agencies with labor, delivery, recovery, postpartum (LDRP) units, mothers are admitted, labor, deliver, recover, and occupy the same room with their infants during the total hospital stay. After the initial bonding period, the nurse caring for the mother–infant couplet conducts a physical assessment of the healthy infant. In agencies in which newborns are admitted to a central nursery, the comprehensive physical assessment may be delayed until admission to the unit. At the end of an initial bonding period, the newborn is transferred to the nursery. The nurse who transports the infant to the nursery is responsible for providing pertinent detailed information about (1) the mother's history; (2) events during labor and delivery; (3) the infant's immediate postdelivery status; (4) initial assessment findings; (5) any treatments implemented, e.g., infant resuscitation; and (6) response to bonding (see Assessment Tool: Newborn Admission to Nursery p. 496). This information provides the initial data base for implementing the nursing process.

Nursery Admission Assessment

MATERNAL HISTORY. Information about the mother's general health, prenatal history, and intrapartum course is essential to effective assessment and management of her newborn. Deviations from expected maternal antepartum and intrapartum patterns and progress should be included in the report. Significant correlations have been identified between maternal risk status and newborn jeopardy.

ANALYSIS OF TOTAL APGAR SCORE. Tallying the points allocated for each of the five Apgar indicators provides a general index of the newborn's physical status at 1 and 5 minutes after delivery. Infants whose total score

Admission to Nursery

Information of particular importance to early identification of potential high-risk infants includes the following:

Antepartum History

Mother's age, gravida, and parity
Estimated date of confinement and duration of gestation at delivery
Mother's general state of health and nutrition
Maternal history of chronic diseases: diabetes, endocrine disorders, cardiac and renal disorders
Severe social problems: adolescent pregnancy, substance abuse
Pregnancy-related disorders: hyperemesis, pregnancy-induced hypertension, hydramnios, abruptio placentae
Results of relevant prenatal diagnostic procedures: blood type and Rh factor, Rh antibody and rubella titers, VDRL, HIV screening, gonorrhea and herpes cultures, nonstress tests, contraction stress tests, ultrasonography, amniocentesis, chorionic villi sampling, estriol levels

Intrapartum History

All information concerning events occurring during the labor and delivery should be considered part of the data base needed to assess the neonate adequately. Of particular importance are the following:

    Time between rupture of membranes and delivery
        History of prolonged rupture of membranes
        Prolonged or difficult intrapartum course
    Time and type of delivery
        Abnormal presentation and/or delivery
        Precipitate delivery
    Type, amount, and time of any medication
    Type and time of any anesthesia
    Any evidence of fetal distress
        Type and results of fetal monitoring
        Meconium-stained amniotic fluid
        Results of any fetal blood gas examinations
    Apgar scores at 1 and 5 minutes
        7-10 Within acceptable normal range
        4-6 Moderately depressed; in need of some assistance to improve transitional status
        0-3 Severely depressed; requires immediate resuscitative efforts
    Any resuscitation efforts
    Any procedures or treatments
    Number of vessels in umbilical cord
    Bonding opportunities and responses
    Other
        Breast-feeding or bottle-feeding
        Any special orders

is less than eight at 5 minutes should be observed closely and reassessed at 10 minutes. Low total Apgar scores at 5 and 10 minutes have been correlated with neonatal morbidity and mortality. However, Apgar scores may overlook subtle effects of intrauterine hypoxia and are not predictive of long-term function.[1,2]

NUMBER OF VESSELS IN UMBILICAL CORD. The normal umbilical cord contains two arteries and one vein. A high incidence of congenital anomalies has been associated with other than the usual three vessels.

GENERAL NEWBORN ASSESSMENT. Immediately after delivery, nursing assessments monitor newborn status and progress through the period of immediate transition. Assessments focus on signs and symptoms that indicate the biophysical changes affecting the newborn's body systems and the infant's response to the physiologic stresses of birth. Initial assessment findings also can identify gross evidence of congenital anomalies or early signs of problems with transition and enable prompt medical and nursing management.[3] While giving immediate newborn care, applying identification bands, and footprinting and wrapping the infant, the delivery room nurse assesses the infant's (1) color; (2) general appearance; (3) respiratory pattern; (4) response to a new environment, e.g., reactivity to stimuli; (5) missing or extra digits; (5) reflexes; (6) birthmarks; (7) foot position; (8) voiding; and (9) defecation and notes any deviations from expected findings. Findings from the immediate postdelivery assessments provide important data for later more comprehensive assessments.

Comprehensive Nursing Assessment

In many health agencies nurses are responsible for the initial and ongoing assessment of the healthy newborn. With the infant under a radiant warmer, the nurse performs an orderly and systematic physical assessment to ensure that all important data are collected. The examiner may use any system of notation that is consistent with agency policy. One suggestion is to use a check ($\sqrt{}$) to indicate that findings are within expected (normal) limits and a plus (+) or minus (−) sign to indicate that something is present or absent. When appropriate, descriptions can be written in the spaces or under "comments." The format presents a comprehensive cephalocaudal nursing assessment. Table 20-1 summarizes usual findings and deviations from normal findings. Assessment begins with an inspection of the infant's general appearance and behavior.

TABLE 20-1

Summary of Newborn Physical Assessment

Assessment Area	Usual Findings	Deviations
General Observations		
Muscle tone	Flexed position; good tone	"Floppy"; rigid or tense
Skin		
Color	Pink tone to ruddy when crying; appropriate to ethnic origin; acrocyanosis	Pallor; cyanosis; jaundice; ecchymosis; petechiae
Texture	Smooth; dryness with some peeling; lanugo on back; vernix	Excessive peeling or cracking; roughness
Rashes and pigmentation	Erythema toxicum; milia; mongolian spots	Impetigo; hemangiomas; nevus flammeus (port-wine stain)
Hydration	Skin pinch over abdomen immediately returns to original state	Skin maintains "tent" shape after pinch
Cry	Lusty	Shrill; weak; grunty
Measurements		
Weight	2700-4000 g (6-9 lb)	
Length	48-53 cm (19-21 in)	
Head circumference	33-37 cm (13-14½ in)	
Chest circumference	31-35 cm (12-14 in)	

Continued

TABLE 20-1

Summary of Newborn Physical Assessment—continued

Assessment Area	Usual Findings	Deviations
Vital Signs		
Temperature	Axillary (preferred method): 36.5°-37°C (97.7°-98.6°F) Rectal: 36.5°-37.2°C (97.7°-99°F)	Hypothermia; fever
Respirations	40-60 respirations/min; quiet and shallow; diaphragmatic; occasional periods of rapid breathing, alternating with short periods of apnea	Prolonged rapid breathing; apnea lasting longer than 10 sec; grunting; retractions; persistent slow rate
Heart rate (apical pulse)	120-160 beats/min; faster when crying (up to 180 beats/min); slower when sleeping (down to 100 beats/min)	Tachycardia: >160 beats/min at rest Bradycardia: <120 beats/min when awake
Head	Vaginal delivery: elongated (molding) Breech or cesarean birth: round, symmetric Size within normal range	Caput succedaneum; cephalohematoma; hydrocephaly; microcephaly
Fontanels	Flat; soft; firm	Bulging; sunken
Anterior	Diamond shaped; 2-3 cm wide; 3-4 cm long; smaller at birth with molding	Small; almost closed; closed (craniostenosis); widened
Posterior	Triangular shape; small; almost closed	Enlarged
Face	Small; round; symmetric; fat pads in cheeks; receding chin	Asymmetric; distorted
Eyes	Edematous lids; usually closed; blue or slate gray color; no tears; red reflex present; pupils equal, round, react to light	Elevation or ptosis of lids; epicanthal folds; absence of red reflex; unequal, dilated, or constricted pupils
	Common variations: subconjunctival hemorrhages; chemical conjunctivitis; occasional slight nystagmus or convergent strabismus	Purulent discharge; frequent nystagmus; constant, divergent, or unilateral strabismus
Mouth	Intact lips, gums, palate; epithelial pearls; "sucking blisters" on lips; tongue midline, mobile, appropriate size for mouth, can extend to alveolar ridge	Cleft lip or palate; white, cheesy patches on tongue, gums, or mucous membrane; large or protruding tongue
Nose	In midline; even placement in relation to eyes and mouth; nares patent; septum intact, midline	Flattened or bruised; unusual placement or configuration; obstructed nares; deviated or perforated septum
Ears	Well-formed cartilage; appropriate size for head; upper attachment on line extended through inner and outer canthus of eye; external auditory canal patent	Floppy, large and protruding; malformed; low set; obstruction of canal
Neck	Short; thick; full range of motion; no masses	Webbing; abnormal shortening; limitation of motion; torticollis; masses
Clavicles	Straight; smooth; intact	Knot or lump; decreased movement of extremity on one side
Thorax	Round; symmetric; protruding xiphoid process	Assymetric; funnel chest
Breath sounds	Loud; bronchial; bilaterally equal	Decreased breath sounds; increased breath sounds
Heart sounds	Regular rate and rhythm; first and second sounds clear and distinct	Murmurs; dysrhythmias
Breasts	Symmetric; flat with erect nipples; engorgement second or third day not unusual	Redness and firmness around nipple

TABLE 20-1

Summary of Newborn Physical Assessment—continued

Assessment Area	Usual Findings	Deviations
Abdomen	Symmetric; slightly protuberant; no masses	Scaphoid or concave shape; distention; palpable masses
Liver	Palpable 2-3 cm below right costal margin	Enlargement
Spleen	Tip may be palpable in left upper quadrant	Enlargement
Kidneys	May be palpable at level of umbilicus	Enlargement
Femoral pulses	Bilaterally equal	Unequal or absent
Umbilicus	No extensive protrusion or herniation; no signs of infection	Umbilical hernia; omphalocele; redness; induration; foul-smelling discharge
	Cord: bluish white, moist → black, dry; three vessels; no oozing or bleeding	Two vessels; bleeding or oozing from stump
Genitalia	Appropriate for gender	Ambiguous genitalia
Female		
Labia	Edematous; labia majora cover labia minora; vernix in creases	Hematoma; lesions; fusion of labia
Vagina	Mucus discharge, possibly blood tinged	
Male		
Foreskin	Adherent to glans penis	
Urethra	Opening at tip of penis	Opening below tip of penis (hypospadias)
		Opening above tip of penis (epispadias)
Testes	Palpable in each scrotal sac	Palpable in inguinal canal; not palpable
Posterior of Body		
Spinal column	Straight, flexible; intact; no masses	Exaggerated curves; spina bifida; any masses; pilonidal cyst
Anus	Patent	Imperforate anus, anal fissures
Extremities	Symmetric in size, shape, and movement	Unequal or abnormal size or shape; asymmetric or limited movement of one or more extremities
Digits	Five on each hand and foot; appropriate size and shape	Missing digits; syndactyly (webbing); polydactyly (extra digits)
Hips	Even leg length, knee height, gluteal folds; no resistance or limitation to abduction	Uneven leg length, knee height, or gluteal folds; uneven or limited abduction; hip "click" or "clunk" on abduction
Feet	Straight, or postural deviation easily corrected with gentle pressure	Structural deformities: talipes equinovarus (clubfoot); metatarsus adductus
Reflexes		
Rooting and sucking	Turns toward object touching cheek, lips, or corner of mouth; opens mouth; begins sucking movements; strong suck, pulls object into mouth	No rooting; weak ineffective, or absent suck
	May be diminished or absent after eating	
Grasp		
Palmar	Fingers grasp object when palm stimulated and hang on briefly	Weak or absent
Plantar	Toes curl downward when soles of feet are stimulated	Weak or absent
Moro	Symmetric response to sudden stimulus: lateral extension of arms with opening of hands, followed by flexion and adduction	Asymmetric; absent; incomplete
Stepping	Stepping movements when infant held upright with sole of foot touching surface	Asymmetric or absent

General Appearance

Immediately on the infant's admission to the nursery, the nurse assesses the newborn's general appearance (see Assessment Tool: Initial Newborn Assessment). A rapid visual appraisal usually notes any gross deviations from expected color, respiratory effort, cry, symmetry of body parts, body attitude (flexion of the extremities), state of awareness, or motility. If any deviations are present, the assessment focus and pattern may be altered. All later contacts with the newborn include an assessment of general appearance (see Assessment Tool: Ongoing Nursing Assessment).

COLOR. The healthy, well-oxygenated, full-term, white or Oriental newborn generally is pink, reddish, or pale. The skin color of black infants may vary but usually has a warm brownish tone. With crying infants become more ruddy. The skin is less pigmented in the neonatal period than later in life, so color changes may be noted even in infants with darker skin. Some transient **acrocyanosis** (blueness of the hands and feet) may be present. Dark-skinned newborns also may be assessed for general

---

ASSESSMENT
TOOL

Initial Newborn Assessment

General Appearance

Color: acrocyanosis, circumoral cyanosis, mottling, harlequin sign
Respiratory effort: nasal flaring, sternal retraction, grunting, excessive mucus
State of consciousness: quiet alert, drowsy, hyperalert, crying, deep sleep, light sleep
Body attitude: flexed, extensions, tonicity
Reactivity: responds to external stimuli, jittery
Symmetry: body structures, facial expression, motility
Vital signs: temperature, pulse, respirations every 30 minutes until stable
Status of umbilical cord stump: clamp in place, bleeding, number of vessels

Measurements

Length and weight
Head and chest circumference

Comprehensive Nursing Assessment

May integrate components of the neurologic (reflexes) and gestational age assessments into comprehensive appraisal of current physical status

---

ASSESSMENT
TOOL

Ongoing Nursing Assessment

In addition to the components of general appearance and vital signs, the nurse assesses the following:
   Skin turgor
   Jaundice
   Feeding: amount and pattern
   Voiding
   Stool
   Sleep patterns

oxygenation status by examining the lips, earlobes, nailbeds, and mucous membranes for pink color.

Other color changes include **mottling** and the **harlequin sign.** Mottling occurs particularly when the infant is cold. Vasomotor fluctuations create a transient, lacy pattern of dark and light areas. The skin color is not uniform and appears mottled. Similarly, a vasomotor disturbance that causes the blood vessels on one side of the infant's body to dilate and those on the other side to constrict results in what is called the harlequin sign. One side of the infant's body appears deep pink, and the other side looks pale; the pattern resembles that of a two-colored clown's suit, i.e., a harlequin.

RESPIRATORY EFFORT. The newborn breathes with the diaphragm and through the nose. Any evidence of nasal flaring, costal breathing and sternal retraction, gasping, or grunting suggests respiratory distress.

SYMMETRY. The shape, size, and relative position of the newborn's body parts, e.g., facial features, arms and legs, should correspond on both sides of the body.

BODY ATTITUDE. After a vertex delivery, the newborn rests in a flexed position with arms and legs adducted and flexed. Newborns who have been in a breech position in utero may rest with thighs adducted and externally rotated.

MOVEMENT. The spontaneous movements of the normal newborn usually involve all extremities. Movements are random, purposeless, and symmetric.

Skin

The skin of the healthy full-term newborn is soft, velvety, and wrinkled. Skin turgor in a well-hydrated term infant is elastic and returns to normal appearance promptly on release.

VERNIX. At birth the skin is covered to varying degrees with vernix caseosa, a white, cheesy material that protects the skin during intrauterine life. On full-term infants vernix is found primarily in the body creases. Postterm infants may have little vernix. Their skin may be dry and peeling, particularly on the palms of their hands and the soles of their feet.

LANUGO. Lanugo is fine, downy hair usually found only on the shoulders, back, and upper arms of the term infant.

MILIA. Milia are pinpoint-sized, pearly-white spots commonly found on the nose, forehead, or chin of the newborn. When touched gently with the tip of a finger, these spots feel like tiny, firm seeds. They are due to retention of sebaceous material within the the sebaceous glands. If they are left alone, they usually disappear spontaneously during the neonatal period.

BIRTHMARKS. Birthmarks are categorized either as vascular nevi or as pigmented nevi. *Vascular nevi* are capillary hemangiomas. Small superficial hemangiomas commonly are called "stork bites." Those located imme-

TABLE 20-2

Birthmarks

Type	Characteristics
Vascular Nevi	
Telangiectic nevi (stork bites)	Tiny pink to red spots found commonly on nape of the neck, eyelids, and bridge of the nose; do blanch on pressure; usually disappear spontaneously during infancy, but some persist into adulthood
Nevus flammeus (port-wine stain)	Flat, purple-red, sharply demarcated areas, often found on the face (on black infants, they are deep purple-black); do not blanch on pressure, increase in size, or fade over time; disfigurement varies with size and placement
	If the infant also displays epileptic-like seizures, may indicate Sturge-Weber syndrome, a serious genetic disorder.
Nevus vasculosus (strawberry marks)	Dark red, rough-textured, sharply demarcated elevations usually found on head or face; continue to grow for several months, then shrink spontaneously and usually disappear by 7-10 yr of age.
Pigmented Nevi	
Mongolian spots	Gray-blue pigmented areas seen most often on lumbosacral region and buttocks of dark-skinned and Asian infants; usually spontanously disappear during late infancy or early childhood; have no relationship to mongolism
Café au lait spots	Patchy, flat, brown areas that are lighter in color than the surrounding skin; commonly found on the face, chest, arms, hands; usually of no significance; however, if spots are >1.5 cm long or more than six are present, they may indicate certain genetic syndromes, e.g., Von Recklinghausen disease

diately below the epidermis are known as "port-wine stains." "Strawberry mark" hemangiomas involve vessels in both the dermal and the subdermal layers of the skin. *Pigmented nevi* are due to either hyperpigmentation **(mongolian spots)** or lack of melanocytes (café au lait spots). Table 20-2 lists differentiating characteristics and possible implications.

ERYTHEMA TOXICUM. **Erythema toxicum** is a nonpathologic newborn rash of unknown etiology that often appears during the first few days of life. It is commonly referred to as "flea-bite" dermatitis because the reddened areas have a small blanched wheal in the center and resemble flea bites (Fig. 20-1).

FIGURE 20-1

Erythema Toxicum. Erythema toxicum develops more frequently on the back, the shoulders, and the buttocks. The rash is transient, likely to change appreciably within a few hours, and usually disappears within a day or so. No treatment is needed.
Courtesy MacDonald House, The University Hospitals of Cleveland, Cleveland, Ohio.

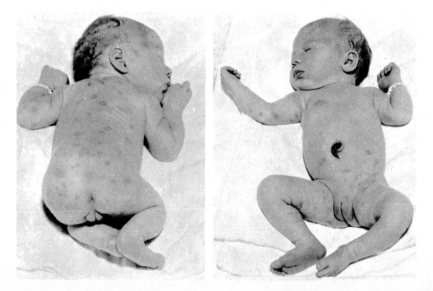

JAUNDICE. Physiologic jaundice (icterus neonatorum) occurs in 40% to 60% of normal full-term newborns. It is thought caused by a high level of serum bilirubin liberated by the destruction of fetal red blood cells (RBCs) (see Chapter 17). Most commonly, it appears 48 to 72 hours after birth. When jaundice is present, blanching the skin on the nose of the newborn produces a yellowish color immediately after release of pressure. Jaundice occurring within the first 24 hours after birth is considered pathologic and should be reported promptly. Pathologic jaundice is discussed in Chapter 26.

Measurements

Expected normal measurements of the full-term infant are listed in Table 20-1. Some variations are anticipated because of the size of the individual infant and events occurring during labor, e.g., molding of the head.

LENGTH AND WEIGHT. Length and weight should be measured soon after birth. These measurements aid in estimating **gestational age.** They also serve as a baseline from which to judge future growth. Since the newborn usually assumes a flexed position, the nurse may experience some difficulty in measuring from the top of the head to the heels accurately. Accuracy is improved by placing the infant on a firm surface and having an assistant hold the infant's head.

HEAD AND CHEST CIRCUMFERENCE. The head is the largest part of the newborn's body. Usually the head is 2 cm larger than the chest. The nurse compares the measurements of the head and chest circumferences to identify signs of microcephaly (small head) or hydrocephaly. Figures 20-2 and 20-3 illustrate the accepted manner of measuring head and chest circumference.

Vital Signs

Vital sign assessment data also suggest and support nursing diagnoses of the newborn's current state of health. The vital signs should be checked every 30 minutes until they are stable or as required by hospital policy. Changes in vital signs may reflect physiologic complications that affect transition.

TEMPERATURE. Newborn body temperature tends to vary with continuing exposure to the environment. Some hospitals require that a rectal temperature be taken on admission to the nursery. Subsequent temperature assessments usually are axillary. The average range of normal newborn rectal temperature is 36.5° to 37.5°C (97.7° to 99.5°F); axillary temperature ranges from 36.5° to 37.2°C (97.6° to 98.6°F).

- Subnormal temperatures may indicate prolonged exposure to low environmental temperatures, respiratory distress syndrome (RDS), sepsis, or prematurity.
- Elevated temperatures may indicate exposure to high environmental temperatures, infection, drug addiction, or dehydration.

PULSE. The nurse should auscultate the apical pulse for 1 full minute (Fig. 20-4). The average newborn apical pulse ranges from 120 to 140 beats/min. Pulse rate also varies with activity, ranging from 100 beats/min during sleep periods to 160 beats/min in crying episodes.

FIGURE 20-2
Measuring Head Circumference. The nurse measures head circumference by placing a nonstretchable tape measure just above the eyebrows and over the most prominent part of the occiput.

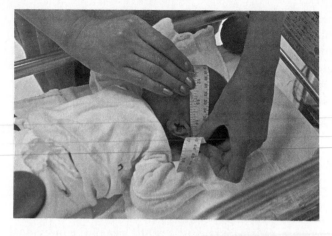

FIGURE 20-3
Measuring Chest Circumference. The chest circumference is measured at or just above the nipple line.

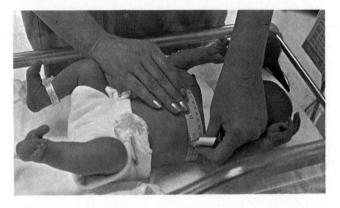

FIGURE 20-4
Auscultating Chest. If the infant is quiet, it is wise to auscultate the chest before beginning any other assessment activities that might cause crying. Because the adult-sized diaphragm may not make complete contact with the infant's chest, the nurse uses the bell or small diaphragm of the stethoscope for auscultating. Warming the diaphragm between the palms before placement on the infant's chest reduces the sensory stimulation that may elicit crying.

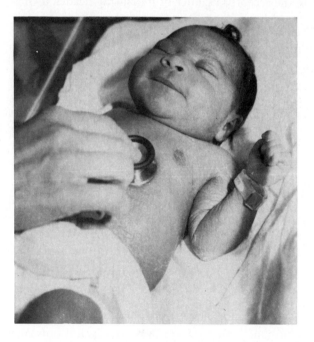

- Persistent **tachycardia** (pulse rate persistently >160 beats/min) is associated with RDS.
- **Bradycardia** (pulse rate <120 beats/min) may indicate congenital newborn heart block.
- Heart murmurs are common in newborns but should be evaluated closely.
- Femoral pulses should be strong and equal. Weak or absent femoral pulses are associated with coarctation of the aorta.[3] Simultaneously palpating the brachial (or temporal) and femoral pulses may identify a pulse lag; femoral pulse lag may indicate obstruction such as coarctation of the aorta.[4]

RESPIRATION. Respirations should be counted for 1 full minute. The characteristic respiratory pattern is diaphragmatic, quiet, shallow, and irregular. Because the infant primarily uses diaphragmatic breathing, the nurse may prefer to count abdominal excursions. An alternate method is to count respirations by auscultation (Fig. 20-5).

The respiratory rate ranges from 35 to 60 breaths/min, with occasional, brief (<15 seconds) periods of apnea.

- **Bradypnea** is identified as a respiratory rate of 25 per minute or less. Bradypnea may indicate newborn narcosis or birth trauma.
- **Tachypnea** is defined as a respiratory rate above 60 per minute. Tachypnea is associated with RDS, atelectasis, meconium-aspiration syndrome (MAS), and diaphragmatic hernia.
- Respiratory distress is accompanied by nasal flaring, sternal retractions, and labored breathing.

BLOOD PRESSURE. Accurate assessment of the blood pressure may be critical for some newborns. To ensure accuracy the width of the cuff used to occlude the arterial circulation must be appropriate to the individual newborn. The cuff should cover approximately two-thirds of the upper

FIGURE 20-5

Breath Sounds. Bronchial breath sounds normally are heard over most of the chest and sound louder and harsher because they are closer. Because breath sounds may be altered with changing positions, auscultation should be done also with the infant in the upright position.

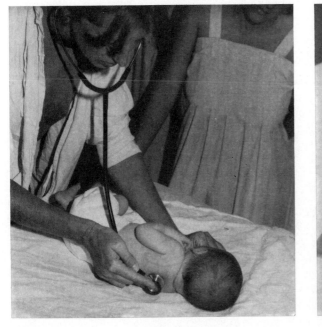
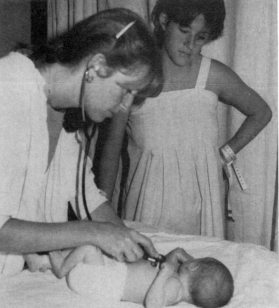

arm or thigh and be 25% greater than the diameter of the limb on which the blood pressure is being taken.[5] Although either the arm or the leg may be used to auscultate the infant's blood pressure, leg pressure will be slightly higher but should be within 20 mm Hg of the arm pressure. The usual range of blood pressure at birth is 60 to 80 systolic and 40 to 45 diastolic.

Assessment of the Head and Neck
Head

In addition to measuring the head circumference, assessment of the head includes inspection and palpation. The infant's head is large and comprises approximately one-quarter of total body size. Usually, the suture lines and fontanels are identified easily by gentle palpation. The fontanels ("soft spots") should be neither depressed nor bulging. At birth the diamond-shaped anterior fontanel usually is 2 to 3 cm wide and 3 to 4 cm long. On initial assessment it may appear smaller if there has been marked overriding of the skull bones during labor and delivery. Closure usually occurs by 12 to 18 months of age.

The smaller posterior fontanel is located between the occipital and parietal bones. It may be almost closed at birth and completely closed by the end of the second month.

The shape and symmetry of the head varies widely in relation to the presentation and position during labor and delivery.[6] Three conditions may contribute to an initial asymmetric appearance in cephalic presentations: (1) molding (Fig. 20-6), (2) **caput succedaneum** (Fig. 20-7), or (3) **cephalohematoma** (Fig. 20-8).

Face

The newborn's face is small and round, and the lower jaw seems to recede. Asymmetry, especially of the chin and mandible, is sometimes seen and

FIGURE 20-6

Head Molding. Molding is due to the overriding of the skull bones that often occurs as the head accommodates to the changing diameters of the birth canal during labor. Although the infant's head appears elongated at birth, the effects of molding subside spontaneously during the first few days after birth.

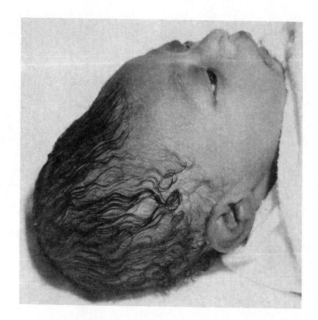

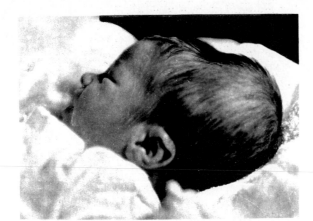

FIGURE 20-7

Caput Succedaneum. Caput succedaneum is a diffuse soft-tissue edema of the scalp caused by extended pressure on the head during labor or delivery or both. The swelling often crosses the suture lines. Scalp ecchymosis may be present. Caput succedaneum usually resolves spontaneously in a few days.

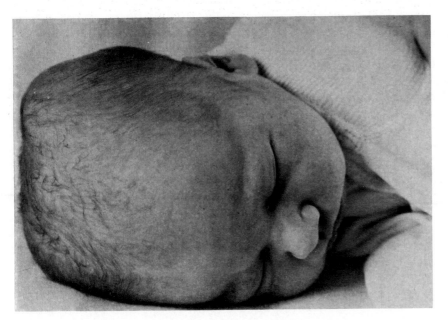

FIGURE 20-8

Cephalohematoma. Cephalohematoma is due to the rupture of blood vessels between the skull and periosteum. This results in a collection of blood between the bone and the periosteum. No ecchymosis is seen on the scalp. Usually the hematoma is unilateral and does not extend across suture lines. Since the bleeding is a slow process, cephalohematomas may not be evident at birth but are obvious between the first and second day after birth. Although some resolve slowly over the first few months of infancy, most resolve within 2 to 6 weeks.

can be caused by the fetal attitude in utero when the flexed head tilts to one side and presses against the shoulder. The nose also may be asymmetric or have a deviated septum resulting from intrauterine pressure.

The scalp, face, and neck are inspected carefully for abrasions, contusions, or lacerations. These can result from application of internal fetal monitor eletrodes, forceps, or vacuum extractors.

Eyes

Although the newborn's eyes are closed much of the time, they may open spontaneously if the infant's head is lifted or rocked gently. From birth the infant can see and discriminate patterns as the basis for form perception. This capacity is limited by imperfect oculomotor coordination and inability to accommodate for various distances. In addition, the eye, the visual pathways, and the visual part of the brain are poorly developed at birth.

Most infants' eyes are blue or slate-gray at birth. Dark eyes are typical of dark-skinned infants. Although iris pigmentation does not occur until the infant is approximately 1 year old, most infants achieve their permanent eye color by 3 months of age. Brushfield's spots (white specks in the periphery of the iris) may be seen.

The eyes are observed for symmetry in (1) size, (2) position, (3) spacing, (4) shape of the inner and outer canthus, and (5) response to light. Deviations from expected patterns may be associated with certain congenital disorders (see Chapter 26).

STRABISMUS (CROSS-EYES). Immature neuromuscular control is responsible for the transient episodes of strabismus in newborns. This usually disappears within 3 to 4 months.

DOLL'S EYES. When the infant's head position is rotated to the left and right, the eyes may move in the opposite direction—like those of a doll. Immature head-eye coordination is responsible for what is known as the doll's eyes phenomenon.

OTHER ASPECTS. The color of the sclera is noted. The expected color is bluish-white. (A yellowish cast suggests jaundice.) Changes in vascular tension during the delivery process may have caused small areas of subconjunctival hemorrhage. In the absence of pathology, these findings are not significant and disappear spontaneously in 1 to 2 weeks.

TEARS. Because the lacrimal glands are immature, tears may not appear for several weeks and sometimes for several months.

CHEMICAL CONJUNCTIVITIS. If prophylactic silver nitrate has been instilled, some edema of the lids or a yellowish discharge may be present.

If an ophthalmoscope is used in examining the eyes, the pupil appears red-orange when the light is directed on it. This is known as the red reflex caused by light shining on the retina. Opacities of the lens are noted and reported. The *blink reflex* occurs in response to shining a bright light in the newborn's eyes.

Ears and Hearing

The ears should be inspected for size, shape, position in relation to the eyes (Fig. 20-9), and anomaly. Abnormal ear position frequently is associated with chromosomal abnormalities or kidney anomalies.

Otoscopic examination identifies patency of the external auditory canal. However, for the first 2 to 3 days of life accumulated vernix caseosa may make the tympanic membranes difficult to visualize. During the first few months after birth the light reflex is diffuse rather than cone shaped.

The ear and nerve tracts for hearing are anatomically mature at birth, and newborns can hear after their first cry. Within several days, as the eustachian tubes become aerated and mucus in the middle ear disappears, the infant's hearing becomes acute. Newborns will turn their heads in the direction of a nearby voice.

Nose and Smell

The nose should be in the facial midline. Because the newborn is an obligate nose breather, the nurse checks for nasal patency. The nurse closes the infant's mouth, occludes one nostril at a time, and observes for any

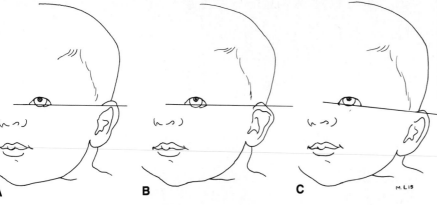

FIGURE 20-9

Ear Attachment. The point at which the top of the ear is attached to the scalp should fall on or above an imaginary line drawn from the inner canthus through the outer canthus of the eye. **A,** Normal ear. **B,** Abnormally angled ear. **C,** Low-seated ear.

signs of respiratory difficulty. Newborns will turn their heads toward the breast or bottle. This demonstrates their ability to perceive and identify a milk odor.

Lips, Mouth, and Cheeks

The rounded, thickened areas often present on the lips are labial tubercles or "sucking blisters." In reality they are not true blisters since they contain no fluid. Sucking (fat) pads are usually present in the cheeks. The buccal mucosa is pink and moist. The lips and gums are inspected and the hard and soft palate palpated to determine if they are intact. **Epstein's pearls** (small, white inclusion cysts) often are noted on the hard palate or gums. These cysts are not clinically significant and usually disappear without consequence. Occasionally, a tooth may be present. Loose precocious teeth are extracted to avoid potential aspiration.

The tongue should be in the midline and mobile. However, because the frenulum normally is short, the tongue does not extend beyond the margin of the gums. The frenulum will lengthen as the infant grows and develops.

Neck

The newborn generally appears to have a short neck. Sometimes this makes it difficult to determine if webbing or other problems are present. To determine the range of motion, the head is rotated gently. The neck muscles are palpated to identify the presence of any masses.

Assessment of the Body

Thorax

The clavicles are palpated to determine intactness and symmetry. The thorax is relatively short compared to the abdomen. The infant's chest is round. The chest wall is thin with little musculature, and the rib cage is very soft and pliant. Often the tip of the xiphoid process protrudes.

SUPERNUMERARY NIPPLES. Occasionally, extra nipples are seen. Usually, they are found along the diagonal "milk line" that extends from the upper outer shoulders to the middle of the pubic bone and are considered within normal limits.

FIGURE 20-10
Breast Hypertrophy. Breast hypertrophy may persist for the first 2 to 3 weeks of infancy but subsides spontaneously without treatment. Witch's milk is the name given the small amount of fluid that may be secreted from the engorged infant breasts.

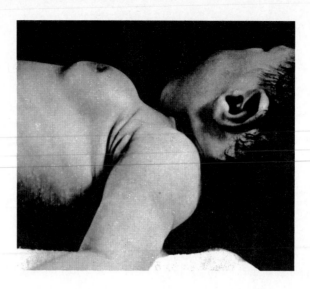

BREAST HYPERTROPHY. Breast enlargement is common in both males and females during the neonatal period (Fig. 20-10). High circulating levels of maternal hormones pass through the placenta during the pregnancy. The endocrine effects on the fetal breasts are similar to the changes that occur in the mother's breasts in preparation for lactation.

HEART SOUNDS. The heart rate is determined by counting the apical pulse (see Vital Signs). The first and second heart sounds should be clear and well-defined. The first heart sound is heard best at the fourth intercostal space. The second sound is heard best at the second intercostal space. Heart murmurs are not unusual in the immediate transitional period. Most commonly, they are related to a closing ductus arteriosus and are not significant. However, because murmurs also are associated with congenital heart defects, they should be recorded, described, and reported. Murmurs may be heard more easily with the bell of the stethoscope held tightly against the chest wall. The areas of cardiac auscultation in which murmurs are most likely to be heard are (1) the right sternal border, (2) the upper left sternal border, (3) the lower left sternal border, and (4) the cardiac apex.

LUNG SOUNDS. Bronchovesicular sounds usually are audible, and inspiration and expiration are equal.[6]

Abdomen

Inspection is a valuable part of the abdominal examination. Sometimes outlines of the anterior organs are seen through the abdominal wall. Normally the abdomen is round, symmetric in contour, and because of the relative size of the abdominal organs and weak muscular structures, slightly protuberant. Often superficial veins are visible. An abdomen that is asymmetric, scaphoid (sunken), or grossly distended is suggestive of abnormalities and is checked carefully. Irregular peristaltic sounds may be heard on auscultation.

ABDOMINAL ORGANS. Palpation is easier if the knees are supported in a flexed position to relax the abdominal muscles. Gentle pressure or upward stroking is followed by deeper palpation. Usual findings are as follows: (1) the liver edge is palpable 1 to 2 cm below the right rib[4] (palpation that is too high or too forceful may fail to identify the liver edge); (2) the top of the spleen sometimes can be palpated at the margin of the left rib; and (3) during the first 4 to 6 hours after birth the lower edges of the kidneys can be palpated at approximately the level of the umbilicus and halfway between the midline and the infant's side (later, they become more difficult to find).

UMBILICAL CORD STUMP. The umbilical cord stump is inspected for bleeding or oozing and the number of vessels recorded. The area surrounding the umbilicus is inspected carefully also. An umbilical hernia (a protruding mass surrounding the umbilicus) may be noted when the infant cries.

GENITALIA. Female genitalia are inspected for presence and size of the labia majora, labia minora, clitoris, and vaginal opening. The labia majora usually cover the labia minora and the vestibule. The clitoris usually is large during the neonatal period. Enlarged labia or vaginal discharge may be present as a result of fetal stimulation by maternal hormones. The discharge may appear bloody **(pseudomenstruation)** but is of no special concern. The labial edema and discharge disappear spontaneously.

In male infants the scrotum usually appears relatively large. Increased pigmentation at birth is due to maternal hormones and disappears spontaneously. In the full-term infant the testes usually can be palpated in the scrotal sac or can be brought down easily. The prepuce (foreskin) covers the glans penis and usually is adherent at birth. When the opening in the foreskin is so small that it cannot be retracted, the condition is called *phimosis*. If it is so tight it interferes with urination, circumcision may be recommended.

The penis is inspected to determine the location of the urinary meatus. It should be in the midline at the tip of the penis. When it is located on the underside of the penis, the condition is called *hypospadias*. When it is located on the dorsum of the penis, it is called *epispadias*. If the meatus is covered by the foreskin, the nurse observes the infant during voiding to determine urethral placement.

Posterior

With the infant in the prone position the entire posterior surface of the body is inspected and palpated. Because the cervical and lumbar curves develop during infancy and the toddler period, the normal spinal curvature is C-shaped.

Any masses or abnormal curvatures of the spine are noted. Tufts of hair or small indentations (particularly in the sacral area) may indicate occult spina bifida.

The perineal area is inspected to determine the location and patency of the anus. Sometimes a pilonidal "dimple" resulting from an irregular fold of skin is seen in the midline over the sacrococcygeal area.

Extremities

The limbs are compared for symmetry of size, shape, and movement. Webbing (syndactyly) or extra digits (polydactyly) are noted. Throughout

FIGURE 20-11

Assessment of Lower Extremities.
A, Infant's legs are extended and compared for symmetry of leg length. **B,** Knees are flexed and compared for equal knee height. **C,** Flexed legs are abducted laterally toward the bed. With congenital dislocation there may be uneven or limited abduction, uneven leg length, or uneven knee height. The examiner also may feel a "hip click" (Ortolani's sign) as the flexed legs are abducted.

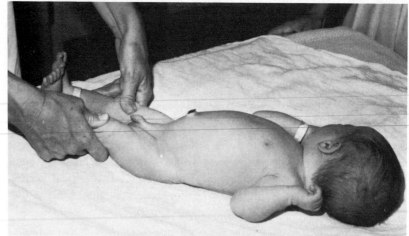

A

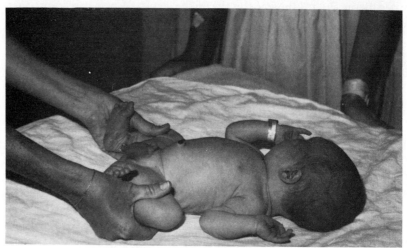

B

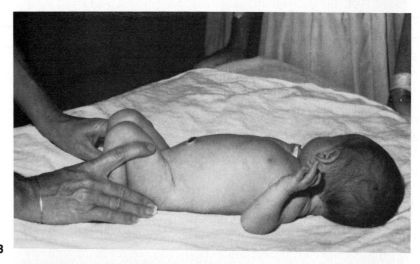

C

the examination the infant's ability to move all four extremities is evaluated.

To check for congenital hip problems the infant is placed in the supine position and the extremities checked for symmetry. Figure 20-11 illustrates assessment of the lower extremities. Asymmetric skin folds on the posterior aspect of the thigh also may alert the nurse to a hip abnormality.

Unusual positions of the feet may indicate congenital clubfoot or other foot and ankle deformities. If the foot can be moved to the normal position with ease, the condition simply may be due to a prolonged fetal position.

Neurologic Assessment

The neurologic assessment focuses on signs that reflect the status and functioning of the infant's nervous system. Posture, movement, muscle tone, and reflexes are important aspects of the neurologic assessment. Accuracy is increased by examining the newborn during the quiet alert period and in an environment of thermal neutrality.[7] The nurse observes the infant's body attitude and movement before beginning assessment activities. Reflex responses and behaviors usually are elicited during the cephalocaudal physical assessment.

Posture, Movement, and Muscle Tone

In the quiet alert state all extremities of the healthy full-term infant are flexed. Spontaneous movements are random, purposeless, and symmetric and involve all extremities. Muscle tone is assessed by passive manipulation of the extremities. Usually strong flexor muscle tone is evident.[8]

TREMORS. Sometimes jitteriness or tremors are noted. Tremors can be differentiated from seizures by the following characteristics: (1) the rhythmic movements of jitteriness or tremors are equal in amplitude, whereas seizures have a fast and slow component to the movements; (2) jitteriness or tremors are provoked by external stimuli such as noise or handling; and (3) movements caused by jitteriness or tremors usually stop when the examiner passively holds the affected limb still.

Reflexes

Several common adult reflexes are present at birth. The same sensory stimuli result in the newborn's blinking, coughing, sneezing, yawning, swallowing, and gagging. The rooting and sucking reflexes enable the infant to seek food. Other reflexes described below reflect the immaturity of the newborn's nervous system. These reflexes usually disappear within the first few months after birth.

ROOTING. When the examiner gently strokes the cheek or corner of the mouth with a sterile nipple or clean finger, a newborn turns toward the stimulus and opens his or her mouth (Fig. 20-12).

SUCKING. Generally newborns spontaneously suck on anything that touches their lips or is placed in their mouths.

TONIC NECK ("FENCING") REFLEX. Turning the infant's head to one side while he or she is lying on his or her back promptly results in extension of the arm and leg on that side. The opposite arm and leg spontaneously flex (Fig. 20-13).

MORO'S ("STARTLE") REFLEX. With the infant lying on his or her back, the head is lifted a few inches and then allowed to drop on the mattress.

FIGURE 20-12
Rooting. When examiner gently strokes cheek or corner of mouth with sterile nipple or clean finger, newborn turns toward stimulus and opens mouth.

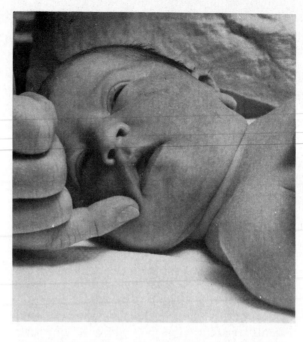

FIGURE 20-13
Tonic Neck ("Fencing") Reflex. Turning the infant's head to one side while he or she is lying on his or her back promptly results in extension of the arm and leg on that side. The opposite arm and leg spontaneously flex.

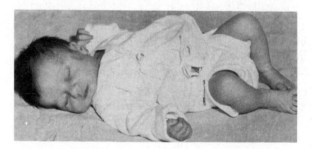

The infant's immediate reaction is rapid symmetric extension of the arms out and to the sides (Fig. 20-14). Simultaneously, the newborn opens the hands and flexes the knees. The reflex ends with flexion and adduction of the arms in an embracing motion.

GRASP. At birth the grasp reflex is present in both the hands and the feet.

Palmar grasp. The infant grasps any object placed in his or her hands, clings briefly, and then lets go. Even at birth the infant may be able to hold onto an adult's forefinger so securely that the infant can be lifted to a standing position (Fig. 20-15). As the newborn grows and develops, the hand grasp soon becomes voluntary and purposeful.

Plantar grasp. When the examiner's thumbs are pressed against the balls of the infant's feet, the toes will curl downward as though trying to grasp.

BABINSKI'S REFLEX. When the examiner strokes the lateral aspect of the sole of the infant's foot upward from the heel toward the little toe, all toes rapidly hyperextend ("fan outward") and then curve inward toward the sole.

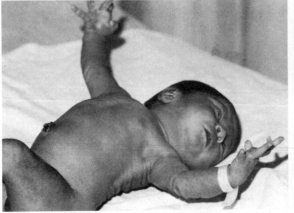

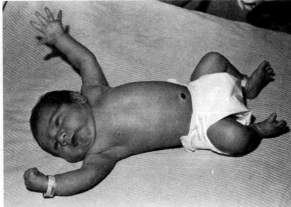

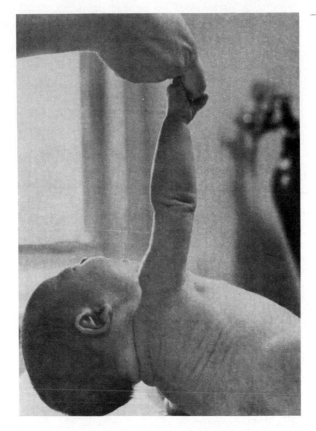

FIGURE 20-14
Moro's ("Startle") Reflex. With the infant lying on his or her back, the head is lifted a few inches and then allowed to drop on the mattress. The infant's immediate reaction is a rapid symmetric extension of the arms out and to the sides. Simultaneously the infant opens hands and flexes knees. The reflex ends with flexion and adduction of the arms in an embracing motion.

FIGURE 20-15
Palmar Grasp. At birth the newborn may be able to hold onto an adult's forefinger so securely that he or she can be lifted to a standing position.
From Reflexes, Vol 2. Evansville, Ind, Mead Johnson & Co, 1974.

STEPPING ("DANCING") REFLEX. When the infant is held in an upright position with the feet touching a firm surface, the newborn makes little stepping or prancing movements (Fig. 20-16).

GALANT'S REFLEX. With the infant in a prone position, the examiner strokes downward from shoulder to buttocks along one side of the spine. In response the infant's trunk curves toward the side stimulated.[6]

BAUER'S (CRAWLING) REFLEX. With the infant in a prone position, the examiner applies moderate pressure to the soles of the feet. The newborn responds by making crawling motions.[6]

FIGURE 20-16
Stepping ("Dancing") Reflex. When infant is held in an upright position with feet touching a firm surface, he or she makes little stepping or prancing movements.

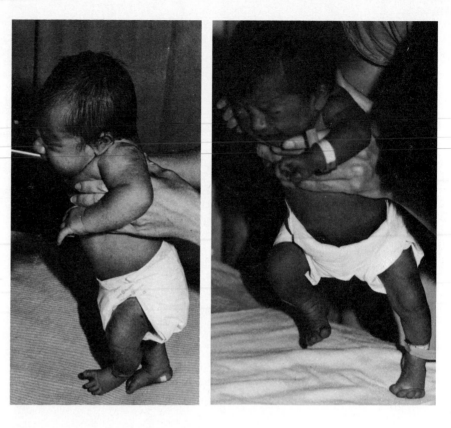

Laboratory Values

Red Blood Cell and Hemoglobin Concentration

The accuracy of laboratory determinations of the RBC count and hemoglobin concentration is determined by the site of blood sampling. Because of peripheral venous stasis, capillary blood samples usually show markedly higher hemoglobin and hematocrit values than venous samples drawn at the same time.[5] Venous samples are considered more accurate. Note: If only heel sticks are used for assessing blood values, anemia can go undetected. The following factors influence these values:

1. Duration of gestation. During the final weeks of intrauterine life, the concentration of hemoglobin increases rapidly. The preterm infant does not have the benefit of this increase and has a low concentration as compared with the full-term infant.
2. Time of cord clamping. Higher hemoglobin and hematocrit levels occur when cord clamping is delayed until the cord has ceased pulsating because the infant receives an (estimated) additional 50 to 100 ml of blood.

Expected laboratory values are described in the margin.[5,9]

Blood Glucose

The energy required for respiration, thermoregulation, and muscle activity rapidly depletes the newborn's limited glycogen stores.[10] Thus many infants are at risk for becoming hypoglycemic in the first hours after birth. Assessment for this condition can now be done by the nursery nurse using a glucometer (Dextrostix or Acucheck) to determine blood sugar levels (see Nursing Procedure).

|||| LABORATORY
|||| VALUES

Expected Values for Full-Term Infant

RBC count	5,000,000-7,000,000/μl
Hemoglobin	14-20 g/dl
Hematocrit	55%
Blood glucose	45-97 mg/dl
Calcium	7.3-9.2 mg/dl

Heel Stick for Blood Glucose

Intervention	Rationale
1. Warm infant's heel by wrapping foot in warm, moist compress for 3 to 5 min.	1. Increases circulation.
2. Cleanse heel with alcohol.	2. Minimizes risk of infection from puncture.
3. Allow to dry.	3. Reduces potential for hemolysis or tissue irritation.
4. Identify site on lateral aspect of heel.	4. Avoids accidental puncture of medial plantar artery or injury to nerves.
5. Rapidly puncture heel with sterile disposable lancet.	5. Minimizes trauma.
6. Remove first drop of blood with sterile gauze.	6. Reduces potential for dilution with tissue fluid.
7. Collect generous sample of blood on test strip. Avoid squeezing foot.	7. Squeezing foot may dilute blood sample with tissue fluid.
8. If using Dextrostix: wait 60 sec before rinsing off blood under steady stream of water.	8. Ensures accurate reading.
9. If using glucometer (e.g., Acucheck): immediately press timer button. At exactly 60 sec lightly wipe off all blood with a clean, dry cotton ball.	9. Ensures accurate reading.
10. Place test strip in meter slot before timer reaches 120 sec.	10. Reading will appear in display window after 120 sec.
11. Apply adhesive bandage to puncture site while waiting.	11. Protects from infection and further trauma.
12. Record results.	12. Enables comparison with preceding and later tests.

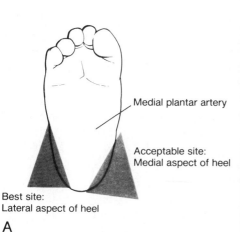

Medial plantar artery

Acceptable site:
Medial aspect of heel

Best site:
Lateral aspect of heel

A

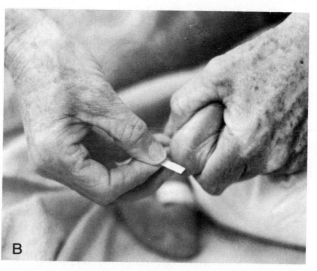

B

Gestational Age Assessment

Gestational age is the estimated age of the fetus or newborn. It is expressed in weeks, counting from the first day of the mother's last menstrual period. Knowing the approximate gestational age helps determine whether the infant was born early (preterm), on time (full-term), or late (postterm). When gestational age is combined with birth weight, infants are designated as small, appropriate, or large for gestational age.

Assessment for gestational age is performed within the first few hours after birth because the extrauterine environment leads to rapid changes in the characteristics of the newborn. Physical characteristics can be used to determine gestational age immediately after birth. Often, however, accurate neurologic data cannot be gathered immediately. The neurologic aspects of gestational age are best evaluated when the infant is in a quiet alert state.[11]

The criteria that have been identified as useful in assessing gestational age are used in a variety of combinations in the different scoring systems that have been suggested. The Dubowitz scoring system[12] uses a combination of physical, neurobehavioral, and reflex criteria to arrive at a gestational age (see Assessment Tool: Dubowitz Scoring System pp. 519-520). It has the disadvantage of being rather long. An abbreviated system, the Ballard score,[13] uses seven physical and six neurologic signs to determine gestational age (see Assessment Tool: Estimating Gestational Age by Maturity Rating p. 521). Other combinations of criteria may be used in different settings.

Physical Characteristics

During fetal growth and development certain external physical characteristics develop and progress in an orderly manner. The presence, absence, or degree of development of these characteristics at birth is used to help determine gestational age.

SKIN AND VERNIX. The skin of preterm infants is (1) thin, (2) pink to red, (3) smooth, (4) almost transparent (blood vessels are visible), and (5) thickly covered with vernix. The skin becomes thicker and more opaque with increasing fetal age. By 40 weeks the term infant is pale, with few visible vessels and sparse vernix; often vernix is found only in skin creases. Postterm infants often have an absence of vernix and extensive desquamation of the skin, particularly on the palms and soles (Fig. 20-17).

HAIR. The hair of the newborn varies in texture and characteristics with race. The nurse assesses the hair after any vernix has been removed. In early gestation the strands of hair are very fine. They tend to mat together like wool, with small bunches sticking out from the head (Fig. 20-18). The full-term infant's hair is silky and lies flat in single strands. The hairline of the postterm infant may recede.

EAR FORM AND CARTILAGE. Infants less than 33 weeks gestation have relatively flat ears. After 34 weeks the upper pinnae begin to curve inward. By 38 weeks the upper two-thirds of the pinnae are incurved. Incurvation extends to the earlobe by 38 to 40 weeks.

Since ear form varies widely from one person to another, the amount of cartilage present provides a more reliable estimate of gestational age.

Dubowitz Scoring System

NAME	D.O.B./TIME	WEIGHT	E.D.D. L.N.M.P.	E.D.D. U/snd.
HOSP. NO.	DATE OF EXAM	HEIGHT		
RACE SEX	AGE	HEAD CIRC.	GESTATIONAL SCORE WEEKS ASSESSMENT	

STATES
1. Deep sleep, no movement, regular breathing.
2. Light sleep, eyes shut, some movement.
3. Dozing, eyes opening and closing.
4. Awake, eyes open, minimal movement.
5. Wide awake, vigorous movement.
6. Crying.

STATE | COMMENT | ASYMMETRY

HABITUATION (≤ state 3)

LIGHT
Repetitive flashlight stimuli (10) with 5 sec. gap.
Shutdown = 2 consecutive negative responses

| No response | A. Blink response to first stimulus only. B. Tonic blink response. C. Variable response. | A. Shutdown of movement but blink persists 2-5 stimuli. B. Complete shutdown 2-5 stimuli. | A. Shutdown of movement but blink persists 6-10 stimuli. B. Complete shutdown 6-10 stimuli. | A. Equal response to 10 stimuli. B. Infant comes to fully alert state. C. Startles + major responses throughout. |

RATTLE
Repetitive stimuli (10) with 5 sec. gap.

| No response | A. Slight movement to first stimulus. B. Variable response. | Startle or movement 2-5 stimuli, then shutdown | Startle or movement 6-10 stimuli, then shutdown | A. B. C. Grading as above |

MOVEMENT & TONE
Undress infant

POSTURE *
(At rest — predominant)

| | | | (hips abducted) | (hips adducted) | Abnormal postures: A. Opisthotonus. B. Unusual leg extension. C. Asymm. tonic neck reflex |

ARM RECOIL
Infant supine. Take both hands, extend parallel to the body; hold approx. 2 secs. and release.

| No flexion within 5 sec. | Partial flexion at elbow >100° within 4-5 sec. | Arms flex at elbow to <100° within 2-3 sec. | Sudden jerky flexion at elbow immediately after release to <60° | Difficult to extend; arm snaps back forcefully |

ARM TRACTION
Infant supine; head midline; grasp wrist, slowly pull arm to vertical. Angle of arm scored and resistance noted at moment infant is initially lifted off and watched until shoulder off mattress. Do other arm.

| Arm remains fully extended | Weak flexion maintained only momentarily | Arm flexed at elbow to 140° and maintained 5 sec. | Arm flexed at approx. 100° and maintained | Strong flexion of arm <100° and maintained |

LEG RECOIL
First flex hips for 5 secs, then extend both legs of infant by traction on ankles; hold down on the bed for 2 secs. and release.

| No flexion within 5 sec. | Incomplete flexion of hips within 5 sec. | Complete flexion within 5 sec. | Instantaneous complete flexion | Legs cannot be extended; snap back forcefully |

LEG TRACTION
Infant supine. Grasp leg near ankle and slowly pull toward vertical until buttocks 1-2" off. Note resistance at knee and score angle. Do other leg.

| No flexion | Partial flexion, rapidly lost | Knee flexion 140-160° and maintained | Knee flexion 100-140° and maintained | Strong resistance; flexion <100° |

POPLITEAL ANGLE
Infant supine. Approximate knee and thigh to abdomen; extend leg by gentle pressure with index finger behind ankle.

| 180-160° | 150-140° | 130-120° | 110-90° | <90° |

HEAD CONTROL (post. neck m.)
Grasp infant by shoulders and raise to sitting position; allow head to fall forward; wait 30 sec.

| No attempt to raise head | Unsuccessful attempt to raise head upright | Head raised smoothly to upright in 30 sec. but not maintained. | Head raised smoothly to upright in 30 sec. and maintained | Head cannot be flexed forward |

HEAD CONTROL (ant. neck m.)
Allow head to fall backward as you hold shoulders; wait 30 secs.

| Grading as above | Grading as above | Grading as above | Grading as above | |

HEAD LAG *
Pull infant toward sitting posture by traction on both wrists. Also note arm flexion.

VENTRAL SUSPENSION *
Hold infant in ventral suspension; observe curvature of back, flexion of limbs and relation of head to trunk.

HEAD RAISING IN PRONE POSITION
Infant in prone position with head in midline.

| No response | Rolls head to one side | Weak effort to raise head and turns raised head to one side | Infant lifts head, nose and chin off | Strong prolonged head lifting |

ARM RELEASE IN PRONE POSITION
Head in midline. Infant in prone position; arms extended alongside body with palms up.

| No effort | Some effort and wriggling | Flexion effort but neither wrist brought to nipple level | One or both wrists brought at least to nipple level without excessive body movement | Strong body movement with both wrists brought to face, or 'press-ups' |

SPONTANEOUS BODY MOVEMENT
during examination (supine).
If no spont. movement try to induce by cutaneous stimulation.

| None or minimal Induced | A. Sluggish. B. Random, incoordinated. C. Mainly stretching. | Smooth movements alternating with random, stretching, athetoid or jerky | Smooth alternating movements of arms and legs with medium speed and intensity | Mainly: A. Jerky movement. B. Athetoid movement. C. Other abnormal movement. | 1 2 |

TREMORS
Mark: Fast (>6/sec.) or Slow (<6/sec.)

| No tremor | Tremors only in state 5-6 | Tremors only in sleep or after Moro and startles | Some tremors in state 4 | Tremulousness in all states |

STARTLES

| No startles | Startles to sudden noise, Moro, bang on table only | Occasional spontaneous startle | 2-5 spontaneous startles | 6 + spontaneous startles |

ABNORMAL MOVEMENT OR POSTURE

| No abnormal movement | A. Hands clenched but open intermittently. B. Hands do not open with Moro. | A. Some mouthing movement. B. Intermittent adducted thumb | A. Persistently adducted thumb. B. Hands clenched all the time. | A. Continuous mouthing movement. B. Convulsive movements. |

Continued

ASSESSMENT
TOOL

Dubowitz Scoring System—continued

						STATE	COMMENT	ASYMMETRY

REFLEXES

						STATE	COMMENT	ASYMMETRY
TENDON REFLEXES Biceps jerk, Knee jerk, Ankle jerk	Absent		Present	Exaggerated	Clonus			
PALMAR GRASP Head in midline. Put index finger from ulnar side into hand and gently press palmar surface. Never touch dorsal side of hand.	Absent	Short, weak flexion	Medium strength and sustained flexion for several secs.	Strong flexion; contraction spreads to forearm	Very strong grasp. Infant easily lifts off couch			
ROOTING Infant supine, head midline. Touch each corner of the mouth in turn (stroke laterally).	No response	A. Partial weak head turn but no mouth opening. B. Mouth opening, no head turn.	Mouth opening on stimulated side with partial head turning	Full head turning, with or without mouth opening	Mouth opening with very jerky head turning			
SUCKING Infant supine; place index finger (pad towards palate) in infant's mouth; judge power of sucking movement after 5 sec.	No attempt	Weak sucking movement: A. Regular. B. Irregular.	Strong sucking movement, poor stripping: A. Regular. B. Irregular.	Strong regular sucking movement with continuing sequence of 5 movements. Good stripping.	Clenching but no regular sucking.			
WALKING (state 4, 5) Hold infant upright, feet touching bed, neck held straight with fingers.	Absent		Some effort but not continuous with both legs	At least 2 steps with both legs	A. Stork posture; no movement. B. Automatic walking.			
MORO One hand supports infant's head in midline, the other the back. Raise infant to 45° and when infant is relaxed let his head fall through 10°. Note if jerky. Repeat 3 times.	No response, or opening of hands only	Full abduction at the shoulder and extension of the arm	Full abduction but only delayed or partial adduction	Partial abduction at shoulder and extension of arms followed by smooth adduction A. Abd>Add B. Abd=Add C. Abd<Add	A. No abduction or adduction; extension only. B. Marked adduction only.	J S		

NEUROBEHAVIOURAL ITEMS

						STATE	COMMENT	ASYMMETRY
EYE APPEARANCES	Sunset sign, Nerve palsy	Transient nystagmus. Strabismus. Some roving eye movement.	Does not open eyes	Normal conjugate eye movement	A. Persistent nystagmus. B. Frequent roving movement. C. Frequent rapid blinks.			
AUDITORY ORIENTATION (state 3, 4) To rattle. (Note presence of startle.)	A. No reaction. B. Auditory startle but no true orientation.	Brightens and stills; may turn toward stimuli with eyes closed	Alerting and shifting of eyes; head may or may not turn to source	Alerting; prolonged head turns to stimulus; search with eyes	Turning and alerting to stimulus each time on both sides			S
VISUAL ORIENTATION (state 4) To red woollen ball	Does not focus or follow stimulus	Stills; focuses on stimulus; may follow 30° jerkily; does not find stimulus again spontaneously	Follows 30-60° horizontally; may lose stimulus but finds it again. Brief vertical glance	Follows with eyes and head horizontally and to some extent vertically, with frowning	Sustained fixation; follows vertically, horizontally, and in circle			
ALERTNESS (state 4)	Inattentive; rarely or never responds to direct stimulation	When alert, periods rather brief; rather variable response to orientation	When alert, alertness moderately sustained; may use stimulus to come to alert state	Sustained alertness; orientation frequent, reliable to visual but not auditory stimuli	Continuous alertness, which does not seem to tire, to both auditory and visual stimuli			
DEFENSIVE REACTION A cloth or hand is placed over the infant's face to partially occlude the nasal airway.	No response	A. General quietening. B. Non-specific activity with long latency.	Rooting; lateral neck turning; possibly neck stretching.	Swipes with arm	Swipes with arm with rather violent body movement			
PEAK OF EXCITEMENT	Low level arousal to all stimuli; never > state 3	Infant reaches state 4-5 briefly but predominantly in lower states	Infant predominantly state 4 or 5; may reach state 6 after stimulation but returns spontaneously to lower state	Infant reaches state 6 but can be consoled relatively easily	A. Mainly state 6. Difficult to console, if at all. B. Mainly state 4-5 but if reaches state 6 cannot be consoled.			
IRRITABILITY (states 3, 4, 5) Aversive stimuli: Uncover, Ventral susp., Undress, Moro, Pull to sit, Walking reflex, Prone	No irritable crying to any of the stimuli	Cries to 1-2 stimuli	Cries to 3-4 stimuli	Cries to 5-6 stimuli	Cries to all stimuli			
CONSOLABILITY (state 6)	Never above state 5 during examination, therefore not needed	Consoling not needed. Consoles spontaneously	Consoled by talking, hand on belly or wrapping up	Consoled by picking up and holding; may need finger in mouth	Not consolable			
CRY	No cry at all	Only whimpering cry	Cries to stimuli but normal pitch	Lusty cry to offensive stimuli; normal pitch	High-pitched cry, often continuous			

NOTES ✱ If asymmetrical or atypical, draw in on nearest figure
Record any abnormal signs (e.g. facial palsy, contractures, etc.). Draw if possible.

Record time after feed:

EXAMINER:

From Dubowitz L, Dubowitz V: The Neurological Assessment of the Preterm and Full-Term Newborn Infant. London, Spastics International Medical Publications, 1981.

Estimation of Gestational Age by Maturity Rating★

Symbols: X - 1st Exam   O - 2nd Exam

NEUROMUSCULAR MATURITY

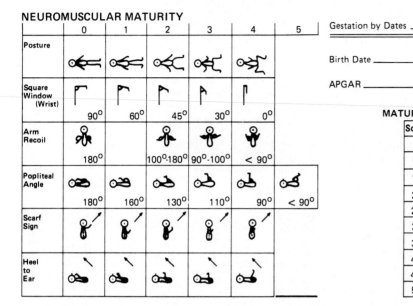

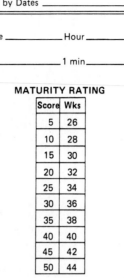

Gestation by Dates _____ wks

Birth Date _____ Hour _____ am/pm

APGAR _____ 1 min _____ 5 min

MATURITY RATING

Score	Wks
5	26
10	28
15	30
20	32
25	34
30	36
35	38
40	40
45	42
50	44

PHYSICAL MATURITY

	0	1	2	3	4	5
SKIN	gelatinous red, transparent	smooth pink, visible veins	superficial peeling &/or rash, few veins	cracking pale area, rare veins	parchment, deep cracking, no vessels	leathery, cracked, wrinkled
LANUGO	none	abundant	thinning	bald areas	mostly bald	
PLANTAR CREASES	no crease	faint red marks	anterior transverse crease only	creases ant. 2/3	creases cover entire sole	
BREAST	barely percept.	flat areola, no bud	stippled areola, 1–2 mm bud	raised areola, 3–4 mm bud	full areola, 5–10 mm bud	
EAR	pinna flat, stays folded	sl. curved pinna, soft with slow recoil	well-curv. pinna, soft but ready recoil	formed & firm with instant recoil	thick cartilage, ear stiff	
GENITALS Male	scrotum empty, no rugae		testes descending, few rugae	testes down, good rugae	testes pendulous, deep rugae	
GENITALS Female	prominent clitoris & labia minora		majora & minora equally prominent	majora large, minora small	clitoris & minora completely covered	

SCORING SECTION

	1st Exam=X	2nd Exam=O
Estimating Gest Age by Maturity Rating	_____ Weeks	_____ Weeks
Time of Exam	Date _____ am Hour _____ pm	Date _____ am Hour _____ pm
Age at Exam	_____ Hours	_____ Hours
Signature of Examiner	_____ M.D.	_____ M.D.

From Ballard J et al: A simplified assessment of gestational age. Classification of the low birth-weight. In Klaus M: Pediatr Res 11:374, 1977. Figures adapted from Sweet A: Classification of the low-birth-weight infant. In Klaus M, Fanaroff A: Care of the High-Risk Infant. Philadelphia, WB Saunders, 1977.

★Ballard score. Gestational age is estimated by adding newborn's scores on each of maturity assessment components and comparing the total score with the maturity rating table.

FIGURE 20-17

Postmaturity. The skin of the postterm infant may be dry and cracked. Desquamation (peeling) often is evident.

From Sullivan R, Foster J, Schreiner RL: Determining a newborn's gestational age. MCN 4:38-45, January/February 1979.

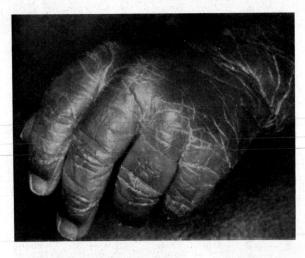

FIGURE 20-18

Comparison of Hairline and Ear of Term and Preterm Infants. Cartilage is well developed in the term infant, **A,** and the ears are erect, away from the head, whereas the ears of the preterm infant, **B,** lie flat against the head. Also note the matted hair of the preterm infant.

From Sullivan R, Foster J, Schreiner RL: Determining a newborn's gestational age. MCN 4:38-45, January/February 1979.

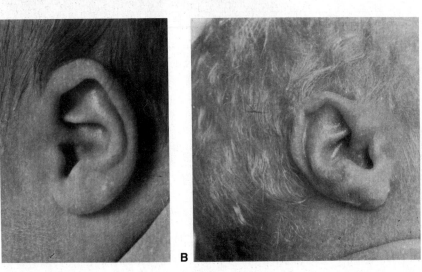

The extremely preterm infant's ear remains folded over if pressed as a result of an absence of cartilage. Cartilage begins to appear at 32 weeks. After that point in gestation, when folded over, the ear gradually returns to its original position. By 36 weeks the pinnae spring back when folded. At term they are firm with the ear standing erect from the head. Figure 20-18 compares the ear of a full-term newborn with that of a preterm infant.

BREAST TISSUE AND AREOLA. The nipples are present early in gestation, but the areolae are barely visible until 34 weeks. After this time the areolae become raised, and hair follicles become evident. Infants of less than 36 weeks gestation have no breast tissue. At 36 weeks a 1 to 2 mm nodule of breast tissue becomes palpable. Under hormonal stimulation the amount of breast tissue increases until it reaches 7 to 10 mm at 40 weeks (Fig. 20-19).

NAILS. The nails appear at approximately 20 weeks and gradually grow to cover the nail bed. At term the nails extend slightly beyond the fingertips. Long nails well beyond the fingertips are characteristic of the postterm infant.

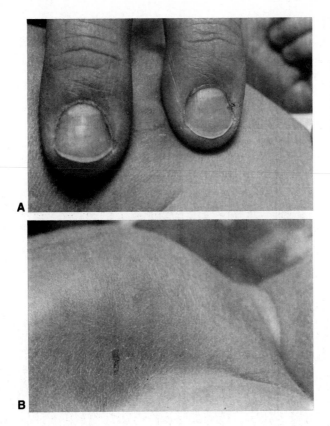

FIGURE 20-19
Comparison of Areola and Lanugo of Term and Preterm Infants. Note the relatively distinct areola of the term infant, **A,** as compared to the preterm infant, **B.** Also note the abundance of the fine hair, lanugo, on the body of the preterm infant.
From Sullivan R, Foster J, Schreiner RL: Determining a newborn's gestational age. MCN 4:38-45, January/February 1979.

GENITALIA. The characteristics of both male and female genitalia change with gestational age.

Female. At 30 to 32 weeks the female displays a prominent clitoris, and her labia majora are small and widely separated. The labia majora increase in size and fullness as gestational age progresses (Fig. 20-20).

Male. At approximately 30 weeks the testes are high in the inguinal canal. They gradually descend and are felt high in the scrotal sac at 37 weeks. Usually by 40 weeks they have descended into the scrotal sac. Rugae appear first on the anterior scrotum at 36 weeks. By 40 weeks the rugae cover the entire sac. The postterm infant often has a pendulous scrotum covered with numerous rugae (Fig. 20-21).

FIGURE 20-20
Labia Majora. The labia majora of the term infant, **A,** completely covers the labia minora and clitoris. However, in the preterm infant, **B,** they are small and widely separated. Also note the loose skin folds on the posterior thighs of the preterm infant.
From Sullian R, Foster J, Schreiner RL: Determining a newborn's gestational age. MCN 4:38-45, January/February 1979.

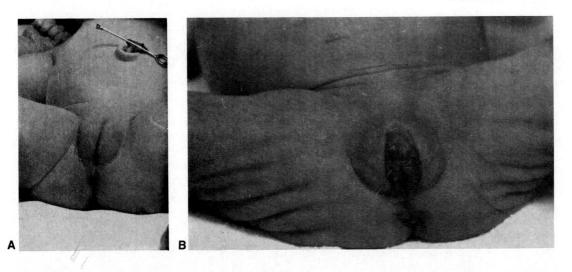

FIGURE 20-21

Comparison of Scrotal Sac and Testes in Term and Preterm Infants. In the term infant, **A,** the testes usually are palpable in the rugae-covered scrotal sac. Depending on gestational age, the preterm infant, **B,** exhibits few rugae, and the testes often cannot be palpated.

From Sullivan R, Foster J, Schreiner RL : Determining a newborn's gestational age. MCN 4:38-45, January/February 1979.

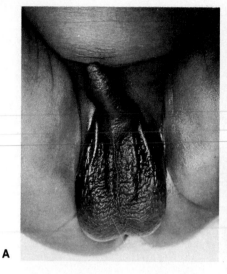
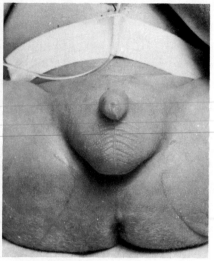

A

B

FIGURE 20-22

Sole Creases. Compare sole creases on the foot of term infant, **A,** with those on preterm infant, **B.** At 40 weeks' gestation the entire foot, including the heel, is crisscrossed with creases.

From Sullivan R, Foster J, Schreiner RL: Determining a newborn's gestational age. MCN 4:38–45, January/February 1979.

A

B

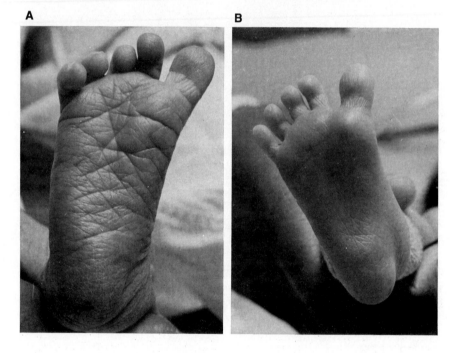

SOLE CREASES. The soles of the feet become wrinkled first on the anterior portion and then, as gestation progresses, in the area extending toward the heel. At 32 weeks one or two creases can be seen. Sole creases become more numerous, crisscrossed, and deeper, and by 37 weeks they cover the anterior two-thirds of the sole (Fig. 20-22).

Neurologic Development

During the first few days of life gestational age may be assessed by a number of neuromuscular responses. Components of the neurologic assessment include the following: (1) posture; (2) passive range of motion of certain parts; (3) righting reactions; and (4) various reflexes. Although frequently the neurologic examination cannot be completed immediately after delivery, posture, recoil, and tonicity are assessed. The remainder of the neurologic assessment may be deferred for a day or so.

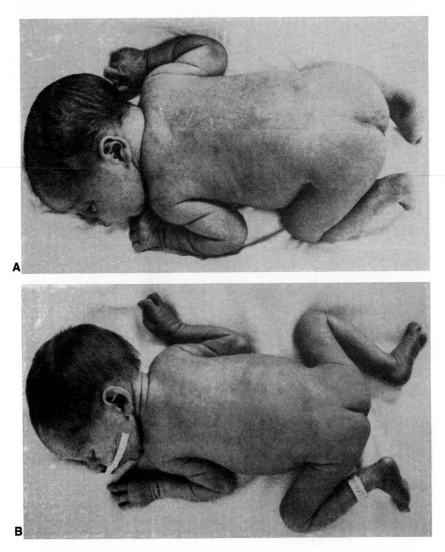

FIGURE 20-23
Resting Posture. Note the flexion of the extremities in the term infant, **A,** as compared to the partial flexion in the preterm infant, **B,** resulting in a froglike resting posture.
From Reflexes, Vol 2. Evansville, Ind, Mead Johnson & Co, 1974.

RESTING POSTURE. In the first hour after birth resting posture and extremity recoil provide a reasonable estimation of neurologic development. The resting posture of the preterm infant is characterized by very little flexion of the upper extremities and only partial flexion of the lower extremities (Fig. 20-23). At approximately 30 weeks there is slight flexion of the feet and knees. At 34 weeks flexion of the hips and thighs results in the characteristic frog position. At 36 to 38 weeks the resting infant exhibits complete flexion of all four extremities.

EXTREMITY RECOIL. To test recoil, the examiner flexes the infant's extremities and maintains the flexed position for approximately 5 seconds. The extremity then is extended, held in position for approximately 30 seconds, and released. Extremity recoil lags behind flexion by approximately 2 weeks. For example, at 36 to 37 weeks the extremities remain extended. At 40 weeks prompt recoil follows passive extension of the extremities.

HEAD LAG. With the infant supine, the hands or arms are grasped, and the newborn is pulled slowly to a sitting position. The position of the head in relation to the trunk is noted (Fig. 20-24).

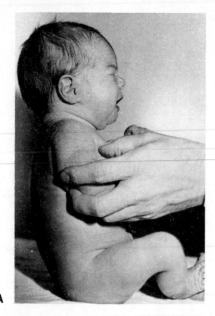

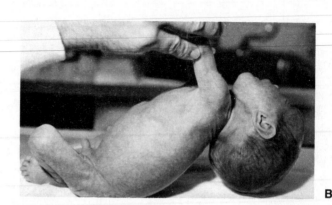

FIGURE 20-24

Head Lag. As the infant is slowly pulled from a supine to a sitting position, the term infant, **A,** holds the head erect, but the preterm infant, **B,** has no flexion in the neck.

VENTRAL SUSPENSION. With the examiner's hand under the chest supporting it, the infant is suspended in the prone position. (For large infants, both hands may be used.) The degree of extension of the head and back, as well as the degree of arm and leg flexion, is noted (Fig. 20-25).

SCARF SIGN. The infant's arm is drawn across the neck and as far across the opposite shoulder as possible (like a scarf). This manuever is best performed by lifting the infant's elbow across the front of the body. The examiner then evaluates how far across the chest the elbow will go (Fig. 20-26). Marked resistance is noted in the full-term infant.

ANKLE AND WRIST FLEXION. The examiner dorsiflexes the foot and measures the angle between the foot and the leg. Figures 20-27 and 20-28 compare the angles produced by dorsiflexion in the term and preterm infants.

POPLITEAL ANGLE. Passive movement of the leg reveals an inverse relationship between muscle tone and popliteal angle. The term infant resists flexion and displays a small popliteal angle (Fig. 20-29).

HEEL TO EAR. With the infant supine and hips flat, the nurse draws the infant's foot as close to the ear as possible without forcing. Figure 20-29 compares the heel-to-ear resistance displayed by the term and preterm infant.

REFLEXES. Although there are differences in reflexes according to the infant's gestational age, these differences are not as age specific as other signs described previously. Thus reflexes are less useful in determining gestational age. The reflexes of the normal newborn are discussed under Neurologic Assessment.

In the preterm infant the following are true. (1) The rooting reflex is less developed as evidenced by the infant's slower response in turning the head toward the stimulus. (2) The sucking reflex, which occurs at ap-

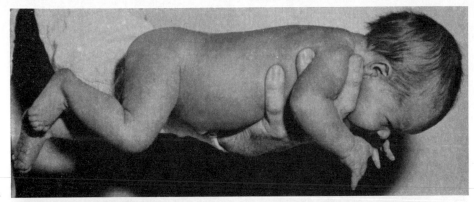

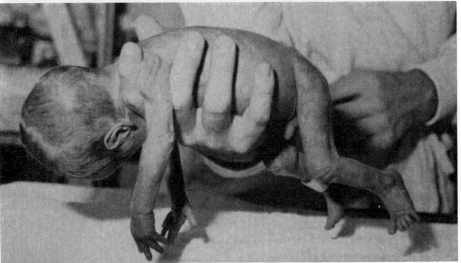

FIGURE 20-25

Ventral Suspension. When suspended in the prone position, the term infant's head,
A, extends, the back is straight, and the arms and legs flex; however, the preterm
infant, **B,** hangs limply with the arms and legs almost straight.

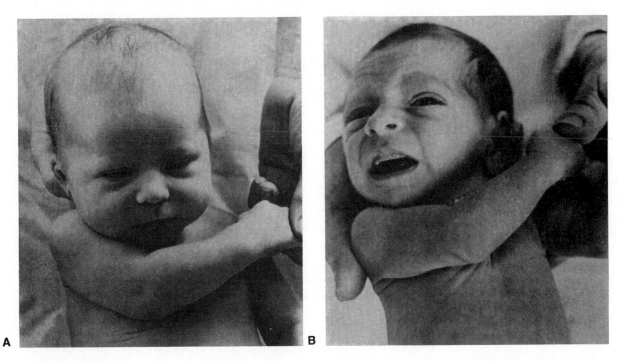

FIGURE 20-26

Scarf Sign. In the term infant, **A,** the elbow will not reach the midline, but in the
preterm infant, **B,** the elbow will reach across the midline.

From Reflexes, Vol 2. Evansville, Ind, Mead Johnson & Co, 1974.

FIGURE 20-27

Wrist Flexion. In the term infant, **A,** the wrist can be flexed onto the arm, but the wrist can only be flexed to an angle of approximately 90° in the preterm infant, **B.**

From Sullivan R, Foster J, Schreiner RL: Determining a newborn's gestational age. MCN 4:38-45, January/February 1979.

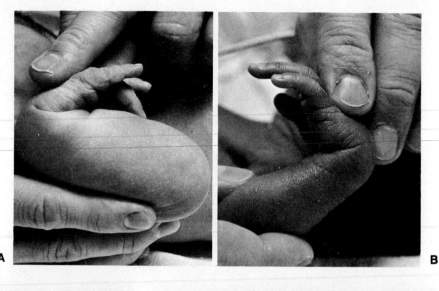

FIGURE 20-28

Ankle Flexion Assessment. To assess the ankle flexion the examiner applies pressure to the foot to push it onto the anterior aspect of the leg and measures the angle between the dorsum of the foot and the leg. In the term infant, **A,** the foot can be flexed until it touches the leg. In preterm infants, **B,** the angle produced is 45 to 90 degrees.

From Sullivan R, Foster J, Schreiner RL: Determining a newborn's gestational age. MCN 4: 38-45, January/February 1979.

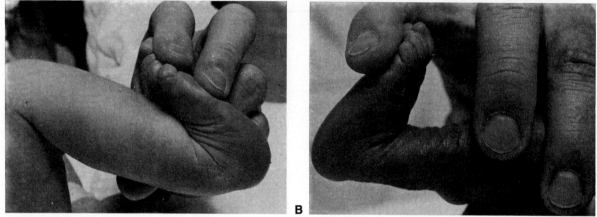

proximately 34 weeks, is weak or absent, depending on the number of weeks of gestation. Sucking is of particular importance because it is related to the infant's ability to take adequate nourishment. (3) The grasp reflex is weak, and the infant cannot be lifted off the bed while grasping the examiner's finger. (4) Moro's reflex also is weak. (5) Often the stepping reflex is absent.

Behavioral Assessment

Healthy infants interact with their environment from the moment they are born. Newborn behaviors provide evidence of cortical control and responsiveness.[2] Assessment is conducted using a behavioral scale.

The Brazelton Neonatal Behavioral Assessment Scale (NBAS) includes aspects of both behavioral and neurologic assessment.[14] The scale can be used as a predictive tool in clinical practice and in research. The NBAS tests a total of 27 behavioral responses.[2] The display on page 529 lists the items in the Brazelton Scale Criteria. The six categories into which these items can be divided are listed in Table 20-3. Each item is scored on a scale of 1 to 9. Each score is based on the infant's best rather than his or

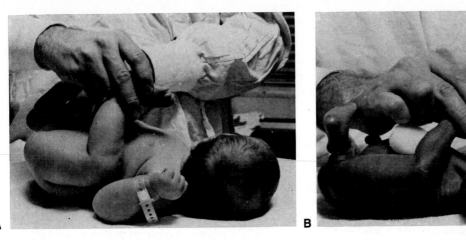

A   B

FIGURE 20-29
Heel to Ear. In the term infant, **A,** there is a marked resistance in the leg as the foot is gently drawn toward the ear, whereas in the preterm infant, **B,** very little resistance is noted. Note the difference in popliteal angle.
From Sullivan R, Foster J, Schreiner RL: Determining a newborn's gestational age. MCN 4:38-45, January/February 1979.

her average performance. The infant's state at the time any given item is tested is an important aspect of the assessment. Some items require that the infant be in a certain state for valid testing. Brazelton has identified six states of consciousness in the newborn. Table 20-4 describes common behaviors exhibited in each state. Figure 20-30 illustrates the quiet alert and hyperalert (crying) states. Self-consoling behavior is illustrated in Figure 20-31. Babies vary greatly in the amount of time they spend in the various states. They also vary widely in the ease or difficulty with which they make the transition from one state to another.

Brazelton Scale Criteria

 1. Response decrement to light
 2. Response decrement to rattle
 3. Response decrement to bell
 4. Response decrement to pinprick
 5. Orientation response—inanimate visual
 6. Orientation response—inanimate auditory
 7. Orientation—animate visual
 8. Orientation—animate auditory
 9. Orientation—animate visual and auditory
10. Alertness
11. General tonus
12. Motor maturity
13. Pull-to-sit
14. Cuddliness
15. Defensive movements
16. Consolability with intervention
17. Peak of excitement
18. Rapidity of buildup
19. Irritability (to aversive stimuli—uncover, undress, pull-to-sit, prone, pinprick, tonic neck response, Moro, defensive reaction)
20. Activity
21. Tremulousness
22. Amount of startle during examination
23. Lability of skin color
24. Lability of states
25. Self-quieting activity
26. Hand-to-mouth facility
27. Smiles

TABLE 20-3

Brazelton Behavioral Categories

Category	Measured Behavior
1. Habituation	How soon the neonate reduces responses to specific repeated stimuli, e.g., light.
2. Orientation	How often and when neonate attends to auditory and visual stimuli.
3. Motor maturity	How well neonate coordinates and controls motor activities
4. Variation	How often neonate exhibits alertness, state changes, color changes, activity, and peaks of excitement
5. Self-quieting behaviors	How often, how soon, and how effectively the newborn can use own resources to quiet and console self when upset or distressed
6. Social behaviors (cuddliness)	How often and how much the newborn smiles and cuddles

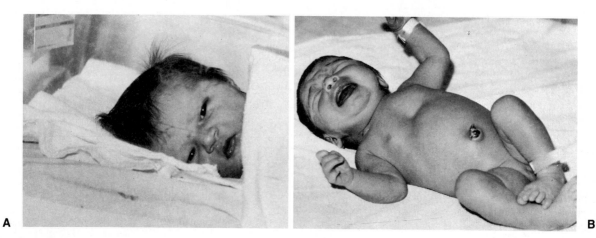

A   **B**

FIGURE 20-30
Quiet Alert and Crying States. **A,** In the quiet alert state the infant's body and face are quiet and inactive. The eyes are bright and shining. **B,** In the crying state the infant exhibits intense motor activity.

FIGURE 20-31
Self-Consoling Behavior. Infants vary in their ability to console themselves. Items under this category are scored when the infant is upset (state 6). Possible self-consoling activities include hand-to-mouth and sucking.

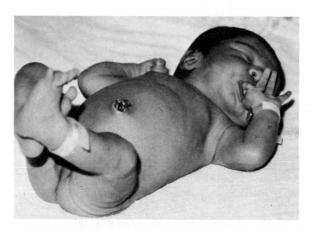

TABLE 20-4

Brazelton States of Consciousness

State of Consciousness	Assessment Findings
Sleep States	
1. Deep sleep	Breathing pattern: regular respirations Eyes: closed; no movements Activity: quiet, only occasional jerky movements or startles Startles: response to external stimuli is delayed and rapidly suppressed, i.e., momentary
2. Light sleep	Breathing pattern: irregular respirations Eyes: closed; rapid eye movements under closed lids Activity: low level; random movements or startles; movements are smoother and more monitored than in state 1 Sporadic sucking movements Startles: responds to internal and external stimuli with startles; state often changes in response to startles
Awake States	
3. Drowsy or semi-dozing	Eyes: may be open or closed; eyelids may flutter Activity: variable with mild startles interspersed with dozing; reactive to sensory stimuli but response often delayed; movements usually smooth; state change following stimulation
4. Quiet alert	Eyes: open with bright look; seems to focus attention on source of stimulation, e.g., visual or auditory stimulus Activity: minimum but impinging stimuli may break through with some delay in response (see Fig. 20-30)
5. Hyperalert	Eyes: open Activity: considerable motor activity with thrusting movements of the extremities Startles: spontaneous Reacts to external stimulation with increased startles or movement; discrete reactions are difficult to identify because of high level of general activity
6. Crying	Intense activity that is difficult to break through with stimulation (see Fig. 20-30)

A trained examiner and considerable time are required to implement the NBAS accurately. However, some aspects of the scale and their findings can be useful to anyone who works with newborns. For example, many people think that all infants are cuddly and that if an infant does not cuddle when held, there is either something wrong with them or with the infant. In fact, infants respond to cuddling in many different ways. Scores on "cuddliness" range from 1, "actually resists being held, continuously pushing away, thrashing or stiffening" to 9, "molds into arms and relaxes, turns toward examiner's body when held horizontally, or leans forward when held on examiner's shoulder, all of the body participates and baby grasps examiner to him." Accurate interpretation of behavioral patterns is important in identifying the needs of the individual newborn and planning effective anticipatory guidance and client teaching for the parents.

Nursing Diagnosis

Clinical judgments and nursing care of the healthy, full-term newborn are based on (1) knowledge of the normal physiologic and metabolic adaptations required for successful transition to independent life, (2) analyses of assessment findings that describe the newborn's health status, and (3) analyses of assessment findings that identify the individual needs of the family unit. Common potential nursing diagnoses are listed below.

Planning and Intervention

Nursing interventions during the neonatal period are designed to maximize the infant's potential for successful transition to independent ex-

---

POTENTIAL NURSING DIAGNOSES

Full-Term Newborn

Ineffective Airway Clearance—related to excessive oropharyngeal mucus
Potential for Aspiration—related to excessive oropharyngeal mucus, regurgitation
Ineffective Thermoregulation—related to limited metabolic ability to compensate for changes in environmental temperature
  Hyperthermia—related to exposure to elevated environmental temperature (e.g., during phototherapy)
  Hypothermia—related to exposure to low environmental temperature (e.g., chilling during bath)
Potential for Infection—related to immature immune system and impaired skin intregrity secondary to umbilical cord stump, circumcision
Potential Fluid Volume Deficit—related to bleeding secondary to marginal coagulability, lack of vitamin K, circumcision
Altered Nutrition: Less Than Body Requirements—related to limited intake, hypoglycemia
Potential for Injury: Cognitive Deficit—related to hyperbilirubinemia
Pain—related to heel stick for diagnostic studies (e.g., blood glucose, hematocrit, PKU) or to circumcision
Knowledge Deficit: Maternal—regarding infant care, diagnostic or therapeutic procedures

---

Focus Assessment

Examine indicators of adaptation status.
  General appearance
  Respiratory effort
  Vital signs
  Level of consciousness and activity
  Response to stimuli
  Weight lose or gain
  Feeding patterns (e.g., frequency, amount, interest, effectiveness)
  Elimination
    Urine: number of wet diapers per shift
    Stool: number and character
Note any evidence of continued bleeding at or from the following:
  Umbilical cord stump
  Heel stick punctures
  Circumcision site
Review findings of diagnostic tests.
  Glucometer
  Bilirubin levels
  Hemoglobin and hemotocrit values
Identify current maternal infant-care competencies and specific learning needs.

trauterine life and to facilitate development of a stable family unit. Nursing care focuses on (1) protecting the newborn from harm, (2) supporting effective physiologic and metabolic adaptations, (3) enhancing family bonding, and (4) enabling clients and families to provide safe, effective newborn care.

Current trends have altered the nurse's role in contemporary maternity care. The shortened hospital stay and mother-baby coupling have reduced the nursing time spent in direct care of the newborn and increased the emphasis on anticipatory guidance and client teaching. Kraybill[15] notes that, as a result of the short hospital stay, common newborn problems (e.g., jaundice, feeding difficulties) often arise after discharge. He states that an informed mother is essential to the newborn's continued well-being. Nurses should maximize teaching opportunities during the hospital stay to enable mothers (1) to provide safe, effective newborn care; (2) to assess their infants and identify danger signs; (3) to develop confidence in their abilities to make informed judgments about the status and care of their infants; and (4) to know how to obtain help promptly. Mother-baby coupling allows maternity nurses to provide the new parents with support and guided learning experiences in caring for their infant during the hospital stay.

Client teaching enables parents to provide safe, effective, efficient care of their newborns. Ongoing discussions and demonstrations and return-demonstrations facilitate development of increasing competence and confidence in their abilities to protect the infant from harm and meet basic newborn needs (see Client Self-Care Education: Providing Protection for and Meeting Needs of Newborn p. 534).

Nurses in LDRP units should explain basic care procedures such as infection prophylaxis (eye care, umbilical cord care) to the parents as they are performed. The nurse then reinforces and augments principles of infection control during daily teaching contacts with the parents.

Immediate Care of the Newborn: The Nurse's Role

From the moment of birth the newborn must be protected from environmental stressors, e.g., cold, infection, trauma.[15] Physiologic and metabolic adaptation also must be facilitated. Nursing interventions during the immediate newborn period include (1) maintaining thermal neutrality, (2) maintaining a patent airway, (3) facilitating family psychosocial adaptation, (4) preventing infection, and (5) performing identification procedures.

Ongoing Care of the Newborn: The Nurse's Role

During the transitional period the nursing focus continues on supporting and maintaining physiologic and metabolic adaptation. Nursing interventions include those listed previously and others specific to the individual infant's needs. The amount of direct care provided by the nurse varies between agencies and depends on the type of maternity unit and the status of the newborn. In agencies with central nurseries most basic care procedures are performed by the nurse. In agencies in which the infant remains with the mother from birth through discharge, basic care is provided by the mother under nursing guidance and supervision. However, the nurse is responsible for ensuring newborn safety throughout the hospital stay. In addition to client teaching and supervision of newborn

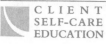

Providing Protection for and Meeting Needs of Newborn

1. Principles of infection control
   a. Modes of transmission of common pathogens
   b. Handwashing
   c. Cover apparel
   d. Masks
   e. Cord care
2. Infant handling and positioning
   a. Lifting
   b. Holding
   c. Carrying
   d. Positioning in crib
3. Oral and nasal suctioning
4. Cord care
5. Circumcision care (if applicable)
6. Diapering
7. General status assessment
   a. Body temperature
   b. Weight gain
   c. Elimination
      (1) Stool
      (2) Urine
   d. Sleeping patterns
   e. Crying
   f. Signs of danger
8. Feeding and burping
9. Bathing and nail care
10. Dressing the infant
11. Importance of follow-up visits
    a. Phenylketonuria (PKU) testing
    b. Immunizations

care, the nurse continuously assesses the newborn's health status and response to care and performs and assists with specific precedures (Fig. 20-32).

Specific Prophylaxis Against Infection

The newborn infant is vulnerable to infection.[16,17] Several routine procedures are implemented to prevent specific types of common infections of the newborn. In agencies that do not offer the LDRP experience, to facilitate bonding these procedures may be delayed until the infant is admitted to the nursery.

EYE CARE. The practice of instilling a 1% solution of silver nitrate in the conjunctival sacs of the newborn's eyes to prevent gonorrheal conjunctivitis (ophthalmia neonatorum) was introduced in 1884 by Credé. Use of the Credé method results in chemical conjunctivitis in more than 50% of newborns.[18] Although in many areas topical erythromycin, penicillin, or tetracycline is used as an alternate therapy, most state laws require implementation of the Credé method of prophylaxis within a few hours after birth.[19] However, silver nitrate is not effective prophylaxis against *Chlamydia trachomatis.* Eye prophylaxis is a nursing responsibility.

   Client teaching. The nurse (1) describes the redness, edema, and yellowish discharge that commonly result from the Credé treatment; (2)

NURSERY FLOW SHEET

TIME	PT. TEMP.	BED TEMP.	H.R.	RESP.	CUFF BP	CENTRAL BP	CHEM-STRIP	SITE	TYPE FEED	AMT. FEED	VOIDS	STOOLS	EMESIS		INITIALS

WEIGHT	
BIRTH	
YESTERDAY	
TODAY	

INITIAL	FULL SIGNATURE	INITIAL	FULL SIGNATURE

DAY OF LIFE _____

DATE _____ MOTHER'S ROOM # _____

Page 1

FIGURE 20-32

Infant Assessment Flow Sheet. The nurse uses an assessment form to record any changes in the newborn's health status.
Courtesy Mease Hospital, Dunedine, Florida.

Continued

NURSERY SHIFT ASSESSMENT AND ROUTINE CARE

Date:	Nurse:	Nurse:	Nurse:
Time:		Time:	Time:

ACTIVITY:
☐ Active ☐ Sleeping ☐ Quiet/Awake
☐ Fussy ☐ Irritable ☐ Lethargic
☐ Jittery ☐ Other _____

COLOR:
☐ Pink ☐ Pale ☐ Dusky ☐ Acrocyanosis
☐ Circumoral Cyanosis ☐ Mottled
☐ Jaundiced ☐ Other _____

SKIN:
☐ Normal ☐ Peeling ☐ Pustules ☐ Edema
Bruises _____
Petechiae _____
Rash _____

RESPIRATORY:
☐ Normal ☐ Tachypneic ☐ Flaring
☐ Clear ☐ Rales ☐ Wheezing
Retractions _____
Grunting _____
Other _____

CARDIAC:
Rhythm: ☐ Regular ☐ Irregular
Murmur: ☐ No ☐ Yes
Pulses: ☐ Normal ☐ Weak ☐ Bounding

ABDOMEN:
Bowel Sounds: ☐ Present ☐ Absent
☐ Soft ☐ Flat ☐ Distended

EYES:
☐ Normal ☐ Drainage ☐ Edema

FONTANELS:
☐ Normal ☐ Bulging ☐ Sunken

CORD:
☐ Moist ☐ Drying
☐ Dry ☐ Other _____

OTHER COMMENTS:
_____
_____

CIRCUMCISION: CARE @
Condition _____
Bath @ _____
Cord Care @ _____
Doctor Visits _____
Parent Visits/Calls _____

(The three columns above — center and right — repeat the same assessment fields: ACTIVITY, COLOR, SKIN, RESPIRATORY, CARDIAC, ABDOMEN, EYES, FONTANELS, CORD, OTHER COMMENTS, CIRCUMCISION.)

	HEAD CIRCUMFERENCE	LENGTH
BIRTH	CM	CM
PREVIOUS	CM	CM
Q. MONDAY	CM	CM

PHOTOTHERAPY

DATE/TIME STARTED _____		7–3	3–11	11–7
DATE/TIME STOPPED _____	BILIMETER READINGS			
	TIME			

LABORATORY RESULTS

INFANT SCREENING   DATE/TIME _____

TIME SENT	TIME REP.		HGB	HCT	WBC	PLAT	NA	K	CL	CO$_2$	BS	BUN	CA	BILI. TOTAL	BILI. DIR.	

REP=REPORTED

FIGURE 20–32—cont'd

Umbilical Cord Prophylaxis: Criteria for Selection of Agent

Agents used for initial cord care must be nontoxic if absorbed through the skin.
They must not have an adverse effect on the skin.
They must not potentiate other infections by destroying normal flora.

From American Academy of Pediatrics (AAP): Guidelines for Perinatal Care, 2nd ed. Chicago, The Academy, 1988.

reassures the parents that the condition is harmless and does not cause the newborn pain; and (3) emphasizes that the reaction is transient and will subside within 24 to 48 hours.

CORD CARE. Initial treatment of the umbilical cord stump and surrounding area with a bacteriostatic agent (e.g., Triple dye) is done to prevent colonization by potential pathogens. Serious local and systemic neonatal infections have been caused by organisms such as *Staphylococcus aureus* and *Escherichia coli*.[18] Seventy percent alcohol commonly is used for umbilical cord stump prophylaxis[20] (see above).

Client teaching. The nurse emphasizes the importance of keeping the umbilical cord stump clean, dry, and free from irritation. Client teaching includes demonstrating appropriate cord care and explaining the rationale for the procedures (see Client Self-Care Education: Care of the Umbilical Cord Stump).

Administration of Prophylactic Vitamin K

Because the newborn has a deficiency of the normal intestinal bacteria needed for synthesis of vitamin K at birth and has a low prothrombin time, the primary health care provider may order an injection of vitamin K to prevent hemorrhage. The medication should be administered within 1 hour of birth.[15] Thus the injection may be given in the delivery or

---

Care of the Umbilical Cord Stump

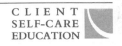

CLIENT
SELF-CARE
EDUCATION

Action

1. Fold and anchor top of diaper below level of cord stump.
2. Use a cotton ball and 70% alcohol to cleanse area between stump and skin. This should be done two to three times daily or with each diaper change. Continue until cord has detached and umbilicus has healed completely.
3. Avoid use of tub baths until umbilical area has healed completely.
4. Avoid dislodging cord before it heals completely.

5. Promptly report any signs of bleeding, inflammation, or discharge from area around stump.

Rationale

1. Avoids irritation and allows air circulation to hasten drying.
2. Hastens drying and sloughing of remainder of cord stump.

3. Further hastens drying; reduces potential for injury.
4. May cause bleeding. Cord usually falls off between day 5 and day 14 after birth.
5. May indicate injury or infection and should be evaluated by primary health provider.

FIGURE 20-33

Intramuscular Injection Technique.
Intramuscular injections for the newborn are
administered in the vastus lateralis muscle
(upper lateral aspect of the thigh muscle).
An acceptable alternative site is the rectus
femoris muscle on the anterior aspect of the
thigh. The nurse uses the nondominant hand
to anchor the leg and prevent inadvertent
movement. The skin is cleansed with an
antibacterial agent, and the needle is inserted
rapidly into the desired site. If aspiration
elicits no blood return, the medication is
injected and the needle withdrawn
immediately.

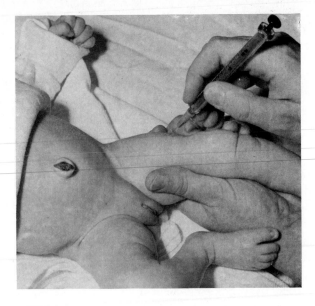

recovery room or on admission to the nursery. Technique for the administration of intramuscular injections to infants is illustrated in Figure
20-33.

Circumcision

Circumcision is the surgical removal of the end of the penile prepuce
(foreskin). Originally, circumcision was a hygienic ritual associated with
the Jewish religion and performed on male infants. The practice achieved
widespread popularity in the United States and was performed almost
routinely on male newborns for decades. Advantages stated by advocates
are that (1) circumcision promotes better hygiene; (2) it prevents inflammation and infection of the penis; and (3) it decreases the incidence of
cancer of the penis in later adulthood. Opponents contend that (1) the
procedure is painful; (2) potential hazards include hemorrhage, infection,
and mutilation; and (3) good personal hygienic practices by uncircumcised
males provide the same benefits.

Since the mid-1960s controversy about circumcision has continued,
and the use of the procedure has declined. In March 1989 the Committee
on Fetus and Newborn of the American Academy of Pediatrics stated
that "newborn circumcision has potential medical benefits and advantages
as well as disadvantages and risks"[21] (see Legal and Ethical Considerations:
Circumcision).

Several techniques have been devised for circumcising newborns. The
most common methods currently use the Gomco clamp (Fig. 20-34) and
the Plastibell (Fig. 20-35).

NURSING CARE DURING CIRCUMCISION. If the parents decide to have
the infant circumcised, the procedure usually is performed 12 to 24 hours
after birth and after the infant has had time to stabilize.[18] Feeding is avoided
just before the procedure to reduce the potential for regurgitation while
the infant is restrained in the supine position for the circumcision.

After checking to be sure the permit for circumcision has been signed,
the nurse assembles the sterile gloves, instruments, and drapes for the

Circumcision is an elective procedure requiring informed parental consent.

The primary health care provider is responsible for explaining the advantages and potential hazards to the parents.

The nurse is responsible for confirming and documenting informed consent. The nurse may serve as a legal witness to the signing of the operative permit.

The nurse provides factual answers to questions asked by the parents and supports them in their decision.

The nurse avoids influencing the parents on the basis of personal or cultural beliefs or values.

Should the parents withdraw consent, the nurse is responsible for informing the provider promptly and documenting the decision in the client's chart.

LEGAL AND ETHICAL CONSIDERATIONS

Circumcision

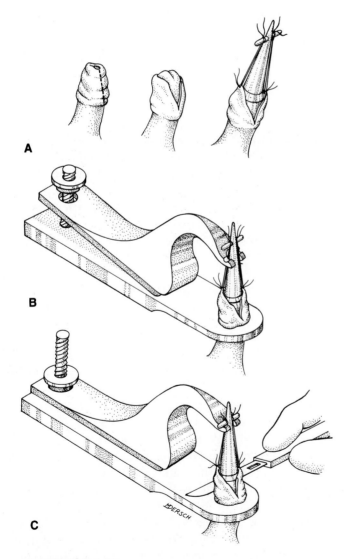

FIGURE 20-34

Circumcision Using Gomco Clamp. **A,** Prepuce is slit and drawn over cone. **B,** Clamp is applied and pressure is maintained for 3 to 5 minutes. **C,** Excess prepuce is cut away.

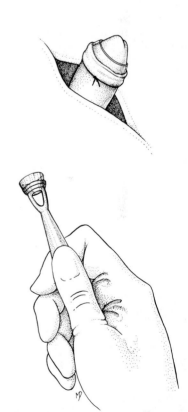

FIGURE 20-35

Circumcision Using the Plastibell. The bell is fitted over the glans. Suture is tied around rim of the bell. Excess prepuce is cut away. The plastic rim remains in place until it falls off after healing has taken place.

FIGURE 20-36

Restraining Infant for Circumcision.
Restraining the infant should be delayed
until shortly before the provider is ready to
perform the procedure. Restraining the
infant's extremities usually results in
immediate anger and complaint from the
newborn. The nurse removes the diaper,
and the infant is placed on a plastic
restraining form. Securing the infant to the
board prohibits his moving during the
procedure. The infant should be kept warm
to prevent cold stress.

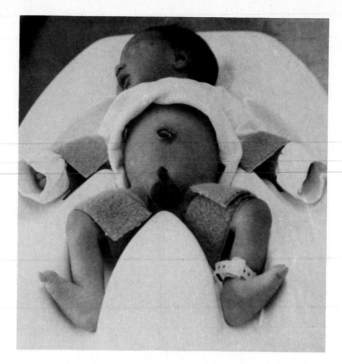

procedure. When the provider is ready, the nurse removes the diaper and
places the infant on the restraint board (Fig. 20-36).

The nurse continuously assesses the infant's condition during the procedure and is alert for any change.[22] Comfort measures such as stroking
his head or talking to him may have a calming effect on the infant's
response to being restrained.

A local anesthetic may be used, or the procedure may be performed
without anesthesia. Studies have identified the infant's physiologic response to pain during unanesthetized circumcision; the infant's respiratory
and heart rates accelerate, and his blood pressure rises.[23] Marchette's
study[23] found that classical music appears to facilitate infant relaxation
during the few minutes wait for hemostasis after the Gomco clamp is
tightened. Further, the infants in the study exhibited no signs of pain or
distress after they were removed from the circumcision board and swad-
dled. Most were alert but quiet.

NURSING CARE AFTER CIRCUMCISION. Postoperative circumcision care
focuses on keeping the wound clean and observing it closely for bleeding
(Fig. 20-37). For the first 24 hours the area is covered with a sterile
petroleum gauze dressing. No dressing is applied if the Plastibell is used.

The infant usually is fed immediately after the circumcision, and both
mother and infant seem to enjoy the comfort that feeding and cuddling
bring. If the infant is left in the mother's room, the nurse periodically
checks the circumcision for bleeding.

Client teaching. If mother-baby coupling is the method of client care
or if the circumcision is performed on the day of discharge from the
hospital, the mother should be instructed and supervised in care of the
circumcision (see Client Self-Care Education: Circumcision Care).

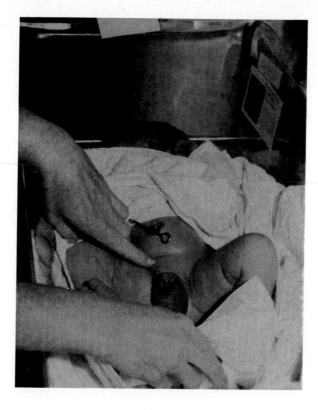

FIGURE 20-37
Nursing Care After Circumcision. To observe the circumcised area the infant is placed in the supine position with his hips abducted. This position also is used postoperatively when cleansing the penis. Gentle cleansing of the circumcised area is done by squeezing a warm, wet, soapy washcloth just above the penis so that the water cascades down on the area, rinsing well using fresh, clear, warm water for the cascade, and gently patting dry. Any signs of bleeding or infection are noted and reported.

Circumcision Care

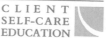

CLIENT
SELF-CARE
EDUCATION

Action

1a. Observe for bleeding at every diaper change.

  b. Report any evidence of bleeding immediately.
2. Plastibell is left in place. Do not attempt to remove.
3. If petroleum gauze has been applied, leave in place unless soiled by urine or stool. A petroleum dressing usually is used for 24 to 48 hours.
4. Monitor voiding for size of stream, amount of urine, and bloody urine.
5. When changing the diaper, hold infant's ankles with one hand.
6. At each diaper change place infant in position for inspection of penis (Fig. 20-37).
   Squeeze a gentle cascade of warm water over penis.
7. Fasten diaper loosely for first 48 hours after circumcision.
8. Yellowish-white exudate may be noted for 2 to 3 days. Do not remove this exudate.
9. During daily bath follow procedure outlined in No. 6. Use warm soapy water for initial cascade. Rinse well with warm water cascades and pat dry.
10. Report promptly any sign of ulceration or difficulty voiding before or after discharge home.

Rationale

1a. Although rare, bleeding is a potential complication of circumcision.
  b. Enables prompt treatment.
2. Does not interfere with voiding or healing. Usually falls off within 3 to 4 days.
3. Protects the surgical site from irritation. Soiling increases potential for irritation and infection.

4. Although rare, damage to urethra is one potential postoperative complication.
5. Prevents infant from kicking against operative site.
6. Facilitates adequate visualization of penis.

   Rinses away urine; reduces potential for irritation.
7. Avoids pressure on the operative area. Reduces discomfort.
8. Signals normal granulation and healing.

9. Cleanses, promotes healing and comfort.

10. Requires evaluation by primary health care provider.

Client Teaching: Care of the Normal, Healthy Newborn

Parents are encouraged to assume increasing responsibility for their infant's care. A growing knowledge and skills base enables them to provide basic care with confidence and to meet the newborn's needs effectively. Client teaching for new parents is designed to meet their individual learning needs. Thus teaching may include all aspects of newborn care or only selected information and skills. Discussions and, when applicable, demonstrations should include the following: (1) actions to minimize newborn hazards, (2) basic supportive and comfort measures, (3) a general newborn status assessment, and (4) identification of danger signs. The nurse serves as role model, guide, instructor, support person, and resource.

Prevention of Infection

The prevention of infection is of paramount importance in caring for the newborn. The newborn comes from the protective intrauterine environment into an outside world containing a wide variety of microorganisms. Although the immune system begins to develop during fetal life, it is still very immature at birth.[16,17] Organisms that pose little threat to adults can cause serious infection in the neonate. Protecting the infant from infection includes minimizing the number of organisms in the infant's immediate environment and using prophylactic measures against specific microorganisms.

MINIMIZING EXPOSURE TO ORGANISMS. Everyone who is in contact with the newborn, including parents, visitors, and hospital personnel, should assume responsibility for protecting the infant from infection. Even infections that seem only minor annoyances to an adult may cause serious problems for the neonate.

Client teaching. Client teaching includes discussing the mode of transmission of common infectious organisms and ways to prevent their transfer to the newborn. Including older siblings in teaching sessions emphasizes their role in protecting the newborn. Parents also may need help in reminding family and friends to postpone visits unless they are well.

Visitors, including the father and other hospital personnel, usually are expected to put cover gowns over their street clothes (or uniforms) before entering the nursery or a mother's room when the infant is there. If these persons are going to touch the infant, they should wash their hands and arms before gowning.

Care is taken to avoid allowing the hair to come in contact with the infant or equipment; long hair should be pulled back and secured. If circumstances require the use of masks, they should cover the nose and mouth. Because masks can become a reservoir for bacteria, they are changed frequently. When removed from the face, the mask is discarded rather than pulled down around the neck.

Handwashing. To reduce potential sources of infection further the nurse discusses handwashing with the family. The nurse (1) explains the rationale for handwashing before handling the infant, (2) discusses the need for handwashing by parents, siblings, and other visitors, (3) demonstrates proper handwashing technique, and (4) reinforces appropriate parental behaviors.

Cord care. The nurse emphasizes the importance of keeping the umbilical cord stump clean, dry, and free from irritation. Client teaching includes demonstrating appropriate cord care and explaining the rationale for the procedures (see Client Self-Care Education: Care of the Umbilical Cord Stump).

Handling the Newborn Infant

LIFTING. Parents often feel insecure about handling their infants. Client teaching emphasizes that, although they are small, newborns are not as fragile as they appear. There is no one correct way of turning, lifting, or holding a newborn, but the following points are emphasized in client teaching: (1) the head and buttocks need to be supported; (2) infants are wiggly and can push themselves out of one's grasp; and (3) picking the infant up from the supine position is easier than from the side-lying or prone position. Figure 20-38 illustrates a suggested way of lifting the infant from a crib or flat surface.

CARRYING. The football hold (Fig. 20-39) is a useful position for holding or carrying an infant. Parents appreciate learning this position because, like the nurse, they often have times when they need to hold the infant and still have one hand free.

HOLDING. Parents most commonly carry and hold their infants in either the cradle position (Fig. 20-40) or the upright (Fig. 20-41) position. These positions provide a sense of security, warmth, and closeness. Cradling permits eye contact and usually is used for feeding the infant. The upright position is used for carrying, comforting, or burping the infant.

POSITIONING. The infant usually is placed in the crib in a side-lying position. To prevent the infant's rolling into the supine position, a blanket roll is placed behind the back. The roll should extend from shoulder to hip. If it is behind the infant's head, it pushes the head forward.

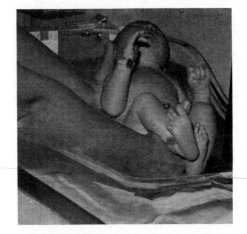

FIGURE 20-38
Lifting the Newborn. When lifting the infant from the supine position, one hand should be placed under the neck to support the head and shoulders. The other hand is placed under the buttocks to grasp the opposite thigh. The infant then can be lifted to a holding position or moved from one place to another.

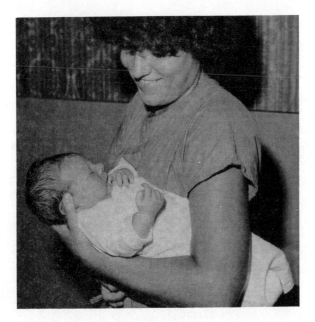

FIGURE 20-39
Football Hold. The football hold provides a safe and secure way to hold and carry infants. Most commonly the client is taught to use the nondominant hand in carrying. This leaves the dominant hand free for other activities. The hand is placed beneath the infant's head and neck and the forearm supports the infant's long axis. In this position the infant is well supported and is locked securely against the lateral aspect of the carrier's waist and hip.

FIGURE 20-40
Cradle Position. The infant is supported as if in a cradle by the parent's arms and abdomen. Cradling allows parent-infant eye contact and provides warmth and a sense of closeness for both parent and newborn. The cradle position often is used for feeding.
Courtesy St. Elizabeth's Medical Center, Edgewood, Kentucky.

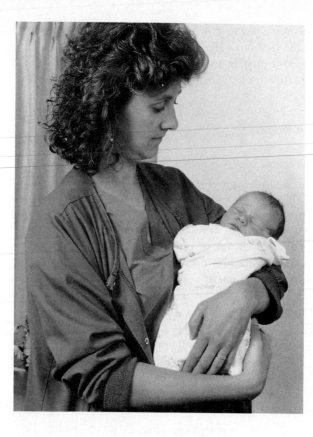

FIGURE 20-41
Upright position. The infant is held with head on the parent's shoulder. One hand supports the infant while the other is placed beneath the buttocks.
Courtesy St. Elizabeth's Medical Center, Edgewood, Kentucky.

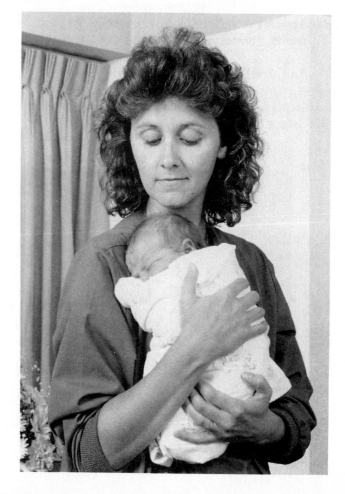

An alternate position is to place the infant on his or her abdomen. Both of these positions allow drainage of secretions such as mucus or regurgitated milk from the infant's mouth. The supine position should be avoided as a sleeping position or when the infant is unattended to reduce the danger of aspiration.

Nasal and Oral Suctioning

Excessive oropharyngeal mucus is a frequent problem during the early transition period. Further, infants may regurgitate feedings and be unable to clear the airway. Gentle suctioning with a bulb syringe (Fig. 20-42) usually removes the obstructing mucus and restores airway patency.

Bathing

The bath demonstration affords an excellent opportunity for teaching general assessment of the newborn. Basic principles of infant safety also are incorporated in discussing and demonstrating the bath procedure (see Client Self-Care Education: Newborn Sponge Bath p. 546). Figure 20-43 illustrates basic bathing techniques. Often the nurse incorporates and reviews elements of previous teaching contacts, e.g., cord care, as an integral part of this teaching episode.

DIAPER RASH. Sometimes, despite good care, the infant's buttocks become reddened and sore. Diaper rash is caused by the reaction of bacteria with the urea in the urine. This in turn causes ammonia dermatitis. The

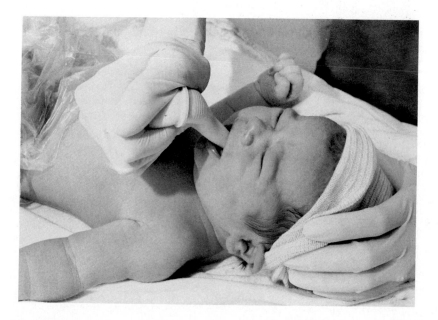

FIGURE 20-42

Nasal and Oral Suctioning.
forcing mucus or emesis into the infant's bronchi and lungs, the bulb syringe should be compressed before insertion into the infant's mouth or nose. Most commonly, the material to be suctioned is in the oropharynx. Therefore the mouth should be suctioned before the nose to avoid involuntary aspiration in case the infant gasps when the nose is suctioned.
Courtesy St. Elizabeth's Medical Center, Edgewood, Kentucky.

CLIENT
SELF-CARE
EDUCATION

Newborn Sponge Bath

Action

1. Prepare environment.
   a. Close windows and doors

   b. Check room temperature (75° to 80°F)
2. Assemble all materials required for care:
   a. Basin
   b. Washcloth
   c. Towels
   d. Cotton balls
   e. 70% alcohol
   f. Fresh diaper
   g. Clean clothes and blanket
   h. Receptacle for soiled clothes and diaper
   i. Unperfumed soap
3. Fill basin with warm water (98° to 100°F).
   NOTE: Test water temperature with elbow;
   temperature should feel comfortable.
4. Maintain hand control of infant at all times.

5. Proceed from clean to soiled area, i.e., face
   and head cleansed first.
6. Begin bath with infant still clothed.
7. Begin by wiping eyes with clean cotton ball
   or washcloth moistened with warm water.
   Wipe from inner canthus to outer canthus.
   Use a fresh cotton ball for each wipe. Report
   any redness, swelling, or discharge from eyes.
8. Cleanse nostrils and outer ear with tip of
   washcloth.

9. Cleanse face with clear warm water.
10. Shampoo hair.
    a. Use football hold

    b. Shampoo hair with mild baby shampoo or
       unperfumed soap.
    c. Rinse well.

    d. Dry thoroughly.
11. Undress infant and wash arms, chest, and
    back with soap and fresh warm water. Rinse
    well and pat dry; may replace shirt. Wash
    legs.
12. Remove diaper and cleanse genital area and
    buttocks.
    a. *Female infants:* Cleanse the labia from front
       to back using a clean, moist cotton ball for
       each stroke. Newborn girls may have a
       white, curdy secretion (smegma) or a slight
       bloody discharge for the first 7 to 10 days.
    b. *Uncircumcised male infants:* Penis should be
       cleansed daily. Avoid any retraction of the
       foreskin.
    c. Circumcised male infants: See Fig. 20-37.
13. Dry well, Apply clean diaper. Wrap in blan-
    ket.

Rationale

1a. Reduces drafts; air flow over wet infant pro-
    motes heat loss, chilling.
  b. Maintains thermal neutrality.
2. Enables effective, efficient care; avoids need to
    stop bath, carry wet baby to get something.

3. Avoids injury from excessive heat or chilling.

4. Minimizes risk of accident or
    injury.
5. Reduces risk of transmitting organisms from
    soiled areas.
6. Avoids chilling.
7. Avoids potential for transmitting organisms
    (crossinfection).

8. Because of potential for injury to the delicate
    tissues, cotton-tipped applicators should not
    be used.

9. —

10a. Affords secure grasp of infant and frees other
     hand for washing.
   b. Avoids irritating sensitive skin.

   c. Removes soap residue; avoids irritation of
      scalp.

11. Minimizes infant exposure and potential for
    chilling.

12. Area considered "soiled" is cleansed last; mini-
    mizes potential for fecal contamination.
    a. Reflects high level of maternal hormones just
       before birth.

    b. Still-developing prepuce is continuous with
       epidermis of the glans and is not retractable.

13. Completes bath.

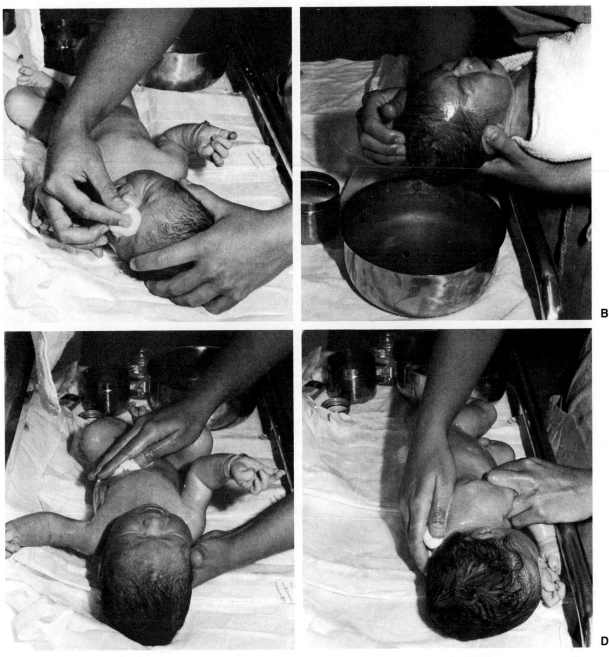

FIGURE 20-43
Bath Procedure. **A,** To avoid transmitting organisms from the hair, face, or opposite
eye, begin by cleansing one eye with a clean, moist cotton ball or washcloth wrapped
around index finger. Wipe from inner canthus to outer canthus. Use fresh cotton ball or
another surface of washcloth for other eye. Note and report any redness, swelling, or
discharge from eyes. **B,** Grasp infant securely in football position to free other hand for
washing hair. Wash hair with mild baby shampoo or unperfumed bath soap. Rinse well
to avoid leaving soap residue. Dry thoroughly. **C, D,** Use fresh water for remainder of
bath. Proceed from clean to soiled areas; wash genital and perianal area last.

best prophylaxis is keeping the diaper area clean and dry. Petroleum jelly,
baby oil, a bland protective preparation (e.g., a vitamin A and D ointment) or a commercial ointment is used to protect the area. The use of
baby powder is not recommended because it may cake with urine and
cause further irritation. Cornstarch also is not recommended because it
may promote fungal infection. Exposing the irritated area to air and heat
several times daily promotes healing (Fig. 20-44).

FIGURE 20-44

Treating Diaper Rash. Exposing skin irritated by diaper rash to air and light several times daily promotes healing. Place the infant in the prone position on a clean diaper and expose to air for 5 to 10 minutes four to six times daily. Protect the infant from drafts during exposure.

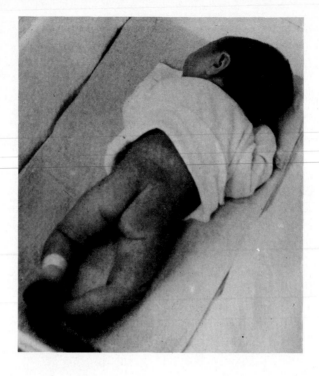

Dressing

The amount of clothing the infant wears is determined by the environmental temperature. Usually the parents are advised to add one layer more of light clothing than they themselves are wearing. The usual clothing worn by the infant includes an undershirt, diaper, and footed sleeper. If cloth diapers are used, plastic pants may be worn to protect other clothing and linens. A blanket may be added for additional warmth if the room is cool. When the infant is taken outside, the head should be covered with a cap or hood.

Nail Care

Because the newborn's nails often adhere to the finger for the first several days after birth, cutting long nails is usually deferred until the infant is 1 week old. If the nails are long and the infant is scratching, the arms of the undershirt may be closed over the hands, or the nails may be trimmed.

Client teaching. Blunt-end infant nail scissors should be used to trim the nails. The nails are trimmed while the infant is asleep and will not resist having his or her hand held down to enable cutting. Long nails are trimmed straight across and slightly above the fingertip to avoid accidental injury to the finger or nail bed.

Parental Assessment of Newborn Health Status

Client teaching focuses on developing the parents' abilities to assess the general health status of the newborn and to perform specific assessment techniques such as taking the newborn's temperature. Emphasis is placed on describing and discussing the signs of danger to the newborn (see display on p. 549).

Signs of Danger to the Newborn

Parents should promptly report the occurrence of any of the following to the primary health care provider:
• Skin color changes: cyanosis around the mouth (circumoral), jaundice
• Periods of apnea lasting longer than 15 sec
• Any change in feeding patterns, i.e., more than one episode of refusing to nurse or feed from the bottle
• Repeated emesis or episodes of projectile vomiting after feeding
• Bleeding from the umbilical cord stump area or circumcision
• Any signs of infection:
   a.   Rectal temperature >101°F (38.4°C) or <97°F (36.1°C)
   b.   Eye redness, swelling, or discharge
   c.   Redness, swelling, or discharge from the umbilical cord stump area
   d.   Excessive crying or fussiness, lethargy, or difficulty in rousing the infant
   e.   Two or more green, watery stools, flatus, and irritability
• Any change in elimination patterns that persists longer than 12 hr, e.g., loose stools or hard, packed stools, decline in number of wet diapers to less than five to eight

---

TEMPERATURE ASSESSMENT. Body temperature is an important indicator of newborn health status. The nurse explains and demonstrates the methods for taking both rectal and axillary temperatures (see Client Self–Care Education: Body Temperature Assessment). Parents need to take the infant's temperature only if the child appears ill. They should report elevations or subnormal temperatures to the primary health care provider promptly (see display on p. 550).

WEIGHT. Accurate weight monitoring is an important assessment component. The infant is weighed daily while in the hospital. The average 5% to 10% reduction from the birth weight during the first few days after birth is explained to the parents. This loss is due to the minimum intake of nutrients and fluid and to the loss of excess fluid. Around the time the meconium begins to disappear from the stools, the weight begins to increase. In healthy newborns weight gain continues, and they regain birth weight in a shorter period of time.

In general, during the first 5 months the average weight gain is 4 to 6 ounces/week. Thereafter the gain usually is 2 to 4 ounces/week. By 6 months of age the infant usually has doubled his or her birth weight, and by the first birthday it has tripled.

Confirming weight gain aids in assessing the infant's general condition and progress. Other signs of general health status include sleeping and crying patterns. A healthy infant should be happy and good–natured while awake and inclined to sleep much of the time between feedings.

Stool Assessment

During fetal life the intestines contain a greenish-black tarlike material called *meconium*. It is composed of lanugo and epithelial and epidermal cells in amniotic fluid swallowed by the fetus. The color is due to bile pigments. Before birth and for the first few hours after birth, the intestinal contents are sterile. Peristalsis apparently begins with birth because, unless the fetus experiences hypoxia, the amniotic fluid is colorless.

Body Temperature Assessment

Action	**Rationale**
Rectal Method	
1. Shake down glass thermometer before beginning procedure.	1. Assures accurate temperature measurement.
2. Remove diaper.	2. Allows access to rectum.
3. Lubricate thermometer with water-soluble lubricant.	3. Allows easier insertion and less discomfort to infant.
4. With the infant in supine position, grasp both his or her ankles with one hand and lift legs.	4. Exposes rectum.
5. Insert thermometer approximately ½ inch, i.e., just until bulb is covered.	5. Minimizes risk of injury to delicate tissues.
6. Hold thermometer in place for 5 full minutes.	6. Ensures accurate measurement.
7. Remove thermometer and, in good light, read temperature recorded. Replace diaper and blanket.	7. Identifies body temperature more accurately.
8. Cleanse thermometer with mild soap and cool water. Shake down and store.	8. Readies thermometer for next use.
Axillary Method	
1. Shake down thermometer as noted above.	1 to 4. Assures accurate temperature measurement.
2. Place bulb of thermometer beneath infant's armpit.	
3. Hold in place for 3 to 4 minutes.	
4. Remove, read, cleanse, and store as above.	

Most newborns pass the first stool within 12 hours of birth; nearly all have a stool in 24 hours. If the infant has not passed a stool by 24 hours after birth, he or she is observed closely for signs of intestinal obstruction or imperforate anus.

The number and type of stools daily can be influenced by the infant's diet. Breast-fed infants usually defecate more often than bottle-fed infants. The newborn passes meconium stools for the first day or two of life. After this period the color and character of the stool changes because of the increasing milk content in the newborn's diet (Fig. 20-45).

Usually by the fifth day after birth the daily number of stools is four to six. As the infant grows, the number of daily stools decreases to one to two each day. Minor variations in the number of stools per day may occur. Usually this variance has little significance if the infant appears comfortable, sleeps, and nurses well. Parents should report loose or hard-packed stools to the primary health care provider (see display p. 549).

Urine Assessment

Fetal urinary activity is evidenced by the presence of urine in the amniotic fluid. The newborn usually voids during delivery or immediately after birth, but voiding may be suppressed for several hours. Failure to void within 24 hours after birth is reported promptly to the primary health care provider, and the infant is evaluated for an imperforate meatus.

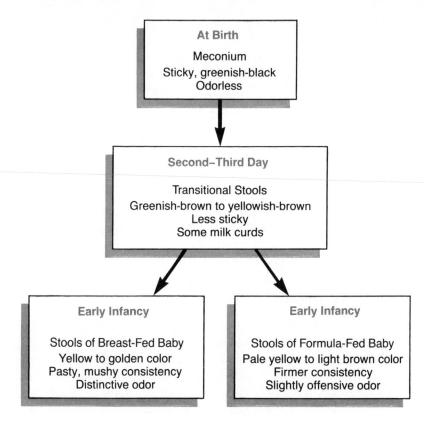

FIGURE 20–45
Newborn Stool Cycle. The character of the newborn stool cycle varies with type of feeding. The daily number of stools usually is four to six by the fifth day after birth. Note and report any deviation from normal pattern: (1) suddenly excessive or reduced number of stools; (2) stools that are watery, green, or contain large amounts of mucus; or (3) hard, packed stools and obvious infant discomfort, e.g., crying, grimacing, straining, passing flatus.

After the first 2 to 3 days, the infant voids 10 to 15 times daily. Parents should be reassured that when the urine is concentrated, rusty stains on the wet diaper are due to uric-acid crystals in the urine. Parents should report promptly to the primary health care provider if the infant has less than five to eight wet diapers daily. The infant should be evaluated by the provider for possible dehydration (see display on p. 549).

Sleeping Pattern Assessment

Infants who are well and comfortable usually sleep much of the day. The amount of sleep required varies between infants. Parents must identify the pattern that characterizes their infant. Many infants sleep as much as 20 out of 24 hours; others require only 12 to 18 hours of sleep. Theirs is not the sound sleep of the adult; rather, they move frequently, stretch, and waken momentarily at intervals. They wake and cry when hungry or uncomfortable. Since they respond so readily to external stimuli (and this may make them restless), clothing and coverings should be light and warm. Infants are placed on their abdomens or sides for sleeping. The supine position is avoided for sleep because of the increased potential for aspiration of any regurgitated fluids.

Crying

Parents usually respond with distress and concern to their newborn's cries. The nurse explains that crying and body posture while crying are the only means by which the infant can communicate needs. After infants are dressed and placed in a warm crib, they usually do not cry unless they are wet, hungry, ill, uncomfortable for some other reason, or disturbed by moving. The nurse describes types of infant cries and helps

---

Interpreting the Infant's Cry

A fretful, hungry cry, accompanied by fingers in his or her mouth and flexed, tense extremities is easily recognized.

A fretful cry, if caused by indigestion, is accompanied by green stools and passing of flatus.

A loud, insistent cry with drawing up and kicking of the legs usually indicates colicky pain.

A whining cry is noticeable when the infant is ill, preterm, or very frail.

A peculiar, shrill, sharp-sounding cry suggests injury, especially to the central nervous system.

---

the parents learn to distinguish their infant's condition and needs from the character of his or her individual cry (see above).

Discharge Teaching

Infant Transportation

Client teaching in anticipation of discharge home includes discussing the use of an infant care seat to safeguard the newborn during travel. Some health agencies loan or rent infant car seats for a minimum fee. The nurse should explain that in an accident infants can be displaced from the parent's arms, causing injury. Because automobile accidents are a leading cause of death in children, many state laws require they be transported in approved car seats. In those states nurses are legally responsible for documenting that the infant was placed in the car seat by the parent (see Legal and Ethical Considerations: Sample Narrative Discharge Note).

Follow-Up Testing

Infants routinely are tested by heel stick sampling on the second day after birth for inborn errors of metabolism, notably phenylketonuria (PKU). In many states this is a legal requirement. However, the accuracy of the test depends on adequate ingestion of protein for 24 to 48 hours. Because full-term infants commonly are discharged 48 hours or less after birth, they may not meet that requirement. The nurse should discuss the importance of a follow-up test 1 to 2 weeks after discharge.

Evaluation

All newborn care skills are evaluated by parental demonstration or return-demonstration. Knowledge is evaluated by requesting that the parent reiterate the new information or correctly respond to questioning. The parent(s) should be able to (1) describe the components of general assessment of newborn status; (2) identify signs of danger that should be reported promptly to the primary health care provider; (3) return-demonstrate appropriate handwashing, assessment, and infant care skills; (4) express and display increasing confidence in their abilities to provide safe, effective newborn care; (5) verbalize their understanding of the rationale for transporting the infant in an approved infant car seat; and (6) actually secure the infant in the car seat for transport home. In addition, parents should be able to (7) explain the rationale for follow-up visits and (8) return for postdischarge assessments. Reassessment of infant status evaluates the effectiveness of both nursing and parental interventions.

LEGAL AND ETHICAL CONSIDERATIONS

Sample Narrative Discharge Note

Newborn status satisfactory. Placed in mother's arms. Client discharged (ambulatory, per wheelchair) with infant. Accompanied by husband to private car. Infant placed and secured in infant seat by father.

NURSING CARE PLAN

Ongoing Care of the Healthy Newborn

Goals (Expected Outcomes)	Interventions	Rationale	Evaluation
Ineffective Thermoregulation—Related to Limited Metabolic Ability to Compensate for Changes in Environmental Temperature			
Infant will experience uneventful thermal adaptation to extrauterine life.	Maintain environmental temperature of 72° to 76°F (22° to 26°C).	Ensures thermal neutrality. Reduces potential for hyperthermia or hypothermia (minimizes energy expenditure).	Infant's vital signs remain within acceptable range.
	Avoid placing infant on cold surfaces.	Minimizes heat loss through conduction.	Infant exhibits no signs of hyperthemia or hypothermia.
	Keep infant dry, warm and covered. Dress in shirt and diaper; wrap in warm blanket; cover with blanket; place cap on head for transport.	Minimizes heat loss through evaporation, radiation, and convection.	
	Avoid placing infant in drafts, near cold walls, or windows. Minimize exposure during infant care, e.g., bath.	Minimizes heat loss through evaporation, radiation, and convection. Protects from air currents.	
	Transport to mother in crib.	Protects from air currents.	
	Client teaching: Explain importance of maintaining thermal neutrality to parents.	Enables parents to understand reasons for dressing infant to minimize environmental stress.	
	Discuss methods of preventing overheating and chilling (see above).	Enables parents to protect newborn from environmental stressors.	
	Describe signs of heat and cold stress.	Facilitates early identification of thermal stress.	
	Discuss immediate treatment: Cold stress—cover, wrap, cuddle. Heat stress—remove coverings; sponge with tepid water.	Enables parents to intervene appropriately to minimize consequences.	
	Demonstrate method of taking axillary temperature.	Enables parents to gather assessment data required.	Parents take and read axillary temperature accurately.
	Emphasize importance of reporting significant changes in infant status and behaviors promptly.	Facilitates prompt and definitive nursing and medical management.	After discharge, parents report elevated or subnormal temperatures promptly to primary health care provider.

Continued

NURSING
CARE
PLAN

Ongoing Care of the Healthy Newborn—*continued*

Goals (Expected Outcomes)	Interventions	Rationale	Evaluation
Potential for Aspiration/Ineffective Airway Clearance—Related to Excessive Oropharyngeal Mucus			
Infant will experience unimpaired gas exchange.	Support newborn in side-lying position with rolled blanket from shoulders to rump.	Facilitates drainage.	Infant's respiratory rate is 30 - 50 per minute.
	Suction mouth and nostrils gently with bulb syringe as needed to remove excess mucus.	Maintains patent airway; reduces risk of aspiration.	Infant has no evidence of nasal flaring, sternal retractions, grunting, or gagging.
	Position infant on right side after feeding.	Encourages escape of air from stomach.	
	Avoid placing unattended infant in supine position.	Minimizes risk of mucus' occluding oropharynx.	
	Withhold feeding immediately before circumcision.	Minimizes risk of regurgitation and aspiration while in supine position.	
	Client teaching:		
	Explain rationale for specific infant positioning and avoiding placing child in supine position while unattended.	Minimizes risk of aspiration.	Parents verbalize understanding signs of respiratory distress; respond accurately to questions. Parents demonstrate appropriate infant positioning.
	Demonstrate proper use of the bulb syringe.	Enables parents to take prompt action if needed.	Parents demonstrate suctioning with bulb syringe. Parents verbalize confidence in own ability to perform procedure safely and effectively.
Potential for Infection—Related to **Immature Immune System**			
Infant will experience minimum exposure to potential pathogens.	Maintain good handwashing technique. Wash hands before and after providing care.	Minimizes risk of transmitting microorganisms from self, environment, or from infant to infant.	Infant's vital signs remain within normal range. Infant is active; responsive; feeds well. Chemical conjunctivitis (if present from eye Credé maneuver) subsides in 3 to 4 days; infant exhibits no purulent drainage from eyes.
Impaired Skin Integrity Secondary to Umbilical Cord Stump			
Infant will remain free of infection.	Apply alcohol to umbilical cord stump with every diaper change.	Hastens drying of cord, closing potential portal of entry.	Exhibits no signs of local infection (redness, swelling, drainage) in area of umbilical stump (or circumcision site if applicable).
	Apply bactericidal preparation to stump as ordered.	Antibiotic ointment or Triple dye reduces risk of infection.	

NURSING
CARE
PLAN

Ongoing Care of the Healthy Newborn—*continued*

Goals (Expected Outcomes)	Interventions	Rationale	Evaluation
Impaired Skin Integrity Secondary to Circumcision			
Infant will remain free of infection.	Minimize potential for irritation or contamination of circumcision site.		Healing progresses without interruption.
	Apply diaper loosely; place infant in side-lying position.	Minimizes irritation from pressure and friction.	
	Change diapers often; cleanse area with warm water cascade; change petroleum gauze if soiled with urine or stool.	Minimizes irritation from urine or stool. Discourages growth of bacterial contaminants.	
	Record and report any signs of infection promptly.	Enables prompt and definitive management.	
	Client teaching: Discuss and demonstrate methods of preventing infection: Handwashing Preventing contact with contaminated surfaces Avoiding contact with persons who are not well Use of masks Cord care	Enables parents to minimize infant's exposure to potential pathogens.	Parents verbalize understanding of basic principles of infection control Parents demonstrate appropriate handwashing technique. Parents demonstrate appropriate care of umbilical cord stump.
	Care of circumcision		Parents demonstrate appropriate care of circumcision.
	Describe signs of infection.	Facilitates early identification.	
	Instruct parent to record and report any signs of infection promptly to health care provider.	Enables prompt and definitive medical management.	After discharge parents promptly report any signs of deviations from expected progress to primary health care provider.

Continued

NURSING
CARE
PLAN

Ongoing Care of the Healthy Newborn—*continued*

Goals (Expected Outcomes)	Interventions	Rationale	Evaluation
Potential Fluid Volume Deficit—Related to Marginal Coagulability Secondary to Lack of Necessary Intestinal Flora and Circumcision			
Infant will experience uneventful postoperative course.	Administer prophylactic vitamin K injection as ordered.	Provides cofactor required for transformation of prothrombin precursor to active prothrombin.[24]	Infant exhibits no evidence of bleeding. Infant heals without incident.
	Avoid pressure, friction, or injury of circumcision site.	Reduces potential for traumatic bleeding.	
	Cover site with petroleum gauze as ordered; remove only when soiled. Cleanse area with warm water cascade.	Minimizes trauma to delicate tissue.	
	Record and report bleeding to primary health provider promptly.	Enables prompt and definitive treatment.	
	In the event of bleeding, apply oxidizing cellulose gauze (Oxycel) as ordered.	Enhances clotting.	
	Client teaching: Discuss the appropriate management of circumcision. Explain rationale for actions.	Enables client understanding. Increases potential for client compliance with behaviors recommended.	Parents demonstrate safe, effective care of circumcision site.
	Demonstrate cleansing of circumcision site (see Client Self-Care Education: Circumcision Care).	Enables parents to participate actively in infant's care; continues safe care after discharge.	
	Describe signs of complications (e.g., bleeding, changes in urinary elimination pattern).	Facilitates early identification and prompt management of problems.	
	Demonstrate assessment of infant hydration status.	Facilitates early identification and prompt management of problems.	
	Instruct parents to report any signs of deviation from expected behaviors.	Enables prompt and definitive management of problems.	

Ongoing Care of the Healthy Newborn—continued

Goals (Expected Outcomes)	Interventions	Rationale	Evaluation
Altered Nutrition: Less Than Body Requirements—Related to Limited Intake, Hypoglycemia			
Infant will exhibit normal fluid and electrolyte balance.	Begin feedings in accordance with protocol or primary health provider's orders.	Newborn has a high metabolic rate; requires glucose to meet energy needs.	Infant feeds well; is active; has lusty cry. Infant exhibits no signs of hypoglycemia (jittery; tremors; irregular respirations, apnea; pallor; cyanosis. Infant has capillary blood glucose level: >45 mg/dl
	First feeding: 15 ml 5% glucose in water.	Water is easily and rapidly absorbed; glucose is rapidly available to meet needs.	
	Offer feedings every 3 to 4 hr or on demand (breast or formula).	—	Infant exhibits weight loss of less than 10% of birth weight during first 3 to 4 days after birth.
	Burp infant frequently during feedings.	Encourages expulsion of air swallowed during feeding; reduces risk of regurgitation.	
	Place infant on right side after feeding.	Facilitates escape of air from stomach; reduces risk of regurgitation.	Infant exhibits no regurgitation of feedings.
	Client teaching: Explain rationale for current nursing management.	Enables parental understanding; reduces anxiety.	
	Demonstrate techniques for burping, positioning.	Allows parents to participate actively in infant care; reduces potential for regurgitation.	

Continued

Ongoing Care of the Healthy Newborn—continued

Goals (Expected Outcomes)	Interventions	Rationale	Evaluation
	Pain—Related to Heel Stick for Diagnostic Studies (e.g., Blood Glucose, Hematocrit, PKU) and to Circumcision		
Newborn will experience minimum procedure-related pain and respond promptly to comforting measures.	*Heel stick* Warm heel with warm compress for 5 min before procedure.	Increases circulation; dilates blood vessels; facilitates adequate sampling.	Infant responds promptly to comforting measures. Quiets Feeds well Exhibits undisturbed sleep pattern
	Cleanse site with alcohol; allow to dry.	Minimizes potential for irritation of puncture site.	
	Grasp heel firmly and puncture with microlancet rapidly.	Facilitates collection of adequate sample; minimizes need for second puncture to obtain sample.	
	Apply cover bandage.	Avoids irritation of puncture site.	
	Circumcision Avoid restraining infant until primary health care provider is ready.	Minimizes discomfort and distress from being confined.	
	Stroke infant's head or cheek; talk to infant during the procedure.	Provides comforting stimuli.	
	Provide pacifier if consistent with agency protocol.	Sucking provides comfort (important to self-consoling).	
	Apply diaper loosely.	Minimizes discomfort from pressure and friction.	
	Wrap infant in blanket.	Increase infant's feeling of security.	
	Cuddle.	Reduces tension.	
	Encourage mother to feed and cuddle infant.	Provides comforting. Reinforces positive parental instincts. Increases infant's sense of security and comfort.	
	Place infant on side in crib.	Minimizes irritation from pressure on circumcision site.	
	Change diapers often. Cleanse area with warm water cascade.	Reduces potential for irritation from urine, stool, or soap.	
	Promptly record and report any signs of bleeding or infection.	Enables prompt and definitive management. Reduces potential for any additional pain.	
	Client teaching: Describe procedure and explain rationale for actions.	Enables parental understanding; Facilitates informed consent; reduces anxiety and guilt.	Parents verbalize understanding of reason for heel stick or advantages and disadvantages or hazards of circumcision.
	Demonstrate care of site (see also Client Self-Care Education: Circumcision Care).	Allows parents to participate actively in infant care; enables safe care. Minimizes risk of inadvertent injury to infant.	Parents demonstrate safe care of site of puncture and circumcision.
	Instruct parent to report any signs of bleeding or infection.	Enables prompt and definitive management of complications.	

NURSING
CARE
PLAN

Ongoing Care of the Healthy Newborn—continued

Goals (Expected Outcomes)	Interventions	Rationale	Evaluation
Knowledge Deficit (Maternal)—Regarding Infant Care			
Mother or parents will gain information and skills needed to provide safe, effective infant care; exhibit growing competence and confidence in providing infant care; and provide safe, effective care appropriate to infant's specific needs.	Target teaching to specific individual knowledge deficits (see preceding information and specific Client Self-Care Education).	Maximizes parental knowledge gain.	Parents actively participate in own learning.
	Demonstrate necessary actions and explain rationale.	Enables parental understanding of need for specific actions; facilitates compliance with nursing recommendations.	Parents seek information and guidance to meet individual learning needs.
	Invite and answer questions as they arise.	Identifies additional learning needs.	Parents verbalize beginning confidence in their knowledge base.
	Provide guidance as needed by parents during return-demonstrations.	Supports parents' growing competence and self-confidence.	Parents demonstrate increasing confidence in ability to provide safe, effective newborn care.
			Parents perform procedures safely and accurately.
			Infant progresses normally without occurrence of common complications of the neonatal period.
			Vital signs stable within normal limits
			Alert, responsive
			Feeds well
			Maintains normal weight gain

REFERENCES

1. Cunningham F, MacDonald P, Gant N: Williams Obstetrics, 18th ed. Norwalk, Conn, Appleton & Lange, 1989
2. Brazelton T: Neonatal behavioral assessment. In Avery G (ed): Neonatology: Pathophysiology and Management of the Newborn, 3rd ed. Philadelphia, JB Lippincott, 1987
3. Coen R, Fanaroff A, Taylor P: A fast, efficient newborn exam. Patient Care, June 15, 1988, pp 192-207
4. Coen R, Fanaroff A, Taylor P: The detailed newborn examination. Patient Care, July 15, 1988, pp 90-112
5. Cabal L et al: Neonatal clinical cardiopulmonary monitoring. In Fanaroff A, Martin R (eds): Neonatal-Perinatal Medicine, 4th ed. St. Louis, CV Mosby, 1987
6. Jones D et al: Health Assessment Across the Life Span. New York, McGraw-Hill, 1984
7. Walsh M: Tables of normal values. In Fanaroff A, Martin R (eds): Neonatal-Perinatal Medicine, 4th ed. St. Louis, CV Mosby, 1987
8. Brann A, Schwartz J: Assessment of neonatal neurologic function. In Fanaroff A, Martin R (eds): Neonatal-Perinatal Medicine, 4th ed. St. Louis, CV Mosby, 1987
9. Volpe J, Hill A: Neurologic disorders. In Avery G (ed): Neonatology: Pathophysiology and Management of the Newborn, 3rd ed. Philadelphia, JB Lippincott, 1987
10. Korones S: The normal neonate: Assessment of early physical findings. In Sciarra J et al (eds): Gynecology and Obstetrics, Vol 2. Hagerstown, Md, Harper & Row, 1985
11. Driscoll J: Physical examination. In Fanaroff A, Martin R (eds): Neonatal-Perinatal Medicine, 4th ed. St. Louis, CV Mosby, 1987
12. Dubowitz L et al: Clinical assessment of gestational age in the newborn infant. J Pediatr 77:1, 1970
13. Ballard J et al: A simplified score for assessment of fetal maturation of newly born infants. J Pediatr 95:769, 1979
14. Brazelton T: Neonatal Behavioral Assessment Scale, 2nd ed. Philadelphia, JB Lippincott, 1984
15. Kraybill E: Needs of the term infant. In Avery G (ed): Neonatology, 3rd ed. Philadelphia, JB Lippincott, 1987
16. Polmar S, Manthel U: Immunology. In Fanaroff A, Martin R (eds): Neonatal-Perinatal Medicine, 4th ed. St. Louis, CV Mosby, 1987
17. Ouimette J: Perinatal Nursing, Care of the High-Risk Mother and Infant. Boston, Jones & Barlett, 1986
18. Pritchard J, MacDonald P, Gant N: Williams Obstetrics, 17th ed. Norwalk, Conn, Appleton-Century-Crofts, 1985
19. Laros R: Care of the infant during pregnancy and labor and after delivery. In Willson R, Carrington E (eds): Obstetrics and Gynecology, 8th ed. St. Louis, CV Mosby, 1987
20. AAP Committee on Fetus and Newborn and ACOG Committee on Obstetrics: Guidelines for Perinatal Care. Evanston, Ill, American Academy of Pediatrics, 1988
21. St. Petersburg Times, March 6, 1989
22. Nurses Association of the American College of Obstetricians and Gynecologists Committee on Practice: Nurse's role in neonatal circumcision (pamphlet). Washington, DC, NAACOG, August 1985
23. Marchette L, Main R, Redick E: Pain reduction during neonatal circumcision. Pediatr Nurs 15(2):207-210, March/April 1989
24. Blanchette, Zipursky A: Neonatal hematology. In Avery G: Neonatology: Pathophysiology and Management of the Newborn, 3rd ed. Philadelphia, JB Lippincott, 1987

SUGGESTED READINGS

Anderson C: Integration of the Brazelton Neonatal Behavioral Assessment Scale into routine neonatal nursing care. Issues Compr Pediatr Nurs 9:341-351, 1986

D'Appolito K: The neonate's response to pain. MCN 9:256-259, July/August 1984

James L, Adamsons K: The newborn infant. In Danforth D, Scott J (eds): Obstetrics and Gynecology, 5th ed. Philadelphia, JB Lippincott, 1986

Judd J: Assessing the newborn from head to toe. Nurs 1985 15:12, 1985

Lincoln G: Neonatal circumcision: Is it needed? JOGN 15(6):463, November/December 1986

Luddington-Hoe S: What can newborns really see? Am J Nurs 83:1286, 1983

NAACOG: Physical assessment of the neonate. Washington, DC, OGN Nursing Practice Resource, 1986

Sheredy C: Factors to consider when assessing responses to pain. MCN 9:250-252, July/August 1984

Tedder J: Newborn circumcision. JOGN, 16(1):42, January/February 1987

Infant Nutrition

IMPORTANT TERMINOLOGY

colostrum Yellowish or creamy fluid, high in protein, fat-soluble vitamins, minerals, and immunoglobulins, secreted by breasts during pregnancy and for 3 days after delivery

engorgement Enlargement of breasts, caused by increase in blood and lymph supply to breasts; occurs in relation to lactation, usually at time milk "comes in"

letdown reflex Contraction of alveoli of mammary gland, pushing milk into larger ducts, which discharge at the nipple; mediated by pituitary hormone oxytocin; initiated by stroking of nipple or crying of baby; may be inhibited by anger, embarrassment, excitement, fear

LaLeche League Voluntary organization that seeks to provide education about breast-feeding and assistance to women who are breast-feeding

prolactin Hormone secreted by anterior pituitary gland; stimulates lactation in mammary glands

oxytocin Hormone secreted by posterior lobe of pituitary gland; stimulates uterine contractions, causes ejection, or letdown, of milk

One vital adaptation the infant makes in the transition to life outside the uterus is to take food into the body orally and digest and assimilate it. The infant sucks and swallows to get food into the stomach. The sucking and swallowing reflexes are present at birth and are quite strong. During the first hour after birth the infant typically swallows mucus and sucks on his or her thumb or fist.

The rooting reflex, which is present at birth, enables the newborn to find food by turning toward anything that touches his cheeks or lips. This reflex allows the infant to "latch on" to the bottle or breast.

Choice of Feeding Method

Choosing the method for feeding is an important and sometimes difficult decision for parents to make. Their choice is influenced by a variety of factors such as personal attitudes, their culture, social pressures, and psychologic needs of the mother.

Information about the differences in available feeding methods can be useful in helping parents make a decision based on facts. Even though the health professional believes breast-feeding is ideal, care must be taken not to force the mother to choose this method, and the mother who chooses to bottle-feed should not be made to feel guilty. Once the feeding method has been chosen, the nurse should focus on providing support to ensure the chosen method is successful.

Advantages of Breast-Feeding

Human milk is the ideal food for the human infant (Table 21-1; display on p. 563). Breast milk is safe because it is not subject to incorrect mixing or contamination. The feeding is immediately available to the newborn at the correct temperature. Human milk contains no bacteria and contains proteins that are nonallergenic to the newborn, and the infant is protected from diarrhea and upper respiratory infections. The milk curd is easily digestible, and overfeeding is much less likely than with bottle-feeding. There are few absolute contraindications to breast-feeding. One is galactosemia, a condition in which affected infants cannot utilize galactose. Breast-feeding by the mother who has diseases such as cancer or infections such as active pulmonary tuberculosis may also be contraindicated.

TABLE 21-1

Composition of Mature Breast Milk, Cow's Milk, and a Routine Infant Formula★

Composition/dl	Mature Breast Milk	Cow's Milk	Routine Formula With Iron†
Calories	75.0	69.0	67.0
Protein (g)	1.1	3.5	1.5
Lactalbumin (%)	80	18	
Casein (%)	20	82	
Water (ml)	87.1	87.3	
Fat (g)	4.0	3.5	3.7
Carbohydrate (g)	9.5	4.9	7.0
Ash (g)	0.21	0.72	0.34
Minerals			
Na (mg)	16.0	50.0	25.0
K (mg)	51.0	144.0	74.0
Ca (mg)	33.0	118.0	55.0
P (mg)	14.0	93.0	43.0
Mg (mg)	4.0	12.0	9.0
Fe (mg)	0.1	Trace	1.2
Zn (mg)	0.15	0.1	0.42
Vitamins			
A (IU)	240.0	140.0	158.6
C (mg)	5.0	1.0	5.3
D (IU)	2.2	1.4	42.3
E (IU)	0.18	0.04	0.83
Thiamin (mg)	0.01	0.03	0.04
Riboflavin (mg)	0.04	0.17	0.06
Niacin (mg)	0.2	0.1	0.7
Curd size	Soft Flocculent	Firm Large	Mod. firm Mod. large
pH	Alkaline	Acid	Acid
Anti-infective properties	+	±	−
Bacterial content	Sterile	Nonsterile	Sterile
Empyting time	More rapid		

From Avery GB, Fletcher AB: Nutrition. In Avery GB (ed): Neonatology, 3rd ed. Philadelphia, JB Lippincott, 1987.
★Composite of a number of sources.
†Enfamil.

Advantages of Breast-Feeding

Breast milk contains ideal nutrients needed for optimum growth of the human neonate.

Breast milk protects the infant against diarrhea. Intestinal flora of the breast-fed infant produces feces with a pH of 5 to 6. This low pH inhibits the growth of bacteria such as *Escherichia coli,* which can cause diarrhea in the infant.

The incidence of respiratory infections is lower in breast-fed infants.

Proteins found in human milk are almost nonallergenic to human infants. The incidence of allergic diseases is lower in breast-fed infants with a family history of allergies.

Breast-feeding promotes uterine involution in the mother, and oxytocin is released when the infant sucks.

Breast milk is readily available at the right temperature.

Advantages of Bottle-Feeding

Women give a variety of reasons for choosing to bottle-feed. Some believe breast-feeding is too tiring, too time-consuming, too confining, or distasteful. Others fear it will disfigure their breasts or that they will fail at breast-feeding. The mores and pressures of the mother's socioeconomic class or peer group or the need or desire to return to work may be significant factors in the decision to bottle-feed.

An important advantage of bottle-feeding is that the father can be an equal partner and can experience the closeness of the feeding experience.

Physiology and Techniques of Breast-Feeding

Mechanisms of Lactation

Two major mechanisms are involved in lactation: the secretion of milk and the milk-ejection reflex.

During pregnancy lactogen, secreted by the placenta, and **prolactin,** secreted by the pituitary gland, prepare the mammary glands for lactation. Estrogen stimulates the growth of mammary tissue, and progesterone stimulates alveolar development in the maternal breasts during pregnancy. After the infant's birth levels of estrogen and progesterone decrease rapidly. Prolactin levels remain high, initiating the onset of lactation. Release of prolactin from the pituitary is also stimulated by the sucking of the infant at the breast. **Colostrum,** present for the first days after birth, is higher in protein and lower in fat, lactose, and immunoglobulins than mature milk.

In the early stages of lactation milk secretion can be stimulated by having the infant nurse every 2 to 3 hours from both breasts at each feeding, generally at least 10 minutes from each breast. This frequent feeding stimulates the production of more milk and helps establish the milk supply. Frequent emptying of the breasts is important for adequate milk production, especially in the early stages of lactation. If the breasts are not entirely emptied and the back pressure in the alveoli is not relieved, milk secretion decreases and eventually stops.

The second mechanism, milk ejection, or **letdown reflex**, is initiated by the infant's sucking. As the infant sucks, **oxytocin** is released from the pituitary gland and stimulates the alveoli to contract and eject milk through the ducts into the lactiferous sinuses. The milk must be in the sinuses before it can be removed by the infant's sucking. The fat-containing hindmilk is not secreted until the foremilk is removed. Failure of the letdown reflex may cause early termination of breast-feeding.

Assessment of Breast-Feeding

Assessment is the first critical step in helping the mother with her goal of successful breast-feeding. A mother who has had a previous successful and rewarding breast-feeding experience often will verbalize and demonstrate confidence in her approach to breast-feeding her newly delivered infant. The nurse must recognize that each mother-infant breast-feeding experience is unique and requires assessment by the nurse. Use of an assessment tool or checklist is helpful in determining the mother's level of knowledge, physiologic status, and any problems or potential problems (see Assessment Tool: Breast-Feeding).

Nursing Diagnosis

Assessment of the mother's ability to feed her infant and of her knowledge about the breast-feeding process and her infant's nursing needs aids the nurse in formulating nursing diagnoses.

ASSESSMENT
TOOL

Breast-Feeding

1. Assess the mother's ability to assume a comfortable position.
2. Assess mother's nipples for the following:
   a. Pliability
   b. Inversion
   c. Cracks
   d. Abrasions
   e. Tenderness
   f. Pain
3. Assess breasts for the following:
   a. Engorgement
   b. Plugged ducts
   c. Tenderness
   d. Pain
4. Is the mother holding the infant correctly?
   a. Supports head and body
   b. Brings infant close
   c. Supports breast with other hand using C hold
5. Is infant sucking correctly?
   a. Lips tightly around the full areola
   b. Jaws moving up and down in a rhythmic pattern
6. Is infant's tongue under nipple?
7. Assess infant's level of activity.
   a. Sleepy
   b. Crying
   c. Sucking on fists

Knowledge Deficit—regarding factors influencing successful breast-feeding, normal newborn behaviors, effective breast-feeding practices
Pain—related to breast engorgement secondary to impending lactation, sore nipples
Ineffective Breast-feeding—related to lack of knowledge, discomfort, stress, maternal ambivalence, nonsupportive family, or sleepy infant
Altered Nutrition (Infant): Less Than Body Requirements—related to ineffective sucking techniques
Fluid Volume Deficit (Infant)—related to inadequate fluid intake

POTENTIAL
NURSING DIAGNOSES

Breast-Feeding Mother and Infant

Focus Assessment

Determine knowledge level regarding breast-feeding.
Determine maternal desire or motivation for breast-feeding.
Observe mother's facial expression and body language during breast-feeding. Monitor mother's state of comfort.
Note position assumed for breast-feeding.
Examine mother's positioning of infant for feeding.
Note infant response to appropriate stimulation, e.g., rooting reflex, sucking pattern and effectiveness.
Examine placement of nipple in infant's mouth.
Monitor indicators of infant intake, e.g., voiding, weight gain, sleep patterns, behaviors while awake.

Planning and Intervention

Many of the problems associated with unsuccessful breast-feeding can be prevented or solved through planning and actions by the nurse.

Preparation of the mother is begun before the hungry newborn is brought for feeding and continues with each feeding. Instructions include information about hospital and home procedures such as handwashing. The mother needs to learn about the infant's behaviors, how to handle the infant, how to interpret cues of hunger and satiety, and how to help the infant grasp the nipple. The nurse should demonstrate ways to elicit feeding reflexes from the infant. The nurse can help the new mother feel confident in her abilities by praising her successes in soothing her infant and praising the mother's care-taking activities or by pointing out the infant's positive responses to her.

Initiation of Breast-Feeding

Initiation of breast-feeding is best accomplished in the first hour after birth. The newborn usually is awake and alert that first hour and is sucking his or her thumb or fist. The mother usually verbalizes confidence and positive feelings after a first successful feeding experience. Even if the infant is too sleepy to nurse well at this time, the closeness to the mother and contact with the nipple may be enough to stimulate release of oxytocin and prolactin. The mother needs reassurance if the infant does not nurse at the first session.

Positioning the Mother

The mother should be encouraged to vary her position from one feeding to the next. Varying the nursing position helps prevent nipple soreness

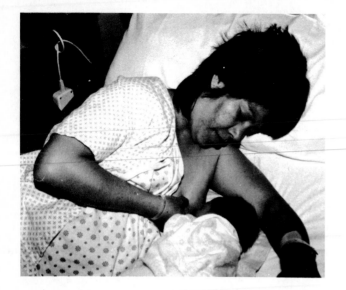

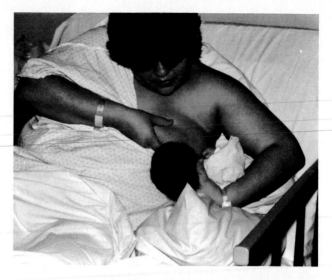

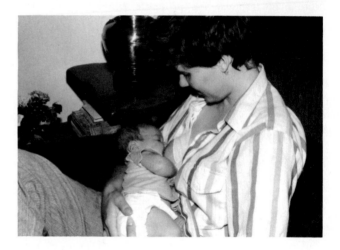

FIGURE 21-1
Positions for Breast-Feeding Infants.
The nurse may have to help the mother find
a comfortable position. The infant is held or
supported by a pillow in position close to
the mother. In each position the mother is
face-to-face with the infant, and she can
determine correct placement of the infant at
her breast.

because it changes the position of the infant's mouth on the nipple. Changing position facilitates thorough breast emptying. See Figure 21-1 for examples of breast-feeding positions. The mother who is in a comfortable position feels more relaxed and milk ejection is facilitated.

Positioning the Infant

After the mother is comfortable, the nurse can assist her in positioning her infant so that he or she can "latch on" to the breast correctly. Although some mothers seem to know how to support an infant at the breast, many are awkward at first and need specific instructions (see Client Infant-Care Education: Positioning the Infant at the Breast).

The Infant's Sucking Behavior

The infant empties the mother's breast through suction and compression. As the infant nurses, he or she moves his or her jaws up and down to compress and empty the sinuses. The infant's tongue suctions the milk from the nipple as it draws the nipple back against the palate (Fig. 21-2).

Positioning the Infant at the Breast

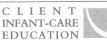

Action

1. Assume a comfortable position.
2. Turn the infant's body toward you.
3. Keep the infant's shoulder and hip in alignment.

4. Support your breast with your hand, with all four fingers below and thumb above. Place all fingers behind the areola.
5. Touch the infant's lower lip with your breast until his or her mouth is wide open.

6. Bring the infant close to your body and your breast (bring the infant to the breast, not the breast to the infant).
7. If breast tissue presses against the infant's nose, lift breast slightly or lift the infant's head and legs slightly so they are more horizontal rather than at a downward angle. This allows more space around the nose.

Rationale

1. Facilitates letdown reflex.
2. Infant should not have to turn head to grasp nipple.
3. Even distribution of infant's weight prevents pull on the breast.
4. Helps the infant grasp the nipple.

5. Stimulates the infant to open his or her mouth. Stroking both cheeks of infant is avoided because to do so stimulates rooting reflex on both sides and confuses the infant.
6. Allows directing the nipple into center of infant's mouth.

7. Breast tissue pressing against the nose causes infant to stop sucking. Changing position of the infant removes breast tissue from against the nose.

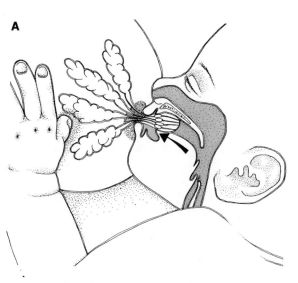
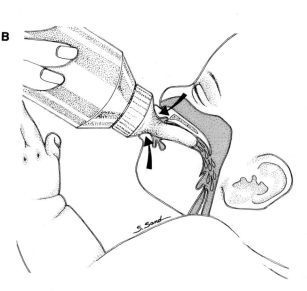

FIGURE 21-2

Comparison of Nipple Placement for Breast-Feeding and Bottle-Feeding.
A, During breast-feeding, the nipple is sucked far back in the mouth. The gums close on the areola while elevation of the tongue, traveling from front to back, presses the nipple against the hard palate, squeezing milk out of the sinuses. **B,** During bottle-feeding the rubber nipple is less pliable, reaches further into mouth, and may strike the soft palate, interfering with normal tongue action. Note the lips flaring outward from pressure of widened area of rubber nipple.

If the infant has a good grasp, his or her jaws will move up and down regularly, and sucking and swallowing movements can be seen in his or her cheeks and throat. Sounds of swallowing, a soft "ka," can be heard. The infant who is sucking ineffectively should be removed from the breast and started again. When removing the infant from the breast, the mother must first break the suction to avoid pain or trauma to the nipple. To break the suction the little finger is inserted in the corner of the infants mouth or the infant's chin is pulled down.

The mother may not realize that infants have different eating behaviors—individual differences do exist. Some, after finding the nipple, suck vigorously without stopping until satisfied. Others appear to sleep or rest at intervals. Some like the feeling of security and may continue to nurse for pleasure. Recognition of these variations may relieve anxiety in the mother.

Breast-Feeding Education

Common concerns of breast-feeding mothers include the following.

Disinterested Infant

Moistening the nipple with a small amount of expressed colostrum or milk may encourage a disinterested infant to suck. Sleepy infants can be awakened by unwrapping or playing with him or her. Sleepy infants will not nurse well and should be allowed to awaken sufficiently by themselves. The mother may request that the infant not be given any feedings in the nursery and be brought to her as soon as he or she awakens. If the infant remains at the mother's bedside, he or she is fed on awakening.

Breast-feeding intervals that are delayed 5 to 6 hours in the first days of the infant's life may interfere with the establishment of breast-feeding. In addition, the infant may become hypoglycemic. The nurse must encourage and assist the mother to feed her infant frequently.

Frequency of Feedings

At first most breast-fed infants want to nurse every 2 to 3 hours. This frequency helps stimulate milk production and helps satisfy the infant's needs.

Following a self-demand schedule is the usual current practice. The infant is fed when he or she indicates hunger by crying and body posture. An infant who waits a long time to nurse may not nurse well because of exhaustion from crying.

Length of Feeding

If positioning and attachment are correct, unlimited nursing has not been found to increase nipple soreness. Limiting the length of breast-feeding to 5 or 10 minutes may actually cause problems such as poor letdown reflex, increased incidence of breast **engorgement,** and reduction in the infant's fluid intake. The letdown reflex in the beginning may take longer than the assigned time. If letdown has not occurred and the breasts cannot be emptied, the breasts become engorged, and the infant's fluid needs are not met.

Both breasts are offered at each feeding. The infant usually gets most of the milk in the first 5 to 10 minutes of sucking. Nursing should begin on the side used last at the previous feeding. A safety pin on the bra strap will help the mother remember which breast should be used first.

Each time the baby has a growth spurt, he or she will want to nurse more frequently for a few days to meet the increased demand for calories.

Use of Bottle-Feedings While Breast-Feeding

If breast-feeding was not begun early and the infant has been fed with a rubber nipple, he or she may be "nipple confused." The milk flows readily from a rubber nipple with little effort by the infant. With a rubber nipple the infant thrusts his or her tongue forward to control the flow of milk instead of using the tongue to extract the milk. Often the newborn has some difficulty switching from bottle to breast, but with time and patience, most infants will do well.

Adequate Intake

An infant is getting enough milk if he or she is wetting four to six diapers a day, sleeping fairly well, and gaining weight at a steady rate. An infant cries for reasons other than hunger. A breast-fed infant will gain weight more slowly than if he or she were bottle-fed. Ways for the mother to increase the milk supply are putting the infant to breast more often, getting more rest, and increasing fluid and protein intake. After a pattern of breast-feeding is established, the breasts will be more normal in size and will feel less full after feedings.

If letdown is not occurring, the mother may need to lie down, have a warm drink, or do things that help her relax. Signs of letdown are a drawing sensation in the breast or dripping of milk from one breast when the infant is sucking from the other.

Breast milk looks different from cow's milk and is "rich enough" even though it normally looks thin and bluish-white in color.

Care of Nipples

The nipples are cleansed with plain water at the time of the daily bath or shower. Use of soap can lead to cracking because it removes the natural protective oils secreted by the nipples. If a commercial ointment or cream is ordered by the primary care provider, the nipples should be dry before its application and the ointment applied very lightly. Nipples are allowed to air dry by leaving the nursing bra flaps open for 15 to 30 minutes between feedings. Another way to keep nipples dry is to use commercial plastic shells that hold the nipples away from clothing between feedings. Plastic liners or thick applications of petroleum jelly (Vaseline) on the nipples are never used because they hold in the moisture and prevent drying of the nipples. Drying the nipples between feedings helps keep the nipples intact and promotes healing.

Expression of Milk

At times the infant cannot be "put to breast" or cannot empty the breast completely. At such times artificial expression of milk is necessary to

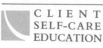

Expression of Breast Milk

Action	Rationale
1. Wash hands with warm water and soap.	1. Removes pathogens and prevents contamination of nipples with pathogens from hands.
2. Prepare equipment; obtain (from nursery) a sterile wide-mouthed container and sterile bottle and cap if milk is to be fed to the infant.	2. Prevents contamination of breast milk with microorganisms.
3. Take a warm shower, have a warm drink, or massage the breasts.	3. Stimulates letdown and flow of milk.
4. Use one hand to support the breast and express the milk; usually the right hand is used for the left breast and left hand for right breast. The other hand is used to hold the container.	4. Helps mother discover the most comfortable position to use.
5. Place forefinger below and thumb above the outer edge of the areola.	5. Places fingers on lactiferous sinuses.
6. Using gentle but firm pressure toward the chest wall, move finger and thumb toward each other; then draw fingers forward with a milking motion.	6. Forces out milk in a stream as the finger and thumb are brought together and released, compressing the area of the lactiferous sinuses between them.
7. Reposition thumb and forefinger, moving in a clockwise direction; then repeat expression of milk.	7. Removes milk from all sinuses.
8. Avoid pulling, pinching, or squeezing motions.	8. Prevents potential damage or bruises to breast tissue.
9. If milk is to be fed to infant, pour into sterile nursing bottle and label with infant's name, the time, and the date. Refrigerate immediately.	9. Breast milk may be refrigerated for up to 48 hours or frozen up to 2 weeks. If a refrigerator is not available, the breast milk can be retained and transported in ice in a small picnic type cooler brought with the mother for this purpose.

relieve maternal discomfort and to preserve the milk supply (see Client Self-Care Education: Expression of Breast Milk). Milk may be expressed manually (Fig. 21-3), by hand pump, or by electric pump (Fig. 21-4). Manual expression more nearly stimulates the action of the infant's jaw, and no special equipment is needed. Mechanical methods have the potential to traumatize breast tissue since they express the milk by suction exerted on the breast tissue. Hand and electric breast pumps are useful if expression of milk is to continue for a longer period of time. Before using any pump, the mother should be given explanations about why it is used, how it works, and how to use it. Clinical agencies provide instructions on correct methods to use for that particular agency's pumps.

Common Problems

The nurse may anticipate that the breast-feeding mother may have problems that can cause her considerable discomfort and that she may discontinue breast-feeding if she cannot receive appropriate help with these

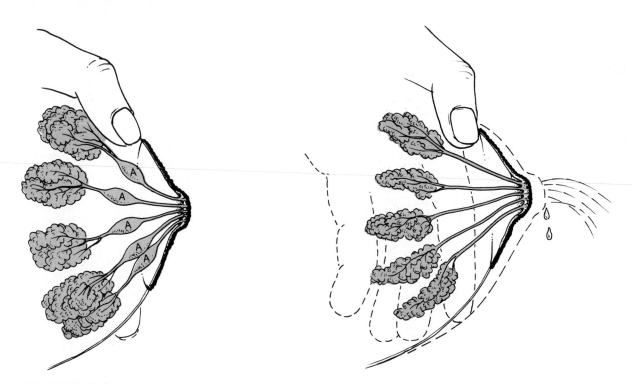

FIGURE 21-3

Manual Milk Expression. Lateral view of left breast shows method of expressing milk from the breast. The thumb and forefinger are placed on opposite sides of the breast just behind the areola. The lactiferous sinuses (*A,* ampulla) are compressed, and milk is forced out as the thumb and forefinger are brought together.

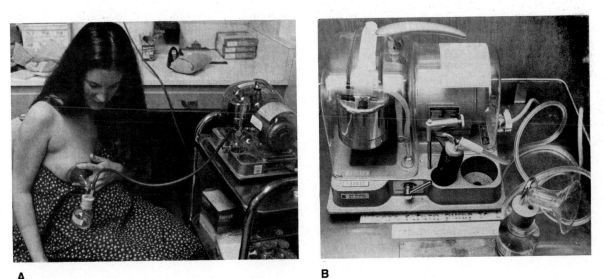

A   **B**

FIGURE 21-4

Electric Breast Pump. A, Mother using electric breast pump. **B,** Close-up of electric breast pump. In the hospital the electric breast pump can be used by more than one mother. Each mother has her own packet of removable parts such as breast pump bottle and cap, breast funnel, and plastic connecter tubing. The mother is taught to wash each part with hot, soapy water, rinse well, and dry after use.

TABLE 21-2

Common Problems With Breast-Feeding★

Problem	Prevention	Treatment
Painful nipples	Make sure most of areola is in infant's mouth so he or she does not chew on the nipple.	If fissures, erosions, or blisters develop, assess mother for proper nipple care.
	Change nursing positions with each feeding so that different areas of the nipple are subjected to the greatest stress from sucking.	Expose nipple to a lamp with 40-watt bulb for 15 to 20 minutes. Ice can be applied to painful nipples just before feeding. Ice may interfere with letdown in some mothers.
	Do not allow breasts to become engorged so that the infant has difficulty grasping the nipple. Feed the infant on demand so he or she does not become overly hungry, causing him or her to suck the nipple too vigorously. Start each feeding on alternate breasts so that both breasts are subjected to vigorous sucking that occurs at beginning of feeding.	If symptoms of breast abscess or mastitis develop, i.e., warmth, tenderness, redness, fever, consult primary care provider for probable antibiotic treatment. If painful nipples burn and itch, assess infant for thrush. Consult primary care provider for medication for mother and infant.
Engorgement	Encourage infant to suck frequently. Encourage letdown reflex (relaxation, warm drinks, warm shower).	Signs and symptoms of engorgement: taut, shiny reddened breasts; pain, which may extend to axillae (usually disappears in 24-48 hr); no fever.
	Empty alveoli of milk at each feeding. Allow infant to nurse in response to filling of mother's breasts as well as when infant is hungry.	If engorgement occurs, massage breasts toward the nipple before feedings to soften breasts and make grasping nipples easier for infant. Applying hot packs or taking hot shower improves flow of milk. Massage different areas of breast without removing infant from breast, especially in areas where lumps are noted.
	Express small amounts of milk to soften the areola enough for infant to grasp nipple.	Wear well-fitting supportive bra. The primary care provider may order aspirin, acetaminophen, or codeine for pain relief.

★Nursing goal is to teach mother about these potential problems and self-care before discharge.

problems. Because of early discharge of the breast-feeding mother, the nurse should instruct the mother about the prevention and treatment of common problems (Table 21-2).

Support for the Mother After Discharge

Most women still need support for breast-feeding after leaving the hospital. In the past information and positive feelings about breast-feeding were passed from mother to daughter. In recent years mothers or grandmothers may not have positive breast-feeding experiences to relate, or family members may not be available to give support to the new mother.

Some sources for help for the new mother are as follows:

1. **LaLeche League,** a voluntary organization that holds classes about breast-feeding both before and after birth. In many communities there are 24-hour phone numbers that nursing mothers may call if they are having problems with breast-feeding.
2. The lactation educator or consultant, a health professional with additional training and experience who presents prenatal classes and is available for counseling and advice. The consultant assists the mother with more serious breast-feeding problems and may work in a clinic or in private practice.
3. The nursery or obstetric unit, which can be called for help or support with problems.
4. Nurses who are hired by some hospitals and private doctors to make follow-up visits or phone calls after the mother leaves the hospital.

Evaluation of Breast-Feeding

Examples of expected outcomes after teaching sessions are (1) the mother verbalizes understanding of the breast-feeding process, (2) the mother assumes a comfortable position, and (3) the mother uses the suggested techniques for positioning the infant at her breasts.

Formula Feeding

Infant Formula

In the hospital nursery the infant will probably receive a ready-to-feed formula in a disposable bottle. Because this form of packaging is expensive, another type is recommended for home use. Formula is available in ready-to-use, concentrated liquid or powdered form.

Human milk is used as the standard in the manufacture of infant formula. Adjustments in formula are continually made as new information about the composition of human milk is discovered.

An infant formula must be free of bacterial contamination and easily digestible and must meet the infant's need for water, energy, vitamins, and minerals. See Table 21-3 for comparison of frequently used milks and formulas.

Assessment of Formula Feeding

Most hospitals have a routine for when the newborn will receive the first water feeding and when formula feedings will start. Indications that the newborn is ready to feed are lusty cry, rooting, sucking, active bowel sounds, and absence of abdominal distention.

During the initial sterile water feeding the nurse assesses the newborn for effectiveness of suck, swallow, and gag reflex. If vomiting or aspiration occurs, sterile water is readily absorbed by lung tissue. During the first feeding the infant is assessed for esophageal atresia or tracheoesophageal fistula. With esophageal atresia the feeding is regurgitated unchanged;

TABLE 21-3

Composition of Frequently Used Milks and Formulas

Milk or Formula	Cal/dl	Percentage Composition			mmol/dl		mg/dl		Type of Carbohydrate	Type of Protein	Remarks
		Pro	Fat	CHO	Na	K	Ca	P			
Human milk	74	1.1	4.5	6.8	0.7	1.3	34	121	Lactose	Human	
Cow's milk	67	3.5	3.7	4.9	2.2	3.5	117	92	Lactose	Cow	
Goat's milk	67	3.2	4.0	4.6	1.5	4.5	129	106	Lactose	Goat	
Enfamil	67	1.5	3.7	7.0	1.2	1.8	55	56	Lactose	Cow	Insufficient folate
Enfamil With Iron	67	1.5	3.7	7.0	1.2	1.8	55	46	Lactose	Cow	
Similac	67	1.6	3.6	7.2	1.1★	2.0★	51	39	Lactose	Cow	
Similac With Iron	67	1.6	3.6	7.2	1.1★	2.0★	51	39	Lactose	Cow	
Similac PM 60/40	67	1.6	3.5	7.6	0.7	1.5	40	20	Lactose	Casein, whey	60/40 lactalbumin; casein
S-M-A	67	1.5	3.6	7.2	0.6	1.4	44	33	Lactose	Whey from cow, cow	60/40 lactalbumin; casein
Advance	54	2.0	2.7	5.5	1.3	2.2	51	39	Corn syrup, lactose	Cow, soy	16 cal/ounce
Isomil	67	2.0	3.6	6.8	1.3	1.8	70	50	Corn syrup, sucrose, corn starch	Soy, methionine	
Soyalac-i	67	2.1	3.8	6.7	1.4	1.9	63	52	Sucrose, tapioca	Soy, methionine	
Nursoy	67	2.3	3.6	6.8	0.9	1.9	64	44	Sucrose	Soy, methionine	
ProSobee	67	2.5	3.4	6.8	1.8	1.9	79	53	Corn syrup solids	Soy, methionine	
Soyalac	69	2.2	3.8	6.6	1.5	2.0	63	52	Dextrose, maltose, sucrose	Soy, methionine	

Adapted from Avery GB (ed): Neonatology, 3rd ed. Philadelphia, JB Lippincott, 1987.
★Slightly higher if made from powder.

with an esophageal fistula the infant chokes and gags and may become cyanotic.

The nurse should assess the mother's level of knowledge and her previous experience with infant feeding and should observe the mother and infant during feeding to assess the mother's handling of the infant and the infant's feeding reflexes. The nurse monitors the amount of formula ingested and notes whether the infant regurgitates or vomits any of the feeding.

Nursing Diagnosis

Nursing diagnoses are based on assessment data that indicate the mother has a knowledge deficit about feeding techniques and about the nutritional needs and feeding behaviors of her newborn. Nursing diagnoses for the infant are directed toward the newborn's inability to ingest, digest, or metabolize an adequate amount of nutrients or fluids to meet nutritional needs for growth.

Planning and Intervention

Some goals useful in planning nursing interventions are as follows:

1. Mother demonstrates effective bottle-feeding techniques after instruction.
2. Infant loses no more than 5% to 10% of birth weight.
3. Infant ingests and retains ½ to 1 ounce of formula every 3 to 4 hours

□ POTENTIAL
NURSING DIAGNOSES

Bottle-Feeding

Maternal Knowledge Deficit—related to lack of information or experience with infant feeding
Altered Nutrition: Less Than Body Requirements—related to inadequate caloric intake
Potential Fluid Volume Deficit—related to inadequate fluid intake

during the first days of life (gradually increased based on size and age of infant).

Mothers who have chosen to bottle-feed their infants need reassurance, support, and information about feeding techniques and infant behavior.

Infant feeding behaviors may be misinterpreted by the mother and may lead to feelings of inadequacy. Many mothers believe that all infants are born knowing how to suck and that if the infant does not suck immediately or is sleepy or groggy, it is because she is doing something wrong. If the mother is helped to understand that newborns are sleepy in the first few days and that some infants do need help in taking a rubber nipple at first, the mother may feel more relaxed with the early feedings.

The new mother may worry about the intake of her infant who is sucking slowly or is sleepy during feedings in the first 24 to 36 hours after birth. The nurse can explain that the infant is born with reserves of water and fat and needs fewer calories during this early period of life. The loss of these reserves leads to the initial expected weight loss of up to 5% to 10% in the newborn.

Immediately before feeding the mother may need help in voiding, washing her hands, and finding a comfortable position. The mother who has had a cesarean section often has pain when the newborn is placed on her abdomen. Placing a rolled pillow under the arm supporting the infant's head helps. She may need assistance in bubbling (burping) the newborn (see Client Infant-Care Education: Feeding Formula to an Infant; Fig. 21-5).

Feeding Formula to an Infant

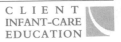

CLIENT
INFANT-CARE
EDUCATION

Action

1. Assume a comfortable position sitting up in bed or in a comfortable chair with adequate arm support.
2. Hold infant close to body in a semireclining position. Tilt bottle enough that milk fills the nipple.
3. If the infant does not open mouth readily, gently stroke the lips with nipple.
4. Place nipple well into mouth on top of the tongue.
5. As infant sucks, note if air bubbles rise in the bottle.

6. Bubble infant after he or she takes approximately ½ ounce of formula. Bubble by holding infant upright on your shoulder or holding infant in a sitting position while stroking or patting his or her back (see Fig. 21-5).

7. Feed for 15 to 20 min.

Rationale

1. A comfortable position helps mother relax and enjoy the feeding.

2. Air that is swallowed can rise to top of infant's stomach and be expelled.

3. Stroking the lips elicits the rooting reflex and stimulates the infant to open his or her mouth.

4. Some infants elevate their tongue when opening their mouths.

5. Indicates infant is getting milk. If there are no air bubbles, check to see if nipple is clogged.

6. Regurgitation is common during first days of feeding. Some causes are mucus in the stomach, feeding too rapidly, or overfeeding. Vomiting more than two feedings in a row or projectile vomiting is reported to the primary health care provider.
Placing infant in a sitting position during bubbling allows better observation of him or her.

7. A longer feeding may tire the infant; a shorter feeding may not satisfy his or her sucking needs.

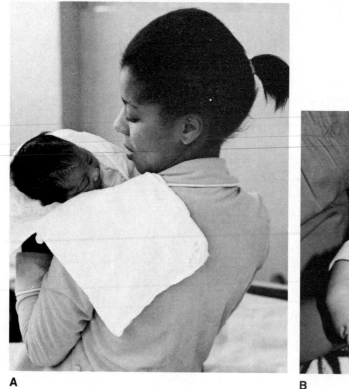

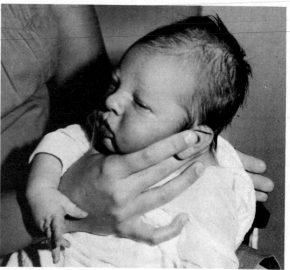

A

B

FIGURE 21-5

Bubbling. **A,** One method of bubbling an infant is to place him or her in an upright position over the shoulder where he or she can be held against the breast. The mother gently pats or rubs the infant's back. **B, An alternate method of bubbling the infant is often preferred because the infant's face is easily observed for color changes or vomiting. The infant is supported in a sitting position in the lap, with his or her chest resting on the mother's hand and his or her chin supported by the mother's thumb and index finger.**

Before discharge the new mother needs instruction on formula preparation. Many physicians no longer insist that bottles or formula be sterilized since a clean technique is proving as safe as sterilization. Requirements of clean technique are an uncontaminated water source, good refrigeration, and proper cleaning of hands and equipment. In addition, formula remaining in a bottle after feeding should be discarded and never saved for a later feeding. There are four methods of formula preparation: the one-bottle method, clean method, aseptic method, and terminal sterilization (see Client Infant-Care Education: Preparation of Formula; Table 21-4).

Evaluation

To evaluate nursing care of the formula-fed infant, the nurse observes the mother during a feeding. The nurse observes the mother-infant interaction and the infant's response to the feeding. The nurse verifies that the infant receives an appropriate amount at an appropriate rate and that the mother bubbles the newborn appropriately.

Education About Infant Feeding

New mothers have some common concerns regardless of the method of feeding.

Preparation of Formula

CLIENT
INFANT-CARE
EDUCATION

Action

1. Wash hands well before starting.
2. If canned formula is used, wash the top of the can with soap and water, using friction, and then thoroughly rinse with hot water.
3. Wash all equipment thoroughly in warm soapy water. A bottle and nipple brush should be used and water squeezed through the nipple to make sure no milk particles or residue remain. Equipment is thoroughly rinsed to remove all traces of soap or detergent.
4. Cover opened cans of formula or milk with foil or plastic wrap and store in the refrigerator. Opened formula must be used within 48 hr.

Rationale

1. Removes pathogens from hands.
2. Removes dust and pathogens from can.

3. Milk particles occlude nipple openings. Using clean dry equipment reduces possibility of growth of bacteria.

4. Covering opened formula protects it from pathogens transmitted through dust or air. Growth of bacteria is likely after milk is open for 48 hr.

TABLE 21-4

*Formula Preparation Using Concentrated Formula**

One-Bottle Method	Clean Method	Aseptic Method	Terminal Sterilization
1. Open can of concentrated formula; pour one-half of total amount desired into bottle. 2. Add equal amount of fresh tap water from safe source. 3. Feed within 30 min of preparation. 4. Discard if not used within 1 hr. 5. Remaining one-half can of concentrated formula is covered with foil and can be stored in refrigerator for 24 hr.	1. Same as one-bottle method, but prepare day's supply at one time. 2. Refrigerate immediately after preparation.	1. Equipment includes glass or enamel pitcher, measuring cup and spoons, mixing spoons, funnel, can opener, tongs. 2. Sterilize bottles, nipples, nipple caps, and all equipment by boiling for 10 min in pan or sterilizer half full of water. 3. Mix formula in pitcher. 4. Pour into bottles. 5. Put on nipples and caps. Refrigerate until needed.	1. Prepare as in clean method. 2. Apply nipples and caps loosely. 3. Place in sterilizer with water in bottom and cover with tight-fitting lid. 4. Boil for 25 min. 5. Tighten nipple collars. 6. Refrigerate until needed.

*For all methods start by washing hands, formula can top, bottles, nipples, and equipment well.
Ready-to-feed and powdered formula can be prepared by any of the above methods.
Ready-to-feed formula needs no water or mixing.
For powdered formula follow directions on can for proportions.

Hunger

The mother may wonder how she can tell if the infant is getting enough to eat. Most infants when awakened from sleep by hunger "pains" will fuss and cry and make sucking movements with their mouths. If the infant awakens a short time after feeding, the mother should try comfort measures such as holding, changing the diaper, and bubbling before as-

NURSING
CARE
PLAN

Infant and Mother Who Are Breast-Feeding

Goals (Expected Outcomes)	Interventions	Rationale	Evaluation
Ineffective Breast-feeding—Related to Lack of Prior Experience and Information			
Mother and infant will demonstrate successful breast-feeding behaviors.	Assist mother with breast-feeding.	Allows nurse to identify and correct errors in breast-feeding techniques.	Mother identifies "hungry" behaviors accurately.
	Discuss feeding behaviors of the term newborn.	Enables mother to identify signs of hunger and respond appropriately to meet infant's needs.	Infant "latches on" correctly, sucks vigorously. Baby empties breasts every 2 to 3 hr.
	Put newborn to breast when he/she demonstrates "hungry" behaviors (e.g., sucking fist).	Increases potential for successful breast-feeding.	Mother expresses satisfaction with breast-feeding.
	Help mother to position self comfortably.	Comfortable position facilitates relaxation; maternal tension or pain inhibits the let-down reflex.	
	Moisten nipple with a small amount of expressed colostrum or milk.	Scent of colostrum stimulates infant rooting.	
	Help mother to position the infant with his/her body turned toward her breast and his/her mouth covering the areola.	Facilitates "latching-on". Allows effective sucking to compress the ducts and eject milk.	
Altered Nutrition: Less Than Body Requirements—Related to Infant's Ineffective Sucking Technique			
Infant will nurse for at least 10 min every 2 to 3 hr.	Assist mother with breast-feeding.	Allows nurse to identify and correct errors in breast-feeding techniques.	
	Verify placement of mother's nipple in infant's mouth.	Facilitates "latching-on" and effective sucking to empty breasts into the infant's mouth.	Infant "latches-on" easily and correctly; sucks vigorously.
	Encourage frequent (every 2 to 3 hr) feedings.	Feeding offered at times when infant usually is hungry.	Infant nurses for at least 10 minutes every 2 to 3 hr.
	Describe signs that infant is receiving adequate nutrition, i.e., voiding, sleeping, weight gain.	Voiding reflects state of hydration. Undisturbed sleep intervals indicate hunger has been satisfied. Weight gain demonstrates nutritional needs are being met.	Infant wets 4 to 6 diapers daily. Sleeps well. Weight loss does not exceed 5% to 10% of birth weight. Regains birth weight within 7 to 10 days after birth.

suming he or she is hungry. If he or she is obviously hungry and crying, the infant may need to eat more frequently for awhile if he or she is breast-fed or may need more in his or her bottle at each feeding if bottle-fed.

Bubbling

In the middle of the formula or when the infant is changed to the other breast and at the end of the feeding, the infant should be held in an upright position and his or her back gently patted or stroked. Milk may be regurgitated with the gas bubbles. Breast-fed infants tend not to swallow as much air as bottle-fed infants. After the feeding the infant is placed in his or her crib on the right side or in a prone position, which helps him or her bring up the air and also prevents choking on any milk that may be regurgitated with the air.

Hiccoughs

The mother may need reassurance that hiccoughs are common and do not seem to bother infants. The infant may be fed again, but hiccoughs usually go away without treatment.

Constipation

Constipation is almost nonexistent in breast-fed newborns and is uncommon in infants fed commercially prepared formulas. Typically, newborns do make grunting noises and may get red in the face with a normal soft stool. Infants may miss having a daily bowel movement. Constipation exists if the stools are hard, formed, and difficult to pass. Breast-fed infants usually have 6 to 10 loose yellow stools per day, whereas formula-fed infants have brown stools once or twice per day.

REFERENCES

1. Reeder S, Martin L: Maternity Nursing, 16th ed. Philadelphia, JB Lippincott, 1987
2. Avery GB (ed): Neonatology, 3rd ed. Philadelphia, JB Lippincott, 1987

SUGGESTED READINGS

Foster RLR, Hunsberger MM, Anderson JJT: Family Centered Nursing Care of Children. Philadelphia, WB Saunders, 1989

Holmes J, Magiera L: Maternity Nursing. New York, Macmillan, 1987

Iyer P, Taptich BJ, Bernocchi-Losey D: Nursing Process and Nursing Diagnosis. Philadelphia, WB Saunders, 1986

Klaus M, Fanaroff A: Care of the High-Risk Neonate, 3rd ed. Philadelphia, WB Saunders, 1986

Waechter EG, Phillips J, Holoday B: Nursing Care of Children, 10th ed. Philadelphia, JB Lippincott, 1985

Whaley L, Wong D: Essentials of Pediatric Nursing, 3rd ed. St. Louis, CV Mosby, 1989

Maternal Disorders

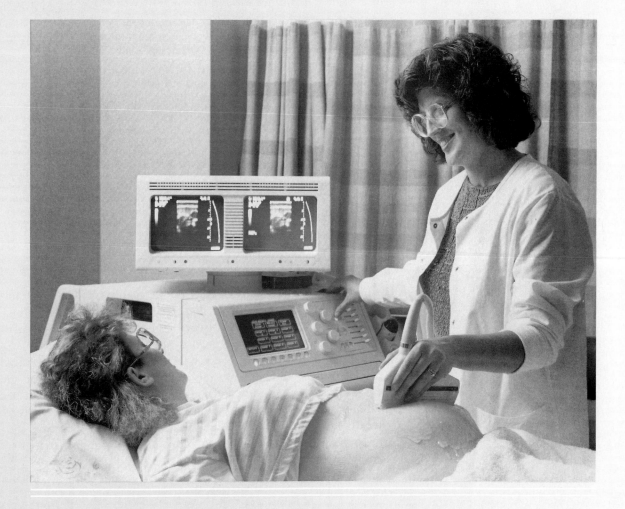

High-Risk Pregnancy

IMPORTANT TERMINOLOGY

biophysical profile Used to assess the fetus at risk for intrauterine compromise; ultrasonography assesses four of five variables: fetal breathing movement, body movement, tone, and amniotic fluid volume (FHR reactivity is assessed with nonstress test); a score of 8 to 10 is considered normal

chorionic villi sampling (CVS) Procedure in which a sample of tissue (chorionic villi) is obtained transvaginally from the edge of the placenta for genetic studies; performed early in the pregnancy at 8 to 12 weeks gestation

estriol determination Test used to determine amount of estriol, a form of estrogen produced by the placenta, in maternal blood plasma or 24-hour urine collection; indication of well-being of maternal-fetal-placental unit

fetoscopy Direct visualization of the fetus through a tiny endoscope introduced through the abdominal wall into the uterus with woman under local anesthesia; a tiny sample of fetal skin or blood is obtained

high-risk pregnancy Pregnancy in which the mother or her fetus or neonate experiences or is at risk for increased morbidity or mortality

hydramnios Excessive amount of amniotic fluid; may be associated with certain congenital anomalies, e.g., tracheoesophageal fistula

late deceleration Periodic decrease in the baseline fetal heart rate occurring after onset of uterine contraction, returning to baseline after contraction, and usually requiring some intervention; indicates uteroplacental insufficiency

In the last 50 years of obstetric care maternal morbidity and mortality have been significantly reduced. Perinatal mortality has not comparably reduced, however, and the fetus or neonate in any given pregnancy is now at greater risk than the mother. A **high-risk pregnancy** is one in which the mother or her baby has an increased chance of death or disability occurring before, during, or after birth. If possible, any factor contributing to mortality and morbidity in a particular pregnancy must be identified and early action taken. Typically, more than one risk factor (multifactorial) is identified in the high-risk pregnancy. For example, the pregnant adolescent less than 15 years old is likely to be unmarried, to have persistent ambivalence about the pregnancy, and to have family conflicts. In addition, the pregnant teenager is likely to have complications of pregnancy.

High-Risk Screening

The nurse, midwife, or physician is responsible for making a careful assessment and evaluating every pregnant woman who presents herself for care at the doctor's office or clinic. A high-risk factor identification tool that includes both social and obstetric facets is found in Table 22-1.

TABLE 22-1

Prenatal Risk Indicator Form

Risk Score*	Risk Indicator
	Demographic Factors
2	Maternal Age: 15 or under, 35 or over
1	Parity: Nulliparous
2	Grand multipara
1	Race: Nonwhite
1	Marital status: Out of wedlock
1	Economic status: Dependent on public assistance
2	Prenatal care: First visit after 27 weeks or less than five visits
	Obstetric Factors
1	Infertility factors: <2 yr
2	>2 yr
1	Previous abortion: One
2	Two or more
	Premature or low birth weight infant:
1	History of one
5	History of two or more
7	This pregnancy
	Previous excessive size infant:
1	One
2	Two or more
5	Previous perinatal loss: One
7	Two or more
7	Postterm, beyond 42 weeks: This pregnancy
5	Previous cesarean delivery
1	Previous congenital anomaly
7	Incompetent cervix
5	Uterine anomaly
2	Contracted pelvis
1	Abnormal presentation: History of
7	This pregnancy
7	Rh negative, sensitized
7	Polyhydramnios
1	Preeclampsia, mild: History of
3	This pregnancy
2	Preeclampsia, severe: History of
7	This pregnancy
1	Multiple pregnancy: History of
7	This pregnancy
	Miscellaneous Factors
1	Nutrition: More than 20% overweight
5	Massive obesity
2	More than 10% under-weight
3	Poor nutrition
5	Inadequate weight gain (<12 pounds)
3	Excessive weight gain (>48 pounds)

Continued

TABLE 22-1

Prenatal Risk Indicator Form—
continued

Risk Score*	Risk Indicator
1	Smoking more than one pack/day
1	Drug or alcohol abuse: History of
	This pregnancy
	Medical Factors
1	Anemia: 8-10 g
2	<8 g
2	Sickle cell trait
7	Sickle cell disease
2	Hypertension: Mild
7	Severe
2	Heart disease: Class I or II
5	Class III or IV
7	Heart failure: History of
7	This pregnancy
3	Diabetes: Gestational
7	Overt
1	Thyroid disease: History of
7	This pregnancy
	Venereal disease
1	gonorrhea or syphilis: History of
5	This pregnancy
3	Cervical neoplasia
	Urinary tract infection
1	afebrile: History of
3	This pregnancy
	Urinary tract infection
2	febrile: History of
5	This pregnancy
	Psychiatric or neurologic problem:
1	History of
1	This pregnancy
	Other medical condition (e.g., pulmonary disease, severe influenza):
1	History of
5	This pregnancy

Risk Score

_____	At first visit
_____	At 36 weeks
_____	On admission to labor and delivery

From Edwards L et al: Simplified antepartum risk-scoring system. Obstet Gynecol 5(2):238, 1979. Reprinted with permission from The American College of Obstetricians and Gynecologists.
*Risk factors have been assigned a weighted number from 7 (highest) to 1 (lowest). A total score of 7 or more places the woman in the high-risk category. Patients identified as high risk should be referred for consultation or intensified prenatal care.

The Pregnant Adolescent

The United States leads the developed countries in the number of pregnancies among adolescents from 15 to 19 years of age. In 1985 there were 51.3 live births/1000 women aged 15 to 19 years in the United States. The rate in the United States is double the rate in England, the country with the second highest rate. There are many theories about the cause of the high pregnancy rates in U.S. teenagers. See display on page 585 for factors influencing the incidence of adolescent pregnancy, which affects the girl, her family, the father of the baby, his family, and the community. A list of family difficulties a teenage pregnancy may cause is found in the display on page 585.

Factors Influencing the Incidence of Adolescent Pregnancy

Developmental Factors

Early physical sexual maturation
Egocentrism
Personal fable (feeling that "it won't happen to me")
Responsiveness to peers' sexual activity
Independence from family
Denial of personal sexuality

Societal Factors

Variety of adult sexual behavior values
Implied acceptance of intercourse outside of marriage
Importance of involvement in heterosexual relationships stressed by the media
Inadequate access to contraception
Access to public financial support for teen parents and offspring

Family and Friends

Difficult mother–daughter relationship
Lack of religious affiliation
Sexually permissive behavior norms of the larger peer group
Sexually permissive values and behavior of close friends
Inadequate communication in heterosexual relationships

From Foster RLR, Hunsberger MM, Anderson JJJ: Family Centered Nursing Care of Children. Philadelphia, WB Saunders, 1989.

Family Difficulties for the Adolescent Parent

Intermittent Crises of Teenage Pregnancy

Recognition of pregnancy
Adolescent crisis
Family crisis

Prenatal Difficulties

Termination or continuation of pregnancy
Special high-risk difficulties
Economic, nutrition, and medication needs
Body image and exercise
Interpersonal relationships

Intrapartum Difficulties

Labor and delivery difficulties
Environmental control and depersonalization problems

Postpartum Difficulties

Possibility of adoption
Body image changes
Breast-feeding
Problems from cesarean section
Environmental restrictions
Bonding
Birth control
Parenting

Adapted from Johnson SH: Nursing Assessment and Strategies for the Family at Risk: High Risk Parenting. Philadelphia, JB Lippincott, 1986.

Assessment

Statistically the teenager and her baby have a higher risk of mortality than the older gravida. Specific health risks of the teenager and her baby are toxemia, preterm or prolonged labor, cephalopelvic disproportion, and low infant birth weight. Some particular factors that indicate the adolescent is at risk for complications are found in the display on page 587. Nursing assessment of the adolescent during pregnancy parallels that of the older woman. In addition, she is assessed in areas in which she is especially vulnerable (see Assessment Tool: Specific Needs of Pregnant Adolescents and Focus Assessment).

Nursing Diagnosis

Nursing diagnoses that may apply to the pregnant adolescent will vary according to her age, social support systems, health, and maturity (see Potential Nursing Diagnoses: Adolescent or High-Risk Pregnancy).

ASSESSMENT
TOOL

Specific Needs of Pregnant Adolescents

1. Ask client to describe or write down her food intake for the past 24 hr or for a typical day.
   a. Type of food
   b. How it was prepared
   c. Amount eaten
2. Evaluate adequacy of diet for sufficient caloric intake to meet needs of pregnancy and the growth and development needs of the nonpregnant female adolescent.
3. Evaluate adequacy of dietary intake of iron (18 mg/24 hr).
4. Assess client's knowledge of what should be included in her diet during pregnancy.
   a. Have you read about the importance of diet in pregnancy?
   b. Have you discussed good nutrition in health class at school?
   c. Describe a "good" diet for a pregnant woman.
5. Assess her knowledge and ability to care for herself during the pregnancy.
   a. Will you need help in keeping your appointments with the doctor?
   b. Do you plan to walk, drive yourself, or will someone accompany you?
   c. When should you call the doctor during your pregnancy?
6. Have you read about the changes that take place in your body? Were they discussed in health class?
7. Are there any changes in your activities at home? At school? On weekends?
8. Will you need help to obtain the foods you will need?
9. Assess her knowledge and ability to care for the baby.
   a. Have you babysat or cared for young babies?
   b. What do you think a newly born infant is like?
   c. Will you need any help to care for your baby?
   d. Who will you ask to help you with your baby?
10. During each visit assess for the following:
    a. Adequate weight gain
    b. Signs of fatigue
11. During last trimester assess for signs of pregnancy-induced hypertension.
    a. Excessive weight gain
    b. Edema
    c. Elevated blood pressure
    d. Proteinuria

Factors Indicating the Adolescent Possibly at Risk for Complications

Age 16 years or less
Anemia
Poor physical state (e.g., obesity, low weight for height)
Any sexually transmitted disease
Use of tobacco, alcohol, or street drugs
Poverty
Lack of social support
Prior medical conditions that pregnancy may complicate (e.g., diabetes, epilepsy, asthma)

From Foster RR, Hunsberger MM, Anderson JJJ: Family Centered Nursing Care of Children. Philadelphia, WB Saunders, 1989.

Ineffective Individual Coping—lack of support system, physiologic changes of pregnancy, developmental tasks
Ineffective Family Coping: Compromised—related to preoccupation with personal reactions secondary to adolescent pregnancy
Altered Health Maintenance—related to inability to assume responsibility for meeting prenatal needs secondary to lack of knowledge regarding the value of prenatal care, access to care, and resources available
Altered Growth and Development—related to psychologic stress secondary to altered self-concept, body image, normal physiologic changes of pregnancy
Altered Nutrition, Less Than Body Requirements or More Than Body Requirements—related to lack of information regarding prenatal nutritional needs, lack of financial resources, developmental tasks of adolescence, substance abuse
Knowledge Deficit—regarding
  Physiologic changes of pregnancy
  Psychologic changes of pregnancy (developmental tasks)
  Available options, i.e., termination of pregnancy, adoption
  Process of labor and delivery
  Self-care
  Infant care
Noncompliance With Recommended Behaviors—related to developmental tasks of adolescence, cultural or value conflicts

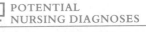

POTENTIAL
NURSING DIAGNOSES

Adolescent or High-Risk Pregnancy

Focus Assessment

Identify current knowledge level regarding:
Potential impact of pregnancy on present and future plans
Options and access to available resources
Common pregnancy-related changes
Anticipated needs and desired pregnancy-related behaviors
Determine current coping behaviors.
Identify current life-style and problem-solving abilities.
Determine adequacy of support system.
Monitor frequency of and interval between prenatal visits.
Monitor pregnancy progress closely (e.g., vital signs, weight gain, fundal height).

Planning and Intervention

The nurse who works with the pregnant adolescent must be open and nonjudgmental so that a trusting relationship can be developed. The nurse plays an important role in the adolescent's decision-making process. A teenage pregnancy may begin a cycle that includes failure to complete educational goals, dependency on the welfare system or low-paying jobs, and a subsequent unwanted pregnancy. The outcome of this cycle may be an unstable family life, neglect, and child abuse. Problems and decisions faced by the pregnant teenager include confirmation of the pregnancy, acceptance of the pregnancy, gaining family support, and whether or not to marry, to continue the pregnancy, and to allow adoption of her baby.

Early and continuing prenatal care must be encouraged. Appointments for prenatal visits may or may not be kept because of denial, ignorance of the value of prenatal care, or availability of prenatal care.

Childbirth preparation and child care classes geared to the teenager's development help prepare her for pregnancy, labor, delivery, and parenting. Because adequate nutrition can prevent or modify some of the hazards faced by the pregnant teenager and her fetus, she must be taught the basics of nutrition.

The nurse must be aware of available community resources and how to use them. Examples of resources available in many communities include prenatal clinics sponsored by health departments or hospitals and childbirth education and child care classes. A program called Women, Infants, and Children (WIC) provides supplemental high-protein foods to the teenager from the prenatal period until 6 months post partum for breast-feeding mothers and to the child until his or her fifth birthday. The program offers nutritional education and requires proof of medical supervision. Financial aid may be available through public funds or Aid to Dependent Children.

The Older Gravida

The optimum age for childbearing is generally recognized as from 20 to 30 years. Childbirth in women over 30 is increasingly common, and many authorities believe that the risks are fewer than previously believed. The firstborn of mothers over 35 is at an increased risk for prematurity, effects of toxemia, and congenital anomalies.[1] The mother over 35 years of age has an increased risk of conceiving a fetus with Down's syndrome, a chromosome abnormality resulting in moderate to severe mental retardation. Pregnant women over 35 are offered **chorionic villi sampling (CVS)** or amniocentesis to identify chromosomal anomalies in the fetus.

After the initial assessment, laboratory screening tests are obtained as early as possible. As the pregnancy advances, ongoing assessment provides the opportunity to discover factors that appear in later pregnancy, e.g., pregnancy-induced hypertension.

Assessment of Fetal Status

Performing a variety of tests is of value in monitoring the gestational age, (appropriateness of) size, well-being of the fetus, and its ability to adapt to extrauterine life. These tests include ultrasonography, computerized tomography, magnetic resonance imaging, **fetoscopy,** percuta-

TABLE 22-2

Summary of High-Risk Screening and Diagnostic Tests

Test Purpose	Test Used	When Test May Be Done
To determine amounts of amniotic fluid present	Ultrasound for gestational sac volume	5 and 6 wk after last menstrual period
To determine how advanced the pregnancy is	Ultrasound: Crown-rump length Ultrasound: Biparietal diameter and femur length	7-10 wk gestation 13-40 wk gestation
To identify normal growth of the fetus	Ultrasound: Biparietal diameter Ultrasound: Head-abdomen ratio Ultrasound: Estimated fetal weight	Most useful 20-30 wk gestation 13-40 wk gestation Approximately 28-40 wk gestation
To detect congenital anomalies and problems	Ultrasound Chorionic villus sampling Fetoscopy Percutaneous blood sampling	18-40 wk gestation 8-12 wk gestation 18 wk gestation Second and third trimesters
To locate the placenta	Ultrasound	Usually in third trimester or before amniocentesis
To assess fetal status	Biophysical profile Maternal assessment of fetal activity Estriol determination Magnetic resonance imaging Nonstress test Contraction stress test	Approximately 28 wk to delivery Approximately 27 wk to delivery During second and third trimesters During second and third trimesters Approximately 30 wk to delivery Last few wk of gestation
To diagnose cardiac problems	Fetal echocardiography	Second and third trimesters

To assess fetal lung maturity	Amniocentesis
	  LS ratio
	  Phosphatidylglycerol
	  Phosphatidylcholine
	  Shake test
		33 to 40 wk
		33 wk to delivery
		33 wk to delivery
		33 wk to delivery
		33 wk to delivery

To obtain more information about breech presentation	Computerized tomography and radiography	Just before labor is anticipated or during labor

neous umbilical blood sampling, CVS, measurement of specific hormones and enzymes in maternal blood and urine, amniocentesis, and fetal stress tests. Each procedure always involves some risk, and the risk must be acceptable to the pregnant woman. The advantages of a given test must outweigh the potential risks and added expense. (For a summary of screening and diagnostic tests, see Table 22-2.) Nursing responsibilities may include (1) providing information about the test, (2) obtaining written informed consent if required, (3) providing support, and (4) providing comfort measures (see Legal and Ethical Considerations).

≡ LEGAL AND ETHICAL CONSIDERATIONS

Wrongful life is the term given to the claim brought against the health care practitioner by the child who has some genetic or other defect. The child is asking the courts to award damages because he or she has been born with a defect because of the health care provider's failure to inform the infant's parents of the availability of amniocentesis, thereby precluding them from aborting the fetus based on test results. Although a number of courts have rejected this claim, California has allowed the child to recover damages for treating the disorder.

From Northrup CE, Kelly ME: Legal Issues in Nursing. St. Louis, CV Mosby, 1987, pp. 161-162.

FIGURE 22-1

Ultrasonography. Woman is positioned comfortably with a small pillow under her head. Display panel is positioned so she can observe images on screen if she wishes (some women do not want to watch).
Courtesy St. Elizabeth's Medical Center, Edgewood, Kentucky.

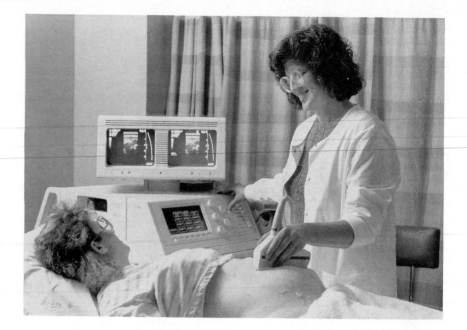

Ultrasonography

Ultrasonography, or ultrasound, is the use of sound waves to visualize outlines of fetal structures within the body (Fig. 22-1). It is used for fetal assessment because it poses minimum risk (see below). Nursing interventions during ultrasound are listed in Nursing Procedure: Ultrasound.

Some Indications for Using Ultrasound in Assessment of the High-Risk Fetus

Estimation of gestational age
Evaluation of fetal growth and development
Evaluation of suspected multiple gestation
Diagnosis of ectopic pregnancy, pelvic mass, or hydatidiform mole
Determination of location of placenta
Evaluation of fetal condition, especially if suspected fetal death
Identification of fetal anomalies
Aid to proper placement of needle in amniocentesis
Aid to special procedures such as fetoscopy or intrauterine transfusion

---

Amniocentesis

Amniocentesis, performed during a high-risk pregnancy to assess fetal status, is the removal of amniotic fluid through a needle inserted into the uterus. The amniotic fluid is then examined for fetal abnormalities (Fig. 22-2). Risks of amniocentesis include amniotic fluid embolism, hemor-

Ultrasound

Intervention	Rationale
1. Explain the procedure to the client.	Ultrasound is a painless procedure that uses sound waves to visualize the baby and placenta. No radiation (or x-ray) is used that could harm the baby. Much information is provided to the doctor about the size, age, growth, and well-being of the baby and the placement and maturity of the placenta.
2. Instruct the woman to drink at least 1 quart of water (4-5 cups) approximately 2 hr before the test if a transabdominal ultrasound is to be performed.	When the bladder is full, other pelvic structures can be identified in relation to the bladder. If a vaginal probe is used, the bladder is emptied.
3. Instruct the woman not to empty her bladder before the test.	The woman may feel discomfort because of the full bladder, so care must be taken so she is not kept waiting.
4. If the bladder is not sufficiently filled, she is asked to drink another quart of fluid and is scanned again 30 to 45 min later.	
5. Gel is spread on the abdomen.	Gel aids transmission of the sound waves.
6. The sonographer moves a transducer across the abdomen for 20-30 min to obtain a picture of the uterine contents.	
7. The woman lies on her back during the test.	If the woman experiences shortness of breath, her upper body may be elevated.
8. Allow the client and her significant other to view the screen during the procedure.	
9. Give verbal explanation and reassurance during the test.	
10. Cleanse gel from the abdomen after the procedure.	Gel is sticky and may adhere to the clothing.

rhage, infection, preterm labor, abruptio placentae, puncture of the intestine or bladder, Rh isoimmunization, and fetal injury or death. Complications occur <1% of the time. Ultrasound is used to locate the position of the fetus and placenta to decrease the potential for fetal injury (see Nursing Procedure: Amniocentesis Under Ultrasound). Before the procedure the woman is instructed to empty her bladder. The mother's vital signs and the fetal heart rate (FHR) are assessed before and after the procedure. Fetal monitoring is preferred for the first 15 to 30 minutes of the procedure. The mother is instructed to report unusual fetal hyperactivity or lack of fetal movement, vaginal discharge, uterine contractions, abdominal discomfort, fever, or chills.

FIGURE 22-2

Amniocentesis. During amniocentesis amniotic fluid is withdrawn for analysis by transabdominal needle aspiration. Early in the pregnancy the test is used to perform genetic studies. Later amniocentesis may be done to determine lung maturity status (lecithin:sphingomyelin ratio and phosphatidlyglycerol). Other tests, e.g., creatinine level, provide additional data about fetal maturity.

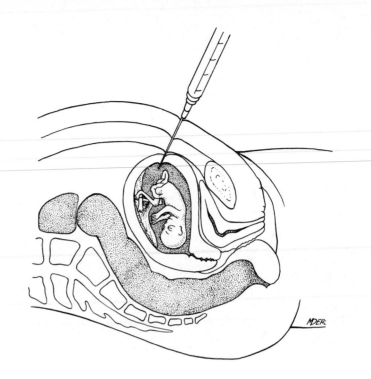

NURSING PROCEDURE

Amniocentesis Under Ultrasound

Intervention	rationale
1. Confirm informed consent.	1. Demonstrates ethical, legal accountability to client, physician, hospital, staff

2. Explain procedure step by step.
  a. Ultrasound
  b. Amniocentesis
  c. Post procedure care
	2. Reduces anxiety; enables cooperation

3. Encourage client to drink three to four glasses of water or other fluids 1 hr before procedure. Instruct client not to void. Inform her she may experience some discomfort from a full bladder.	3. Fills bladder to enhance transmission of sound waves and visualization of uterus
4. Assemble all equipment; prepare labels for specimen containers.	4. Facilitates effective, efficient completion of procedure
5. Immediately before procedure, take blood pressure and fetal heart rate.	5. Provides baseline for comparison

6. Place client in supine position.
  a. Instruct client to fold her hands on her chest or place them over her head.
 	
  b. Remind client to remain still throughout the procedure.
  c. If procedure is performed in later pregnancy, may elevate right hip on small pillow.
	6. Facilitates locating placenta and fetus with Doppler
	  a. Reduces risk of accidental contamination by client
	  b. Reduces risk of injury to client or fetus
	
	  c. Minimizes the potential for supine hypotensive (vena caval) syndrome

7. Ultrasonographer will coat abdomen with conductive gel.	7. Enables transmission of sound waves
8. Transducer is passed vertically and horizontally across the client's abdomen.	8. Locates position of fetus, placenta, and pocket(s) of amniotic fluid; verifies fetal life; minimizes risk of injury to fetus, placenta, or maternal organs

Amniocentesis Under Ultrasound—continued

Intervention	Rationale
9. If assisting with the procedure, mask, scrub, gown, and glove while ultrasound is in progress.	9. This is a sterile procedure
10. Cleanse abdomen with antiseptic solution.	10. Removes surface microorganisms; reduces risk of infection
11. Drape client's abdomen.	11. Maintains sterile field
12. Assist as directed, maintaining sterile technique.	12. Facilitates effective, efficient completion of sterile procedure
a. If requested, prepare sterile syringe with local anesthetic.	a. Physician may use local anesthetic to reduce client discomfort from needle insertion
b. Provide sterile 20- or 22-gauge spinal needle with stylette in place. Ready sterile 20 to 30 cc syringe for use.	b. Size appropriate to aspirate fluid with minimum tissue trauma
c. Open sterile specimen tubes; prepare to receive specimen.	c. Contamination can cause chromosomal aberrations
d. Physician will discard first 5 ml of fluid.	d. May contain maternal cells
e. Collect sterile specimen; cap tubes tightly.	e. Protects specimen from contamination or spilling
13. When physician withdraws needle, remove drapes and apply adhesive bandage over insertion site.	13. Protects puncture wound
14. Complete laboratory request slips; send specimen to laboratory immediately.	14. Assures prompt, appropriate treatment of specimen
15. Monitor maternal vital signs and fetal heart rate every 15 min for 30 min or for 1 to 2 hr (according to hospital protocol).	15. Detects changes from baseline; identifies early signs of complications; ensures prompt treatment
16. Instruct client to notify physician promptly of	16. Assures prompt evaluation of maternal and fetal status
a. Vaginal discharge of fluid or blood	
b. Decreased fetal movement	
c. Contractions	
d. Fever, chills	
17. Complete client record.	17. Documents procedure instructions given and client status at discharge

Sample Narrative Charting: Postamniocentesis. Alert and responsive. No complaint of pain. Bandage applied to site. Bandage dry and intact. Resting on examining table. Temperature 98.8°F (oral), BP 110/76, P 68, R 16. FHR LLQ 136. Instructions reviewed regarding reporting of bleeding, fever, or leakage of amniotic fluid. Verbalized understanding of how to contact Dr. Edmiston.

Fetoscopy

Direct visualization of the fetus can be accomplished by the use of a tiny endoscope. With the client under local anesthesia, the fetoscope is inserted into the uterus through the abdominal wall (Fig. 22-3). Small amounts of fetal blood and skin can be obtained from the placental vessels during fetoscopy. Diseases with blood abnormalities such as hemophilia can be diagnosed. This procedure is performed in large perinatal centers.

Nonstress Test

The nonstress test (NST) evaluates changes in the FHR in response to fetal movements with an external fetal monitor (see display on p. 594). The fetus is normally active, and its movement results in an increase of the FHR. This FHR acceleration implies the central nervous system is

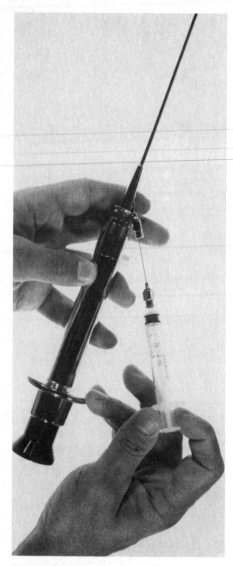

FIGURE 22-3

Fetoscope. Direct visualization of the fetus is achieved by introducing a fine-caliber endoscope through the abdominal wall and into the amnionic sac.

Nonstress Test

Purpose

Demonstrates that FHR increases normally with movement.

Results

Reactive: FHR accelerations are present, indicating a healthy fetus.
Nonreactive: Normal accelerations are not present with movement, or lack of fetal movement may mean the fetus is sleeping or compromised. Further evaluation is indicated.

---

responsive and not affected by hypoxia. The NST is performed by applying two straps around the woman's abdomen. One strap holds a tocodynamometer, which detects fetal movement or uterine contractions. The other is the ultrasound transducer, which monitors the FHR in response to fetal movement.

The test is read as reactive or nonreactive. A reactive test demonstrates two FHR accelerations >15 beats/min above the baseline and lasting 15 seconds or more, with fetal movement in a 10-minute period. Failure to demonstrate a reactive pattern owing either to lack of accelerations with movement or to lack of fetal movement is taken as an indication for further evaluation of the fetus by a contraction stress test.

Contraction Stress Testing

The contraction stress testing (CST) (see below) is used to identify the fetus at risk for intrauterine hypoxia by observing the response of the FHR to uterine contractions. Contractions are stimulated by infusing intravenous oxytocin or by nipple stimulation. Many hospitals require performance of the test in or near the labor and delivery unit. The nurse ascertains that the infusion is running at the prescribed rate and reports any changes in maternal or fetal condition immediately. An infusion pump is used so that the amount of oxytocin can be measured accurately. Uterine contractions and fetal heart tones are monitored electronically and are assessed by the nurse at least every 15 minutes. After obtaining a 10-minute baseline FHR, contractions are stimulated. Oxytocin is administered until three uterine contractions lasting 40 to 60 seconds occur in a 10-minute period. If **late decelerations** occur more than three times or if contractions last longer than 60 seconds or occur closer than every 5 minutes, the infusion should be discontinued.

Contraction Stress Test

Purpose

Evaluates the reaction of the FHR to induced or spontaneous contractions.

Results

Negative (desired test outcome): No late deceleration of the FHR when an adequate frequency of three contractions in 10 min has been established.
Positive: Occurrence of late decelerations with three contractions in 10 min.
Unsatisfactory test: Inadequate contractions or FHR records.

In a positive stress test late FHR decelerations are present with at least 50% of uterine contractions. The fetus is identified as potentially unable to tolerate uterine contractions. Determining if the woman with a positive CST should have a cesarean delivery depends on how quickly the baby must be delivered to avoid severe fetal distress, the fetal maturity of the lungs, and how close the mother is to vaginal delivery at the time the decision is made.

Maternal Assessment of Fetal Movement

A simple, inexpensive, and noninvasive method of assessing fetal health is the maternal monitoring of fetal movements during the third trimester. Some health care providers recommend that all pregnant women, starting with the 28th week of gestation, count fetal movements and complete a chart. The count is done two to three times a day for 30 minutes each time or just once each day. Most women report perceiving 10 movements in 20 minutes to 2 hours. The nurse instructs the mother that her activity, e.g., eating a meal, walking, or smoking, may increase the fetus' movements. Babies have periods of sleep that will decrease fetal activity. The woman is instructed what to report and the value of reporting.

In addition, fetal monitoring can be done using an attached monitoring device that permits the mother to go about her daily activities (Fig. 22-4).

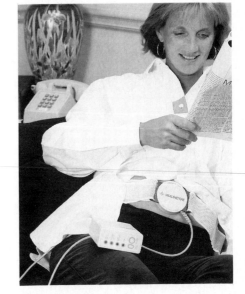

FIGURE 22-4

Home Monitoring. A woman using a home uterine monitor, which can store data and transmit it over telephone lines. The purpose of home monitoring is to detect signs of uterine activity in the woman who is at risk for preterm labor.
Courtesy Health Dyne Prenatal Services, Marietta, Georgia.

Concurrent Maternal Diseases
Diabetes Mellitus

Women with diabetes mellitus are able to conceive and maintain pregnancies because of modern management, although perinatal morbidity and mortality remain significantly higher in diabetic pregnancies than in normal pregnancies. Maternal fetal complications are increased for women with a longer history of diabetes or poor control of diabetes before pregnancy.

Gestational Diabetes

Diabetes has been classified in several ways. The currently accepted classification is found in the display below. Gestational diabetes mellitus (GDM) is a carbohydrate intolerance that is diagnosed during pregnancy

---

Classification of Diabetes by the National Diabetes Data Group of National Institutes of Health (1979)

Type I: insulin dependent (IDDM)
Type II: noninsulin dependent (NIDDM)
   Nonobese
   Obese
Secondary diabetes
Impaired glucose tolerance or subclinical diabetes (IGT)
Gestational diabetes (GDM)

From National Diabetes Data Group: Classification and diagnosis of diabetes mellitus and other categories of glucose intolerance. Diabetes 28:1042, 1979.

TABLE 22-3

Effects of Diabetes Mellitus on Pregnancy

Effects on Mother	Effects on Fetus or Neonate
Fourfold increase of pregnancy-induced hypertension	High perinatal mortality rate
Infection, commonly severe	Birth trauma caused by large size
Dystocia caused by large baby	Fourfold increase of congenital, especially cardiac, anomalies
Hydramnios	Postnatal hypoglycemia
Increased frequency of cesarean section	Polycythemia
Postpartum hemorrhage	Hyperbilirubinemia

and disappears after delivery. Perinatal mortality rates are approximately doubled in pregnancies complicated by undiagnosed gestational diabetes.[1]

Effects of Pregnancy on Diabetes

During the course of pregnancy the maternal requirements for insulin increases. The placenta produces human placental lactogen (hPL), which is an insulin antagonist. Estrogen and progesterone also counteract the influence of insulin. A placental enzyme, insulinase, accelerates the breakdown of insulin. The glomerular filtration rate of glucose in the kidneys is increased, resulting in a reduction of the renal threshold for glucose from normal nonpregnant levels. These physiologic alterations in insulin and carbohydrate metabolism cause pregnancy to be a diabetogenic condition.

During the pregnancy the fasting blood sugar is lower. In the first trimester the caloric intake may be decreased because of anorexia, nausea, or vomiting. At the same time there is a significant transfer of glucose to the embryo or fetus. The pregnant diabetic is at risk for hypoglycemia (Table 22-3).

As insulin requirements rise and insulin antagonist factors rise during the second half of pregnancy, the pregnant woman is prone to hyperglycemia and may develop ketoacidosis. After delivery and during the early postpartum period insulin demands drop dramatically because of the rapid clearance of hPL. Insulin administration is greatly reduced or discontinued.

Therapeutic Management

In any client who has glucosuria, diabetes should be suspected, and the diagnosis should be established or ruled out by evaluation of glucose blood levels (see display on p. 597). The glucose tolerance test (GTT) administered orally (50 g or 100 g) or intravenously (25 g) is primarily used to screen potential diabetes during pregnancy. An oral GTT is considered abnormal if two of the client's blood glucose values are elevated or if one blood glucose value is exceeded in two successive tests.

Medical care of the client with diabetes includes dietary regulation, glucose monitoring, insulin administration, evaluation of mother and baby for complications, and education of the couple (see display on p. 597).

Assessment

Prenatal assessment should include obtaining a careful nursing history and performing an analysis of predisposing factors in the client's prenatal

Blood Tests Used in Diagnosing Diabetes

Fasting blood sugar (FBS): Test used to determine the amount of glucose remaining in the blood after a period of fasting. Two elevations >140 mg/dl are indicative of diabetes mellitus.

Two hour postprandial test: A more sensitive test but not considered totally diagnostic of diabetes.

Oral glucose tolerance test (OGTT): Considered positive if plasma glucose concentration is 200 mg/dl or higher 1 to 2 hr after a measured intake of oral glucose.

Intravenous glucose tolerance test (IGTT): Preferred test in pregnancy because glucose absorption from the intestinal tract may vary and alter findings of OGTT.

Principles of Management of Diabetes During Pregnancy

Principle 1: Strict control of maternal glucose levels
Principle 2: Prompt detection and treatment of maternal complications
Principle 3: Fetal surveillance, including diagnosis of fetal macrosomia
Principle 4: Avoidance of unnecessary premature delivery

Modified from Gibbons JM: Diabetes in pregnancy. In Schnatz JD (ed): Diabetes Mellitus: Problems in Management. Menlo Park, Calif, Addison-Wesley, 1982.

and family history (see Assessment Tool: Diabetes in Pregnancy). Prenatal assessment includes observing for signs and symptoms that may indicate gestational diabetes or complications in the preconceptional diabetic. A steady rise in blood pressure or a sudden increase in weight may be a sign of pregnancy-induced hypertension, a frequent complication of diabetes. The presence of bacteriuria is a forerunner of pyelonephritis, to which the diabetic is prone. The client's need for teaching about her disease and self-care is assessed.

Diabetes in Pregnancy

ASSESSMENT
TOOL

Ask client while obtaining nursing history if she has any of the risk factors for diabetes:
   Previous infant weighing more than 9 pounds
   Previous pregnancy loss
   Previous neonatal death, stillbirth, anomaly, or premature infant
   Family history of diabetes mellitus or previous gestational diabetes
   History of hypertension or recurrent urinary tract infections or candidiasis
At each prenatal visit observe client for the following:
   Weight gain
   Glucosuria on two or more visits
   Fundal height greater than expected for gestation
   Signs of diabetes
      Polyuria beyond first trimester and before third trimester
      Polydipsia
      Polyphagia
      Weight loss
If diabetes is diagnosed, assess client's knowledge of the following:
   Signs and symptoms of hypoglycemia
   Signs and symptoms of hyperglycemia
   Signs and symptoms of urinary tract infections or candidiasis
   Self-care, including diet and insulin if needed

The woman may be concerned about the well-being of her baby, the high cost of hospitalization, and antepartum testing procedures for herself and her baby. The nurse must be aware of these and other possible causes of anxiety produced by a diagnosis of diabetes.

Nursing Diagnosis

Potential nursing diagnoses for the pregnant diabetic are related to fear, lack of self-care information, potential for fetal effects, importance of adequate nutrition, and infection susceptibility.

Planning and Intervention

During pregnancy nursing care is focused on assessment of the diabetic mother and fetus using tests that screen and verify maternal and fetal well-being. Teaching the diabetic mother and her family about diet, glucose testing, and other aspects of self-care is another important aspect of antenatal nursing care. The woman and her fetus are monitored closely during the last 8 to 10 weeks of pregnancy. For more precise monitoring of mother and fetus, the mother may require hospitalization, usually at a level III facility.

During labor the mother's blood glucose level is monitored carefully. Regular insulin is usually added to the intravenous infusion of glucose. The intravenous insulin is discontinued with the third stage of labor. The

---

POTENTIAL NURSING DIAGNOSES

Pregnant Diabetic

Fear—related to impact of disorder (diabetes) on pregnancy outcome

Knowledge Deficit—related to effects of pregnancy on diabetes, effects of diabetes on pregnancy, and required behavioral alterations, e.g., diet, exercise, prenatal evaluation of fetal status

Potential for Injury (Maternal or Fetal)—related to ketosis secondary to nausea and vomiting

Potential for Injury (Fetal)—related to effects of prolonged hyperglycemia or inadequate uteroplacental function

Altered Nutrition: More Than Body Requirements—related to hyperglycemia secondary to the action of placental hormones and enzymes on levels of circulating insulin

Altered Nutrition: Less Than Body Requirements—related to hypoglycemia secondary to increased metabolic rate of pregnancy and imbalance between food intake and insulin availability

Potential for Infection—related to diminished resistance to disease secondary to diabetes, elevated blood glucose, and decreased tissue perfusion

---

Focus Assessment

Identify when client first developed symptoms.

Determine current management of disorder and effects on symptoms.

Determine specific learning needs, e.g., prenatal diabetic diet, capillary blood glucose testing (CBG), signs and symptoms of hyperglycemia and hypoglycemia.

Monitor blood glucose levels (client report, lab report, CBGs)

Explore complaints that suggest complications of pregnancy, e.g., hyperemesis, threatened abortion, premature labor, or infection.

As pregnancy progresses:

Monitor fundal height for indications of fetal macrosomia, hydramnios.

Monitor fetal status, e.g., nonstress testing.

laboring woman is encouraged to lie on her left side to promote placental perfusion.

After birth diabetes control and establishment of parent–child relationships are priorities of care. During the first 24 hours the mother requires much less insulin because the levels of hPL fall after placental separation. Insulin needs are determined by blood sugar testing.

Since the newborn usually is placed in a special care nursery, the mother needs support and information about her infant's condition. Infants of diabetic mothers (IDM) are at risk for being large for gestational age (LGA) and for hypoglycemia, birth trauma, and respiratory distress.

Breast-feeding is supported if it is the mother's chosen feeding method. The postpartum diabetic must be frequently assessed for vaginal bleeding and fundal firmness because of the increased incidence of postpartum bleeding with an LGA infant or with **hydramnios.**

Evaluation

Expected outcomes of nursing care are as follows:
1. The client verbalizes understanding of her condition and its impact on pregnancy.
2. The client demonstrates self-care techniques such as testing of blood for glucose.
3. The client demonstrates care of her newborn, including feeding, diapering, bathing.

Cardiac Disease

Approximately 1% of all pregnant women have some type of cardiac disease. The majority of these women is able to complete a pregnancy successfully. Common types of heart conditions seen during pregnancy are congenital heart disease, a heart defect that has been surgically repaired, and rheumatic heart disease. The likelihood of a favorable perinatal outcome depends on the functional capacity of the heart and the presence or absence of other complications that increase cardiac load. See Table 22-4 for classification of heart disease. The presence of cardiac disease

TABLE 22-4

Classification of Heart Disease

Class	Description
I	Cardiac disease with *no* limitation of physical activity. Absence of symptoms of cardiac insufficiency and anginal pain.
II	Cardiac disease with *slight* limitation of physical activity. Comfortable at rest. Experiences fatigue, palpitation, dyspnea, or anginal pain with *ordinary* physical activity
III	Cardiac disease with *moderate* to *marked* limitation of physical activity. Comfortable at rest. Experiences excessive fatigue, palpitation, dyspnea, or anginal pain with *less* than ordinary physical activity.
IV	Cardiac disease with *inability* to perform any physical activity without discomfort. Symptoms of cardiac insufficiency or of the anginal syndrome may occur *at rest* and with *any* physical activity.

Adapted from The Criteria Committee of New York State Heart Association: Nomenclature and Criteria for Diagnosis of Diseases of the Heart and Blood Vessels, 6th ed. Boston, Little, Brown, 1964.

Heart Disease in Pregnancy

1. Ask client to describe the following:
   a. Ability to perform various types of physical activities before pregnancy
   b. Dyspnea on exertion
   c. Coughing
   d. Palpitations
2. At each prenatal visit assess the following:
   a. Heart and breath sounds
   b. Edema and tenderness of extremities
   c. Baseline vital signs and FHR
   d. Symptoms of cardiac decompression: coughing and hemoptysis, dyspnea or orthopnea, edema, heart murmurs, palpitations, rales
3. Note results of tests and report to physician:
   a. Chest x-ray examination
   b. Electrocardiogram

---

increases the risk for a low birth weight infant, premature labor, and intrauterine fetal hypoxia.

Assessment

The stress of pregnancy on the functional capacity of the heart is assessed initially and during each antepartum visit (see Assessment Tool: Heart Disease in Pregnancy). Some signs to assess are the same as ones in a pregnant woman without cardiac problems. The woman with cardiac problems is observed for the appearance and progression of the signs of congestive heart falure (CHF). These cardiac assessments are particularly important at 28 to 32 weeks gestation when the blood volume reaches its maximum. If CHF signs appear, prompt medical therapy is required. Delivery is not attempted until cardiac status improves. (See Focus Assessment.)

Nursing Diagnosis

Potential nursing diagnoses that may apply to the pregnant woman with heart disease include activity intolerance, anxiety, lack of information, and changes in cardiac output.

Planning and Intervention

ANTEPARTUM INTERVENTIONS. All women with heart disease require additional rest during pregnancy. A minimum of 10 hours of sleep per night plus morning and afternoon rest periods is recommended. The diet should be well balanced, including approximately 2200 calories, large amounts of high-quality protein, and no salt added to food. Excess weight gain places additional stress on the heart and circulation. The gravida may require specific drug therapy. CHF may be treated with digitalis, thiazide, and diuretics, e.g., furosemide (Lasix). Both maternal and fetal heart rates are slowed by the administration of digitalis, which crosses the placental barrier. Dysrhythmias may be safely treated with quinidine. Coagulation problems are treated with the anticoagulant heparin, which does not cross

POTENTIAL
NURSING DIAGNOSES

Fluid Volume Excess—related to normal physiologic changes of pregnancy
Activity Intolerance—related to cardiac overload secondary to the normal physiologic changes of pregnancy
Anxiety—related to the effect of cardiac condition on perinatal outcomes
Knowledge Deficit—Regarding maternal or fetal implications of cardiac disorders in pregnancy, protective self-care activities
Decreased Cardiac Output—related to cardiac decompensation during pregnancy

Focus Assessment

Determine current cardiac status and management.
Identify number of weeks gestation.
Monitor vital signs closely.
Explore complaints of fatigue with usual activities, dyspnea, sleep pattern disturbance, signs of infection.

the placental barrier. Penicillin may be used as prophylaxis for women with valvular disease and congenital heart disease.

INTRAPARTUM INTERVENTIONS. The laboring woman with heart disease must be relieved of discomfort, anxiety, and fatigue. Relaxation is encouraged and administering a systemic analgesic and sedatives may be useful early in labor. To facilitate cardiac circulation and maximum oxygenation, the client is placed in a semi-Fowler's or side-lying position with her head and shoulders elevated. Oxygen administration may be indicated. Vaginal deliveries are preferable to cesarean births. In the second stage of labor forceps are often applied to avoid maternal pushing.

POSTPARTUM NURSING INTERVENTIONS. After delivery the mother is observed for cardiac decompensation, particularly in the first 24 hours. She may remain in the hospital longer than others to rest and recover. Her activities should be gradual and progressive. Depending on the mother's cardiac status, the nurse may provide care for the newborn for the first few days. The mother needs support and information about her infant during this time.

Evaluation

Anticipated outcomes are as follows:
1. The client shows no signs of congestive heart failure.
2. The client verbalizes the signs and symptoms of possible complications during the pregnancy and during the postpartum period.
3. The client verbalizes her understanding of her condition and its possible impact on her pregnancy.
4. The client verbalizes components of self-care, including rest, diet, medications, and need for decreased activity.
5. The client demonstrates care of her infant.

Iron Deficiency Anemia

Iron deficiency anemia is the most common hematologic disorder in pregnancy. Pregnancy increases maternal plasma volume and lowers the total number of red blood cells. Hemodilution with a fall in hemoglobin concentration occurs. In addition, the developing fetus requires iron. Many American women begin pregnancy with depleted iron stores from menstrual blood loss and low dietary intake. Overt anemia may develop, especially in the socioeconomically deprived woman with poor general health.

Therapeutic Management

A hemoglobin level <11 g/dl or a hematocrit level <35% is suggestive of anemia. Iron deficiency anemia renders the pregnant woman susceptible to fatigue and postpartum hemorrhage. Severely or chronically anemic women (hemoglobin <8 g/dl) are symptomatic and risk abortion, premature birth, and small-for-gestational-age (SGA) infants because oxygen is limited for fetal exchange. Treatment is administration of oral ferrous sulfate (200 mg to 300 mg three times per day) or ferrous gluconate (320 mg three times per day). These drugs should be ingested with meals to decrease gastrointestinal side effects. The absorption of iron and the metabolism of folic acid are enhanced by administration of vitamin C. Folic acid deficiency may also occur. Foods high in folic acid (uncooked green, leafy vegetables, red meats, fish, legumes, and poultry) should also be included in the diet. Symptoms of this type of anemia are glossitis, sore tongue, and anorexia. Both folic acid and vitamin C are included in prenatal vitamin-mineral supplements. Some supplements do not include iron, which is taken separately.

Urinary Tract Infection and Renal Disease

The most common renal problem in pregnancy is urinary tract infection (UTI). Anatomic changes and hormonal effects cause narrowing of the lower ureter and renal pelvis, with dilation of the upper ureter. These changes result in stasis of urine, delayed emptying, and increased risk of infection. Pregnant women with asymptomatic bacteriuria (100,000 organisms in a urine culture) should be treated to prevent UTI and pyelonephritis. Renal disease may be a factor in premature labor.

The nurse should teach the pregnant woman personal hygiene practices, how to collect a midstream urine specimen, and the importance of maintaining an adequate fluid intake of 3 to 4 L/24 hours (see Client Self-Care Education: How to Prevent Urinary Tract Infections). Tetracycline, vancomycin, and gentamicin are contraindicated in pregnancy. They cross

---

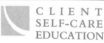

CLIENT
SELF-CARE
EDUCATION

How to Prevent Urinary Tract Infections

Action	Rationale
1. Drink eight 8-ounce glasses of fluid a day.	1. Increased fluid intake helps dilute the urine and lessen irritation and burning.
2. Void frequently.	2. Emptying the bladder helps prevent stasis of urine.
3. Void before and after intercourse.	3. Voiding removes bacteria from lower urethra.
4. Wear cotton underpants.	4. Wearing cotton underpants prevents irritation of the perineum.
5. Practice good personal hygiene.	5. Wiping perineum from front to back helps prevent contamination of the meatus with bacteria from anus.
6. Seek immediate treatment for recurrent symptoms.	6. Early treatment helps prevent complications of a more serious nature.

the placental barrier and potentially can cause congenital malformations. Hospitalization is recommended for clients with pyelonephritis because intravenous therapy and bed rest in the left-lateral position are prescribed.

Thyroid Disease

Thyroid conditions are a risk to pregnancy if the pregnant woman is untreated. The goal of treatment is to keep the client's thyroid hormone levels normal with use of a minimum of medication. Regular evaluations of thyroid function are needed to determine daily maintenance doses. Hypothyroid women have a high stillbirth rate and have low birth weight infants.

Methimazole and propylthiouracil are drugs commonly used in therapy. Dosages are reduced because the drugs easily cross the placenta and can cause fetal goiter or cretinism.

Infectious Diseases

Although most infectious diseases have no established specific effects on the mother or newborn, some do produce serious effects. The effects on the fetus are related to the gestational age at which infection occurs. Early infections might precipitate spontaneous abortion. Others may cause deafness or cataracts. Infections during the birth process can cause neonatal sepsis. See Table 22-5 for some commonly occurring infections, maternal assessment, effects on fetus, and treatment.

TORCH Diseases

More than 1 dozen viral infections can be contracted by a newborn during the prenatal, intrapartum, and postpartum periods. An acronym, TORCH, is used to designate some of these viral diseases,

TABLE 22-5

Sexually Transmitted Diseases in Pregnancy

Infection	Assessment of Mother	Fetal Effects	Treatment
Gonorrhea caused by *Neisseria gonorrhoeae,* a gram-negative coccus	Mucopurulent vaginal discharge Pelvic infection	Can infect infant's eyes during birth, causing ophthalmia neonatorum	Penicillin may be used in pregnancy Prophylactic administration of erythromycin to eyes at birth
Genital herpes type II caused by a virus	Painful vesicles in the vulva, perineal areas, and buttocks Cesarean birth recommended if viral cultures positive or disease active; may be performed even if herpes not currently active	If infected during birth, central nervous system damage, death	Topical acyclovir Sitz baths two or three times per day
Chlamydia caused by *Chlamydia trachomatis,* a parasite	Inflammation of cervix Mucopurulent discharge Pelvic infection	Premature birth, stillbirth, ophthalmia neonatorum, pneumonia	Tetracycline, but usually contraindicated in pregnancy Tetracycline ophthalmic ointment applied to infected newborn's eyes for several weeks

Continued

TABLE 22-5

Sexually Transmitted Diseases in Pregnancy—continued

Infection	Assessment of Mother	Fetal Effects	Treatment
Syphilis caused by a spirochete, *Treponema pallidum*	Primary lesion a chancre, a deep painless lesion found in genitalia, lips, or rectal area Secondary stage: macular rash over entire body Latent: no symptoms Third stage: neurologic symptoms	Congenital anomalies Congenital syphilis	Penicillin
Trichomoniasis vaginitis caused by a protozoa, *Trichomonas vaginalis*	White to gray-green, frothy vaginal discharge Pruritus, irritation	No effect on fetus	Metronidazole (Flagyl) in the last half of pregnancy Cotton underpants Good perineal hygiene
Listeriosis caused by a gram-positive bacteria, *listeria monocytogenes*	May be asymptomatic or have fever of unexplained origin	Respiratory distress at birth Skin lesions Meningitis	Ampicillin or penicillin with gentamicin
Candidiasis caused by a fungus, *Candida albicans*	Thick, curdy white discharge Vulvar pruritus	Oral infection during birth called thrush	Vaginal cream or tablet of micronazale, chlordantoin, or nystatin for 7-10 days
Acquired immune deficiency syndrome (AIDS) caused by the retrovirus, HTLV III	Susceptible to opportunistic infections such as pneumonia caused by *Pneumocystis carinii* or Kaposi's sarcoma	May acquire AIDS transplacentally or during breast-feeding	Drug zidovudine (AZT) apparently delays disease process
Hepatitis B caused by the hepatitis B virus	Nausea and vomiting Jaundice in 25% Enlarged liver	May acquire hepatitis at birth Associated with abortion, premature labor, stillbirth	Passive immunization of mother if exposed Bed rest Good nutrition

including *t*oxoplasmosis (a protozoal disease), *r*ubella, *c*ytomegalic inclusion disease, and *h*erpes. Other infections such as hepatitis, varicella, syphilis, and AIDS are included in the *O* category. Because the mother may be asymptomatic, the disease process may be unsuspected. Some problem TORCH infections are listed in Table 22-6.

TABLE 22-6

Congenital Disorders Caused by Maternal TORCH Diseases

Disease	Transmission	Mother	Fetus or Infant	Medical Intervention	Nursing Interventions
Toxoplasmosis caused by a protozoa, *Toxoplasma gondii*	Placental transfer Handling cat litter contaminated with feces containing oocytes (from unconfined cats) Eating poorly cooked or raw meat	Generally asymptomatic Primary infection acquired just before or during early pregnancy May result in congenital infection May result in spontaneous abortion	Death in 10% to 15% Classic congenital defects: chorioretinitis, microcephaly, hydrocephalus, cerebral calcifications	IgG and IgM antibody testing in cord and neonatal blood; drugs of choice: pyrimethamine, sulfadiazine	Counsel pregnant woman to avoid emptying cat litter from unconfined cats and to avoid ingestion of partially cooked or raw meat. Special isolation precautions are not needed.
Rubella caused by a virus	Across the placenta Fetus vulnerable during first trimester and early second trimester if mother contracts rubella	Spontaneous abortion in 33% of pregnant women with rubella in first trimester	Cardiac defects, cataracts, deafness	Testing for rubella-specific IgM from cord or neonatal serum; immediate serologic testing for exposed women Perinatal rubella rare in United States because of immunization programs; nonimmune women followed carefully for clinical rubella or development of antibodies Immunization and gamma globulin not recommended	Affected babies and their placentas are highly infected. Nonimmune personnel, especially pregnant women, should avoid contact. Immunity status of all personnel is determined and vaccination administered at the time of employment. Provide strict isolation for affected infants. Infants may be isolated with their mothers in a private room.
Infection caused by cytomegalovirus (CMV)—most common of perinatal viruses	Across the placenta Contaminated vaginal or nasopharyngeal secretions, urine, or feces Less frequently, blood transfusions or breast milk	Asymptomatic	Many asymptomatic Bone lesions, low birth weight, anemia, jaundice, hepatosplenomegaly	Diagnostic studies: viral cultures of amniotic fluid or neonatal serum; anti-CMV IgM antibodies in cord or neonatal serum; CMV inclusion in urine or cerebrospinal fluid Treatment is supportive	Counsel pregnant women to avoid close contact with known cases. Counsel parents that CMV may be found in affected infant's urine for a number of years. Teach parents appropriate disposal of diapers and handwashing after diapering.

Continued

TABLE 22-6

Congenital Disorders Caused by Maternal TORCH Diseases—continued

Disease	Transmission	Mother	Fetus or Infant	Medical Intervention	Nursing Interventions
Hepatitis B caused by specific hepatitis B virus	Infection of infants during last trimester or during delivery During postpartum period through infected maternal saliva, urine, feces, serum, breast milk	Malaise, fever, jaundice, dark urine, light stools, anorexia	Low birth weight if affected in utero May be asymptomatic if infected at time of delivery	Diagnostic studies: hepatitis B virus cultured from amniotic fluid; IgM in cord blood or neonatal serum Administration of hepatitis B immunoglobin to infants of infected mothers	Follow enteric, blood, and secretion precautions.
Fifth disease (erythema infectiosum, slap-cheek disease) caused by human *Parvovirus 19*	Through air from person to person Infectious period uncertain, probably only in prodromal period	Rash, fever, chills, joint pain	Increased incidence of stillbirth and abortion in women with this disease during pregnancy	Detected by specific antigen-antibody testing No vaccine available Identification of recent infections through IgM tests No specific treatment	Counsel pregnant women to avoid persons with febrile diseases, especially if known outbreak. Counsel pregnant women to report febrile diseases with rashes.

REFERENCE

1. Knuppel R, Drukker I: High-Risk Pregnancy. Philadelphia, WB Saunders, 1986

SUGGESTED READINGS

Foster RLR, Hunsberger MM, Anderson JJJ: Family-Centered Nursing Care of Children. Philadelphia, WB Saunders, 1989

Hogge JS et al: Chorionic villus sampling. J Obstet Gynecol Neonat Nurs 15(1):25, January/February 1986

Koehl L, Wheeler D: Monitoring uterine activity at home. Am J Nurs 89:200-203, February 1989

Northrop CE, Kelly ME: Legal Issues in Nursing. St. Louis, CV Mosby, 1987

Sever J: TORCH infections: The list keeps growing. Contemp OB/GYN (March):65-72, 1989

Antepartum Complications

IMPORTANT TERMINOLOGY

abortion Termination of pregnancy before fetus attains stage of viability (i.e., before it is capable of extrauterine existence); lay term is *miscarriage* and denotes occurrence of a spontaneous abortion

abruptio placentae Separation of placenta (part or all) from uterine wall

cerclage Surgical procedure in which purse-string suture is placed at cervical internal os for treatment of cervical incompetence

disseminated intravascular coagulation Widespread clotting in all the body's arterioles and capillaries

eclampsia Development of convulsion or coma by the preclampsic client (one who has hypertension with proteinuria or edema after 20 weeks gestation)

ectopic pregnancy Pregnancy located outside the uterine cavity (often in a fallopian tube)

hydatidiform mole Benign neoplasm of the chorion in which chorionic villi degenerate and become transparent vesicles containing clear, viscid fluid having a grapelike appearance

hyperemesis gravidarum Excessive, severe vomiting during pregnancy

incompetent cervix Mechanical defect in cervix that causes it to efface and dilate prematurely

placenta previa Implantation of placenta low in uterus

preeclampsia Hypertension with proteinuria or edema after 20 weeks gestation

pregnancy-induced hypertension Hypertension with proteinuria or edema after 20 weeks gestation; also called *preeclampsia*

Pregnancy-related maternal disorders are divided into two broad categories: (1) complications related to the pregnancy itself and not seen at other times and (2) diseases that are not pregnancy related but occur coincidentally. The latter may arise in the nonpregnant woman as well, but when they occur during pregnancy, they may complicate the pregnancy and influence its course or may be aggravated by the pregnancy. There are only a few major complications that result from pregnancy, but may present serious health hazards.

Complications Early in Pregnancy

Complications occurring early in pregnancy include **abortion, incompetent cervix, ectopic pregnancy, hyperemesis gravidarum,** and **hydatidiform mole.**

Abortion

Manifestations and Cause

Abortion is the medical term for what the lay public calls a miscarriage. It indicates loss of pregnancy before 20 weeks gestation. Most abortions occur during the first trimester of pregnancy. The two most common of the many types of abortions are spontaneous and therapeutic (see below).

Spontaneous abortion occurs in 15% to 20% of pregnancies. It is believed that many of these abortions occur because of some inherent imperfection of the embryo. The client has a history of menstrual-like cramping (uterine contractions) and bleeding. This cramping causes cervical softening and dilation, which result in complete or incomplete loss of the products of conception. The client aborts the products of conception at home and often has been unaware that she was pregnant.

When the spontaneous abortion occurs quickly, hospitalization is necessary if severe, excessive cramping and bleeding are present.

The second common type of abortion is therapeutic, or induced. This abortion is performed by a physician to sacrifice the pregnancy for the sake of the mother's well-being. It is important to differentiate between an abortion (occuring at less than 20 weeks gestation) and a fetus (more than 20 weeks gestation) because some states require a birth certificate for any pregnancy terminating beyond 20 weeks or for a fetus weighing greater than 500 g. When the pregnancy is near 20 weeks gestation but the actual fetal age is unknown, fetal age can be determined based on fetal weight. The usual weight for classifying the pregnancy as an abortion is 500 g or less.

Types of Abortion

Spontaneous: Process occurs through natural causes.
Therapeutic: Artificially induced for medical or other reasons.
Threatened: Bleeding and/or cramping occurs, but cervix is closed. Pregnancy may or may not be lost.
Inevitable: Bleeding and cramping with dilating cervix.
Incomplete: Part of products of conception are passed, but part are retained. Bleeding usually persists until uterus is empty.
Complete: Expulsion of all products of conception.
Missed: Fetus dies in utero but is retained.
Habitual: Three or more pregnancies are lost in succession.
Illegal: Termination of pregnancy outside of appropriate medical facilities, generally by nonphysician abortionists. Each state has statutes that define the parameters that constitute an illegal abortion in that particular state.

Diagnosis and Prognosis

The signs and symptoms of abortion are uterine bleeding and cramping. When the client experiences these manifestations she must be examined by a primary health care provider to determine if the cervix is dilated. When bleeding is scant and does not last for more than 3 days and the ultrasound results are normal, the risk of abortion is lower.[1]

Ultrasonography can differentiate between a live fetus and a pregnancy with a blighted ovum. If the ovum is blighted, there is an empty gestational sac because a fetus never formed. Studies have shown that threatened abortion is significantly correlated with preterm birth or term delivery of a low birth weight infant.[2]

Therapeutic Management

Clients with severe pain or excessive bleeding or both may experience a life-threatening situation requiring hospitalization. They are assessed for hypovolemia and receive fluid replacement as indicated and oxytocics to control bleeding and support homeostasis. It may be necessary to perform dilatation and curettage (D and C) or vacuum extraction to empty the uterus before bleeding can be controlled. If the client is Rh(D) negative, immunoglobulin is given within 72 hours to prevent Rh sensitization.

Uncomplicated D and C is an outpatient surgical procedure. Recovery after D and C requires 2 to 3 hours; then the client is discharged from the hospital or outpatient surgery center.

Assessment

When the client is admitted to the hospital, the nurse obtains a history of the client's pain, bleeding and last menstrual period (LMP) to determine the length of gestation. Vital signs, pain, and bleeding are assessed. The client may be anxious because of the severe bleeding and hospitalization and may be fearful of what this symptom means to her pregnancy. An assessment tool for bleeding in early pregnancy is shown on p. 610.

Nursing Diagnosis

Potential nursing diagnoses pertinent to bleeding include both biophysical and psychosocial aspects of abortion (see Potential Nursing Diagnoses: Spontaneous Abortion on p. 610). Immediate nursing care focuses on the biophysical aspects of stabilizing and maintaining maternal homeostasis. The psychosocial aspects to address relate to what this loss means to the client. Effective nursing care must address both of these aspects. At all times the family must be encouraged to communicate and resolve crises that arise.

Planning and Intervention

Findings from the admission assessment are reported to the client's physician. Orders will be received to start an intravenous line, obtain laboratory work (complete blood count [CBC], type, and crossmatch). If a D and C is scheduled, the nurse reinforces the explanation given by the physician and ensures that all client issues and questions are addressed.

LEGAL AND ETHICAL CONSIDERATIONS

The nurse's obligation after the physician has obtained consent to perform surgery is to ensure that all further client questions and issues about the surgery are communicated to the physician. The nurse documents in the nurses' notes that the physician was notified about the client's additional questions or need for further clarification about the pending procedure.

ASSESSMENT
TOOL

Bleeding in Early Pregnancy: Initial Data Base

The initial data base should be completed at time of admission to the hospital.
  Chief complaint: Why are you here?
  Vital signs:
  Gravida and parity:
  Date of last menstrual period:
  Estimated date of confinement:
  Pregnancy history (previous abortion, ectopic, etc.):
  Allergies:
  Current pregnancy confirmed:
  Nausea and vomiting:
  Type of pain: contractions, cramping backache, abdominal pain (dull or
      sharp)
  Onset of pain:
  Previous bleeding or coagulation problems:
  Quantity of bleeding: (e.g., teaspoon, ½ cup)
  Nature of blood loss: bright red to dark brown (with or without tissue
      fragments)
  When bleeding began: intermittent or continuous
  Dizziness:
  Client anxiety:
  Emotional status: What does the loss mean to you?

Sample Narrative Charting: Admitted per stretcher complaining of severe
cramping and excessive bleeding since early this morning. Has saturated 9
maxi pads (¾ of pad each time) in past 6 hours and has passed several 50-cent
piece size clots. No tissue seen. Presently there is a large amount of bright red
bleeding (2 pads thoroughly soaked in 20 minutes). Cramping is intermittent
at 3- to 4-minute intervals. Feels some rectal pressure. Nothing seen at
introitus. Temperature 97.6° F. Blood pressure 80/40, pulse 120 and thready,
respirations 24 and shallow. Skin is clammy and perspiring. States "Every
time I lift my head I feel very dizzy." Dr. Edmiston called and given report.

POTENTIAL
NURSING DIAGNOSES

Spontaneous Abortion

Fluid Volume Deficit (2)—related to excessive bleeding secondary to spontaneous in-
    terruption of pregnancy, i.e., abortion
Pain—related to uterine contractions, cramping
Anticipatory Grieving—related to expected pregnancy outcome
Fear, Anxiety—related to unfamiliarity with hospital procedures
Knowledge Deficit—regarding surgical procedure and postoperative activity restric-
    tions
Potential for Infection—related to bacterial invasion of uterus secondary to trauma to
    endometrium from currettage.
Situational Low Esteem—related to inability to carry pregnancy to term successfully
Altered Parenting—related to feelings of inadequacy, disappointment, and grief over
    loss of pregnancy

Maternal status is monitored during preparation for medical or surgical
management and the surgical procedure. Both the physical and emotional
aspects of care are monitored and supported. A support person should
remain at the bedside with the client as much as possible.

The client should receive follow-up care after she leaves the hospital
to ensure that she is recovering physically and emotionally. Some hospitals
send a letter after discharge to extend sympathy for the loss of the "hoped-
for child" and to inform the would-be parents of local support groups.

Focus Assessment

Estimate number of weeks gestation.
Monitor vital signs closely.
Monitor vaginal bleeding:
   Maintain perineal pad count.
   Note degree of saturation.
   Identify signs of increasing or decreasing bleeding.
Examine any clots or tissue discharged.
Elicit description of pain (type, persistence); note any changes.
Elicit information describing perception of self.
Explore nonverbal indicators of emotional status, e.g., irritability, inability to
   concentrate, withdrawal.

Incompetent Cervix

Manifestations and Cause

Incompetent cervix is a mechanical defect of the cervix that causes premature dilatation. The cause is unknown. Cervical incompetence is suspected if there has been a prior second trimester spontaneous abortion, cervical trauma, or surgical procedures that have left scarring or shortening of the cervix. Signs of incompetent cervix are (1) painless cervical softening, (2) effacement and dilatation, (3) premature rupture of membranes, and (4) spontaneous abortion.

Diagnosis and Prognosis

Serial vaginal examinations early in the second trimester reveal the cervical changes indicative of possible cervical incompetence. The cervix may be scarred or stenosed from a previous difficult delivery or previous surgery. The membranes may be bulging through the cervical os. The client has a history of repeated termination of pregnancy in the second trimester.

Therapeutic Management

Some physicians believe that performing **cerclage** (purse-string suture in cervical os; McDonald and Shirodkar's procedure) is helpful if there are no contractions. The success rate for the procedure is approximately 40%. Others believe that surgery is not indicated and use conservative measures including bed rest, hydration, and use of drugs (ritodrine, magnesium sulfate) to decrease or inhibit uterine activity, to manage the client.

Assessment

The nurse assesses how the client feels about her pregnancy. Evaluating the availability of the client's support systems is also important. Finally, it is important to determine the client's understanding about an incompetent cervix.

POTENTIAL NURSING DIAGNOSES

Pregnancy Loss

Situational Low Self-Esteem—related to inability to carry pregnancy successfully to term

Ineffective Individual Coping—related to potential or actual loss of pregnancy

Dysfunctional Grieving—related to potential or actual loss of pregnancy

Altered Family Processes—related to loss of pregnancy

Knowledge Deficit—regarding cervical incompetence, procedures for management

Focus Assessment

Elicit information describing perception of self.

Explore nonverbal indicators of emotional status, e.g., affect, mood, inability to concentrate.

Identify previous patterns of coping with crisis.

Determine current support system.

Nursing Diagnosis

Potential nursing diagnoses that relate to incompetent cervix deal with the client's self-concept, ability to cope with possible loss of pregnancy, and information level (see margin).

Planning and Intervention

Clients who do not need hospitalization must understand the importance of bed rest at home and the need for close observation and supervision by the nurse and physician. If labor-inhibiting drugs are prescribed, she must understand the importance of taking the medication exactly as instructed and how it will make her feel. She should be taught when to call her doctor and what to report. Sometimes a "home-monitoring" program is begun. The client is taught to apply a contraction monitor (Fig. 23-1) several times a day and to transmit the monitor tracing by telephone. Nurses on the receiving end assess the tracing for contractions, answer questions, provide emotional support and education, and report information to the client's physician. These nurses also call her with orders about medication and instructions if she should need to go to her physician or to the hospital for immediate treatment.

FIGURE 23-1
Home Contraction Monitor.
Courtesy Health Dyne Prenatal Services, Marietta, Georgia.

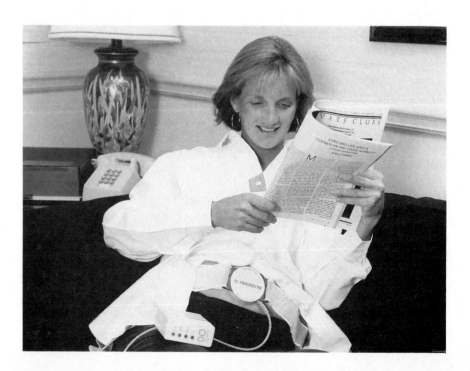

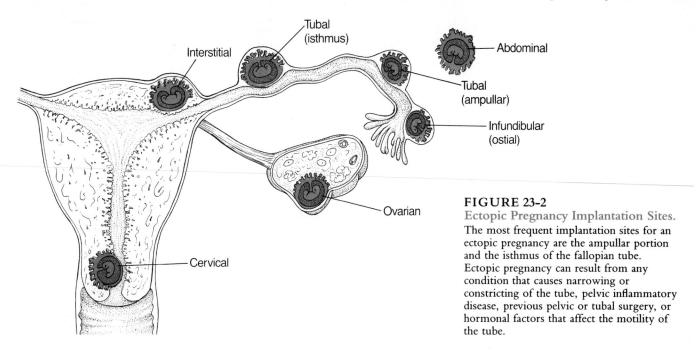

Interstitial

Tubal
(isthmus)

Abdominal

Tubal
(ampullar)

Infundibular
(ostial)

Ovarian

Cervical

FIGURE 23-2
Ectopic Pregnancy Implantation Sites.
The most frequent implantation sites for an
ectopic pregnancy are the ampullar portion
and the isthmus of the fallopian tube.
Ectopic pregnancy can result from any
condition that causes narrowing or
constricting of the tube, pelvic inflammatory
disease, previous pelvic or tubal surgery, or
hormonal factors that affect the motility of
the tube.

When the client approaches her due date, a decision is made about the
route of delivery. If management is unsuccessful and the fetus delivers
before viability, grief support should be provided.

Ectopic Pregnancy

Manifestations and Cause

Ectopic pregnancy is an implantation of the fertilized ovum in a site other
than the uterine cavity. The most frequent implantation sites are the
ampullar portion and the isthmus of the fallopian tube (Fig. 23-2). Clients
relate a history of a missed period and normal symptoms of pregnancy,
followed by spotting or irregular vaginal bleeding and lower abdominal
pain.

Diagnosis and Prognosis

Physical examination reveals pain on one side over the tube and ovary
(adnexa), and often an adnexal mass can be palpated. Laboratory testing
reveals a low human chorionic gonadotropin (hCG) level. Ultrasonography visualizes a gestational sac if the tube is intact. Laparoscopy reveals
an extrauterine pregnancy and may help prevent tubal rupture. Performing a laparotomy will confirm the diagnosis and permit immediate treatment.

Ectopic pregnancy is a significant cause of maternal death (15%), and
three-fourths of these deaths are preventable. If a woman has one ectopic
pregnancy, the recurrence risk is 10% to 20%.

Therapeutic Management

Management focuses on establishing homeostasis and combating shock.
Surgery is done to remove the affected tube (salpingectomy) and some-

times the ovary (oophorectomy). The tube and ovary are saved if possible. Rh_o (D) immune globulin is given to Rh_o (D) negative clients to prevent Rh sensitization.

Assessment

Assessment involves obtaining a history from the client or significant other (see Assessment Tool: Bleeding in Early Pregnancy: Initial Data Base on p. 610). Bleeding, pain, vital signs, and emotional status of the client are also important considerations when preparing her for surgery.

Nursing Diagnosis

Major nursing diagnoses for this client may include comfort issues, tissue perfusion, and coping (see Potential Nursing Diagnoses: Ectopic Pregnancy).

Planning and Intervention

Performing preoperative and postoperative care is often critical in saving the life of the mother. As in caring for a client with abortion or incompetent cervix, providing emotional support is an important task for nurses caring for women who have suffered a pregnancy loss and a physiologic insult to her body.

Nursing care is aimed at combating the shock that is frequently present in clients with a rupture. An intravenous infusion should be maintained so that blood or plasma expanders can be administered as needed to replace losses from the hemorrhage and surgery.

During the postoperative period vital signs are carefully monitored, fluid replacement is continued, and intake and output are recorded. The nurse should accurately record the perineal pad count. The surgical site may require special care and dressings.

Emotional care is directed toward facilitating effective coping through a critical complication of pregnancy, death of the fetus, and possibly altered fertility. The client is assisted in resolving feelings of guilt, self-blame, and despair as previously described for abortion clients.

☐ POTENTIAL NURSING DIAGNOSES

Ectopic Pregnancy

Fluid Volume Deficit (2)—related to excessive bleeding secondary to tubal rupture

Altered General Tissue Perfusion—related to hypovolemia shock secondary to tubal rupture

Pain—related to distention (or rupture) of fallopian tube

Ineffective Individual Coping—related to personal perception of inability to become a parent

Knowledge Deficit—regarding hospital procedures and outcome of surgery

Dysfunctional Grieving—related to loss of pregnancy

Focus Assessment

Monitor vital signs closely.
Identify nonverbal signs of pain, anxiety, fear.
Elicit description of pain (type, persistence); note any changes.
Examine intake and output balance.
Indentify individual teaching or learning needs.
Monitor response to analgesia and anesthesia.
Elicit information describing perception of self.
Explore nonverbal indicators of emotional status, e.g., irritability, inability to concentrate, withdrawal.

Hyperemesis Gravidarum

Manifestations and Cause

Vomiting is a common complaint in pregnancy. Approximately 60% to 80% of pregnant women in the United States experience some nausea and vomiting during pregnancy. Women reporting vomiting are less likely to experience miscarriage or stillbirth and delivery before 37 weeks gestation.[3]

Hyperemesis gravidarum refers to persistent, intractable vomiting that begins in early pregnancy and results in fluid and electrolyte imbalance and eventual weight loss. It occurs more often in first pregnancies and is more likely to recur in the subsequent pregnancies of clients experiencing it in the first pregnancy. The cause of this ailment is unknown, but it is more common in the United States than in the rest of the world. Rates do seem to vary with life-styles and with the presence of stress, leading to the belief that psychologic determinants are a predisposing factor.

Diagnosis and Prognosis

Diagnosis of hyperemesis gravidarum is not simple. When a client reports excessive nausea and vomiting, careful evaluation is crucial. Laboratory assessment is performed to determine electrolyte values, ketosis, and acidosis. Performing a urinalysis is also helpful.

Typical findings include hyponatremia, hypochloremia, and metabolic acidosis. If the hyperemesis is long-standing, the kidneys may lose their ability to concentrate urine effectively. Hyperemesis gravidarum usually is self-limiting, but death and serious complications can occur.

Therapeutic Management

HOME CARE. The mainstays of home-care treatment are hydration and eating small, frequent high-carbohydrate meals that are easily digested. Clients with hyperemesis gravidarum also need much reassurance and empathy. Antiemetics are often ordered.

Symptoms of heartburn and reflux esophagitis are treated symptomatically. Identifying and reducing sources of stress are helpful.

HOSPITAL TREATMENT. Hospital treatment includes correction of dehydration, electrolyte replacement, nutritional support, and antiemetic therapy. The use of hyperalimentation and parenteral nutrition may be necessary in severe cases. Psychotherapy and hypnosis have provided good results.[4] Behavioral modification is a coping skill that may assist clients to cope with hyperemesis.

Assessment, Nursing Diagnosis, Planning, and Intervention

Nursing assessment addresses obtaining information about onset, frequency, duration, and amount of emesis. Assessment of the client with signs and symptoms of hyperemesis gravidarum may lead to diagnoses that focus on nutrition, problems with vomiting and dehydration, maternal coping, and fetal nutrition (see Potential Nursing Diagnoses: Hyperemesis Gravidarum). It may be necessary to infuse intravenous fluids

POTENTIAL NURSING DIAGNOSES

Hyperemesis Gravidarum

Alteration in Nutrition—related to pernicious vomiting

Potential Impairment in Skin Integrity—related to excessive vomiting and dehydration

Ineffctive Individual Coping—related to the psychologic tasks of pregnancy and motherhood

or monitor hyperalimentation if the client's intake is inadequate. Nursing care should always by nonjudgmental, tactful, and understanding. These clients need much reassurance.

Hydatidiform Mole

Manifestations and Cause

Hydatidiform mole is another complication of pregnancy that causes bleeding (Fig. 23-3). Initially the pregnancy may appear normal. If the client has a complete (or classic) mole, no fetal tissue is present; if a partial (incomplete) mole exists, embryonic or fetal tissue is present. In approximately 50% of clients with hydatidiform mole, the uterus enlarges more rapidly and is larger than expected for gestation. Bleeding is a usual sign, varying from brownish-red spotting to a heavy bright red bleeding, and produces suspicion of a threatened or inevitable abortion. The bleeding may persist intermittently for several weeks. If abortion does not occur, the uterus continues to grow rapidly, and profuse hemorrhage is likely. Blood loss commonly leads to iron deficiency anemia. Vomiting may be severe and begin early in pregnancy. **Pregnancy-induced hypertension** (PIH) can occur before the 20th week of pregnancy. The exact cause of hydatidiform mole is unknown.

Diagnosis and Prognosis

Suspicion of hydatidiform mole is based on persistent bleeding, a uterus larger than expected for dates, and absence of fetal parts. Ultrasonography

FIGURE 23-3

Hydatidiform Mole. Hydatidiform mole is an abnormal placenta, usually without a fetus or fetal tissue. The chorionic villi form into an overgrowth of transparent vesicles that resemble a cluster of grapes.

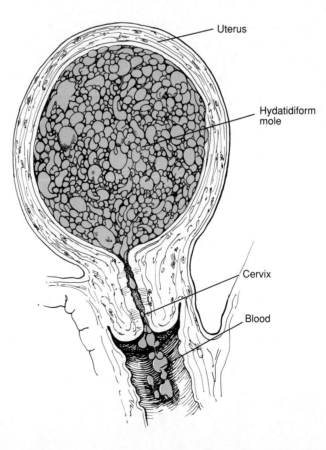

Uterus

Hydatidiform mole

Cervix

Blood

reveals no fetal parts. In addition to anemia and hypertension, a malignancy, choriocarcinoma, is a threat after the pregnancy is terminated if any placenta is retained.

Therapeutic Management

The hydatidiform mole may be aborted spontaneously but it is often removed surgically by curettage. These clients should be followed for a year, and pregnancy should be avoided during that time. Elevated chorionic gonadotrophins (hCG) levels associated with pregnancy can cause confusion about whether choriocarcinoma has developed. If hCG levels remain normal for a year, the client can be assured of a low probability of recurrent hydatidiform mole.

Assessment, Nursing Diagnosis, and Planning and Intervention

See Table 23-1.

Hemorrhagic and Hematologic Complications

Approximately 3% of pregnancies are complicated by bleeding in the third trimester. Bleeding disorders still represent one of the three leading causes of maternal and fetal mortality. Clients with these disorders must be assessed quickly and be given supportive care while a diagnosis is being determined. Interventions provide maximum safety for the mother and her fetus.

Two placental problems, **placenta previa and abruptio placentae,** cause bleeding during late pregnancy and may jeopardize fetal well-being and maternal health. Bleeding that results from these conditions is the primary problem because the placenta is very vascular and receives a significant blood supply. The most common cause of bleeding in later pregnancy is placenta previa. Abruptio placentae is a major emergency. Other hematologic complications include **disseminated intravascular coagulation** (DIC), sickle cell anemia, and Rh sensitization.

Placenta Previa

Manifestations and Cause

The placenta should be attached high in the upper part of the uterus. In placenta previa implantation of the placenta is lower than normal. When implanted low in the uterus, the placenta may partially or completely cover the os (Fig. 23-4). This is considered a serious complication of pregnancy. The result is painless bleeding that begins when the lower uterine segment becomes thinner as the cervix softens and begins to efface and dilate. When the placenta is low, its size and margins are affected by the changes in the lower uterine segment. Bleeding occurs as a result of some separation at placental margins. Placenta previa occurs in approximately 1:200 pregnancies.

TABLE 23-1

Summary of Bleeding in Early Pregnancy

Condition	Manifestations	Causes	Medical Diagnosis and Prognosis
Abortion	Bleeding and cramping Softening and dilation of cervix	Abnormal embryo or trophoblast Infection (acute) Abnormalities of generative tract (e.g., uterine malformations)	If bleeding is scant and lasts no longer than 3 days and result of ultrasound is normal, pregnancy failure is lower than if bleeding lasts for >3 days and ultrasound result is abnormal. Clients who continue pregnancy have a greater risk of preterm birth or low birth weight baby.
Hydatidiform mole	Early normal or greater-than-normal uterine enlargement Vomiting Early bleeding (brownish-red spotting to heavy) Late rapid uterine enlargement Profuse hemorrhage Possible preeclampsia	*Unknown* Apparent association with age, multiparity, and dietary factors	Diagnosis is based on following symptoms: Persistent bleeding Uterus larger than expected for dates Absence of fetal parts Confirmation by ultrasonography Elevated levels of human chorionic gonadotropin (hCG) Prognosis is not associated with maternal mortality. Chance of advancing to metastatic choriocarcinoma is 10% to 20%.

Diagnosis and Prognosis

Placenta previa should always be suspected in clients experiencing bleeding during the last half of pregnancy. A definitive diagnosis can be made using ultrasonography to locate the placenta. The potential for hemorrhage represents a serious complication to the client and a threat of premature delivery for the baby. Advances in technology and management have reduced maternal mortality. The fetus may still be compromised by hypoxia related to maternal blood loss, decrease in uteroplacental perfusion, and prematurity when early delivery is necessary.

Medical Management	Nursing Assessment	Nursing Diagnoses	Nursing Interventions

Home care instructions:
  Call physician if bleeding recurs
  Rest in bed
  Abstain from sexual intercourse
Hospital care for excessive bleeding:
  Intravenous fluids
  Oxytocic therapy
  Blood replacement
  Surgery:
    Dilation and curettage
    Vacuum extraction
  Antibiotics for infection
	Assess for the following:
	  Bleeding (amount and type)
	  Shock
	  Pain (type, onset, duration)
	  Emotional state
		Fluid Volume Deficit, Active—related to excessive bleeding secondary to retention of some products of conception
		Fear, Anxiety—related to invasive procedure and loss of pregnancy
			Count perineal pads; estimate blood loss.
			Place client in Trendelenburg position.
			Monitor vital signs.
			Assist with drawing blood for determining CBC, hemoglobin and hematocrit levels, Rh factor, type, and crossmatch.
			Give paid medication if ordered.
			Keep client and support person together.
			Explain what is happening, what is being done, and why.
			Provide reassurance and support.
			Use therapeutic touch as appropriate.
			Encourage verbalization of questions and feelings.

Empty the uterus:
  Perform suction curettage if uterus <10 wk size.
  Induce labor with oxytocin if uterus larger; perform curettage after uterus is partially emptied.
Obtain tissue examination from pathologist.
Perform follow-up care:
  Assess for changes suggestive of trophoblastic malignancy.
  Follow hCG levels for 1 yr (normally negative levels within 6 wk).
  Administer prophylactic chemotherapy (controversial).
  Advise client to postpone another pregnancy for up to 1 yr.
	Assess for the following:
	  Bleeding
	  Shock
	  Pregnancy-induced hypertension (PIH)
	  Client's understanding of problem
	  Client's physical or psychologic emotional state
	  Client's preparation for surgery
		Knowledge Deficit—regarding effects of hydatidiform mole, complications, and surgery
		Grief—related to loss of pregnancy
			Monitor vital signs.
			Provide preoperative and postoperative care and instructions.
			Provide educational follow-up.
			Stress importance of follow-up care by physician.
			Keep client and significant other together as much as possible.
			Encourage the client and significant other to express their feelings.
			Be a good listener; be empathetic.
			Express own grief at the loss.
			Explain the grief process.
			Give information about support groups.

Therapeutic Management

Treatment is based on the client's condition, the degree of obstetric hemorrhage, the fetal condition, and gestational age. The main cause of prenatal loss is prematurity. The aim is to delay delivery until the fetus is mature without increasing the risk to the mother. Bed rest and observation often result in cessation of bleeding. The client may be managed at home if bleeding stops, if there is no anemia, and if transportation to the hospital is always available.

Delivery is necessary if the fetus is mature, active labor begins, excessive bleeding occurs, the fetus dies (or has anomalies incompatible

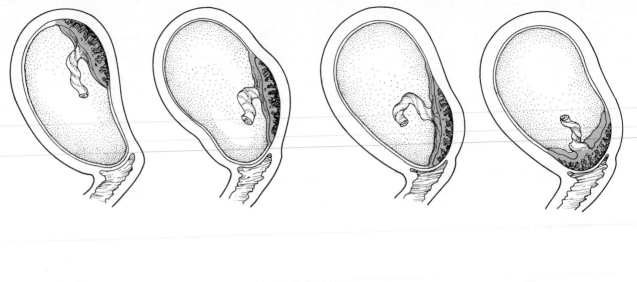

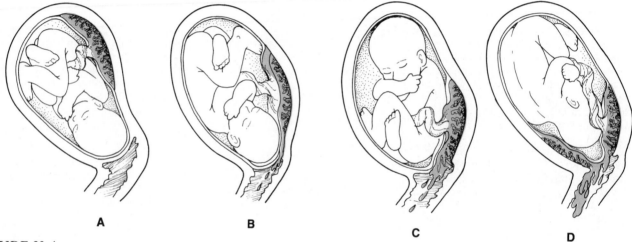

| | | | |
| A | B | C | D |

FIGURE 23-4

Placenta Previa. There are four categories of placenta previa. **A,** Normal placental attachment is in the upper part of the uterus. **B-D,** Abnormal placental sites of attachment. **B,** Low implantation is lower than normal placental attachment but does not cover the cervical os. Some bleeding can be observed as the lower uterine segment thins, causing some separation at the placental margin. **C,** Partial placenta previa is low placental attachment that partially covers the cervical os. Observable bleeding is caused by partial separation. **D,** In total placenta previa the placenta completely covers the cervical os, making vaginal delivery an impossibility. Massive hemorrhage can occur.

with life), or there is another obstetric complication necessitating termination of the pregnancy. Cesarean section has become the method of choice for delivery with placenta previa. This approach has significantly lowered maternal and perinatal mortality rates.

Assessment

When the client is admitted to the hospital, the nurse begins the assessment process. History includes how and when bleeding began and the client's estimate of how much bleeding has occurred (see Assessment Tool: Bleeding in Late Pregnancy).

Nursing Diagnosis

Nursing diagnoses for placenta previa are concerned with alteration in cardiac output, tissue perfusion, knowledge deficits about placenta previa, fears about mother and newborn, and the effects on the family.

Bleeding in Late Pregnancy

Gravida, para, abortion:
Estimated date of confinement:
LMP:
Quantity of bleeding: (e.g., teaspoon, ½ cup)
What precipitated bleeding:
Pain associated with bleeding: (uterine contractions, backache)
Amniotic sac: (ruptured, intact)
Uterine activity and condition: (size, contour, irritability, relaxation)
Abdominal pain: (dull, sharp, knifelike)
Vital signs:
Fetal activity:
Fetal heart rate:
General status: (level of consciousness, dizzy, apprehensive, anxious)

Fluid Volume Deficit (2)—related to excessive bleeding secondary to premature separation of the placenta or placenta previa

POTENTIAL
NURSING DIAGNOSES

Bleeding in Late Pregnancy

Decreased Cardiac Output—related to excessive blood loss (hypovolemia)
Altered General Tissue Perfusion—related to hypovolemia secondary to premature separation of the placenta or abnormal placental attachment (placenta previa)
Potential for Injury (Fetal)—related to decreased placental perfusion secondary to excessive maternal blood loss
Pain—related to bleeding between placenta and uterine wall secondary to abruptio placentae
Fear—related to concerns about condition of self and fetus, pregnancy outcome
Knowledge Deficit—regarding hospital procedures and management of condition
Altered Family Processes—related to mother's condition
Diversional Activity Deficit—related to need for bed rest secondary to placenta previa

Focus Assessment

Monitor vital signs and fetal heart rate closely.
Estimate amount of blood loss. Identify signs of increase or decrease in bleeding.
Monitor level of consciousness.
Identify presence or absence of pain.
When pain is present, note changes in character, amount, site, and response to pain.
Explore nonverbal indicators of emotional status, e.g., affect, mood, appearance, irritability, inability to concentrate, sleep patterns.
Identify expectations of pregnancy outcome.
Determine individual teaching or learning needs.
Observe family interactions.

Planning and Intervention

Plans for nursing intervention are dependent on whether conservative or active medical management is necessary. If the client is managed at home, referral is made for homemaking services and child care. Both home and hospital assessment and care focus on changes in perinatal status (Table 23-2).

TABLE 23-2

Summary of Bleeding in Late Pregnancy

Condition	Manifestations	Causes	Medical Diagnosis and Prognosis

Placenta previa	Painless bleeding at end of second trimester or in third trimester (usually bright red)
	 Soft uterus
	 Observed blood loss with signs of shock
		Unknown
		 Contributing factors:
		   Damaged endometrium
		   Advancing maternal age
		   Multiple pregnancies
		   Previous cesarean births
			History of painless bleeding
			 Speculum examination of cervix
			 Definite diagnosis with ultrasonography
			 Maternal mortality—0.1%
			 Major problem—prematurity

Abruptio placentae	Bleeding—may or may not be external (often dark brown)
	 Uterine rigidity and tenderness
	 Shock out of proportion to blood loss
		Unknown
		 Frequently associated with:
		   Hypertension
		   Sudden intrauterine decompression
		   Folic acid deficiency
		   Chronic smoking
		   Multiple pregnancy
		   Hydramnios
		 Other contributing factors—short umbilical cord, trauma
			Increase in contraction frequency and duration
			 Suspicion related to abdominal pain and/or vaginal bleeding
			 Ultrasound scan to visualize abruption
			 Maternal mortality—0.5%-5%
			 Perinatal mortality—15%
			 Major problem—prematurity

Abruptio Placentae

Manifestations and Cause

Abruptio placentae is another complication of the last half of pregnancy in which a normally located placenta separates from its uterine attachment. Bleeding, apparent or concealed, is always present (Fig. 23-5). The placental separation causes an increase in contraction frequency, resting tone, and tonus of the uterus (often resulting in tetany) and is accompanied by pain.

When separation occurs at the placental margin, blood passes between the uterine wall and fetal membranes, creating external bleeding. This is called an *overt* or partial abruption. *Covert* abruptio placentae is charac-

Medical Management	Nursing Assessment	Nursing Diagnosis	Nursing Interventions
Based on client's condition, degree of hemorrhage and fetal age; aim is to delay delivery until fetus is mature. Bed rest and observation may occur at home or in the hospital. Hospitalization and delivery are required if (when) bleeding recurs. Complications: 　Hemorrhage 　Hypovolemic shock 　Thrombocytopenia 　Anemia 　Premature rupture of membranes and labor 　Fetal malposition 　Air embolism 　Postpartum hemorrhage 　Uterine rupture	Assess: 　Bleeding 　For shock 　For presence or absence of uterine contractions 　Presentation, position, and lie of fetus 　For pain	**Potential Fluid Volume Deficit**—related to bleeding **Potential Alteration in Cardiac Output**—related to hypovolemia	Monitor vital signs Monitor fetal heart rate (FHR) Perform perineal pad count Provide diversional activities Assist with amniocentesis (for fetal maturity) Prepare client for surgery Give emotional support Provide up-to-date information
Treatment depends on condition of fetus and client at time diagnosis is made. If fetus is alive and at or near term, prompt delivery is in order for moderate-to-severe abruptions and should be by cesarean birth unless vaginal delivery can be accomplished quickly. If fetus has already died, uterus may contract intermittently; therefore labor and vaginal delivery are possible. Complications: 　Couvelaire uterus (bleeding into myometrium and serosa) 　Hemorrhage 　Coagulation defects (e.g., DIC) 　Renal failure 　Anemia	Assess: 　For signs and symptoms of external blood loss (amount, color, consistency) 　For pain (onset, duration, location) 　Uterine irritability 　Fetal status Provide emotional support	**Potential Alteration in Tissue Perfusion**—related to hypovolemia **Potential for Injury to the Fetus**—related to uteroplacental insufficiency **Potential for Fetal Injury**—related to prematurity	Monitor vital signs Draw line on abdomen (at top of fundus) Monitor uterus for tenderness or contractions Monitor FHR Explain procedures Keep client and significant other together Assist with drawing blood for laboratory studies (CBC, type, Rh, crossmatch, coagulation studies) Prepare client for surgery

terized by central separation that entraps lost blood between the uterine wall and the placenta. This is termed a *retroplacental bleed*. When this occurs, the bleeding is concealed and may mask the amount of blood loss. The most common and consistent symptom of covert abruption is continuous uterine pain that is described as knifelike.

If blood accumulates between the separated placenta and the uterus, it may produce a Couvelaire uterus. The term *Couvelaire* is used to describe the damage to the uterine muscle resulting from extensive myometrial bleeding. The uterus appears purplish and copper colored and is ecchymotic, and contractility is lost. Shock may occur and is often out of proportion to blood loss. Shock is manifested by rapid pulse, dyspnea, restlessness, pallor, syncope, cold and clammy perspiration, and hypotension.

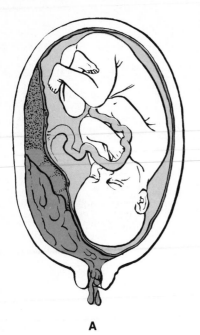

A   B   C

FIGURE 23-5

Abruptio Placentae. Abruptio placentae can occur at various sites. **A,** External hemorrhage is due to marginal separation of the placenta. Shock is in proportion to observable blood loss. **B,** Concealed, or "covert," abruptio placentae is central separation that entraps blood between the uterine wall and the placenta. The greater the separation, the greater the blood loss and shock in the mother and hypoxia in the fetus. Fetus is in jeopardy and may die. **C,** Complete separation of the placenta increases maternal morbidity and fetal mortality.

Although the precise cause of abruptio placentae is unknown, it is frequently noted in association with hypertension, sudden intrauterine decompression, folic acid deficiency, chronic smoking, multiple pregnancy, hydramnios, and cocaine abuse. Other contributing factors are short umbilical cord and trauma.

Diagnosis and Prognosis

Abruptio placentae should be considered in a client who develops sudden, intense, usually focalized uterine pain with or without vaginal bleeding. Although the clinical picture is usually clear-cut, ultrasonography may be used to demonstrate the site of retroplacental hematoma formation. DIC can develop in more severe cases.

The maternal mortality rate from abruptio placentae has declined significantly, ranging from 0.5% to 5% in the world. A high degree of suspicion, early diagnosis, and management should reduce this maternal mortality rate to 0.5% to 1%. Perinatal mortality rates vary with the type and degree of abruption, ranging from 15% to 100% (Table 23-3).

Therapeutic Management

It is useful to manage cases of abruptio placentae according to severity (Table 23-4). In mild cases maternal and fetal conditions are good, so no special intervention is necessary. In moderate cases there are uterine irritability and possible maternal cardiovascular instability. Fetal distress is not present, so vaginal delivery may be possible. If the fetus or mother develops further problems, an emergency cesarean delivery is performed. With severe abruption the maternal condition may be unstable with hypotension, tachycardia, coagulopathy, and even renal failure. Providing blood and fibrinogen replacement may be necessary before cesarean delivery is performed. Loss of blood, increased uterine activity (or tetany), and maternal shock can severely distress the fetus or cause fetal death.

TABLE 23-3

Comparative Overview of Placenta Previa and Abruptio Placentae

	Placenta Previa	Abruptio Placentae
Etiology	Unknown	Unknown
Associated risk factors	Multiparity, multiple gestation, advancing age (over 35), uterine incisions, previous cesarean section	Multiparity, chronic hypertension, PIH, uterine trauma, short umbilical cord, uterine anomaly, (perhaps) folic acid deficiency
Frequency	1:167 deliveries	1:77 to 1:200 deliveries
Symptoms	Painless bleeding, soft uterus, observable blood loss comparable to that with signs of shock	Sudden, intense, localized uterine pain with or without bleeding Shock out of proportion to observable blood loss
Prognosis	Maternal mortality: 0.1% Major problem: prematurity Perinatal mortality: 15%–20%	Maternal mortality: 0.5%–5% Perinatal mortality: 15%
Recurrence	1:17	1:6 to 1:18
Complications	Hemorrhage Hypovolemic shock Thrombocytopenia Premature rupture of membranes Fetal malposition Air embolism Postpartum hemorrhage Uterine rupture	Hemorrhage DIC Renal failure Anemia Pulmonary embolus

TABLE 23-4

Classification of Abruptio Placentae According to Placental Separation

Mild	Moderate	Severe
Minimum placental separation (less than one-sixth of placenta is separated) Bleeding: less than 500 ml Maternal condition: good Fetal condition: good No special intervention	Bleeding: 500–1000 ml Maternal condition: cardiovascular instability Fetal condition: FHR may or may not be present	Bleeding: hemorrhage (overt or covert) Placental separation: more than two-thirds Maternal condition: unstable (hypotension, tachycardia, DIC, renal failure) Fetal condition: distress or intrauterine death

Assessment

The nursing assessment includes all of the components described for clients with spontaneous abortion and placenta previa. In addition, the nurse must carefully assess for an increase in fundal height, indicating probable concealed bleeding. Initial laboratory test results to review and monitor include fibrinogen levels, fibrin degradation products (FDP), thrombin time, prothrombin time (PT), and partial thromboplastin time (PTT).

Nursing Diagnosis

Assessment of the client for signs and symptoms of abruptio placentae may lead the nurse to some of the previously described nursing diagnoses for placenta previa.

Planning and Intervention

During labor the nurse must be alert to any sudden change such as aching or knifelife pain in the abdomen that may signal separation of the placenta. Additionally, the uterus is assessed for irritability and to ensure there is good relaxation between contractions. A line marked on the skin at the fundus assists in determining if fundal height has increased. The nurse should also be alert to signs of increased bleeding and symptoms of shock (Table 23-5). At all times the nurse should be truthful and realistic about the client's health situation when providing psychologic support to the family. After delivery the nurse should continue assessing fluid volume balance, vital signs, firmness of the uterus, and excessive blood loss.

Disseminated Intravascular Coagulation

Manifestations and Cause

Disseminated intravascular coagulation (DIC) is a blood clotting disorder that occurs when the balance between factors favoring clotting and factors opposing clotting become unbalanced. DIC may occur after abruptio

TABLE 23-5
Clinical Staging of Hemorrhagic Shock by Volume of Blood Loss

	Mild (20%-25% Loss)	Moderate (25-35% loss)	Severe (>35% loss)	Irreversible
Respirations	Rapid, deep	Rapid, becoming shallow	Rapid, shallow, may be irregular	Irregular or barely perceptible
Pulse	<100 bpm Rapid; tone normal	100-120 bpm Rapid; tone may be normal but is becoming weaker	>120 bpm Very rapid; easily collapsible; may be irregular	Irregular apical pulse
Blood pressure	Normal or hypertensive	80-100 mm Hg systolic	<60 mm Hg systolic	None palpable
Skin	Cool and pale Peripheral vasoconstriction	Cool, pale, moist; knees cyanotic	Cold, clammy; cyanosis of lips and fingernails	Cold, clammy, cyanotic
Urinary output	No change	Decreasing to 10-22 ml/hr	Oliguric (<10 ml) to anuric	Anuric
Level of consciousness	Alert, oriented; diffuse anxiety	Oriented, mental cloudiness, or increasing restlessness	Lethargy; reacts to noxious stimuli; comatose	Does not respond to noxious stimuli
Central venous pressure	May be normal	3 cm H$_2$O	0-3 cm H$_2$O	

bpm = beats per minute.

placentae, pregnancy-induced hypertension (PIH), infection, or amniotic fluid embolism. These complications hasten and intensify the blood clotting process to the point that subsequent bleeding may be life threatening. Once the coagulation process has been initiated, massive clotting occurs rapidly. Fibrinogen becomes depleted. Four common predisposing factors are involved in DIC: arterial hypotension (often associated with shock), hypoxemia, acidemia, and stasis of capillary blood.

Diagnosis and Prognosis

With DIC the stage has been set for crisis. When the clotting factors are depleted and excessive anticoagulants are present, the client begins to bleed either occultly or overtly. The client is at risk for tissue damage from multiple thrombi and hemorrhagic death.

Therapeutic Management

Management of DIC begins with identifying and correcting the underlying cause(s), preventing or managing hemorrhage or shock, and managing the consequences of tissue necrosis. If the precipitating factors can be eliminated, the acute DIC episode should subside within 24 hours. Blood or blood products are given to replace factors that are deficient.

Assessment

The nurse assesses for obvious signs and symptoms of bleeding. Signs and symptoms of occult hemorrhage include abdominal distension, guaiac-positive stool, cloudy urine, changes in skin and scleral color, malaise, weakness, altered sensorium, vision changes, headaches, air hunger, and tachycardia.

Nursing Diagnosis

As assessment is performed, nursing diagnoses are developed that relate to the severity of the client's condition and the anxiety and fear of the family. DIC is a critical condition that requires skill in medical and nursing care and psychologic support of the client and her family (see Potential Nursing Diagnoses: Disseminated Intravascular Coagulation).

Planning and Intervention

The six major interventions in caring for a client with DIC are (1) to detect occult bleeding; (2) to prevent further bleeding; (3) to monitor

---

POTENTIAL NURSING DIAGNOSES

Disseminated Intravascular Coagulation

Fluid Volume Deficit (2)—related to excessive blood loss, i.e., hemorrhage

Altered General Tissue Perfusion—related to hypovolemia and decreased cardiac output

Decreased Cardiac Output—related to excessive blood loss and hypovolemia

Altered Family Processes—related to woman's condition

Anxiety, Fear—related to woman's condition

Knowledge Deficit—regarding high-risk situation, implications, management

---

Focus Assessment

Monitor vital signs and fetal heart rate closely.
Estimate amount of blood loss. Identify signs of increase or decrease in bleeding.
Monitor level of consciousness.
Identify presence or absence of pain.
Determine individual teaching or learning needs.
Observe family interactions.

NURSING
CARE
PLAN

Hemorrhage Occurring in Late Pregnancy

Goals

Goals (Expected Outcomes)	Interventions	Rationale	Evaluation
Decreased Cardiac Output—Related to Hypovolemia			
Alterated Placental Tissue Perfusion—Related to Separation From Uterine Wall			
The client will maintain adequate cardiac output so perfusion is maintained to brain, kidneys, liver, and uteroplacental unit.	Assess maternal blood loss and vital signs every 15 min to every 1 hr.	Hypotension indicates a large amount of blood loss.	Client's blood loss is controlled, and vital signs are stable.
	Maintain bed rest with client in left-lateral position.	Ensures best blood supply to uterus, placenta, and kidneys.	Client rests comfortably in bed.
	Initiate and monitor intravenous fluids to restore circulating volume (use at least 18-gauge needle).	Restores circulation volume.	Client received adequate fluid intake.
	Type and crossmatch two (or more) units of whole blood.	Replaces blood immediately as needed.	Client returns to normal urinary output.
	Review results of serial CBC, hemoglobin, and hematocrit values.	Indicates amount of blood lost.	Homeostasis is achieved.
	Administer oxygen as needed for client and infant.	Increases oxygen saturation.	Both are well-oxygenated; maternal vital signs are normal; and baseline fetal heart rate (FHR) in normal range of 110-160.
	Monitor and record intake and output.	Promotes and maintains fluid electrolyte balance.	Fluid and electrolyte balance is maintained.
	Count and weigh perineal pads; inspect contents for tissue.	Estimates blood loss.	Homeostasis is achieved.
	Report change in level of consciousness.	May occur with shock.	Client is alert and visiting with mate.
	Report presence of pallor, cyanosis, coolness, dampness.	Occurs with shock and loss of hemoglobin.	Color is good; skin is warm and dry with good turgor.
	Report change in uterine contractions for frequency, duration, intensity, and resting tone.	Increase may be due to placental separation (no increase with placenta previa).	Contraction pattern is normal, with good relaxation between contractions.
	Report change in fundal height.	Concealed bleeding may cause increase in fundal height.	Fundal height is unchanged.
	Monitor CVP for vital functioning.	Monitors adequate return of blood to maternal heart.	Homeostasis is achieved.
	Apply fetal monitor; assess FHR.	Assesses fetus for stress or distress (possibly death).	Fetus has normal baseline FHR (110-160); with good variability and no accelerations and decelerations.
	Prepare for delivery.	Optimizes fetal outcome and controls hemorrhage.	All equipment for initial care and resuscitation is ready and checked.
	Notify neonatologist or pediatrician of impending delivery.	Infant may require care and resuscitation.	Neonatologist or pediatri-

NURSING
CARE
PLAN

Hemorrhage Occurring in Late Pregnancy—*continued*

Goals (Expected Outcomes)	Interventions	Rationale	Evaluation
Knowledge Deficit—Regarding Physiologic Alterations in the Reproductive System			
Client will verbalize understanding of performed procedures.	Instruct client about "danger signals" in early pregnancy and what actions to take.	Encourages early recognition and reporting of danger signals.	Client verbalizes danger signals and what to do.
	Instruct client about limiting activity, getting bed rest, and abstaining from sexual activity.	Enables active client participation in own health maintenance.	Client verbalizes why interventions are necessary.
Dysfunctional Grieving—Related to Actual or Threatened Loss of Pregnancy			
Client feels comfortable to grieve as she wishes.	Provide opportunities for expression of grief, anger, loss.	Provides understanding of grieving process.	Client is resolving grief appropriately.
	Allow client to be with supportive family members.	Individuals derive support from family or significant others.	Grief is being shared with supportive individuals.
Client believes support is available in a nonjudgmental atmosphere.	Accept client's feelings of grief and associated behaviors in nonjudgmental manner.	Anger is part of grieving.	Client understands anger in the context of grief.
	Provide factual information about abortion (or ectopic pregnancy or hydatidiform mole) and possible future reproductive capacities.	Fear is greater with unknown.	Client understands information about bleeding.
	Initiate referral for genetic counseling if appropriate.	Information related to recurrence rates is provided.	Client makes arrangements for counseling (genetic) if appropriate.
	Initiate referral for support services if desired.	Follow-up with support services helps resolve grieving process.	Client is resolving grief process.
Infection—Related to Ruptured Membranes, Procedures			
Client recovers without complications of infection.	Provide education about perineal hygiene.	Proper cleansing helps prevent infection.	Client demonstrates proper cleansing technique after voiding.
	Assess vital signs (especially temperature).	Infection usually causes fever.	Vital signs remain within normal limits.
	Assess for local tenderness.	Sign of postpartum endometrial infection.	Client states has no tenderness or pain.
	Assess for malodorous vaginal discharge.	Sign of infection.	Client has no odor with vaginal discharge.

blood loss; (4) to administer blood products and medication and maintain fluid and electrolyte balance; (5) to administer oxygen to prevent or treat hypoxia; and (6) to assess vital functions carefully and continuously through central venous pressure (CVP) monitoring or use of a pulmonary artery catheter (see Nursing Care Plan).

Sickle Cell Anemia

Manifestations and Cause

Sickle cell anemia is a genetic disorder that occurs most frequently in blacks. It is characterized by an abnormal hemoglobin molecule, hemoglobin S, which causes red blood cells (RBC) to become sickleshaped. Approximately 8% to 10% of blacks in the United States carry the sickle cell trait, and 1:500 to 1:625 has sickle cell disease. It is an autosomal-recessive inheritance disease. If both parents have the sickle cell gene, 1:4 of their children will inherit the disease, and 2:4 will be carriers.

Diagnosis and Prognosis

Prenatal genetic counseling is important since sickle cell disease is inherited. Antepartum diagnosis can be made by testing amniotic fluid. Pregnancy complicates sickle cell disease. The increased rates of maternal morbidity and mortality are due to hemolytic and folic acid deficiency anemias, frequent crises, infection, PIH, and **eclampsia,** pulmonary complications, and congestive heart failure. Maternal mortality rates are as high as 4% to 5%. Morbidity and mortality rates of the fetus are also increased due to spontaneous abortion, stillbirth, preterm delivery, and intrauterine growth retardation.

Therapeutic Management

The keys to the successful management of clients with sickle cell anemia are early detection, good prenatal care, and prompt, effective management of complications. Folic acid and iron supplements are prescribed, and ultrasonic and biophysical evaluations are done to assess fetal growth and well-being. Close monitoring of maternal and fetal progress is necessary during labor. The client must receive adequate pain relief. She and her fetus must be watched closely for signs of hypoxia. If there are any signs of fetal distress, a cesarean delivery is performed. If the client develops acidosis or hypoxia, the sickling increases, which obstructs the capillaries and causes increased blood viscosity in the capillaries, resulting in more sickling and further deoxygenation and a vasoocclusive crisis. Its symptoms include (1) pain crisis, which is bone and joint pain precipitated by dehydration, acidosis, or infection and (2) aplastic crisis, in which there is a rapidly developing anemia caused by cessation of RBC production.

The management of crises is based on eliminating and treating the precipitating factors. Pain management includes administering intravenous fluids and analgesics. If the hematocrit level falls to <25%, providing a blood transfusion may be necessary.

Assessment

The nurse assesses the client's understanding about sickle cell disease and pregnancy. During the client's pregnancy the nurse should be alert for signs and symptoms of sickle cell crisis, as well as problems that may precipitate crisis (see display on p. 631). Urinary tract infection is more common in clients who have sickle cell disease. The nurse reviews signs and symptoms indicative of infection with the client so she can notify her physician about their occurrence and receive early intervention.

Sickle Cell Crisis

Signs and Symptoms

Joint pain
Laboratory verification of RBC sickling
Temperature elevation
Petechiae
Jaundice
Abdominal pain
Hematuria/hemoptysis
Chills

Precipitating Factors

Infection
PIH
Hemolytic and folic acid deficiency anemia
Eclampsia
Dehydration

Timely treatment can prevent a pain crisis. Vital signs are monitored for signs of infection and the skin observed for petechiae and jaundice caused by anemia. How the client feels in general is also helpful in recognizing symptoms of anemia. Signs and symptoms of crisis include severe bone and joint pain, abdominal pain, hemoptysis, hematuria, and chills and fever.

Nursing Diagnosis

It is imperative to identify nursing diagnoses that relate to the individual needs of clients with sickle cell disease. Some clients understand the implications of their disease during pregnancy and need minimum help. Others need several nursing diagnoses and in-depth teaching, care, and understanding to accept the added responsibilities of pregnancy and the risks to herself and her fetus (see Potential Nursing Diagnoses: Sickle Cell Anemia on p. 632).

Planning and Intervention

Nursing interventions are directed toward client education about protecting against infection, maintaining good nutritional intake, taking the prescribed vitamins and iron, and getting proper rest. The nurse also assists with administering blood transfusions and oxygen and arranging for help at home as indicated. Vital signs and laboratory values are monitored. The client and her family are kept informed of the pregnancy prognosis and are taught the signs and symptoms to report to the physician.

Rh Sensitization (Hemolytic Disease)

Manifestations and Cause

Hemolytic disease is another complication of pregnancy in which there can be devastating fetal effects. There is no risk to the mother. Attention has been focused on the Rh factor as a cause, but the ABO blood groups also can cause a milder form of hemolytic disease.

□ POTENTIAL
NURSING DIAGNOSES

Sickle Cell Anemia

Knowledge Deficit—regarding implications of disease for pregnancy and outcome, diet, self-care
Fear—related to impact of maternal disease on the fetus
Pain—related to sickle cell crisis secondary to physiologic stress of pregnancy
Altered Tissue Perfusion—related to low oxygen-carrying capacity of blood secondary to sickle shape of red blood cells
Potential for Injury (Maternal; Fetal)—related to decreased perfusion of maternal liver, kidneys, and placenta
Situational Low Self-Esteem—related to altered body image secondary to perception of potential effects of sickle cell anemia on pregnancy

Focus Assessment

Determine current level of knowledge regarding her disorder, effects of pregnancy on the disorder, effects of the disorder on pregnancy, and prenatal management.
Explore nonverbal indicators of affect, mood.
Elicit information regarding self-image.
Monitor hemoglobin and hematocrit values.
Explore complaints that suggest
   Complications of pregnancy, e.g., threatened abortion, pregnancy-induced hypertension, premature labor, or infection.
   Complications of sickle cell anemia, e.g., renal dysfunction, cardiovascular instability.
Monitor fetal status, e.g., nonstress testing, contraction stress testing, ultrasonography.

The incidence of hemolytic disease is most prevalent in white people with 15% Rh negative. Rh problems can occur with an Rh-negative mother and Rh-positive father (Fig. 23-6). Fetal involvement with hemolytic disease has been reduced by prophylactic use of Rh_o (D) immune globulin (RhoGAM), which suppresses the immune response of the Rh-negative mother to the Rh-positive RBCs of the fetus.

The maternal and fetal circulations are separate. Rh hemolytic disease occurs when a break in the barrier between the maternal and fetal circulations permits entry of some fetal RBCs into the maternal circulation. This can occur during the second and third trimesters and at delivery. Such breaks also occur with abortions beyond 6 to 8 weeks of pregnancy and during or after some procedures such as amniocentesis or external version.

If the mother and fetus possess the same Rh factor, a break in the barrier between maternal and fetal circulation is uneventful. But if the mother is Rh negative and the fetus is Rh positive (containing the Rh-positive, or D, antigen), she will have a reaction to the mismatched "minitransfusion" of fetal blood, and protective antibodies will be formed (Fig. 23-7). The mother who is pregnant for the first time usually is not sensitized, so this problem is rarely encountered with the first pregnancy. Antibodies formed as a result of that first reaction persist throughout the woman's life. Once the antibodies are formed, all subsequent pregnancies with Rh-positive fetuses will have problems. When the woman becomes pregnant again and the fetus is Rh positive, she will respond with rapid antibody formation as soon as she is exposed again to Rh-positive cells.

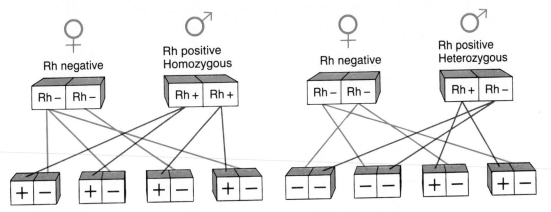

FIGURE 23-6

Rh Blood Type Inheritance. Inheritance of Rh blood type follows dominant-recessive rules, with Rh positive dominant. If the mother is Rh negative (carries two Rh negative genes) and the father is Rh positive, it is important to determine if the father is heterozygous or homozygous positive. If he is heterozygous positive, there is a 50-50 chance the fetus will be Rh negative with an unaffected pregnancy. If the father is homozygous, he will always transmit the Rh-positive gene, with the potential for pregnancies affected by hemolytic disease.

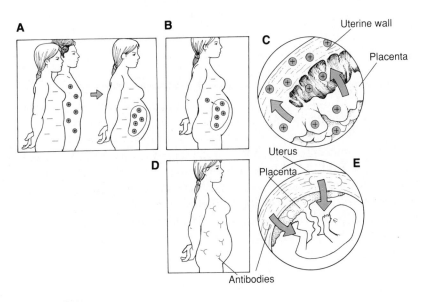

FIGURE 23-7

Rh Isoimmunization. **A,** Rh-negative woman before pregnancy. **B,** Pregnancy with Rh-positive fetus. Some Rh-positive blood passes into mother's blood. **C,** During separation of placenta a massive inoculation of mother by Rh-positive red blood cells occurs. **D,** Approximately 72 hours after delivery, mother becomes sensitized to Rh-positive blood and develops anti–Rh-positive antibodies. She now has titer, or positive Coombs' test. **E,** During subsequent pregnancy with Rh-positive fetus maternal anti–Rh-positive antibodies enter fetal circulation, attached to fetal Rh-positive red blood cells, and subject them to hemolysis.

Diagnosis and Prognosis

On the first prenatal visit, the client's blood group, Rh type, and indirect antiglobulin (Coombs' test) antibody screen are identified. Prognosis depends on prenatal surveillance as noted in the display on page 634. If no sensitization has occured and Rh_o (D) immune globulin is administered, there is little or no risk to the mother and her fetus.

Management of Unsensitized Rh-Negative Client

Initial Visit

Blood group, Rh type, and indirect Coombs' test antibody screen are determined.

At 28 Weeks Gestation

Indirect Coombs' test is repeated. If there are no Rh antibodies, 300 µg of Rh_o (D) immune globulin are administered to provide protection for 12 weeks.

At 35 Weeks Gestation

An anti-D (Rh_o) titer is done. If titer is 1:4 or greater, it could mean there is active immunization.

At Delivery

The anti-D (Rh_o) titer is repeated. A titer greater than 1:4 means the client has active immunization and the client is *not* a candidate for Rh_o (D) immune globulin.

Lower titers indicate client *is* a candidate for Rh_o (D) immune globulin.

Blood grouping, Rh typing, and direct Coombs' test are determined on cord blood.

A Betke-Kleihaner test is ordered if a transplacental bleed is suspected, and its results are used to determine if additional Rh_o (D) immune globulin is required.

Therapeutic Management

If the initial and 28-week antibody screens are negative, 300 µg of immune globulin is given intramuscularly to protect the client from any possible feto-maternal bleeding episode (see Drug Guide: Rh_o Immune (D) Globulin). If the indirect Coombs' test exceeds the critical titer (a 1:8 to 1:16 dilution), an amniocentesis is done to determine the quantity of bilirubin in the amniotic fluid. The higher the bilirubin in the amniotic fluid, the lower is the fetal hemoglobin value, indicating anemia in the fetus. The bilirubin is analyzed by spectrophotometry and is plotted on the Liley graph (Fig. 23-8). Another purpose of amniocentesis is to identify the need for intrauterine transfusion of the immature anemic fetus.

Assessment

Much of nursing assessment is directed toward determining the client's understanding of Rh disease and her psychologic and emotional status resulting from concern for fetal welfare.

Nursing Diagnosis

Nursing diagnoses are formulated to meet the client's need for procedures and continuing management of the pregnancy and for preparation for delivery (see Potential Nursing Diagnoses: Hemolytic Disease).

Planning and Intervention

Nursing interventions focus on educating the parents about Rh hemolytic disease so they can understand what it is, why it occurs, the diagnostic tests that must be performed, and other interventions that will be done.

◻ POTENTIAL NURSING DIAGNOSES

Hemolytic Disease

Knowledge Deficit—regarding hemolytic disease and procedures used in management

Altered Parenting—related to feelings of inadequacy and concern about outcome of pregnancy and health of the fetus

Anxiety, Fear—related to outcome for the fetus

Potential Injury to Fetus—related to prematurity or effects of maternal sensitization (anemia, heart failure, and intrauterine fetal death are possible)

Rh₀ (D) immune globulin (human) (RhoGAM): A sterile concentrated solution of specific immunoglobulin (IgG) containing anti-Rh₀ (D) prepared from human fractionated plasma.

Obstetric Action: Immune globulin acts by suppressing the specific immune response of unsensitized Rh-negative mothers to Rh-positive red blood cells (RBCs). It prevents hemolytic disease in their Rh-positive newborns.

Administration: Rh₀ (D) immunoglobulin is administered intramuscularly.

1. One vial (300 μg) is given for antepartum prophylaxis (at approximately 28 wk).
2. One vial (50 μg) is given after amniocentesis, miscarriage, abortion, or etopic pregnancy or beyond 13 weeks of gestation. If pregnancy terminates before 13 weeks, a vial of MICRhoGAM may be used.
3. One vial is given for postpartum prophylaxis within 72 hr of delivery if tests indicate no sensitization has occurred.

Potential Side Effects and Complications: Reactions are infrequent and mild and are confined to the area of injection. Systemic reactions are rare.

Nursing Implications:

1. The nurse is responsible for checking the blood types and Rh status of every pregnant client.
2. The nurse will have a standing order or will obtain an order from the primary physician to do all of the following unless the father is known to be Rh negative.
   a. Give one dose of prophylactic Rh immunoglobulin (RhIG) (300 μg) to every unsensitized Rh-negative client at 28 weeks gestation unless the father of the fetus is known to be Rh negative.
   b. Do an Rh blood workup on both mother and infant at the time of the delivery to determine the blood type and Rh of the neonate, and give one prophylactic dose of RhIG as soon as possible after delivery to affected mothers.
   c. Give every Rh-negative unsensitized woman who aborts at least 50 μg of RhIG.
   d. Administer RhIG (300 μg) to every Rh-negative, unimmunized woman undergoing amniocentesis.
3. The nurse will be asked to order a Betke-Kleihauer stain to assess the amount of fetal blood in the maternal circulation; this result will assist the physician in adjusting the dosage of Rh₀ (D) immune globulin.

◯ DRUG
◯ GUIDE

FIGURE 23-8

Liley Graph. Modified Liley graph for relating the optical density peak at 450 (ΔOD_{450}) to weeks of gestation in determining severity of hemolytic disease.

American College of Obstetrics and Gynecologists: Management of Isoimmunization in Pregnancy. (ACOG Tech Bull 80.) Washington DC, ACOG, September 1984.

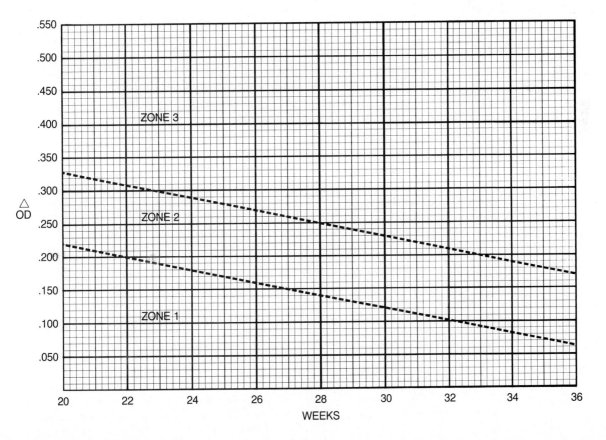

This information can lower their anxiety and apprehension. The nurse should also encourage the parents to verbalize their fears and be together when diagnostic tests are performed.

Hypertensive Disorders of Pregnancy

Hypertensive disorders include a variety of vascular disturbances. Because of its many cardiovascular alterations, pregnancy can induce hypertension in women who have been normotensive before gestation or can aggravate existing hypertensive conditions.

Previously, *toxemia* or **preeclampsia** were the terms used to describe the type of hypertension particular to pregnancy. The term *pregnancy-induced hypertension* (PIH) is currently used to describe the syndrome of hypertension, edema, and proteinuria seen in some pregnant women.

PIH (preeclampsia) concerns the hypertension that develops as a direct result of pregnancy and is characterized by hypertension with proteinuria or edema that develops after the 20th week of gestation. Eclampsia develops when the preeclamptic woman develops convulsions or coma that is unrelated to any other cerebral conditions. The preeclamptic client becomes eclamptic when she has a convulsion or becomes comatose.

The hypertensive disorders of pregnancy are considered in two broad classifications: (1) PIH, including preeclampsia and eclampsia, and (2) hypertensive disorders not confined solely to pregnancy but that can occur during pregnancy.

Pregnancy-Induced Hypertension

Manifestations and Cause

PIH is the occurrence of hypertension with proteinuria or edema or both after the 20th week of pregnancy. Its cause is unknown. Risk factors before and during pregnancy are listed in Table 23-6. Hypertension is defined as being 30 mm Hg systolic or 15 mm Hg diastolic above the baseline pressures recorded before pregnancy or during the first prenatal visit. The elevated blood pressure must be present on two occasions 6 hours apart.

Edema associated with PIH is excessive and generalized and weight gain caused by edema is generally rapid. Proteinuria is the last sign of the three (hypertension, edema, and proteinuria) to occur. Proteinuria is revealed by readings of more than 1+ or 2+ by dipstick on two occasions 6 hours apart.

TABLE 23-6

Predisposing Conditions for PIH

Before Pregnancy	During Pregnancy
Diabetes mellitus	Primigravida age extremes (<20 yr or >35 yr)
Hypertension	
Renal disease	Hydramnios
Low income	Multiple gestation
Family history of PIH	Hydatidiform mole
Family history of hypertension or vascular disease	Large fetus
	Glomerulonephritis

TABLE 23-7

Laboratory Data Related to PIH

	Normal Pregnancy	Pregnancy with PIH
Hemoglobin and hemat-ocrit	12.1-12.7 g/dl 35%-42%	Elevated due to hemoconcentration
Plasma volume	Increased by 45%-50%	Reduced
Uric acid	6 mg/dl	Usually elevated
Serum creatinine	0.6-0.8 mg/dl	Elevated in severe PIH
Blood glucose	70-110 mg/dl	Normal
Electrolytes	Normal	Normal
Glomerular filtration rate	Increases by 50%	Decreased

PIH occurs as a result of widespread, generalized vasospasms, which cause decreased blood flow to the uterus, placenta, kidneys, and brain. Blood volume decreases, and systemic vascular resistance increases, resulting in elevated blood pressure.

Vasospasms in renal blood vessels cause a decreased glomerular filtration rate, which results in proteinuria. Laboratory data related to PIH are included in Table 23-7. Vasospasms also cause decreased blood flow to the brain, resulting in visual disturbances and headache. A complication of PIH is seizures. The exact cause of the seizures is unknown.

Vasospasms cause progressively decreasing blood flow to the utero-placenta unit, resulting in an abnormally small placenta, intrauterine growth retardation, and chronic hypoxia of the fetus.

Diagnosis and Prognosis

PIH is one of the three major complications (along with hemorrhage and puerperal infection) of the woman and her fetus. In recent years the combination of timely delivery and use of magnesium sulfate and hydralazine has almost eliminated maternal mortality. The perinatal mortality is higher for infants of mothers with PIH and is caused by placental insufficiency and abruptio placentae, which cause death before or during labor, and prematurity. Fetal growth retardation is another common complication. The prognosis depends on the severity and time of onset of PIH.

Therapeutic Management

Management objectives for PIH are (1) to protect the mother from the effects of high blood pressure (especially cerebral hemorrhage) and prevent seizures and other complications; (2) to improve uteroplacental blood flow to decrease the risks of intrauterine growth retardation and placental abruption until fetal maturity is achieved and delivery can be safely done; and (3) to deliver the fetus when mature by the safest and most expeditious means or, if the fetus is immature, deliver the premature fetus when to do so is safer than its remaining in the uterus.

Complete recovery from PIH occurs only after delivery. All signs usually are gone within 10 to 14 postpartum days. If blood pressure elevation continues after delivery, it may indicate chronic hypertension (see display on p. 638).

Signs of Recovery from PIH After Delivery

Urinary output of 4–6 L/day for first 2 days
Resolution of edema within 4–5 days
Rapid weight loss
Resolution of proteinurea in approximately 1 wk
Normotensive in approximately 2 wk

If all signs are not absent 4–6 wk after delivery, chronic hypertension is suspected.

Assessment

Assessment for PIH begins during the first prenatal visit. Signs must be recognized early to optimize the outcome for mother and fetus. During the first prenatal visit baseline data is obtained and recorded. Data is updated at each subsequent visit. When PIH is diagnosed but remains mild, home care is possible with client education (see Client Self-Care Education: PIH: Home Care). When symptoms require intensive management, the client is admitted to the hospital. Assessment of the client admitted to the hospital with severe PIH is shown in Assessment Tool: PIH. Table 23-8 shows progression of severe PIH to ecalmpsia.

Fetal assessment is based on the client's perception of fetal movement and electronic fetal monitoring is done to determine the fetus' stable baseline, reactivity, and presence or absence of periodic fetal heart rate (FHR) changes. This data indicates how well the fetus is responding to the plan of care. The fetus is assessed for well-being and for maturity (see display on p. 641).

Finally, it is important to assess the understanding of the client about PIH and its management.

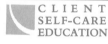

CLIENT SELF-CARE EDUCATION

PIH: Home Care

Intervention

1. Explain necessity of *rest* in left-lateral recumbent position.

2. Explain diet modification: high in protein, avoidance of high-sodium foods, 6–8 glasses of water daily.
3. Instruct client to weigh self daily.

4. Instruct client to report *signs* and *symptoms* of increased severity of PIH.
   a. Decreased urinary output
   b. No weight loss
   c. No decrease or minimum decrease in blood pressure
   d. Headaches, blurred vision, or epigastric pain
   e. Decreasing fetal movement

Rationale

1. This position improves blood flow to kidneys and results in improved glomerular function and placental perfusion.
2. Replaces protein lost in urine and increases urinary output.

3. Determines if amount of edema is changing.
4. Home care is no longer sufficient with increased severity, and hospitalization with more aggressive management is necessary. Depending on gestation, response to medical management, client's well-being or decreasing uteroplacental perfusion, hospitalization may be brief.

PIH

Gravida, para, abortions:
Estimated date of confinement:
LMP:
Gestation:
Age:
Marital status:
Prenatal history: (complications of previous pregnancy; complications of
 present pregnancy)
Previous and present medications and reasons for use:
Prepregnant weight:
Present weight:
Pattern of weight gain:
Fetal activity: (active, decreased fetal movement)
Subjective signs of elevated blood pressure: (frontal headache, blurred vision,
 seeing spots of flashes of light, muscle twitching, vomiting, epigastric pain)
Vital signs: (blood pressure taken in sitting or left-lateral position)
Edema: (location and amount)
Dipstick results for urinary protein:
Review of laboratory results: (electrolytes, blood urea nitrogen, creatinine, uric
 acid, aspartate transaminase, magnesium sulfate, CBC, platelets, PT, PTT)
Lung sounds: (rales present, absent)
Central nervous system status: (jittery, muscle twitchings)
Level of consciousness:
Psychologic status: (apprehensive, anxious)
Fetal assessment: (nonstress test for fetal reactivity, contraction stress test for
 placental-respiratory reserve, amniotic fluid volume [stable, decreased])

TABLE 23-8

PIH Progression

Mild PIH	Severe PIH	Eclampsia
Manifestations		
Blood pressure (BP) 140/90 or +30/+15 × 2, 6 hr apart (diastolic most important) Proteinuria: in clean catch specimen on 2 successive days Edema of face or hands (no diagnosis based on edema only) Weight gain of 2 pounds or more in 1 wk or >6 pounds in 1 mo	BP 160/110 × 2, 6 hr apart with patient at rest Proteinuria: 5 g/24 hr or 3+ or 4+ protein on dipstick Oliguria: urinary output <400 ml/24 hr Cerebral or visual disturbances Pulmonary edema or cyanosis Epigastric pain	Progression of disease to one or more convulsive seizures followed by coma Not attributable to other conditions such as epilepsy or cerebral hemorrhage
Medical Diagnosis and Prognosis		
Prenatal care Perform early examination for dating of pregnancy. Obtain first trimester BP. Note rising or elevated BP after 20th week of pregnancy. Check for protein in urine. Note presence of edema above waist and weight increase of >2 pounds/wk. *Sequence of occurrence* 1. Edema 2. Elevated BP 3. Proteinuria	Any of the above criteria meets diagnostic criteria for severe PIH. *Prognosis* Depends on severity. Depends on gestation at onset. Perinatal loss relates to prematurity, labor, and delivery factors. Maternal condition depends on response to care and labor and delivery without significant complications (e.g., abruption).	Same as above.

Continued

TABLE 23-8

PIH Progression—continued

Mild PIH	Severe PIH	Eclampsia
Medical Management		
Regular visits to physician; early detection of PIH	Objectives:	Observe.
Resting in left-lateral recumbent position	Prevent eclampsia and intracra-nial hemorrhage.	Protect from injury.
Increased intake of salt free fluids if output is normal	Limit progression of severity, maternal mortality.	Deliver fetus.
High protein diet; avoidance of salty foods (particularly empty calorie snacks)	Reduce fetal mortality and morbidity.	
Daily weights	Client resting in left-lateral re-cumbent position	
Office visits as prescribed	Monitoring of intake and output; fluids may be oral or intrave-nous, output may be measured using Foley catheter, and CVP may be used to assess volume deficit	
Kick counts; monitoring time required to count 10 kicks		
Reporting of any of the following:		
Decreased urinary output		
Swelling (edema) that does not recede with rest		
No decrease in weight	High protein diet; avoidance of salty foods (particularly empty calorie snacks)	
Headaches, blurred vision, epigastric pain		
Indications for Delivery	Daily weights	
Maternal indications	Monitoring of vital signs (blood pressure and pulse every 1-4 hr except at night [may or may not be ordered at night])	
Deterioration or failure to improve		
Ripe cervix		
Fetal indications	Biweekly nonstress or contrac-tion stress testing or both; nonstress test may be done daily	
Mature lecithin/sphingomyelin ratio		
Results from oxytocin challenge test and nonstress test		
Poor fetal growth	Monitoring of deep tendon re-flexes	
Route of delivery	Ophthalmic examination to as-sess ocular fundi for choked discs (indicating arteriolar con-striction of vessels behind eyes in optic chiasma)	
Vaginal		
Cesarean section		
Note: Avoid supine hypotension; avoid volume depletion		
	Laboratory evaluations: *blood* for hematocrit, hemoglobin, blood urea nitrogen, uric acid, creati-nine, and creatinine clearance; *urine* for protein (24 hr)	
	Seizure precautions	
	Drugs: magnesium sulfate for depression of central nervous system; antihypertensives to decrease blood pressure (used for diatolic blood pressure >100 mm Hg)	
	Assessment for coagulation changes	
	CVP monitoring	

Nursing Diagnosis

Nursing diagnoses to consider for the client with PIH are related to cardiovascular instability, potential central nervous system involvement, potential fetal injury, and knowledge deficit (see Potential Nursing Diagnoses: PIH).

Focus Assessment

Closely monitor: vital signs, weight gain or loss, presence and amount of protein in urine, digital and periorbital edema, fetal heart rate, results of nonstress tests. (Frequency varies with severity of previous assessment findings and change in maternal or fetal status.)

Observe for signs of pathologic progression: deep tendon reflexes, emergence of complaints of headache or epigastric pain, level of consciousness.

Monitor for signs of medication effects: vital signs, deep tendon reflexes, intake and output, weight loss.

Determine current level of knowledge regarding disorder, status, management.

Explore nonverbal indicators of emotional status, e.g., affect, mood, appearance, inability to concentrate, sleep patterns.

Identify expectations of pregnancy outcome.

POTENTIAL
NURSING DIAGNOSES

PIH

Potential for Injury (Maternal)—related to central nervous system irritability secondary to cerebral edema, vasospasm, decreased renal perfusion

Potential for Injury (Fetal)—related to diminished uteroplacental perfusion, intrauterine hypoxia, anoxia, or asphyxia, preterm delivery

Altered General Tissue Perfusion—related to vasospasm, hypertension, and loss of fluid to extravascular spaces

Fluid Volume Deficit (1)—related to loss of intravascular volume to extravascular spaces secondary to decreased serum albumin

Altered Health Maintenance—related to cardiovascular instability secondary to hypertension, edema, and proteinuria

Anxiety, Fear—related to maternal or fetal condition

Knowledge Deficit—regarding the disorder, medical management, diet

Self-Care Deficit—related to severity of disorder, e.g., eclampsia

Powerlessness—related to personal inability to prevent or control condition and outcome

Fetal Assessment

For Well-Being

Fetal movement (mother records interval of time it takes for 10 fetal movements)

Nonstress testing

Contraction stress testing

Biophysical profile

Ultrasonography for placental grading

For Maturity

Amniocentesis for lecithin / sphingomyelin ratio or phosphotidyl glycerol

Ultrasonographic measurements

Planning and Intervention

Interventions are directed at improving cardiovascular instability, providing a safe environment, administering ordered medications (see Drug Guide: Magnesium Sulfate on p. 642), preventing seizures, and being prepared for emergency treatment.

⊖ DRUG
⊖ GUIDE

Magnesium sulfate (50%): Primary action is to compete with calcium to block the reuptake of acetylcholine at the synapses. Its anticonvulsant mechanism of action is still not understood and is controversial.

Obstetric Action: To control seizure activity.

Preparation and Administration:
Intravenous route
1. Prepare *loading dose:* 4 g magnesium sulfate added to 240 ml D_5W. Administer by piggyback method (using an infusion pump or controller) over a 15- to 20-min period.
2. Maintenance of a therapeutic level requires an intravenous (IV) infusion of 3 g/hr. (Effects of drug last 30 min if given intravenously and 3-4 hr if given intramuscularly).
Combination of intramuscular (IM) and intravenous (IV) routes
1. Administer the *loading dose* of 4 g magnesium sulfate IV over 20 min and simultaneously administer 10 mg magnesium sulfate IM (5 g deeply into each buttock). If drug is injected into subcutaneous tissue, necrosis will occur.
2. Give 5 g of magnesium sulfate every 4 hr (deep IM). The IV dose is given to obtain therapeutic levels rapidly (4-7 mg/dl).

Maternal Contraindications: Magnesium sulfate should be withheld if the patellar reflex disappears, respirations are <12-14 per minute, or if urinary output is <30 ml/hr.

Potential Side Effects and Complications: *Early signs* of magnesium intoxication include the following:

Hot all over	Depression of reflexes
Flushing	Hypotension
Thirst	Muscle flaccidity
Sweating	

Later signs of hypermagnesemia are as follows:
Central nervous system depression (respirations <12, decreased reflexes)
Respiratory paralysis (magnesium, 10-12 mg/dl)
Circulatory collapse (dose >15 mg/dl)
Note: If the above occur, calcium gluconate is the antidote.

Nursing Implications:
1. Assess deep tendon reflexes hourly (if client receiving continuous infusion).
2. Monitor client's blood pressure, pulse, and respiration every 15-30 min; report if respirations <12-14 or hypotension occurs.
3. Monitor intake and output every hour; if output is <30 ml/hr, notify physician and anticipate decreasing or discontinuing the magnesium sulfate.
4. Continuously monitor client's orientation to person, place, and time.
5. Assess client for complaints of headache, nausea, vomiting, or epigastric pain.
6. Monitor fetus intermittently or continuously as indicated by physician's order.
7. Continue seizure precautions (e.g., padded side rail, quiet environment).
8. Keep the antidote, calcium gluconate (10% solution), at client's bedside.

As PIH becomes more severe, the intrauterine environment become hazardous to the fetus. Because of decreased uteroplacental perfusion, the fetus becomes chronically hypoxic. Interventions focus on maintaining a safe environment for the fetus.

The FHR monitor assists in assessing the oxygenation status of the fetus. Reassuring FHR patterns include stable FHR in the normal baseline range (110 to 160 beats/minute) and accelerations of the FHR during movement or other stimulation, indicating reactivity and thus well-being. A reassuring sign is absence of decelerations, specifically no variable or late decelerations.

The client's knowledge deficit can be addressed by teaching her about PIH and the importance of compliance in managing the disease process (see Client Self-Care Education: PIH: Hospital Care).

PIH: Hospital Care

Intervention

1. Explain why hospitalization is necessary.

2. Explain the special diet (70-100 g protein, balanced amount of sodium, and 6-8 glasses of water if urinary output is sufficient).
3. Explain drugs:
   a. Phenobarbital

   b. Magnesium sulfate

   c. Hydralazine
4. Explain why weight is checked daily.

5. Check fluid intake and output daily; give client cups or glasses marked with measures of volume and graduated for measuring output so that she can help in maintaining accurate measurements.
6. Explain need for checking blood pressure, pulse, and respiration every 4 hr or as ordered.
7. a. Explain need for fetal movement counts and nonstress testing daily.
   b. Explain need for contraction stress testing by nipple stimulation at least biweekly.
8. Explain use of 24-hr urine sample for protein and creatinine determination; explain need to measure and save every voiding.
9. Explain need for drawing blood for laboratory analysis.

10. Explain ultrasound scan.

11. Explain amniocentesis.
12. Explain drug betamethasone.

13. Explain checking of reflexes.

14. Explain ophthalmoscopic examination.

15. If client not too ill, take her by stretcher or wheelchair to newborn intensive care nursery and explain how her infant will be cared for (may explain and use pictures if she is too ill).

Rationale

1. Home care is no longer possible if blood pressure continues to rise; proteinuria and edema continue.
2. Special diet will replace protein being lost in urine (must not cheat)

3. a. Barbiturate provides relaxation and rest (in left-lateral position), which are important to facilitate increased blood flow return to client's heart and her cardiac output and uteroplacental perfusion and oxygenation to fetus; also helps mobilize edema.
   b. Decreases brain stimulation to reduce possibility of seizures.
   c. Decreases blood pressure.
4. Determines whether edema is decreasing or increasing or disease is improving or worsening.
5. Ensures intake and output are appropriate, edema is not increasing, and diuresis is occurring.

6. Determines progress or improvement of PIH.

7. a. Determines fetal well-being

   b. Determines respiratory function of placenta and fetal well-being.
8. Determines kidney function (helps assess deterioration or improvement of disease process).

9. All laboratory work gives critical information about functioning capacity of maternal kidneys, electrolytes, hemostats, and homeostasis.
10. Determines fetal age and estimates fetal weight.
11. Determines pulmonary lung maturity of fetus.
12. This drug is used to accelerate pulmonary maturity; if fetal lungs are immature but fetus must be delivered, the benefits of delivery outweigh the risks of prematurity.
13. Determines excitability of central nervous system.
14. Shows normal or decreased blood flow to part of brain behind eyes.
15. Helps her know what to expect if infant is born prematurely or requires intensive care and reduces her anxiety and apprehension.

Eclampsia

Manifestations and Cause

Severe PIH sometimes progresses to the point of convulsions, coma, or both. The term used to described this condition is *eclampsia*. Signs and symptoms suggesting impending convulsions are increasing blood pressure with increasing central nervous system involvement (headache, vision disturbances, hyperreflexia, confusion and disorientation, jitteriness) and epigastric pain caused by congestion of the liver.

Diagnosis and Prognosis

Diagnosis is based on the presenting signs and symptoms. When the PIH client convulses or becomes comatose, the diagnosis is changed to eclampsia. After delivery the signs and symptoms of PIH often resolve quickly as the physiology of the mother's body returns to prepregnant status.

Therapeutic Management

The initial objectives of management are to protect the client from injury, to maintain or manage her airway, and to prevent or control the seizures. Magnesium sulfate is the drug of choice. It is given intravenously or intramuscularly to decrease central nervous system irritability and thus prevent a seizure. Hydralazine (Apresoline), an antihypertensive drug, is used to lower diastolic pressure if it is greater than 110. The woman is delivered as soon she as is stabilized. Labor may be induced using oxytocin (Pitocin) if the cervix is ripe.

Continuous monitoring of the fetus before and during labor is necessary since decreasing placental circulation and perfusion cause increasing fetal hypoxia. Often a cesarean delivery is done to ensure expedient rescue of the fetus.

Postpartum management includes continuing the administration of magnesium sulfate, monitoring intake and urinary output, and administration of antihypertensive medication for a minimum of 24 hours.

Assessment

Assessment focuses on intense surveillance to detect signs of impending seizure activity (see below). Vital signs are monitored hourly or more frequently if the client is not responding to treatment. Hourly urinary volume per indwelling catheter is recorded. Laboratory data is reviewed for signs that PIH is increasing in severity. The nurse also observes for increased irritability or other central nervous system signs indicative of impending seizure activity.

Clinical Signs and Symptoms of Impending Eclampsia

Progression of PIH
Headaches, visual disturbances, epigastric discomfort
Apprehension, excitability
Tachypnea (respiration of 50)
Temperature elevation (103° F)
Increasing proteinuria
Oliguria (less than 30 ml/hr)
Acidosis

Focus Assessment

Closely monitor vital signs, fetal heart rate, level of consciousness, deep tendon reflexes, intake and output.

Identify signs of impending convulsions: vacant stare, lack of response to verbal stimuli, twitching of facial muscles.

Closely monitor number and severity of convulsions, length of apneic period, depth and duration of coma, return to consciousness.

Identify signs of labor: restlessness at regular intervals during coma, contractions, rupture of membranes, vaginal bleeding.

Explore complaints of abdominal pain.

Closely monitor FHR since convulsions decrease O_2 to fetus already experiencing hypoxia.

Nursing Diagnosis

Assessment of the eclamptic client assists the nurse in formulating nursing diagnoses aimed at protecting the mother and fetus from injury (see Potential Nursing Diagnoses: Eclampsia).

Planning and Intervention

Both the mother and fetus require 1:1 nursing care and emotional support. A detailed nursing care plan for the client with severe PIH is provided on pages 646–647.

HELLP Syndrome

Manifestations and Cause

Another often life-threatening complication of severe PIH is the HELLP syndrome. HELLP is an anachronym for the problems comprising this syndrome: hemolysis, elevated liver enzymes, and low platelets. Just as venous vasospasm is the underlying factor in PIH, arterial vasospasm is the underlying factor in the development of the hemolysis that occurs in the HELLP syndrome. The incidence is highest among older, white multiparous women. Severity is greatest when the diagnosis of PIH is delayed or management is too conservative.

Diagnosis and Prognosis

Hemolysis of RBCs is confirmed by abnormal morphology on peripheral blood smears. It may be accompanied by hemoglobinemia and hemoglobinuria. RBCs are damaged and develop irregular shapes when they pass through blood vessels that are damaged by vasospasm and contain fibrin deposits. The result is progressive anemia. Damage to the vessel walls causes adherence of platelets to the damaged site, resulting in consumption of platelets and development of thrombocytopenia. As the hemolytic process continues, the hematocrit level falls, and the woman develops hyperbilirubinemia. The platelet consumption with HELLP syndrome is similar to that with DIC except that maternal coagulation factors, prothrombin time (PT), and partial thromboplastin time (PTT) are nor-

---

◻ **POTENTIAL NURSING DIAGNOSES**

Eclampsia

Potential for Injury (Maternal)—related to convulsions

Potential for Injury (Fetal)—related to hypoxia secondary to decreased placental perfusion during mother's convulsions

Fluid Volume Deficit (2)—related to excessive bleeding secondary to abruptio placentae

Potential for Injury (Fetal)—related to preterm delivery and immaturity

Self-Care Deficit—related to pregnancy complicated by eclampsia

NURSING
◤ CARE
◤ PLAN

Client With Severe Pregnancy-Induced Hypertension

Goals (Expected Outcomes)	Interventions	Rationale	Evaluation
Potential for Injury (Maternal)—Related to CNS Irritability			
Client will respond to treatment without further complications.	Decrease environmental stimuli and limit visitors.	Reduces CNS stimulation.	Client is quiet and relaxed.
	Organize care to minimize disturbing client's rest and quiet.		
	Administer medications as ordered.		
	Phenobarbital	Encourages rest and relaxation.	Client states she rests well.
	Magnesium sulfate	Is a CNS depressant; inhibits convulsions; causes vasodilation and diuresis.	Client exhibits increased urinary output, decreased BP, and normal deep tendon reflexes.
	Apresoline	Causes vasodilation; increases cardiac output and renal flow.	Client exhibits decreased BP.
	Perform client teaching: report any headache, visual disturbances, epigastric pain.	Requires prompt evaluation; may indicate pathologic progression.	Client presents no new signs of progression; all assessment findings are within normal limits.
Potential for Injury (Fetal)—Related to Diminished Uteroplacental Perfusion, Hypoxia/Anoxia/Asphyxia, Preterm Delivery			
Client experiences a successful gestational outcome.	Encourages woman to rest on left side.	Promotes placental perfusion; protects fetal status.	FHR remains stable between 120 and 160.
	Perform client teaching: Explain rationale and anticipated benefits of bed rests, diagnostic tests (nonstress test [NST], contraction stress test [CST], ultrasonography. Explain diagnostic procedures (nonstress tests, ultrasonography).	Monitor fetal and placental status. NST records fetal heart rate response to activity. CST shows fetal response to imposed stress of contractions. Ultrasonography allows evaluation of fetal size and growth, amniotic fluid volume, and placental grading (including degree of calcification and placental age).	Fetal monitor consistently records reactive NST and reassuring pattern on oxytocin challenge test (OCT), i.e., lack of repetitive late decelerations. Ultrasonography reveals normal fetal growth, normal amniotic fluid volume, and placenta free of signs of aging.
	If monitor reveals fetal tachycardia, bradycardia, late decelerations, loss of baseline variability, provide (1) position change, (2) bolus of IV fluids, and (3) provide oxygen at 6 to 10 L/min by face mask (intrauterine resuscitation).	Increases level of circulating oxygen available to fetus.	FHR returns to normal baseline rate and variability; late decelerations disappear.

NURSING
CARE
PLAN

Client With Severe Pregnancy-Induced Hypertension—*continued*

Goals (Expected Outcomes)	Interventions	Rationale	Evaluation
Altered General Tissue Perfusion—Related to Vasospasm, Hypertension, and Edema			
Client will experience no alteration in thought processes, blurred vision, increased CNS irritability.	Encourage bedrest in left lateral position.	Promotes increased circulatory volume, renal flow, and diuresis.	Reports no episodes of visual disturbances or altered sensorium. Deep tendon reflexes (DTRs) are normal.
Fluid Volume Deficit (1)—Related to Loss of Intravascular Fluid to Extravascular Spaces			
Client will re-establish normal fluid distribution between intravascular and extravascular compartments.	Encourage high protein intake; reduce intake of foods and fluids that are high in sodium; 6 g sodium allowed per day.	Replaces protein lost in the urine; increases serum albumins; restores normal blood osmolality.	Urine tests negative for protein; edema subsiding; BP and DTRs are within normal limits.

TABLE 23-9

Changes in Laboratory Data with HELLP Syndrome

Test	Result in Healthy Pregnancy	Result With HELLP Syndrome
Liver Function Tests		
AST	4–20 (1 U/L)	Increased
ALT	3–21 (1 U/L)	Increased
Other Laboratory Values		
Platelets	150,000–400,000/mm³	Decreased
PT	10.2–13.8 sec	Unchanged
PTT	20–31 sec	Unchanged
Fibrinogen	150–400 mg/dl	Increased
Clotting time	Normal	Normal
Total bilirubin	0.2–0.9 mg/dl	Increased
Burr cells	Absent	Present

Adapted from Poole JH: Matern Child Nurs J 13: 432–437, November/December 1988.

mal. Hepatic dysfunction is confirmed by liver function tests: elevated aspartate transaminase (AST) and alanine transaminase (ALT) (Table 23-9). Hepatic dysfunction produces symptoms of nausea and vomiting, malaise, and right upper quandrant (RUQ) pain.

Therapeutic Management

Antepartum care for clients with HELLP syndrome focuses on stabilizing and preparing the mother for delivery. The only definitive management of HELLP is delivery, regardless of fetal gestational age.

Assessment

Assessment includes doing all that has been suggested for the client with PIH. The nurse also observes for signs and symptoms indicative of anemia: fatigue, pallor, anorexia, weakness, lassitude, dyspnea, edema, nausea and vomiting, and RUQ pain caused by liver involvement. The nurse closely monitors the client for hematuria, ecchymosis, petechiae, nose bleeds, or oozing from puncture sites.

In addition to these signs and symptoms, monitoring laboratory values is important (Table 23-9).

Nursing Diagnosis

Nursing diagnoses and interventions include all those listed for PIH and DIC.

Planning and Intervention

Required nursing interventions are discussed in sections dealing with PIH and DIC. A care plan for ineffective individual coping related to both PIH and the HELLP syndrome may need to be developed. The client may be fearful for her safety and for the well-being of her fetus. Inter-

---

POTENTIAL NURSING DIAGNOSES

HELPP

Potential for Injury (Fetal)—related to diminished uteroplacental perfusion, malnutrition, intrauterine hypoxia, anoxia, or asphyxia, preterm delivery
Potential for Injury (Maternal)—related to effects of pathophysiology of the HELPP syndrome
Altered General Tissue Perfusion—related to diminished intravascular volume secondary to hemolysis and obstruction of blood vessels by fibrin deposits
Decreased Cardiac Output—related to diminished intravascular volume secondary to hemolysis and edema
Knowledge Deficit—regarding the disorder, implications for maternal and fetal status, pregnancy outcome, and management
Anxiety, Fear—related to concern regarding disease process, hospitalization, pregnancy outcome
Situational Low Self-Esteem—related to guilt feelings and shame regarding high-risk pregnancy, threat to fetal status, and uncertain pregnancy outcome
Altered Family Processes—related to maternal hospitalization and severity of disease processes

---

Focus Assessment

Estimate number of weeks' gestation.
Note complaints of nausea and upper abdominal discomfort (epigastric pain).
Review findings of diagnostic studies: AST, platelet count, total bilirubin, hemoglobin and hematocrit, blood glucose, uric acid level.
Monitor closely vital signs, fetal heart rate, intake and output, results of nonstress testing.
Observe for signs of bleeding, fetal distress, labor, severe preeclampsia.
Elicit information describing prerception of self.
Explore nonverbal indicators of emotional status, e.g., affect, mood, appearance, irritability, inability to concentrate, sleep patterns.
Identify expectations of pregnancy outcome.
Determine individual teaching or learning needs.
Observe family interactions.

ventions should be instituted to meet the biophysical and psychosocial needs of these clients.

Chronic Hypertensive Vascular Disease

Manifestations and Cause

Chronic hypertensive vascular disease includes (1) hypertension that exists before pregnancy, (2) hypertension occurring before the 20th week of pregnancy, and (3) hypertension secondary to maternal disease (discovered after the 20th week of pregnancy). These hypertensive problems persist beyond 6 weeks post partum. Primary hypertension may also be compounded by superimposed PIH. Sometimes the client with chronic hypertension is warned to avoid pregnancy. Although the cause is unknown, primary renal disease may be a factor.

Diagnosis and Prognosis

The diagnosis is made by excluding other diseases. Fetal effects resulting from hypertension are related to duration and severity of the process. Perinatal mortality can be 30% if PIH is superimposed. Maternal mortality is rare but can result from cerebral hemorrhage or heart failure by worsening of the initial hypertensive disease.

Therapeutic Management

For clients who have chronic hypertension, with or without superimposed PIH, management is directed toward maintaining the best possible environment for the fetus in utero. Chronic placental dysfunction causes fetal growth retardation and hypoxia.

Assessment

Client assessment is described in the section on PIH. In addition, the nurse assesses the client's feelings about this pregnancy and her compliance with the medical management plan.

Nursing Diagnosis

Nursing diagnoses for the client with HELLP syndrome highlight problems relevant to the client's disease process and her coping ability and provides information about tests for assessing maturity and well-being of the fetus (see Potential Nursing Diagnoses: Chronic Hypertensive Vascular Disease on p. 650).

Planning and Intervention

Interventions are discussed in detail in earlier sections.

POTENTIAL
NURSING DIAGNOSES
Chronic Hypertensive Vascular Disease

Altered Tissue Perfusion—related to hemolysis and anemia
Decreased Cardiac Output—related to decreasing intravascular volume and edema
Altered Family Processes—related to severity of client's illness and confinement in the
  hospital
Anxiety, Fear, Powerlessness—related to concern about fetal outcome
Potential for Injury to the Client—related to pathophysiology of HELLP syndrome
Potential for Injury to the Fetus—related to prematurity, chronic hypoxia, and malnu-
  trition
Guilt, Shame—related to high-risk pregnancy and uncertain outcome for the fetus
Knowledge Deficit—regarding the HELLP pathology

Prolonged Pregnancy

The average duration of pregnancy is roughly 280 days from the first day of the last menstrual period, or 267 days from the time of conception if the menstrual period is of average length. Only 5% of women deliver on the actual due date, although most deliver within 10 to 14 days in either direction from the date. Since the placenta has a normal life span equal to the duration of pregnancy, one may be justifiably concerned that if the due date is exceeded by more than 2 weeks, the aging placenta may no longer be able to support the fetus adequately. Fortunately, in most instances the placenta is capable of such support. In fact, in a great number of women who are postdates, the date has been miscalculated or based on faulty memory. In addition to these postmature pregnancies in which there is placental insufficiency, there is another group of late pregnancies in which the placenta functions well and the fetus becomes oversized, creating potential mechanical problems in labor and delivery.

Manifestations and Cause

Prolonged pregnancy is defined as one that has reached 42 weeks of gestation from the first day of the LMP or 40 weeks gestation from the time of conception. The cause of postmaturity is unknown in most cases.

Diagnosis and Prognosis

Diagnosis of this complication of pregnancy is usually aided by the use of ultrasonography and one frequent finding is decreased amniotic fluid volume. To assess risk it is important to confirm gestational age, perform nonstress tests two or three times per week, use ultrasound monitoring at least twice a week to obtain a biophysical profile, and assess amniotic fluid volume. The client should also report any decrease in fetal activity.

Therapeutic Management

Some physicians will not allow a pregnancy to continue after 42½ weeks gestation. If the pregnancy is allowed to continue and the fetal activity is decreased, a nonstress test should be done immediately. If the nonstress test is nonreactive, a contraction stress test is done. A decision to deliver (vaginally or by cesarean section) is made if any nonreassuring signs are noted. Nonreassuring signs include a positive contraction stress test, decreased amniotic fluid volume, abnormal biophysical profile, and presence of meconium in the amniotic fluid. Labor may be induced if the cervix is ripe and the FHR is reassuring. Continuous fetal monitoring should be done.

Assessment

Nursing assessment includes determining if the client perceives a decrease in fetal movement, verbalizes signs of beginning labor, and can state when to go to the hospital. The nurse should also assess how the client is coping with the prolonged pregnancy, which can cause her to be apprehensive.

Nursing Diagnosis

Nursing diagnoses should be identified to address the client's feelings of fatigue, frustration, anger, and disappointment, as well as her feelings of loss of control and fear about the fetal condition (see Potential Nursing Diagnoses: Prolonged Pregnancy).

POTENTIAL NURSING DIAGNOSES

Prolonged Pregnancy

Anxiety, Fear—related to prolonged pregnancy, concern over potential outcome
Self-Esteem Disturbance—related to delayed birth plans
Ineffective Individual Coping—related to emotional stress of prolonged pregnancy

---

Focus Assessment

Monitor closely vital signs, fetal heart rate, results of nonstress tests and contraction stress tests.
Elicit information regarding self-image.
Explore nonverbal indicators of emotional status, e.g., affect, mood, appearance, inability to concentrate, sleep patterns.

Planning and Intervention

The family may also be worried, and tensions may increase. Interventions by the nurse should be directed toward providing support for the woman and her family.

Infectious Diseases

Although most infectious diseases have no established specific ill effects on the woman or her fetus, some do produce profound effects. Two categories of infectious diseases complicate pregnancy: (1) sexually transmitted diseases and (2) other diseases that are not sexually related but that cause unique problems.

Sexually Transmitted Diseases

Manifestations and Cause

Sexually transmitted diseases (STDs), also called venereal diseases, are spread through sexual contact. They include a variety of conditions that range from ones that are mild and easily treated to potentially fatal ones for both mother and fetus. Initial infection does not produce immunity.

Diagnosis and Prognosis

Some STDs are incurable, whereas others may cause repetitive episodes of outbreaks.

Therapeutic Management

During the first prenatal visit clients are screened for evidence of STD. Serology testing for syphilis is done on all pregnant women, using either the VDRL test or the rapid plasma reagin (RPR) test. Other STDs can be diagnosed through a positive culture or blood testing. Women with negative VDRL and gonorrhea test results are assessed again in the eighth or ninth month of pregnancy if risk factors continue. It is common for clients with a history of herpes type II to receive periodic culturing during pregnancy.

A physical examination is done during the first prenatal visit. The external genital area is inspected for lesions or other skin eruptions. Vaginal discharge is assessed for color, odor, and quantity. A pelvic examination is performed, the cervix is inspected, and a cervical smear is collected.

Assessment

The client is assessed for risk factors, particularly if there has been no prenatal care. Assessment includes asking questions about multiple sex partners, a history of known or suspected lesion(s), and if there has been a sexual partner with a known or suspected past sexually transmitted disease. The client should be questioned about dysuria or systemic symptoms (headache, fever, chills, malaise), urinary incontinence or pain, and itching of the vulva.

Focus Assessment

Explore history of past STD and treatment.
Observe for signs of substance abuse. Elicit history as possible.
Elicit information regarding sexual partner(s).
Screen for specific STD (e.g., serologic test for syphilis; culture for gonorrhea)
Determine level of discomfort (may use a 0 to 10 rating scale to measure pain)
Observe response to diagnosis.
Elicit information describing perception of self.
Note nonverbal signs of emotional distress (e.g., hostility, inability to concentrate, withdrawal).
Determine past patterns of coping with crisis.
Identify current support system.

POTENTIAL NURSING DIAGNOSES

Sexually Transmitted Disease

Knowledge Deficit—regarding the complications, treatment, and prevention of sexually transmitted diseases
Pain—related to inflammation, itching, open sores, involvement of pelvic organs
Situational Low Self-Esteem—related to personal perception of the stigma of sexually transmitted disease

Nursing Diagnosis

After the assessment process is finished, nursing diagnoses are developed to assist in planning care for the woman and the fetus who have an increased perinatal risk for mortality and morbidity related to STD and its complications (see Nursing Care Plan: Client With a Sexually Transmitted Disease).

NURSING
CARE
PLAN

Client With a Sexually Transmitted Disease (STD)

Goals (Expected Outcomes)	Interventions	Rationale	Evaluation
Knowledge Deficit—Regarding Complications, Treatment, and Prevention of Sexually Transmitted Diseases			
Client will verbalize understanding of how to prevent infection. Remain free of sexually transmitted diseases. OR Client will verbalize understanding of the disease and its treatment.	Teach client cause, mode of transmission, and rationale for treatment	Assists in understanding how to practice preventive health	Client discusses basic facts about STDs. Client's secretions are cultured, or client has necessary test for diagnosis.
Client will comply with the recommended therapeutic management.	Teach the warning signs of complications: fever, increased pain, bleeding, urinary retention, adenopathy, infection of fetus and inflammation.	Urges client to seek health care.	Client verbalizes warning signs or complications.
Client will recover form the infection.	Refer sexual partner for appropriate treatment.	Imperative to treat all partners.	Sexual partner(s) seeks and receives treatment.
	Teach how and when to take medication and about side effects.	Ensures that infection is properly treated.	Client verbalizes understanding of how and when to take medication.
	Emphasize the importance of taking all prescribed medication	Maximizes treatment.	Client takes all medication.
	Explain importance of follow-up care.	Begins preventive health measures.	Client returns for follow-up care
Pain—Related to Inflammation, Itching, Open Sores, Involvement of Pelvic Organs			
Client will experience relief of symptoms	Administer medication or analgesics as ordered.	Medication used must be safe for mother and infant.	Client has no verbal complaints of pain or verbalizes intensity of discomfort or pain using rating scale.
	Recommend warm sitz baths three to four times a day for genital pain or discomfort.	Warm heat is very soothing for genital or perinatal pain.	Client takes all medication as given or ordered.
	Apply heating pad to client's abdomen (if ordered) for abdominal pain.	Decreases abdominal pain.	Client states warm moist heat or heating pad relieves pain.
	Advise client to wear cotton underwear and loose clothing and leave open sores exposed to air.	Keeps genital area clean and dry, promotes healing.	Genital lesions are dry and healing.
	Wear gown (impervious) and gloves when in contact with infected area.	Prevents spread of infection	Client has no spread of infection.
	Teach client importance of personal hygiene.	Decreases chance of spread of infection and secondary infection.	Client verbalizes and demonstrates good feminine hygiene.

Continued

NURSING
CARE
PLAN

Client With a Sexually Transmitted Disease (STD)—*continued*

Goals (Expected Outcomes)	Interventions	Rationale	Evaluation
Situational Low Self-Esteem—Related to Personal Perceptions of the Stigma of Sexually Transmitted Disease			
Client will work through emotions and accept the disease and its treatment.	Encourage and assist client to verbalize positive and negative feelings toward self.	Feelings must be explored to have insight and understanding of self.	Client expresses feelings about self.
	Clarify misconceptions.	Client must deal with truth, not misconceptions.	Client calmly verbalizes correct information about infection.
	Encourage client to explore and verbalize feelings about her own sexuality.	Feelings are clarified; normal grieving process about STD occurs.	Client speaks about infection and treatment.
	Encourage expressions of anger.	Feelings must be expressed before they can be dealt with.	Client verbalizes angry feelings about infection.
	Encourage verbalization of understanding of connection between life-style and STD.	Must alter life-style to prevent future infections.	Client verbalizes understanding of life-style changes that are necessary.

Planning and Intervention

Universal precautions, including careful attention to handwashing and wearing impervious gown and gloves when providing any care that involves contact with the genital area or body secretions (e.g., amniotic fluid), should be followed when caring for all clients.

Client education is an essential component in the care of pregnant women with a potential or active STD. Client teaching is specific for the particular STD. The teaching includes information about the signs and symptoms of the specific infection; its incubation period, transmission, and methods for prevention; treatment and basic comfort measures; follow-up assessment; perinatal implications, including method of delivery; and neonatal implications.

Because there is such a great volume of information to present, it is necessary to give small amounts of information over several teaching sessions. The nurse remains nonjudgmental in attitude while presenting the information. The atmosphere must be positive and therapeutic so the client can feel free to express emotions and anxieties and ask questions. If possible, the client's sexual partner should be invited to attend the education sessions so that he may also be informed. A discussion with the couple about the possible need for modification in sexual behavior and for using other methods of expressing sexuality may be necessary. The precise information given varies with the specific STD. Sometimes abstinence is recommended until a negative culture or blood test is obtained or symptoms have resolved for a minimum of 7 to 10 days (herpes).

To relieve local discomfort the client may be told to take sitz baths two or three times per day, to expose the infected area to a heat lamp, or to apply wet compresses. All lesions must be kept clean and dry and good personal feminine hygiene maintained. Douching should be avoided by women with most STDs. Topical antibiotics or steroid creams may be applied if prescribed by the physician. Intramuscular antibiotics such as penicillin are necessary for treating some STDs. See Table 23-10 for a summary of STDs.

TABLE 23-10

Sexually Transmitted Diseases

Syphilis	Gonorrhea	Chlamydia Trachomatis Infection	Genital Herpes
Manifestation			

Latent stage
  Diagnosis based on serology
Primary stage
  Classic lesions called chancres
  Deep, painful ulcers on genitalia, lips, or rectal area
Secondary stage
  Macular rash over body
Third stage
  Neurologic symptoms
	Nonspecific vaginal discharge	Becoming the most dominant sexually transmitted disease in United States.
		Cervical infection; sometimes urinary tract infection
		Vaginal ulcers, cervicitis
			1%-2% incidence in pregnant women
			Painful vesicles in area of vulva and perineum
			Flu-like symptoms
			May have inguinal adenopathy

Cause			
Treponema pallidum Affects socioeconomically disadvantaged	Gram-negative coccus, neisseria gonorrhoeae Affects mucous membrane of symptomatic carrier (5%-10%)	*Chlamydia trachomatis*	Herpes Type II
Diagnosis			
Positive serology (RPR, VDRL)	Gram-negative coccus, N. gonorrhoeae	Smear and stain examined microscopically Antibody titer (not always accurate) Papanicolaou smear (not specific)	Cytologic smears: reveal large multinucleate cells with eosinophilic inclusion bodies Papanicolaou smear
Prognosis			
If detected and treated, no danger to fetus Contagious in all stages Transmitted to fetus through placenta after 18th wk of pregnancy	Risk of permanent injury to infant's eyes at birth Can cause serious postpartum infection (pelvic inflammatory disease)	Preterm labor Endometritis postpartum Conjunctivitis in infant with use of tetracycline or erythromycin ophthalmic ointment; *also* pneumonia	Abortion in early pregnancy Preterm labor Microcephaly, microophthalmia in infant Fetus delivered through active lesions has 50% chance of developing
Medical Management			
Penicillin G (benzathine) Penicillin G or penicillin G procaine Erythromycin if allergic to penicillin Infection may recur (must treat sexual partner also) Follow client and infant by postpartum serology Unaffected infant will have positive test if mother is positive	Single injection of aqueous procaine penicillin preceded by 1 g of probenecid orally	Erythromycin, 500 mg q.i.d. × 7 days Male simultaneously treated with tetracycline	Disseminated herpesvirus infection Topical acyclovir Oral acyclovir if taken 4-6 mo, prevents or reduces frequency, duration and severity of recurrence

Continued

TABLE 23-10

Sexually Transmitted Diseases—continued

Listeriosis	HIV/AIDS	Candidiasis	*Trichomonas vaginalis*
Manifestation			
Possible fever of unknown origin	*Early* Initially asymptomatic *More advanced* Termed AIDS-related complex *Lymph adenopathy* Severe immune deficiency *Full-blown AIDS* Pneumocystitis carinii pneumonia, Kaposi's sarcoma, and other severe sexually transmitted infections	Present in 20%-25% of pregnant women Especially prevalent in diabetic pregnant women Increased incidence in pregnant women taking antibiotics or steroids Thick, white, cottage cheese-like appearance to vaginal discharge Burning and itching	Present in approximately 20% of pregnant women (many asymptomatic) White to gray-green foamy discharge Possible inflammation and irritation of vagina and cervix and vulvitis
Cause			
Gram-positive bacillus, Listeria monocytogenes	Human immunodeficiency virus (HIV); also called human T-cell lymphotropic virus (causes loss of immunity)	*Candida albicans,* a fungus	*Trichomonas vaginalis*
Diagnosis			
Blood and urine cultures	Serologic studies for detection of HIV detection of HIV antibodies or virus	Microscopic examination of vaginal discharge or vaginal culture (culture takes longer)	Microscopic examination of vaginal discharge
Prognosis			
50% mortality rates for infected infants *Early onset* clinical signs at birth—respiratory distress, cyanosis, skin lesions, hypothermia *Late onset* (1-6 wk) Meningitis, causing central nervous system damage	Risk of perinatal transmission: 20%-50% Infants with perinatal infection become ill during first 2 yr of life Eventual death for symptomatic clients Concern that pregnancy accelerates AIDS	Possible acquisition of thrush by fetus during delivery process	Medication used for treatment not used during first half of pregnancy because of possible teratogenic effects
Medical Management			
Combination of ampicillin or penicillin with gentamicin		Topical miconazole (Monistat) cream or nystatin vaginal suppositories	Metronidazole (Flagyl) orally or vaginally Oral use is avoided during first trimester because of possible teratogenic effects

Acquired Immunodeficiency Syndrome

Manifestations and Cause

Most individuals infected with the human immunodeficiency virus (HIV) are asymptomatic carriers. The exact incubation period is unknown but may be as short as 2 months or as long as 5 years.[5] As the disease continues, manifestations gradually appear. All clients do not progress at the same rate, and not all progress from the asymptomatic phase to develop the full-blown clinical picture of AIDS.

In early stages of the disease clients remain asymptomatic, but abnormalities are noted on laboratory studies. More advanced disease is called AIDS-related complex, and lymphadenopathy, weight loss, fever, fatigue, arthralgia, maculopapular rash, diarrhea, anorexia, and night sweats are present. Full-blown AIDS (severe immune deficiency) includes *Pneumocystis carinii* pneumonia, Kaposi's sarcoma, and various severe sexually transmitted infections such as herpes, cytomegalovirus, *Candida albicans,* and toxoplasmosis. T-cell lymphocytes may disappear from the circulation.

Diagnosis and Prognosis

The causative agent is believed to be an HIV called human T-cell lymphotropic virus (HTLV-III, ARV). The virus infects the lymphocytes and destroys immunocompetence, causing the person's inability to fight off immune challenges. Laboratory studies detect circulating antibodies to HIV and the lymphocyte ratio.

AIDS is a terminal illness. It is suspected that women carrying HIV spread the virus to sexual partners. There is a 50% risk of perinatal spread to the newborn. If this occurs, the newborn is at risk for death within a few years.

Therapeutic Management

At present there is no vaccine for AIDS and no way to correct the immunodeficiency. The prognosis is bleak. After the client with AIDS has developed infections, the mean survival time is 11 to 15 months.

Assessment

Assessment for AIDS begins with screening prenatal clients to determine if they are in a high-risk group, which includes IV drug abusers, prostitutes, women with sexually transmitted infections, or women with sexual partners who are in a high-risk group for HIV.[6]

Nursing Diagnosis

A predominant nursing diagnosis for clients in high-risk groups is a knowledge deficit regarding their lack of understanding about AIDS and its relationship to them and their pregnancy (see Potential Nursing Diagnoses: AIDS).

Planning and Intervention

The primary intervention for these high-risk clients is education. They must be taught that HIV is transmitted through sexual intercourse, by sharing equipment used for injecting drugs, and through blood products or artificial insemination. They must be taught that there is a 20% to 50% probability that an infected woman will transmit the infection perinatally to her fetus or newborn. Infected women should also be taught the importance of informing physicians, dentists, and other appropriate health care professionals about their antibody status, in addition, they should never donate blood or plasma and should avoid pregnancy.

POTENTIAL
NURSING DIAGNOSIS

AIDS

Knowledge Deficit—regarding lack of understanding about AIDS and its relationship to her and her pregnancy

Viral Hepatitis

Manifestations and Cause

The hepatitis viruses are the most common causes of liver disease during pregnancy. All are similar clinically during the acute attack. Signs and symptoms range from mild to severe. The most characteristic symptoms are anorexia, nausea, and vomiting. Most affected women have no sign of jaundice, so the diagnosis may be missed or delayed. Because of the symptoms, the client may be diagnosed as having hyperemesis gravidarum.

Diagnosis and Prognosis

The diagnosis of hepatitis B is confirmed by the appearance of circulating hepatitis B surface antigen (HB$_s$Ag) in the blood. The risk of transmission of the disease to the fetus is small. It is important, however, to determine if the hepatitis B antibody (HB$_s$Ab) is present. If the antibody is not present, the neonate must receive an injection of hepatitis B immune globulin (0.5 ml intramuscularly) immediately after birth and again at 3 and 6 months of age. If the mother is infectious (HB$_s$Ab is present), the neonate must receive active immunization with hepatitis B vaccine in addition to the immune globulin. The immune globulin is very effective and has few side effects.

Hepatitis B is transmitted by infected blood or blood products but may also be present in saliva, vaginal secretions, and semen. Untreated hepatitis is associated with an increased incidence of abortion, premature labor, and stillbirth. There is no evidence that the viruses are teratogenic. Maternal mortality rates vary from 1% to 17%. Nutritional status of the mother influences course of the disease. There is greater maternal mortality in the poorer countries of the world.

Therapeutic Management

There are four types of hepatitis, and all are similar clinically during the acute attack. Acute viral hepatitis is a systemic infection that affects the liver. Viral agents that cause hepatitis types A and B are diagnosed by testing for the immunologic response to hepatitis A virus (HAV) and hepatitis B virus (HBV). A third type of hepatitis, hepatitis C, was formerly called non-A/non-B hepatitis and is diagnosed by excluding HAV and HBV. Hepatitis C is transmitted most often by transfusion but also may be transmitted sexually. An even newer type, hepatitis D, requires the presence of hepatitis B to replicate and causes severe, progressive active disease and cirrhosis. These four types of hepatitis vary in occurrence during pregnancy and in the effects on the mother, fetus, and newborn. Clients with hepatitis A are given supportive care with careful monitoring of liver enzymes and are placed in enteric isolation. Clients exposed to hepatitis A may be given gamma globulin.

Exposure of the fetus to hepatitis B is rare but exposure may occur at delivery. The neonate who breast-feeds can also be exposed to the virus. Treatment for the mother is supportive. It is important that the infant's physician be notified when a mother with hepatitis B delivers so that the newborn can receive hepatitis B vaccine. Hepatitis B immunoglobin and hepatitis B vaccine can prevent vertical transmission to the fetus.

Assessment

Early in the pregnancy the nurse obtains a complete client history to assess for potential risk for hepatitis. Assessment is done at each prenatal visit.

Nursing Diagnosis

If assessment indicates the client is at risk for hepatitis, nursing diagnoses should be developed to increase her knowledge about the disease in relation to care of and effect on the fetus or newborn. Her knowledge deficits may relate to her nutritional status, general hygiene, and rest (see Potential Nursing Diagnoses: Hepatitis).

Planning and Intervention

Interventions are aimed at educating the client about hepatitis. The nurse must understand the effects of the disease on the client's body and on the fetus.

☐ POTENTIAL
☐ NURSING DIAGNOSES

Hepatitis

Potential for Injury (Maternal)—related to hepatitis secondary to exposure to high-risk sexual partners or sharing articles used for substance abuse (e.g., needles)
Potential for Injury (Fetal)—related to maternal hepatitis secondary to exposure to high-risk sexual partners or sharing articles used for substance abuse
Knowledge Deficit—regarding hepatitis B as a sexually transmitted disease
Knowledge Deficit—regarding the implications of hepatitis during pregnancy, transmission to the fetus, effects on the newborn
Knowledge Deficit—regarding the risk of AIDS and its relationship to them and their pregnancy

---

Focus Assessment

Note complaints of anorexia, fatigue, nausea, right abdominal discomfort.
Observe for jaundice.
Closely monitor pregnancy progress (weight gain, vital signs, fundal height).
Closely monitor fetal status (fetal heart rate, results of nonstress testing).
Identify current individual teaching or learning needs.

REFERENCES

1. Mantoni M: Ultrasound signs in threatened abortion and their prognostic significance. Obstet Gynecol 65(4):471-475, 1985
2. Hert JD, Heisterberg I: The outcome of pregnancy after threatened abortion. Acta Obstet Gynecol Scand 64:151-156, 1985
3. Klebanoff MA et al: Epidemiology of vomiting in early pregnancy. Obstet Gynecol 66(5):612-616, November 1985
4. Long MA et al: Outpatient treatment of hyperemesis gravidarum with stimulus control and imagery procedures. J Behav Ther Exp Psychiatry 17(2):105-109, 1986
5. Cunningham FG et al; Williams' Obstetrics. Norwalk, Conn, Appleton & Lange, 1989
6. Sweet RL, Gibbs RS: Maternal and fetal infections: Clinical disorders. In Creasy RK, Resnik R (eds): Maternal-Fetal Medicine: Principles and Practice. Philadelphia, WB Saunders, 1989
7. Morrison JC, Palmer SM: General medical disorders during pregnancy. In Pernoll ML, Benson RC (eds): Current Obstetric and Gynecologic Diagnosis and Treatment. Norwalk, Conn, Appleton & Lange, 1987

SUGGESTED READINGS

Callahan EJ et al: Behavioral treatment of hyperemesis gravidarum. Psychosom Obstet Gynecol 5:187-195, May 1987

Graber EA: Dilemmas in the pharmacological management in preterm labor. Obstet Gynecol Surv 44(7):512-517, 1989

Main DM et al: Can preterm deliveries be prevented? Am J Obstet Gynecol 151:892-898, 1985

Pool JH: Getting Perspective on HELLP Syndrome. Matern Child Nurs J 13:432-437, November/December 1989

Shannon DM: HELLP Syndrome: A severe consequence of pregnancy-induced hypertension, JOGN, November/December:295-402, 1987

Intrapartum Complications

IMPORTANT TERMINOLOGY

amniotic fluid embolism Occurs when a large amount of amniotic fluid is infused into the maternal circulation; multiple tiny emboli are formed and occlude the pulmonary arteries

cephalopelvic disproportion Discrepancy between size of the fetal head and size of the pelvis

dystocia Difficult labor

dysfunctional labor Abnormal uterine contraction patterns

external version Turning fetus externally to a vertex presentation

Friedman labor curve Graph used to assess progress of labor

hypertonic labor Inefficient uterine contractions that may be perceived by the client as stronger than the amount of work that the contraction accomplishes; resting tone of uterus is elevated

hypotonic labor Contractions of very poor tone intensity — not strong enough to dilate the cervix

persistent occiput posterior Back of infant's head (occiput) is against mother's sacrum instead of directed toward the symphysis pubis

premature rupture of membranes Rupture of the amniotic sac before the onset of labor

prolapse of umbilical cord Umbilical cord precedes the presenting part, resulting in pressure on the cord as it is trapped between the presenting part and the pelvis

prolonged active phase Dilatation and descent or both that occurs more slowly than usual

prolonged latent phase Abnormally long period of early labor from onset (of labor) to active (phase of) labor

psyche Soul, mind; all that constitutes the mind and its processes

tonus State of muscle tone

transverse arrest Fourth mechanism of labor, "internal rotation" is incomplete; occiput rotates from posterior to transverse (L.O.T.) or (R.O.T.); should rotate an additional 45 degrees to occiput anterior (O.A.)

uterine inversion Rare occurrence of uterus turning inside out because of laxity of uterine wall and undue tension on the umbilical cord

uterine resting tone (tonus) Baseline tone of uterus between contractions; complete relaxation is necessary to maximize blood flow through uterine vessels to placenta

Throughout the labor and delivery process, the nurse is vigilant in assessing and evaluating the client's progress. When labor and delivery fails to proceed as expected or signs and symptoms indicative of other complications occur, the primary care provider is notified. Management of complications of emergency delivery and uterine tetany, rupture, and inversion as well as amniotic fluid embolism, cord prolapse, and multiple pregnancy are discussed.

Dystocia

Dystocia literally means "difficult labor" and is characterized by a labor that is abnormally slow. Abnormalities that can cause dystocia include:

1. Uterine factors: Uterine contractions may be too weak, short, irregular, or infrequent to cause cervical effacement and dilatation, or expulsive forces, both involuntary and voluntary, are insufficient to cause fetal descent.
2. Pelvic factors: The size and shape of the bony pelvis can interfere with the mechanisms of engagement, descent, and expulsion of the fetus.
3. Fetal factors: Excessive fetal size, abnormal presentation or position, or abnormalities of the fetus may prevent entrance or passage through the bony pelvis.
4. Psychologic factors: Psychologic factors can influence the mechanism or progression of labor. Maternal factors such as anxiety, lack of preparation, and fear can cause a prolonged labor. It has been suggested that this phenomenon occurs because pain and stress can stimulate sympathetic activity, which in turn decreases uterine activity.[1]
5. Position factors: Maternal position can affect the length of first and second stages of labor. The supine position can cause contraction frequency to increase, but contraction intensity decreases. This position also can cause the heavy pregnant uterus to compress the inferior vena cava and aorta. The results are decreased blood flow to the uterus ("colicky" contractions), potential maternal hypotension, and fetal hypoxia.

Uterine Dystocia Factors and Complications
Dysfunctional Labor
Etiology and Pathophysiology

Dysfunctional labor is abnormal uterine contraction patterns. Any of the following can cause dysfunctional labor: (1) **premature rupture of membranes** before the onset of labor (cervix is firm and uneffaced), (2) analgesia or anesthesia given during the latent phase, (3) overdistention of the uterus (multiple pregnancy, large fetus, or polyhydramnios), (4) grand multiparity, (5) **cephalopelvic disproportion,** (6) false labor, or (7) uterine abnormalities.

Uterine dysfunction can result in maternal exhaustion and dehydration. Risk for intrauterine infection increases if there is accompanying prolonged rupture of membranes. Maternal hemorrhage from uterine atony after delivery is another complication.

≡ LEGAL AND ETHICAL
≡ CONSIDERATIONS

Labor and delivery is a high-risk area for potential law suits. Dysfunctional labor, electronic fetal monitoring, and oxytocic drugs are frequently the focus of today's malpractice suits.

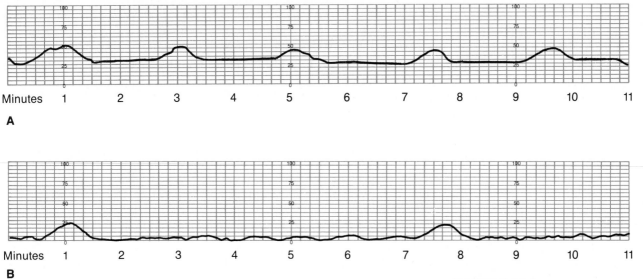

Minutes 1 2 3 4 5 6 7 8 9 10 11

A

Minutes 1 2 3 4 5 6 7 8 9 10 11

B

FIGURE 24-1

Hypertonic and Hypotonic
Contractions. **A,** Hypertonic contractions
are frequent but poor in quality. Note the
elevation in resting tone. This can be
described as a colicky uterus. Over some
time the fetus may develop a nonreassuring
pattern as a result of a decrease in
oxygenation caused by decreased
uteroplacental blood flow. Mother becomes
fatigued, has increased perception of pain,
and may become dehydrated. **B,** Hypotonic
contractions may occur in the active phase
of first stage or in the second stage of labor.
Contractions are irregular and farther apart,
and uterine resting tone is lower than
normal. Labor will not progress, and mother
and fetus are at increased risk for
complications.

There are five categories or classifications of dysfunctional labor patterns: **hypertonic labor, hypotonic labor,** uterine tetany, arrest disorders,
and precipitious labor.

Hypertonic Labor (Prolonged Latent Phase)

The first stage of labor is divided into two phases: latent and active. The
latent phase of the first stage of labor begins with the onset of contractions
and continues until there is a stable contraction pattern and the cervix
effaces and dilates between 3 and 4 cm. The major work of this phase is
cervical effacement. The latent phase is prolonged if it exceeds 20 hours
in the primigravida and 14 hours in the multigravida.

Hypertonic uterine contraction prolong the latent phase (Fig. 24-1,
A). These contractions occur frequently and are cramp-like, ineffective,
and stronger in the midportion (body) of the uterus than in the fundus.
Tonus (between contractions) is greater than normal. Hypertonic contractions are more likely to occur in the latent phase of labor (see display
below).

Signs and Symptoms of Hypertonic Labor

History

Usually occurs in primigravidas
Occurs early in labor during latent phase
Client complains that contractions are extremely painful
Palpated contractions of poor quality (intensity)

Physical Examination

Frequent contractions
Stronger contractions in midportion of uterus than in fundus
Hypertonus

Pelvic Examinations

Lack of progress in cervical effacement, dilatation, and station

---

ETIOLOGY AND PATHOPHYSIOLOGY. Causes of **prolonged latent phase** are false labor, a long and firm cervix not softened and thinned prior to onset of labor, analgesia given too early in labor, and dysfunctional uterine contractions. A prolonged latent phase results in client exhaustion before active labor begins.

THERAPEUTIC MANAGEMENT. The two modes of management used for prolonged latent phase of labor are client sedation and uterine stimulation. Sedation may be used first to help the client rest. This 8 to 12 hour rest period is often followed spontaneously by normal active labor. If active labor does not occur after the sedated rest, stimulation of uterine contractions using an oxytocin infusion may be tried.

Hypotonic Labor (Prolonged Active Phase)

The active phase of labor begins when the cervix is 4 cm dilated and ends with complete cervical dilatation. During this phase dilatation occurs rapidly at a rate not less than 1.2 cm/hour for a primigravida and 1.5 cm/hour for a multigravida. The transition phase occurs during the latter part of the active phase. Transition is abnormally prolonged if descent is less than 1 cm/hour for primigravidas and 2 cm/hour in multigravidas.

As rapid cervical dilatation occurs, the fetus begins a progressive descent through the pelvis requiring stronger and more frequent contractions. When cervical dilatation fails to progress at the usual rate, there is an abnormal prolongation of the active phase of the first stage of labor. Uterine activity characteristic of this labor disorder are hypotonic contractions (Fig. 24-1, *B*), which are too weak, short, irregular, and too far apart to cause progress in dilatation and descent (see below).

ETIOLOGY AND PATHOPHYSIOLOGY. The cause of delayed dilatation and descent is often unknown, but cephalopelvic disproportion, occiput posterior or occiput transverse position, artificial or spontaneous rupture of membranes before the onset of labor, and excessive medication or anesthesia given during the latent phase of labor may be factors. It has been noted that about 70% of clients experiencing hypotonic labor will develop an arrest disorder.

THERAPEUTIC MANAGEMENT. Neither rest nor stimulation with oxytocin are effective in this abnormal labor pattern. The end result of hy-

---

Signs and Symptoms of Hypotonic Labor

History

Client is comfortable during contractions
Progress is normal until active phase of first stage of labor or second stage
Progress ceases

Physical Examination

Contractions are infrequent, of short duration, and of mild intensity

Pelvic Examination

No further progress in cervical dilatation or descent occurs

---

potonic labor is operative delivery, particularly cesarean section. Both cesarean delivery and operative vaginal deliveries increase perinatal mortality.

Uterine Tetany

Etiology and Pathophysiology

A contraction that lasts longer than 90 seconds is a tetanic contraction. It is important to intervene quickly because uterine tetany interferes with uteroplacental blood flow and causes fetal hypoxia. Oxytocin use and abruptio placentae are the most common causes.

Nursing Interventions

Interventions include decreasing uterine activity by turning off the oxytocin infusion, turning the mother onto her left side, increasing intravenous fusion rate, notifying the primary health care provider, and starting oxygen at 6 to 8 L by face mask. The nurse should have available and be prepared to administer a tocolytic drug (usually Brethine 0.25 ml, subcutaneously or intravenously). If the uterine tetany is not resolved, the client should be prepared for an immediate emergency cesarean section.

Arrest Disorders

Etiology and Pathophysiology

An arrest in dilatation occurs when there has been no progress in labor for 2 hours or longer. Arrest in descent occurs when no descent has occurred for at least 1 hour. Dilatation and arrest disorders complicate about 5% of primigravida labors, and arrest in descent occurs in 3% of all clients.[2] Causative factors include abnormal fetal positions (O.P. and O.T.) in 70% of clients as well as dystocia, inadequate pelvis, and excessive sedation or anesthesia.

Therapeutic Management

These clients' labors do seem to respond to oxytocin augmentation, and most do deliver vaginally. If dilatation and descent remain arrested, delivery is usually accomplished with midforceps or by cesarean section. There is an increased perinatal mortality because of this traumatic delivery.

Precipitate Labor Disorder

Etiology and Pathophysiology

A precipitous labor is an abnormally rapid, intense labor characterized by rapid cervical dilatation and descent of the presenting part. The entire labor lasts only 2 to 4 hours. Precipitous labor tends to occur in multiparas with a history of rapid labor and delivery, adolescents who are not aware of the signs of active labor, and in clients who experience a minimum of pain with labor. The frequency, duration, and intensity of the contractions

Do's and Don'ts of Emergency Childbirth

Do

Remain calm and confident.
Give clear, positive, repeated directions.
Control the delivery of the infant's head.
Clear the infant's airway.
Dry the infant off.
Hold infant at or slightly above level of introitus.
Place infant next to the mother's skin and cover.
Put the infant to breast (if the newborn can reach).
Wait for the placenta to separate.
Inspect placenta for intactness.

Don't

Put fingers into birth canal.
Force rotation of infant's head after head is delivered.
Put traction on cord or pull on cord.
Allow newborn to get cold.
Push on uterus to try to deliver placenta.

---

may cause decreased uteroplacental perfusion, thus compromising the fetus by hypoxia.

Precipitate delivery can cause trauma to maternal soft tissues and traumatic damage to the fetal head. Precipitous labor occurs because contractions are frequent, very intense, and there is minimum maternal soft tissue resistance.

Nursing Interventions

It is important for maternity nurses to be prepared to assist in providing a physically and psychologically safe childbearing experience. The nurse must manage the birth calmly and with an attitude of confidence so that the family can trust that everything is under control (see above). As the nurse takes charge of the emergency, he or she should explain to the couple what is happening and what they can do to help. Team work is important.

If delivery is imminent, the mother must never be left alone. The nurse can use the mother's call light to get assistance and to ensure that the primary care giver is being contacted.

An emergency delivery pack should be available (see below). The mother is assisted into a comfortable position (usually a high Fowler's) while the nurse continues to be calm and reassuring, talking and in-

---

Contents of Emergency Delivery Pack

Gloves
Bulb syringe to clear infant's mouth and nose
Two sterile Kelly clamps (to clamp umbilical cord)
One sterile cord clamp
Several 4 × 4 gauze pads for wiping off face and removing secretions from the mouth
Two baby blankets to wrap infant to prevent cold stress
One small round basin for placenta

structing confidently. If there is time, the nurse should wash her hands and put on a pair of gloves. Clean, dry linen or a sterile drape should be placed under the mother's hips. If the intact membranes become visible outside the vagina, they should be opened (with a finger) so that the newborn will not aspirate amniotic fluid. The nurse may massage the perineum as the head crowns to aid in stretching the tissues to help prevent lacerations.

When the head is ready to deliver, the mother must be coached to stop pushing and breathe to keep the head from "popping" out too quickly. She can be coached to pant (short, shallow breaths) until the head is delivered. The ideal situation would be to deliver the head between contractions because contractions are very intense. Delivery between contractions, or at least without the added pressure from pushing, minimizes the quick changes of pressure on and in the fetal head. As the head delivers, the nurse places one hand over the head. A small amount of counter pressure is applied (do not restrain the delivery) as the head emerges under the symphysis and is born across the perineum. This maneuver will control the delivery of the head, minimizing pressure changes, and will also minimize or prevent trauma to the perineum (vaginal or perineal lacerations).

As soon as the head is delivered, it is important to check for the presence of the cord, which may be looped around the neck (nuchal). It may be possible to slip the loop over the infant's head or loosen it so that the loop is large enough for the infant to slide through without causing tension on the cord. After the head is delivered, the nurse should suction the mouth and then the nose so that when the shoulders and chest deliver and the infant takes the first breath, the airway will be clear.

After the head is out, it will turn (restitution). This is so that the shoulders can slip by the ischeal spines in the anterior-posterior position. Delivery may occur very quickly at this time. If not, the nurse should place one hand on each side of the infant's head and apply gentle traction downward. This will assist the anterior shoulder to deliver under the symphysis. Applying gentle traction upward will permit the posterior shoulder to slip out over the perineum. A firm hold on the infant is now very important, since the infant will deliver very quickly once the shoulders are out. Newborns are wet and slippery.

The newborn is held at the level of the uterus to avoid gaining or losing volume to the placenta until the cord is clamped and cut.

As soon as the nurse determines that the newborn is breathing, the infant can be placed on the mother's abdomen with the head slightly lower than the body to facilitate drainage of fluid and mucus. The weight of the newborn on the mother's abdomen stimulates uterine contractions, which aids separation of the placenta. When the newborn is stable, breast-feeding can be initiated. Suckling of the infant at the breast will also initiate uterine contractions, which will expedite placental separation.

The nurse will assess for signs of placental separation: a brief gush of blood, lengthening of the cord, and change in uterine shape from discord to globular.

The mother will feel another uncomfortable contraction as the placenta passes through the cervix. The mother should be asked to give a little push, and the placenta will usually deliver. If the placenta does not deliver, it should be left until the primary health care provider arrives.

After the placenta is out, the nurse should gently massage the fundus to ensure it is contracting well. After the placenta is expelled, it should be inspected to make sure it is intact.

IMMEDIATE CARE OF THE INFANT. Care of the infant includes ensuring a patent airway by using a bulb suction to clear the oral airway and then the nares (infants are obligatory nose breathers). The infant is then assessed for breathing. If breathing does not occur, resuscitation is done. Apgar scoring is done at the end of 1 and 5 minutes of age. If the infant is vigorous and stable, breast-feeding can be initiated.

CONTINUED CARE OF MOTHER AND INFANT. The mother's response to delivery (and the father's, if present) should be assessed. A note should be made regarding how she acted, what she said, and what she did when the infant was born.

The mother's fundus should be assessed for consistency and location. Her bleeding should be assessed as well as her pulse, respirations, color, and general condition. She needs to be reassured about how well she handled the delivery. The father should be praised also. If the fundus is not firm, it will require some massage. The perineum and the area under the buttocks should be cleaned and dry linen applied. Her perineum can be inspected for obvious lacerations, a sanitary napkin applied, and then the mother instructed to keep her thighs together to decrease bleeding from possible lacerations. The infant is again assessed to ensure that no problems are overlooked. If there is any respiratory distress, the infant should be transferred to the nursery. It is also important to remember to be sensitive to the parents' feelings about their childbearing experience. Some parents will grieve over their powerlessness, loss of control, and their unfulfilled birth plans. They need reassurance and encouragement that their feelings are normal and understood. Important information to be recorded is included in the display below.

Assessment

The graphic recording **(Friedman labor curve)** of cervical dilatation and descent of the presenting part provides a concise guide for assessing normal vs. abnormal progress in labor.

The graph identifies problems with cervical dilatation and descent of the presenting part of the fetus (Fig. 24-2). Assessment of contractions by the electronic fetal monitor for frequency, duration, intensity, shape, and resting tone helps to identify hypertonic, hypotonic, prolonged, and precipitous labor patterns. If an internal monitor is used, more precise information about **uterine resting tone** and contraction intensity can be

---

Important Information to Be Recorded

1. Time of delivery.
2. Exact position of the cord if it was around the neck (called a nucal cord)
3. Appearance of the amniotic fluid, especially if it was green or brown
4. Time when the placenta was expelled and its condition
5. Condition of mother and newborn
6. Estimation of the Apgar score
7. Mother's blood type and Rh factor, if she knows it

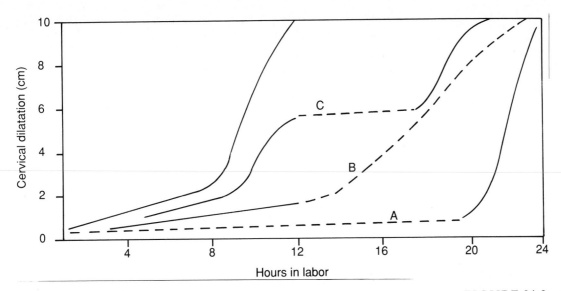

FIGURE 24-2

Friedman Labor Graph. Friedman has plotted cervical dilatation and degree of descent against lapsed time on a graph. Categories of delayed progression are seen. *A* = prolonged latent phase (hypertonic labor); *B* = protracted active phase (hypotonic labor); *C* = secondary arrest of dilatation.

Friedman E: Greenhill Obstetrics, 13th ed. Philadelphia, WB Saunders.

measured in mm Hg. If external monitoring is done, the nurse must palpate the uterus for resting tone and contraction intensity.

The progress of contraction frequency, duration, intensity, shape, and resting tone help cue the nurse to perform vaginal examinations to assess progress. Additionally, the monitor tracing will aid in assessing the fetal heart rate response to labor.

It is also important to assess how the mother is handling labor and managing pain. Are the mother and father working together? Is she moaning and groaning or very quiet and withdrawn? Behaviors exhibited by the mother may contribute to dysfunctional labor (see below).

Nursing Diagnosis

Nursing diagnoses are concerned with comfort, anxiety, infection, and fetal injury (see Potential Diagnoses: Dysfunctional Labor p. 670).

Planning and Intervention

Interventions include assisting the mother to utilize relaxation techniques and breathing exercises, maintaining a quiet, restful environment, and

Focus Assessment

Monitor vital signs and fetal heart rate closely.
Note frequency, duration, strength, and interval between contractions.
Identify response to pain.
Monitor intake and output.
Determine current knowledge level regarding condition, implications, and
     management.
Explore nonverbal indicators of emotional status, e.g., irritability, inability to
     concentrate, withdrawal.
Explore individual concerns.

POTENTIAL NURSING DIAGNOSES

Dysfunctional Labor

Potential for Infection (Maternal)—related to prolonged rupture of membranes
Potential for Infection (Fetal)—related to prolonged rupture of membranes
Altered Uteroplacental Perfusion—related to hyperstimulation of the uterus
Potential for Injury (Fetal)—related to hypoxia secondary to interruption of uteroplacental circulation by abnormal uterine contractions
Fluid Volume Deficit (1)—related to prolonged labor and restricted fluid intake
Pain—related to uterine contractions
Anxiety—related to unexpected length of labor
Knowledge Deficit—regarding dysfunctional labor

explaining about the process and progress of labor. The mother and her support person are given explanations about the need for: (1) pelvic examinations to determine effacement and dilatation progress, (2) contraction pattern monitoring, and (3) monitoring fetal response to labor.

Universal precautions must be followed as the labor and delivery area is an area of increased risk for organisms transmitted by blood and body secretions (see below).

In addition to administering ordered medications and monitoring their effects, the nurse also provides comfort measures and emotional support. The nurse should be warm and caring and attend to the needs of both the mother and the support person. Working through the "coach," the nurse can assist in promoting relaxation techniques to help conserve the mother's energy.

COMFORT MEASURES. Comfort measures that promote relaxation include changing gowns and underpads as often as necessary after rupture of membranes. Frequent emptying of her bladder, positional changes, back rubs, quiet conversation, and a restful environment are all helpful interventions.

Walking can be helpful, since perception of pain is usually decreased when ambulating. After the membranes rupture, the client can ambulate

Principles of Body Substance Isolation

Body substance isolation (BSI) provides a consistent approach to managing body substances from *all* clients. It focuses on isolating body substances from staff. Body substances include, but are not limited to, blood, urine, feces, wound drainage, oral secretions, vomitus, sputum, amniotic fluid, and vaginal secretions. BSI is accomplished by wearing gloves when caring for clients and by following the handwashing procedure.

BSI includes the following elements and should be followed by *all* personnel at *all* times, regardless of the client's diagnosis.
1. Wash hands often and thoroughly. Handwashing is the most effective method of reducing the spread of infection.
2. Wear gloves when there is *any possibility* that your hands will come in contact with body substances (see above listing).
3. Hands *must* be washed following the removal of the gloves.
4. *Always* change gloves before caring for another client.
5. Protect your clothing by wearing an impervious gown when there is *any possibility* that your clothing could be contaminated with a client's body substance.
6. Wear a mask or eye protection or both when there is *any possibility* that a body substance from a client could be splashed into your mouth, nose, or eyes.

if the presenting part is engaged. If it is not engaged, the client is to remain in bed.

The support person should be encouraged to take breaks, eat, and rest when the client rests to continue being an effective assistant.

EMOTIONAL SUPPORT. Dysfunctional labors are extremely discouraging for both the mother and the support person. It is important for the couple to understand what is happening, and the plan of care as explanations can reduce their anxiety. Feedback assists the nurse in determining their level of understanding and acceptance. Both mother and the support person should receive generous amounts of encouragement about how well they are doing.

See Nursing Care Plan: Client with Dysfunctional Labor.

NURSING
CARE
PLAN

Client With Dysfunctional Labor

Goals (Expected Outcomes)	Interventions	Rationale	Evaluation
Potential for Infection (Maternal)—Related to Prolonged Rupture of Membranes			
Client will experience a progressive labor without an infection.	Record temperature and pulse every 2 hours after rupture of membranes (ROM).	Identifies early signs of infection.	Temperature and pulse normal.
	Keep perineum clean and as dry as possible.	Minimizes or prevents contamination from wet bed.	Client remains free of infection.
	Minimize frequency of vaginal exam.	Reduces the risk for vaginal infection.	Progress is assessed by assessing contractions and response to labor.
	Cleanse perineal area after exams.	Keeps perineal area clean, dry and free of infection.	Perineal care given and taught to client. No signs of infection seen.
	Wash hands before and after client care.	Protects client and self from risk of infection.	Client is free of infection.
Potential Altered Uteroplacental Perfusion—Related to Hyperstimulation of the Uterus			
Client will have a progressive labor without hyperstimulation and the fetus will be free of distress.	Run monitor strip on fetus to determine baseline FHR before starting oxytocin infusion.	Ensures fetal heart rate pattern is reassuring.	Baseline fetal heart pattern is normal.
	Ensure that physician is readily available while oxytocin infusion is used.	Is available for emergency delivery if there is fetal intolerance to oxytocin.	Physician is present in the hospital.
	Always piggyback oxytocin solution into mainline IV line (in port closest to client).	Quickly halts drug absorption and reduces drug-related stimulation of contractions.	Infusion is started with oxytocin piggybacked into mainline.
	Increase rate of oxytocin as ordered to elicit effective uterine contractions; discontinue if contractions occur more often than every 2 minutes and last longer than 60 seconds.	Establishes effective uterine contractions; minimizes risk of decreased uteroplacental perfusion and fetal hypoxia.	Monitor records normal pattern of contractions. Labor progresses at normal rate.

Continued

NURSING
■ CARE
■ PLAN

Client With Dysfunctional Labor—continued

Goals (Expected Outcomes)	Interventions	Rationale	Evaluation
Potential Altered Uteroplacental Perfusion—Related to Hyperstimulation of the Uterus—continued			
	Clients with external monitor: note and record uterine response to oxytocin as identified by palpation, i.e., frequency, duration, intensity of contractions, and resting tone.	Distinguishes normal labor pattern from hypertonic pattern and frequency.	Client's labor progresses at normal rate without hypotonic or hypertonic contractions.
	With internal monitor: record intrauterine resting tone and intensity.	Identifies presence of normal vs. hypertonic vs. hypotonic contractions.	Normal contraction pattern is occurring.
	Change position every 30 minutes from sitting upright vs. up and walking (if presenting part well engaged).	Offers more positions for fetal descent and internal rotation to anterior.	Normal patterns of fetal descent in anterior position.
	Encourage client to avoid supine position.	Avoids aortocaval compression and interruption of blood flow to uterus and through placenta.	Client has normal blood pressure; fetal monitor records normal baseline FHR; fetus is reactive with good baseline variability and reassuring fetal heart patterns.
	Encourage emptying bladder every 2 hours. Record intake and output.	Full bladder may impede labor failure to progress. Adequate circulatory volume maintains cardiac output and adequate uteroplacental perfusion.	Client voids and empties bladder every 2 hours. Client takes ice chips and voids clear urine every 2 hours.
	Initiate intrauterine resuscitation if there is hyperstimulation or a nonreassuring pattern noted:	Improves uteroplacental blood flow.	Normal contraction pattern; fetus has normal baseline FHR, reactivity, variability, and no periodic fetal heart tones.
	Turn off oxytocin.	Decreases stimulation of uterine activity.	
	Turn to side.	Prevents aortocaval compression.	
	Speed up mainline infusion.	Increases blood flow to heart and therefore to uterus, placenta, and to baby.	
	Give oxygen 6-8 L/m by tight face mask.	Assists maternal oxygenation.	
	Report and record.	Documents nursing care.	

NURSING
CARE
PLAN

Client With Dysfunctional Labor—continued

Goals (Expected Outcomes)	Interventions	Rationale	Evaluation
Fluid Volume Deficit—Related to Prolonged Labor and Restricted Fluid Intake			
Client will exhibit normal state of hydration.	Offer ice chips.	Decreases thirst and dryness of mouth which accompanies labor.	Client states ice quenches her thirst and adds to her comfort.
	Check urine for acetone.	Identifies signs of dehydration.	Urine is negative for acetone.
	Encourage to void about every 2 hours.	Assesses hydration.	Client voids clear, straw- or amber-colored urine every 2 hours.
	Give IV fluids as ordered.	Ensures hydration.	Client retains normal fluid volume as evidenced by vital signs and intake-output ratio.
Pain—Related to Uterine Contractions			
Client will experience relief of pain; verbalize sense of control of situation, and make informed choice among available alternatives.	Review comfort measures and pain relieving techniques.	Provides choices for pain relief and enables selection of method appropriate to individual needs and desires.	Client uses breathing and relaxation techniques very·effectively.
	Assist with relaxation techniques.	Relaxation decreases perception of pain and increases the efficacy of analgesia/anesthesia.	Client relaxes easily; states pain is tolerable.
	Explain options for pain relief (analgesic, anesthesia).	Involves client in decision making regarding analgesia/anesthesia.	Client verbalizes understanding of options available for pain relief and remains calm and responds to nursing interventions.
	Encourage mother and father and provide positive feedback.	Parents need encouragement and praise for their efforts; supports positive self-image and coping abilities.	Client and husband effectively work together and display no evidence of panic and discouragement.
	Encourage client to utilize alternate positions to assist progress.	Upright or left lateral and change of position every 30 minutes often will improve contraction effectiveness.	Client remains relaxed with position changes. Fetal monitor records normal baseline FHR.
	Record and report characteristics of uterine contractions, i.e., frequency, duration, intensity, and resting tone.	Determines efficient vs. incoordinate contractions.	Contractions are effective and there is good oxygenation of fetus.

Continued

NURSING
CARE
PLAN

Client with Dysfunctional Labor—*continued*

Goals (Expected Outcomes)	Interventions	Rationale	Evaluation
Anxiety—Related to Lack of Labor Progress			
Client's feelings of anxiety will by allayed by explanation.	Listen, take time to touch, and show concern.	Helps client to feel situation is under control and people are concerned and want to help.	Client states she is more relaxed.
	Explain reasons for dysfunctional labor and what plan of care will be.	Fear of unknown is greater than having some understanding of what is happening.	Client verbalizes understanding of dysfunctional labor and management.
Knowledge Deficit—Related to Dysfunctional Labor and Intravenous Oxytocin for Augmentation of Labor			
Client and family will verbalize understanding of reason for oxytocic augmentation and effects expected.	Reinforce physician's explanations of oxytocin augmentation of labor.	Increases understanding of procedure; reduces anxiety and fear; increases cooperation.	Couple reports they are less fearful and anxious.
	Explain how procedure will be done.	Increases knowledge and allays fear of unknown.	Couple verbalizes understanding and readiness to begin.
	Explain what to expect from oxytocin drip.	Prepares for contractions that can effect progress.	Couple verbalizes their desire for labor to progress and their infant to be born.

Uterine Rupture

Etiology and Pathophysiology

Rupture of the uterus is a rare intrapartum complication. The incidence is 1:1500 deliveries. Uterine rupture can occur during pregnancy but usually occurs during labor. Maternal mortality is about 5%. Fetal mortality is about 50%[3] and is due to hypoxia caused by placental separation.

The most common cause of uterine rupture is rupture of a scar from a previous cesarean section, particularly if there was a classic incision. The second cause is injudicious use of oxytocin for induction or augmentation of labor. Other contributing factors include previous uterine surgery, prolonged or obstructed labor, abnormal fetal positions or fetal abnormalities, excessive fetal size, thinned lower uterine segment in multiparity, and traumatic delivery, such as version and extraction, or injudicious use of forceps.

Presenting Signs and Symptoms

Signs and symptoms of uterine rupture can either be dramatic (complete rupture) or quiet (incomplete rupture). The dramatic (complete) rupture extends through the entire uterine wall, and the uterine contents are expelled into the abdominal cavity (Fig. 24-3). In dramatic rupture the most common presenting sign is pain (see display on p. 675). At the

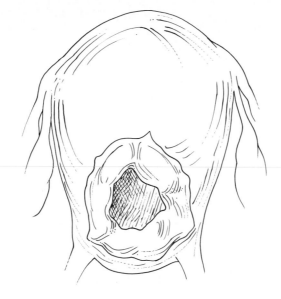

FIGURE 24-3
Complete Uterine Rupture. Complete uterine rupture extends through the entire myometrium, and hemorrhage is the major problem. Rupture of the uterus results in fetal death and may be a threat to the mother's life.

Signs and Symptoms of Dramatic and Quiet Uterine Rupture

Dramatic Rupture

Sharp shooting pain in lower abdomen at height of severe contraction
No further uterine contractions
Feeling of great relief from previous intense pain
Vaginal bleeding (slight amount of hemorrhage) followed by signs of shock

Quiet Rupture

Client may vomit
Increased tenderness of abdomen
Severe suprapubic pain
Hypotonic uterine contractions
No further progress in labor
Feeling of faintness
Eventual signs of shock
FHR may be lost

height of an intense contraction the client complains of a sudden, sharp, shooting abdominal pain. She may say, "Something ripped or tore inside." This is followed by immediate cessation of uterine contractions, which produces a feeling of great relief from the intense pain. Vaginal bleeding may be slight, or hemorrhage may occur. Excessive bleeding into the abdominal cavity and sometimes into the vagina may result in the signs and symptoms of shock. Additional signs and symptoms are feelings of apprehension, impending doom, restlessness, air hunger (shortness of breath), and visual disturbances.

A quiet rupture is the dehiscence of a lower segment scar, which may cause no bleeding or shock, and the rupture is discovered when cesarean section is performed because labor fails to progress (Fig. 24-4). With a quiet rupture (see above), the mother may vomit, feel faint, and have abdominal tenderness with severe suprapubic pain. Uterine contractions become hypotonic, and there is no further progress in labor.

FIGURE 24-4
Rupture of Lower Uterine Segment
Into Broad Ligament.

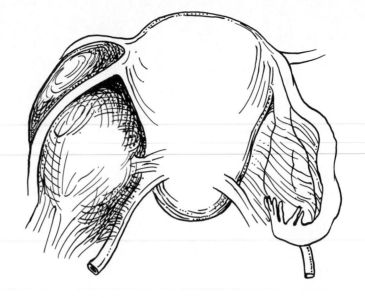

Pain and abdominal tenderness commonly occur in both quiet and dramatic rupture. These signs should raise suspicion that rupture of the uterus may have occurred.

Therapeutic Management and Nursing Intervention

The nurse must review the client's history and initial data base to identify high-risk factors, that indicate potential for uterine rupture. The nurse is very often the one to identify the signs and symptoms of uterine rupture. The primary care provider must be notified immediately and staff personnel informed to prepare for emergency surgery. Vital signs are monitored and bleeding evaluated. The nurse assists in preparing the client for surgery, which usually includes insertion of intravenous line as ordered for fluids and blood.

The emotional needs of the client's family also need attention. The primary care provider is responsible for providing the client with the information about what is happening, the surgery to be performed, and its implication on future childbearing. If fetal death has occurred, grief support will be needed.

Emergency surgery is initiated after definitive diagnosis has been made. Usually a hysterectomy is performed. However, depending on the type, location, and extent of the laceration the uterus may be repaired.

Uterine Inversion

Etiology and Pathophysiology

Inversion of the uterus is an extremely rare, potentially life-threatening complication of labor that occurs after the birth of the infant. This complication is associated with umbilical cord traction and fundal pressure. The uterus may be partially or completely inverted so that the fundal portion of the endometrial cavity protrudes through the cervix into the vagina (incomplete inversion) or outside the introitus (complete inversion). If the placenta is still attached, it can be felt in the lower vagina with the inverted uterus above it (Fig. 24-5).

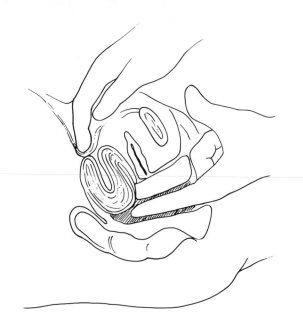

FIGURE 24-5
Complete Uterine Inversion. Uterus literally turns inside out. It may occur spontaneously or can occur because of application of too much fundal pressure (with hand) or pulling on cord or placenta. Abdominal-vaginal palpation is used to diagnose uterine inversion. There are various degrees of inversion ranging from slight to complete.

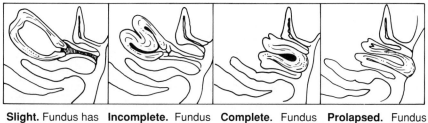

Slight. Fundus has slight indentation.

Incomplete. Fundus protrudes through cervical os.

Complete. Fundus inverted to level of introitus.

Prolapsed. Fundus extends beyond the vulva.

Pain, bleeding, and shock develop rapidly. Shock can be profound, and hemorrhage can result in death if not quickly managed. Hemorrhage is the result of (1) attempted manual placenta removal while the placenta is still attached and (2) uterine atony.

Presenting Signs and Symptoms

Observable phenomena and symptoms such as profuse vaginal bleeding and shock after delivery, excruciating abdominal pain, inability to palpate the fundus abdominally, and protrusion of the inverted uterus out of the vagina indicate uterine inversion.

Therapeutic Management

The key to management of an inverted uterus is to act quickly. Two intravenous infusions are started, one for blood and one for fluids. This fluid and blood replacement attempts to combat the blood loss and hypovolemic shock.

As fluids are being replaced, general anesthesia is given and then the placenta is removed. After the removal the primary health care provider places the palm of the hand on the fundus with the fingers extended to identify the margins of the cervix. Then the fundus is pushed upward through the cervix. After the uterus is restored to its normal placement, oxytocin is administered. If the uterus cannot be reinverted by this method, a laparotomy will be necessary to reposition the uterus.

Nursing Interventions

The nurse has available lactated Ringer's solution for emergency volume replacement. The laboratory is notified to be on standby for possible tests that will need to be done STAT. Blood transfusion will be ordered.

The nurse assists in keeping the family informed about what is happening. Additional responsibilities include providing care for the infant until it can be transferred to the newborn nursery and to provide recovery care for the client after the procedure has been completed. An important part of recovery care is to continue monitoring vital signs as ordered for possible shock, ensure consistent uterine firmness, and evaluate blood loss.

Pelvic Dystocia Factors

Variations or abnormalities in the pelvic structure can cause dystocia. The pelvis may be contracted (smaller than usual) at the inlet, the midpelvis, or the outlet (Fig. 24-6). Disproportion between the size of the fetus and the size of the pelvis is the most common pelvic dystocia factor.

Inlet Contraction

The inlet is said to be contracted when the anterioposterior diameter is decreased (10 cm or less) or the greatest transverse diameter is decreased (12 cm or less). Either of these contracted (decreased) diameters increases the potential for labor difficulties. When both diameters are decreased, there is an increased incidence of dystocia.

FIGURE 24-6

Variations in Pelvic Structure That Cause Dystocia. The major planes of the bony pelvis are the inlet, the midpelvis, and the outlet. When the diameter or shape of any of these planes is abnormal, the pelvis is said to be *contracted*. A contracted pelvis can mean prolonged and ineffective labor.

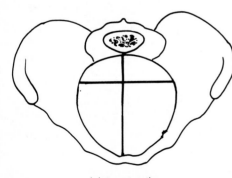

Inlet contraction

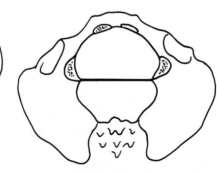

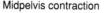

Midpelvis contraction

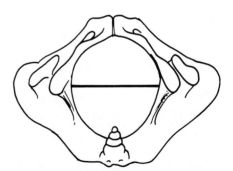

Outlet contraction

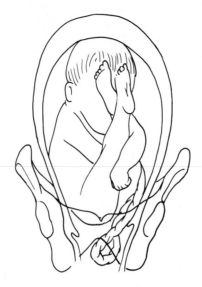

FIGURE 24-7
Inlet Contraction. When the measurements of the inlet are smaller than normal, engagement of the presenting part may be difficult. Breech presentation is common.

When the inlet is contracted, the presenting part of the fetus may not engage (Fig. 24-7). Risk of **prolapse of umbilical cord** is increased since the presenting fetal part does not fit the inlet well. Also there is increased incidence of fetal malposition, deflexed attitude, and extreme molding of the presenting fetal part.

Pronounced inlet contraction prevents engagement of the head. Labor is prolonged and effective labor is never achieved. Maternal complications from inlet contraction include (1) early spontaneous rupture of membranes, (2) weak contractions, (3) lack of progressive cervical dilatation, (4) infection, and (5) potential thinning of the lower uterine segment, which can result in uterine rupture. Fetal implications from pelvic inlet contraction include (1) infection (causing increased risk for mortality), (2) swelling or molding of the fetal head, (3) skull fractures, and (4) prolapse of the umbilical cord (which may cause irreversible fetal damage or death).

Midpelvis Contraction

The midpelvis is considered to be contracted when the transverse diameter between the ischial spines is less than 9.0 cm (normal is 10.5 cm) (see Fig. 24-6) and the widest diameter of the fetal head does not descend below 0 station. When arriving at the level of the ischeal spines, the fetal head must rotate to the occiput anterior (O.A.) position so the smallest diameter can pass, and then the head must curve forward as it continues to descend (Fig. 24-8). Molding (Fig. 24-9) occurs to accommodate the fetal head to this curvature in the pelvic canal. When the transverse diameter is contracted, internal rotation may not occur, resulting in a persistent posterior position or a **transverse arrest.** Both of these malpositions can require a difficult and traumatic forceps delivery or a cesarean delivery.

Outlet Contraction

If the distance between the ischial tuberosities is less than 8 cm, the pelvic outlet is contracted. When the outlet is contracted, the pubic arch is high and narrow and the fetal head does not fit under the symphysis pubis

FIGURE 24-8
Mechanism of Labor. The mechanism of labor is initiated when fetal head reaches ischial spines and consists of a combination of movements. The head must rotate and extend backward to be delivered. *A* = flexion; *B* = internal rotation; *C* = extension. (External rotation not shown.)

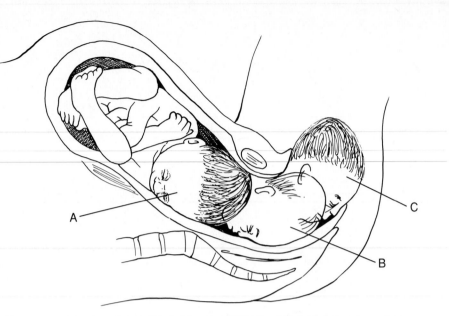

FIGURE 24-9
Effects of Labor on Fetal Head. **A,** As labor progresses, fetus descends so that head becomes more and more firmly applied to dilating cervix causing molding and swelling of soft tissue (caput succedaneum). **B,** Cephalic presentation determines which area of fetal head is molded. *1* = occiput anterior; *2* = occiput posterior; *3* = brow; *4* = face.

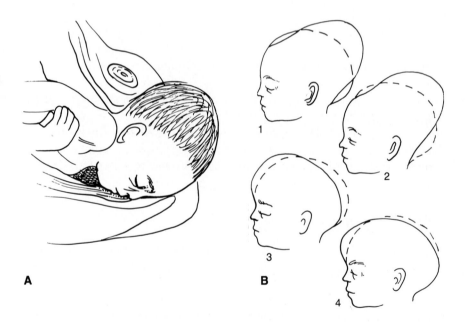

(Fig. 24-10). The decreased distance between the ischial tuberosities forces the fetal head backward against the sacrum and coccyx, causing progress to be impeded.

Cephalopelvic Disproportion

The term *cephalopelvic disproportion* (CPD) implies a discrepancy between the size of the fetal head and the size of the pelvis. The problem could originate with the pelvic size or shape, the fetal head size, or both. Whether the fetus will descend, rotate internally, and then be expelled depends on several factors: (1) efficiency of uterine contractions, (2) elasticity and

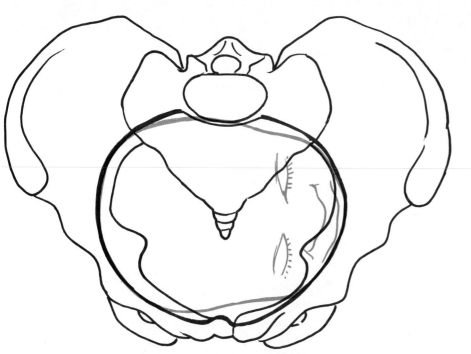

FIGURE 24-10

Outlet Contraction. Delivery is most difficult because the fetal head is under the pubic arch and forced backward against the sacrum and coccyx. Extreme molding and caput succedaneum formation are common in the infant, and formation of fistulas on the mother's vaginal wall may occur. Cesarean delivery may be necessary if forceps delivery is considered unsafe.

stretchability of maternal soft tissues, (3) attitude, presentation, and position of the fetus, and (4) fetal head moldability.

Therapeutic Management

An extreme degree of pelvic contraction can sometimes be detected during antepartum care. Early detection provides the physician with an opportunity to educate the mother about the necessity for a cesarean delivery. When the degree of pelvic contraction is less obvious, a trial labor is needed to determine if the uterine contractions are sufficient to propel the fetus through the contracted bony pelvis.

Nursing Interventions

Mothers with pelvic disproportion experience greater anxiety. Their level of anxiety is determined partly by the support and information they have received. If cesarean delivery is the eventual outcome, there may be a great deal of disappointment and perhaps a feeling of failure for not being able to deliver vaginally. The warm empathetic attitude of the nurse is greatly needed by these clients. Frequent reports about the progress of labor should be given to the couple even if the labor progress is not favorable.

Fetal Dystocia Factors and Complications

Fetal position and presentation influence progress of labor. Deviations of fetal position and presentation can adversely affect uterine contractions or prevent the fetus from passing through the birth canal.

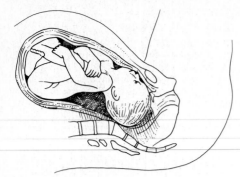

FIGURE 24-11

Persistent Posterior Position. When fetal head rotates to posterior position instead of anterior, second stage of labor is usually prolonged and mother experiences "back labor" because of fetal head being pressed into sacrum during each contraction.

Abnormal Positions

Persistent Occiput Posterior and Transverse Arrest

Persistent occiput posterior presentation is a common cause of lack of progress during the second stage of labor. The fetal head usually enters the pelvic inlet transversely and makes a 90 degree turn (internal rotation) to the O.A. position (see display p. 282 for key to abbreviations).

In about 25% of labors the head enters the pelvis in the L.O.P. or R.O.P. position. During internal rotation, the head that enters in the L.O.P. or R.O.P. must rotate 135 degrees instead of 90 degrees to be in the O.A. position. If the uterine contractions are efficient, if the fetal head is adequately flexed, and if the passenger is of average size, the 135 degree rotation occurs spontaneously as soon as the head is on the pelvic floor. When the fetal head is posterior (O.P. position) (Fig. 24-11), labor may be prolonged and the majority of mother's pain is felt in the low back ("back labor"). This back pain is due to the fetal head being rammed into the sacrum with each contraction. Ramming causes fetal head compression, which stimulates the fetal vagus nerve and in turn slows the baseline fetal heart rate.

In a minority of cases fetal head rotation does not occur and the head becomes stationary (or arrested) in the transverse position (transverse arrest) (Fig. 24-12). The head does not descend below 0 station.

NURSING INTERVENTIONS. Nursing interventions for persistent occiput posterior and transverse arrest are aimed at improving contractions. Changing the client's position to left lateral prevents inferior vena cava and aorta compression and ensures blood flow and oxygenation to the uterus, placenta, and fetus. Adequate uterine oxygenation is necessary for good contractions. Other positions can also facilitate contractions. Standing, sitting, squatting, and on hands and knees maximize uterine contractions, descent, and bearing down during labor.

FIGURE 24-12

Tranverse Arrest of Fetal Head. **A,** Neck is not well flexed so descent is not progressive and labor is prolonged. **B,** Depicts fetal head and fontanels showing what landmarks to assess when determining fetal position.

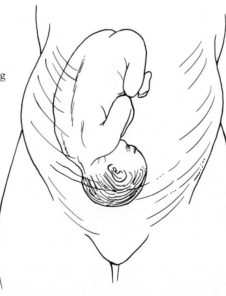

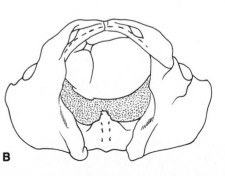

A   B

The nurse should praise the couple for all their efforts. Both are likely to become discouraged because of the lack of labor progress. Discouragement can increase their exhaustion and decrease their ability to cope. They should be kept informed of the labor progress or lack of progress.

If rotation of the fetal head does occur, it will be followed by spontaneous delivery. Occiput posterior and transverse arrest can be overcome by improved contractions and maternal pushing, but delivery with forceps, vacuum extractor, or cesarean section may be necessary.

Abnormal Presentations

Breech Presentation

Breech presentation means that the fetal buttocks rather than the fetal head is the presenting part. Breech presentation is categorized by the position of the presenting part as it enters the pelvic inlet. Categories include frank breech, incomplete breech, and complete breech (Fig. 24-13).

Breech is the presenting part in 3% to 4% of single births. The most frequent causes of breech presentation are fetal prematurity, multiple gestation, hydramnios, placenta previa, uterine fibroids, hydrocephalus, or fetal congenital anomaly.

Breech delivery presents no increased risk to the mother, although there may be increased risk of perinatal morbidity and mortality. A high percentage of breech presentation is delivered by cesarean section even though this increases the risk for maternal morbidity.

Shoulder Presentation

Shoulder presentation occurs when the fetus lies crosswise in the uterus (Fig. 24-14). It is also referred to as a "transverse lie." The shoulder is

FIGURE 24-13

Classification of Breech. **A,** Frank — buttocks present with hips flexed and legs extended against abdomen and chest. This is most common type of breech presentation. **B,** Incomplete — one or both feet or knees extend below buttocks. This type of presentation is also known as single or double footling breech. **C,** Complete — buttocks present with feet and legs flexed on thighs and thighs on abdomen.

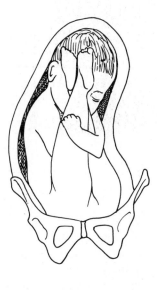
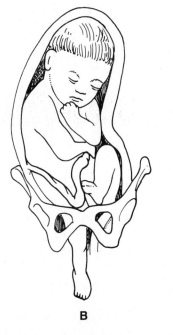
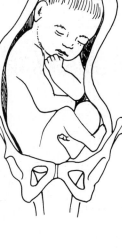

A   B   C

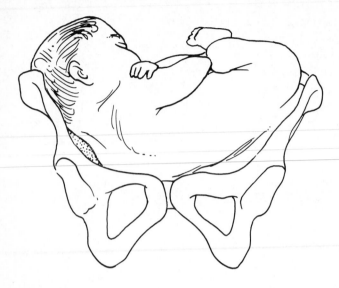
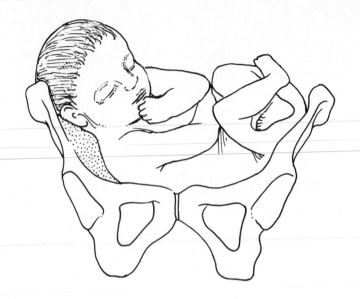

FIGURE 24-14

Shoulder Presentation (Tranverse Lie). In transverse lie or oblique lie long axis of fetus is perpendicular to or at angle to long axis of mother. This fetal position has 20 times greater incidence of cord prolapse.

often the fetal presenting part, although it can be the back, abdomen, or flank. If the diagnosis is made before labor begins, **external** cephalic **version** enables most of these clients to have a vaginal delivery. If diagnosis is made at the time of labor, a cesarean delivery is mandatory.

Brow Presentation

Brow presentation occurs when the fetal head enters the pelvis with the neck extended (Fig. 24-15). As descent continues, the head may become flexed, resulting in an occiput presentation, which is the smallest diameter of the fetal head. If, however, the head becomes hyperextended, the widest diameter of the head, the face (mentum), will present.

Face Presentation

Face presentation occurs when the vertex enters the pelvis with the neck hyperextended (Fig. 24-16). Face presentation poses a high risk for the umbilical cord to drop between back of head and the shoulders. This could result in compression of the cord during descent. Face presentation can cause trauma to the fetal soft tissues of the face, cerebral and neck compression, and damage to the trachea and larynx.

Other Fetal Dystocia Factors

Shoulder Dystocia

Shoulder dystocia (shoulder arrest) (Fig. 24-17), or difficult delivery of the shoulders after the fetal head is delivered, is an obstetric emergency. The mother's legs should be sharply flexed against her abdomen. This changes the incline of the pelvis and provides more room so the anterior shoulder can slide under the symphysis. The primary care provider may apply external suprapubic pressure in an attempt to free the wedged anterior shoulder.

The time between delivery of the head and delivery of the body must be short, since the fetal head may not receive oxygen as long as the

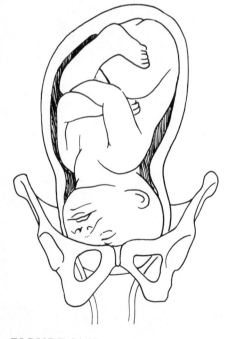

FIGURE 24-15

Brow Presentation. Note extension of neck. Further descent may cause flexion resulting in occiput presentation or hyperextension, which will result in face presentation.

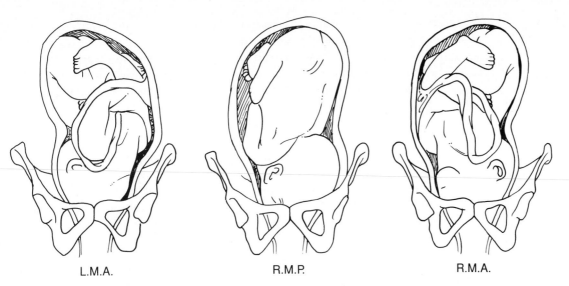

L.M.A. R.M.P. R.M.A.

FIGURE 24-16

Face Presentation. Note hyperextension of neck. This position represents largest diameter of vertex presentation. Chin (mentum) is presenting part of fetus. Cord may drop between back of head and shoulders, resulting in cord compression and fetal distress. *L.M.A.* = left mentum (chin) anterior; *R.M.P.* = right mentum (chin) posterior; *R.M.A.* = right mentum (chin) anterior.

shoulders are undelivered. This may occur because the broad shoulders of the fetus fills the pelvis and can compress the umbilical cord so that blood flow to the fetal head is dramatically reduced. Fetal brain damage or death can occur. Other potential complications resulting from shoulder dystocia include nerve damage to brachial plexus (Erb's palsy) and fractured clavicles. Maternal complications include extensive perineal and vaginal lacerations and emotional trauma in response to a traumatic delivery. Additional emotional trauma and grief occur if the baby is damaged or dies.

Fetal Macrosomia

Macrosomia is defined as fetal weight greater than 4000 g (about 9 lb). Associated factors for macrosomia are maternal obsesity, maternal dia-

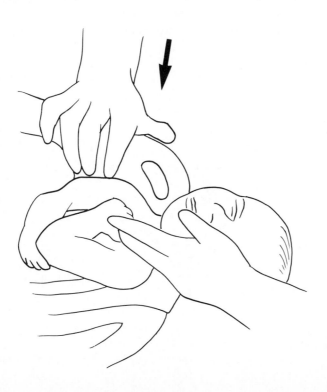

FIGURE 24-17

Shoulder Dystocia. After infant's head is delivered, sometimes broad shoulders become impacted against symphysis pubis (shoulder dystocia). Shoulder must be dislodged and delivery completed to avoid damage to neonate. Fingers of one hand are placed in vagina while opposite hand exerts light suprapubic pressure to force shoulder down in attempt to dislodge anterior shoulder.

betes, post date pregnancy, multiparity, and previous delivery of a macrosomic infant. Perinatal mortality for fetuses weighing more than 4500 g (about 10 lb) is about five times higher than in normal term and average weight infants. The size of these unusually large neonates causes dystocia, as they are too large to be pushed through the birth canal.

Fetal Anomalies

Any fetal anomaly that increases the size of a fetal part or parts can cause dystocia. The most common fetal anomaly causing dystocia is hydrocephalus. Other fetal anomalies that may inhibit progress of labor are enlargement of fetal abdomen caused by distended bladder, or ascites, or other fetal masses, including meningomyelocele. Other rare problems such as incomplete twinning resulting in conjoined (Siamese) twins also cause dystocia.

Other Fetal Complications

Prolapse of the Umbilical Cord

ETIOLOGY AND PATHOPHYSIOLOGY. The three types of umbilical cord prolapse are occult, frank, and complete (Fig. 24-18). In occult cord prolapse the cord slips down alongside the presenting part but is not visible through the cervix. In frank cord prolapse the cord slips through the cervix ahead of the presenting part. The cord protrudes from the vagina in complete prolapse. The danger from cord prolapse is fetal hypoxia secondary to compression of the cord between the presenting part and the pelvis. Hypoxia is manifested by slowing of the fetal heart rate.

The incidence of cord prolapse is about 1:400. The primary precipitating cause of cord prolapse is spontaneous or artificial rupture of membranes before the presenting part is engaged at the pelvis inlet. When the amniotic sac ruptures, the sudden rush of fluid carries the cord along with it as it rapidly flows out through the vagina.

Other reasons for cord prolapse are fetal prematurity, abnormal presentations (breech, transverse), placenta previa, cephalopelvic disproportion, hydramnios, and multiple gestation.

FIGURE 24-18

Types of Prolapsed Cords. All these may precipitate life-threatening crisis. **A,** Occult prolapse. Cord is compressed between fetal head and side of uterus. Fetal heart rate will probably speed up initially. As labor progresses and water breaks, more compression occurs. Severe hypoxia may occur. **B,** Frank cord presentation. Umbilical cord is presenting in front of vertex. Fetal jeopardy increases as labor progresses. **C,** Complete prolapse of umbilical cord. Cord presents in front of fetal head and is visible in vagina.

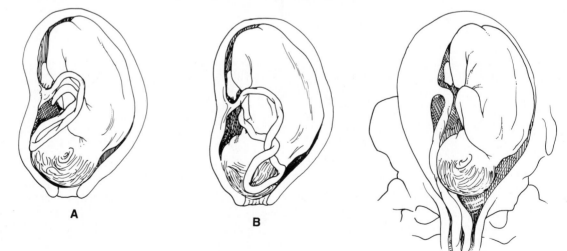

A   B   C

The incidence of frank umbilical cord prolapse is greater when fetal position is in the breech or transverse lie. When the fetus is vertex, the incidence of cord prolapse is 0.5%.[4] With frank umbilical cord prolapse, perinatal mortality is near 20%.

THERAPEUTIC MANAGEMENT AND NURSING INTERVENTIONS. Prolapse of the umbilical cord is an emergency situation requiring prompt recognition and intervention to ensure oxygenation of the fetus. When the bag of waters ruptures, the first action is to check the fetal heart rate for deceleration. If the fetal heart rate is electronically monitored, variable decelerations indicate cord compression.

As soon as the primary care provider determines there is a prolapsed umbilical cord, attempts are made to maximize blood flow (oxygenation) to the fetus. The mother is positioned in a knee-chest position (Fig. 24-19) or a modified Sims' position and the hips elevated as high as possible using pillows (Fig. 24-20) to decrease pressure on the cord and facilitate adequate blood flow to the fetus. The primary care provider inserts two to three fingers into the vagina to elevate the presenting part of the cord (Fig. 24-21). The fingers continue to relieve the pressure on the cord until the infant is delivered. Delivery room staff is quickly alerted to prepare for an immediate cesarean delivery if the cervix is not completely dilated. A completely dilated cervix can permit a vaginal delivery, but internal podalic version, mid forceps, or any operative technique is a greater risk than a cesarean delivery. If the fetus is dead, it will be delivered vaginally.

Prognosis depends on the degree and duration of cord compression before the prolapse is discovered. If discovery occurs early and compression duration is less than 5 minutes, the prognosis is good. If compression has lasted longer than 5 minutes, fetal brain damage or death will occur. Gestational age and trauma during delivery also affect outcome.

The mother and her support person should be informed about what has happened about what the plan of care will be. Both require psychologic and emotional support. It is important for them to know what they can do to help themselves and to remain together as much as possible to experience the birth together, not separately.

> ≫ EMERGENCY NURSING INTERVENTION

Cord Prolapse

1. Place mother in Trendelenburg or knee-chest position.
2. Call for assistance.
3. Do vaginal examination, elevate presenting part, and assess cord pulsation.
4. Notify primary care provider STAT.
5. Increase IV fluids.
6. Administer O_2 (6-8 L) by tight face mask.
7. Prepare for delivery.

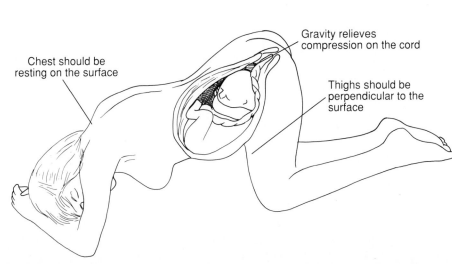

FIGURE 24-19
Position for Prolapsed Cord. Knee-chest position for prolapsed cord may reduce cord compression. Dilatation and station is assessed by nurse or primary care provider, and high concentration of oxygen is administered. Intravenous infusion rate is increased and client prepared for delivery.

Chest should be resting on the surface

Gravity relieves compression on the cord

Thighs should be perpendicular to the surface

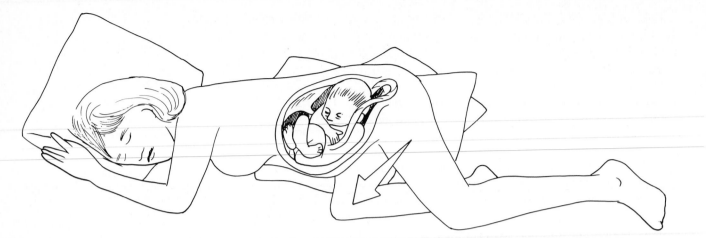

FIGURE 24–20

Alternate Position for Prolapsed Cord.
When there is prolapse of umbilical cord, it
is important to try positioning mother in
effort to alleviate cord compression.
Repositioning mother may eliminate
pressure on cord and maintain umbilical
cord circulation.

||| **LABORATORY**
||| **VALUES**

Amniotic Fluid Embolism

Tests	Results
Fibrinogin	Decreased
Fibrin split products	Elevated
Partial thromboplastin time (PTT)	Prolonged
Platelets	Decreased

Amniotic Fluid Embolism

ETIOLOGYAND PATHOPHYSIOLOGY. Amniotic fluid embolism (AFE) is
another extremely rare and potentially fatal complication for the mother
and her infant. Amniotic fluid embolism occurs when a large amount of
amniotic fluid is infused into the maternal circulation. Predisposing factors
for development of AFE are multiparity, hypertonic uterine contractions,
induction or augmentation of labor with oxytocin, and traumatic delivery.
Fifty percent of all clients with AFE die within 1 hour after onset of the
symptoms, and approximately 50% of survivors subsequently die.

For amniotic fluid embolism to occur there must be a connection between the amniotic fluid sac and the maternal venous system. Amniotic
fluid is able to get into the maternal circulation when there is a tear through
the amnion and chorion. The pressure created by the contracting uterus
forces the amniotic fluid through the entry site into the maternal circulation. The most likely sites of entry are the endocervical veins and the
uteroplacental area. This condition usually follows a tumultuous labor.

The debris in the amniotic fluid (vernix caseosa, lanugo, meconium)
is what causes the emboli to form in the maternal circulating blood. These
emboli occlude the pulmonary vessels and result in pulmonary embolism,
which in turn creates acute cor pulmonale. The emboli (debris) in the
maternal vessels also initiate an abnormal blood–clotting mechanism (disseminated intravascular coagulation, or DIC) which causes rapid, massive
hemorrhage and loss of clotting factors.

Cardinal signs and symptoms (see below) of AFE are respiratory distress as a result of the debris in the pulmonary capillaries, which prevent

Premonitory and Cardinal Signs and Symptoms of Amniotic Fluid Embolism

Premonitory	Cardinal
Shaking, chills	Chest pain
Sweating	Dyspnea
Anxiety	Tachypnea
Coughing	Hemorrhage
Vomiting	Hypotension
Convulsions	Cardiovascular collapse
	Coma

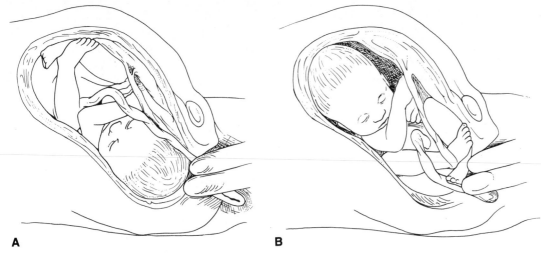

A   **B**

oxygen transfer to the blood. Respiratory distress symptoms include chest pain, dyspnea, tachypnea, cyanosis, apprehension, and restlessness. Decrease in the blood flow to the heart precipitates hypotension and cardiovascular collapse. Lack of cerebral circulation and the resulting hypoxia cause coma.

THERAPEUTIC MANAGEMENT AND NURSING INTERVENTIONS. Three goals of treatment for amniotic fluid embolism are (1) oxygenation, (2) maintenance of cardiac output and blood pressure, and (3) combating coagulopathy (DIC). Management includes initiation of cardiopulmonary resuscitation if needed. If the mother is apneic, oxygen at 100% concentration is given using bag, mask, and positive pressure ventilation. When the physician or anesthesiologist arrives, the client may be intubated and ventilated with 100% oxygen. If the client is undelivered, the nurse monitors the fetal heart rate to detect signs of fetal distress.

Hypotension is usually secondary to cardiogenic shock, so the intravenous fluids are increased as ordered to expand volume and increase blood flow to the heart. A pulmonary artery catheter will be placed to guide hemodynamic management. The nurse collects the necessary equipment for this procedure and assists with the insertion. If hypotension continues, a dopamine infusion may be ordered by the primary health care provider. Clients who do not become severely hypoxic or hypotensive are assessed for congestive heart failure. The primary health care provider may give instructions for digitalization. The nurse maintains accurate records of intake and output to minimize risks for development of pulmonary edema.

Blood samples collected from the pulmonary artery catheter are sent to the laboratory to determine which coagulation factors are depleted so they can be replaced and the DIC managed. Fibrogen or cryoprecipitate may be administered as well as fresh whole blood, packed red blood cells, or fresh frozen plasma. The nurse continues to monitor and record vital signs, bleeding, response to treatment, and administration of drugs and blood and blood products.

Multiple Pregnancy

ETIOLOGY AND PATHOPHYSIOLOGY. Women who are a dizygotic twin tend to have multiple pregnancies. Increased age, parity, and infertility drugs also increase the probability of multiple pregnancy.

FIGURE 24-21
Relieving Pressure on Prolapsed Cord. When there is umbilical cord prolapse, mother's position is changed to help relieve pressure on cord. Additionally, vaginal exam is done to determine if cord can be palpated. Examiner will elevate presenting part (vertex, **A**, or breech, **B**) in attempt to decrease pressure on cord so that blood flow through cord is maximized.

Multiple pregnancy is a high-risk pregnancy because of increased frequency of anemia, urinary tract infection, pregnancy-induced hypertension, hemorrhage (before, during, and after delivery), and uterine inertia. The fetuses are at risk for preterm delivery, abnormal presentation and position, and hydramnios. There is a threat of prolapsed cord for both twins, and the second may be at risk for premature separation of the placenta, hypoxia, dystocia, operative delivery, and prolonged anesthesia. Monozygotic twins are less hardy than dizygotic twins, as their weight differences are more pronounced, and they have a higher incidence of congenital anomalies and neonatal mortality. A monochorionic (single chorion) placenta is thought to be less competent than the dichorionic (two chorions). An incompetent placenta can cause placental vascular disorders. The most serious of these is the shunting of blood from twin to twin due to vascular anastomosis or communication between the fetuses. This can result in disparity in size and appearance in the fetuses. The donor twin is pallid, anemic, dehydrated, growth retarded, and hypovolemic. The recipient twin appears healthy, larger, and ruddy (polycythemic) (hematocrit greater than 65). This appearance is due to edema, plethora (ruddy color), and hypertension. The larger twin is at great risk for death in the first 24 hours of life.

TYPES OF TWINS. Twins may occur as a result of one of two processes, dizygotic or monozygotic. In the first, fertilization of two separate ova by two different sperm results in dizygotic or fraternal twins (Fig. 24-22, *A*). These do not share identical genetic material but do resemble one another, yet they have significant differences. About two thirds of twins are dizygotic.

FIGURE 24-22
Multiple Gestation. A, Monozygotic twins (identical) result from single fertilized ovum and single sperm. **B,** Dizygotic twins (fraternal) are product of two ova and two sperm.

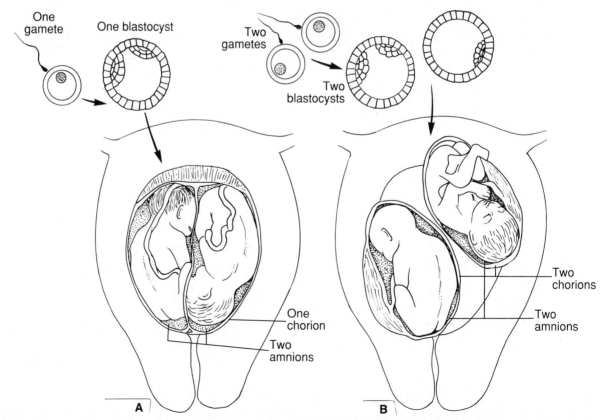

One gamete   One blastocyst

Two gametes

Two blastocysts

One chorion

Two amnions

Two chorions

Two amnions

A

B

The remaining one third of twins are the result of a single ovum that is fertilized by a single sperm and at some point in early embryonic development splits into two separate but genetically similar structures to become monozygotic or identical twins (Fig. 24-22, *B*). Identical twins may appear dissimilar because of asymmetric intrauterine growth caused by placental abnormalities or shared intervascular communication.

Examination of the fetal membranes assists in diagnosing identical and fraternal twins.

CONFIRMATION AND MANAGEMENT OF MULTIPLE PREGNANCY. Twins may be suspected when uterine size is greater than expected for gestation. Twins have been diagnosed as early as the 10th week. Ultrasonography is the preferred diagnostic tool. At present there is no biochemical test that clearly differentiates between multiple and single pregnancies.

All the maternal systems are subject to additional stress in multiple pregnancy. Physical discomforts are more extreme, body image is more distorted, preparation for infant care is greater, and the financial costs will be increased.

Early identification of multiple pregnancy and more frequent visits to the obstetrician result in better maternal support, particularly in the area of nutrition. If there are no complications, visits are usually scheduled every 2 weeks during the second trimester and weekly during the third trimester. Calories, protein, iron, folic acid, and vitamin supplements are increased. Rest in the left lateral position should be encouraged to maximize gestation, uteroplacental circulation, and fetal oxygenation.

Psychologic Dystocia Factors
Etiology and Pathophysiology

There is a relationship between anxiety and uterine dysfunction. Studies have suggested the possibility of an interrelationship between difficulty during labor and delivery and sociocultural or psychologic factors.

Various factors influence a client's reactions to the childbearing experience. Significant factors include how the tasks of pregnancy have been accomplished, her usual coping mechanisms in response to stress, her support systems, childbirth preparation, and cultural influences.

The same coping mechanisms used by the mother in everyday life will be used during pregnancy, labor, and delivery. Her comfort in the role of female, wife, and mother and her relationship with her own mother and the child's father are all important factors. Preparation for childbirth is also an important factor. Preparation tends to increase perceived satisfaction with the childbearing experience.[5]

Nursing Interventions

Therefore, it is very important to assist mothers psychologically during their labors. This can be done by supporting and encouraging both the mother and her coach and by providing information to reduce anxiety.

Physical care, a sustaining human presence, relief from pain, acceptance of attitudes and behaviors, and information and reassurance of a safe outcome for herself and her infant dramatically affect the mother's **"psyche"** and help her to cope and have self-confidence and a satisfying childbearing experience.

CULTURAL IMPLICATIONS

If a woman perceives the time of pregnancy as an illness, there may be the likelihood of a longer labor.

Position Dystocia Factors
Etiology and Pathophysiology

The functional relationships between the uterine contractions, the fetus, and the mother's pelvis are altered by maternal positioning. Position can provide a mechanical advantage or disadvantage to the mechanisms of labor.[6]

1. The supine position causes gravity to work against alignment of the uterus with the pelvic canal. The presenting part is directed in an S-shaped curve, first to the symphysis, then to the sacrum, and finally forward again.

2. The supine position results in the uterus lying on the inferior vena cava and the aorta, causing compression and possible maternal hypotension and fetal distress. This position causes contractions to be inefficient because of uterine muscle hypoxia.

3. Higher levels of stress-related hormones (β-endorphin, ACTH, cortisol, and epinephrine) are produced when clients are supine, which may be associated with dystocia patterns.

4. Restriction to one position may prolong a poor fit and poor alignment between the fetal head and maternal pelvis, which can slow labor.

5. When the mother remains in a semisitting or in a modified lithotomy position, her weight is largely on the sacrum and coccyx, which reduces the joint-softening effect of the sacrum and reduces pelvic outlet dimensions.

6. The direction of uterine force when the mother is supine encourages extension of the fetal neck and deflexion of the fetal head, causing a larger diameter to present in the pelvis. Uterine contractions cause the head to become wedged in the pelvis in an abnormal position.

Nursing Interventions

The nurse instructs her clients about the value of movement during labor. Movement is encouraged as one means to seek comfort during labor. The positions that the mother chooses for comfort may also reduce the length of labor, which can decrease dystocia and the need for labor augmentation, forceps delivery, and cesarean delivery.

The nurse explains to the mother the importance of the lateral and upright positions for labor. It should be suggested that the laboring woman try alternative positions such as standing, sitting, squatting, and on hands and knees to maximize uterine contractions, descent, and bearing down in labor.

REFERENCES

1. Bonica JJ: Obstetric Analgesia and Anesthesia. Amsterdam, World Federation of Societies of Anaesthesiologists, 1980
2. Schalteer S, Pernoll ML: Dystocia. In Pernoll ML, Benson RC (eds): Current Obstetric and Gynecologic Disorders. Norwalk, Conn, Appleton & Lange, 1987
3. Herrera E, Pernoll ML: Complications of labor and delivery. In Pernoll ML, Benson RC (eds): Current Obstetric and Gynecologic Disorders. Norwalk, Conn, Appleton & Lange, 1987
4. Collen JA: Malpresentation and cord accidents. In Pernoll ML, Benson RC (eds): Current Obstetric and Gynecologic Disorders. Norwalk, Conn, Appleton & Lange, 1987
5. Humenick S: Mastery: The key to childbirth satisfaction? A review. Birth Fam J 8:79-83, 1981
6. Fenwick L, Simkin P: Maternal positioning to prevent or alleviate dystocia in labor. Clin Obstet Gynecol 30(1):83-89, March 1987

SUGGESTED READINGS

ACOG Technical Bulletin: Induction and Augmentation of Labor. No. 110, November 1987.

Bowes WA Jr: Clinical aspects of normal and abnormal labor. In Creasy RK, Resnik R (eds): Maternal-Fetal Medicine: Principles and Practice. Philadelphia, WB Saunders, 1989

Kelpatrick SJ, Laras RK: Characteristics of normal labor. Obstet Gynecol 74(1), July 1989

Kentz DL: Nursing support in labor. JOGN (March/April):126-130, 1987

Lesser MS, Keane VR: Nurse-Patient Relationships in Hospital Maternity Nursing. St. Louis, CV Mosby, 1956

MacLennan AH: Multiple Gestation: Clinical characteristics and management. In Creasy RK, Resnik R (eds): Maternal-Fetal Medicine: Principles and Practice. Philadelphia, WB Saunders, 1989

Murray M: Essentials of Fetal Monitoring: Antepartal and Intrapartal Monitoring. NAACOG, 1989

NAACOG: The Nurse's Role in the Induction/Augmentation of Labor. OGN Nurs Prac Resource, January 1988

NAACOG: Statement: Nurses' Responsibilities in Implementing Intrapartum Fetal Heart Rate Monitoring, October 1988

O'Driscoll K, Foley M, MacDonald D: Active management of labor as an alternative to cesarean section for dystocia. Obstet Gynecol 63(4), April 1984

Price TM, Cefalo RC: Saving the patient who has amniotic fluid embolism. Contemporary OB/Gyn March 1988

Pritchard JA, MacDonald PC, Gant NF: Williams Obstetrics, 17th ed., Chapter 29. New York, Appleton-Century-Crofts, 1985

Rossi MA, Lindell SG: Maternal Position and Pushing Techniques in a Nonprescriptive Environment. JOGN (May/June): 203-208, 1986

Schlateer S, Pernoll ML: Common obstetric problems. Part I: Labor disorders. The Female Patient 9, March 1984

Postpartum Complications

IMPORTANT TERMINOLOGY

embolus Mass of undissolved matter present in a blood or lymphatic vessel (may be solid, liquid, or gaseous)

endometritis Localized infection of lining of uterus

mastitis Inflammation of breast

pelvic cellulitis or parametritis Infection extending along lymphatics to loose connective tissue around uterus

peritonitis Infection (local or general) of peritoneum

pulmonary embolism Embolus (thrombus fragment) carried by venous circulation to right side of heart

pyelonephritis Infection involving ureters and kidneys

salpingitis Infection of fallopian tubes

subinvolution of uterus Retarded uterine involution with delay in return to normal size and function

thrombophlebitis Infection of endothelial lining of vessels with clot formation attached to vessel wall

thrombus Blood clot obstructing a vessel or cavity of the heart

vulvar hematoma Blood in connective tissue under the skin that covers the external genitalia or beneath the vaginal mucosa

Post partum is a time of increased physiologic and psychologic stress for the family as the mother's body returns to a nonpregnant state and new family roles are assumed. Many complications can occur during the postpartum period, but only three are serious or life-threatening: hemorrhage, infection, and embolism. The nurse must be familiar with the normal anatomy and physiology of the puerperium to identify the deviations from normal as soon as possible. All information collected about the client from prenatal visits, during admission, and through labor and delivery must be reviewed to identify risk factors that would produce complications.

LEGAL AND ETHICAL CONSIDERATIONS

Postpartum conditions most frequently involved in litigation are hemorrhage (before, during, or after delivery) and infection.

Hemorrhagic Complications

Hemorrhage

Etiology and Pathophysiology

Immediate postpartum hemorrhage is defined as blood loss of more than 500 ml during the first 24 hours after delivery. The most common cause of immediate postpartum hemorrhage is uterine atony caused by "overstretching" during pregnancy. In addition, lacerations of the perineum, vagina, and cervix and sometimes hematomas that develop in the areas of these lacerations can result in rapid, profuse blood loss.

Hemorrhage is the third leading cause of maternal mortality with an incidence of 5% to 8% after vaginal delivery. Predisposing factors are listed in Table 25-1.

Hemorrhage can be classified as immediate, delayed, or late. Delayed hemorrhage, occurring more than 24 hours after delivery, is usually caused by retention of placental fragments or abnormal involution of the placental site. Late hemorrhage can occur as much as 6 weeks after delivery but often occurs between the 5th and 15th postpartum day.

Shock

Etiology and Pathophysiology

Hypovolemic shock is the leading cause of maternal mortality in the United States. Hypovolemia may not be recognized until it becomes life-threatening because of the process of compensated shock. Shock is compensated because pregnancy increases the blood volume and the vasoconstriction initiated by the sympathetic nervous system maintains a normal rate of blood flow to the head. Orthostatic signs and symptoms may be masked by the compensated shock mechanism. Signs and symptoms of hemorrhage and shock depend on both the quality and the rate of blood loss (see Assessment Tool: Shock p. 696). A review of the signs and symptoms of shock and the priorities of management are listed in Table 25-2.

TABLE 25-1

*Conditions Predisposing for
Postpartum Hemorrhage*

Antedating Pregnancy	Arising During Pregnancy and Labor
Previous postpartum hemorrhage	Placenta previa
Grand multiparity	Abruptio placentae
Fibroids	Multiple pregnancy
Idiopathic thrombocytopenia purpura	Polyhydramnios
Von Willebrand's disease	Precipitate labor
Leukemia	Prolonged labor
	Chorioamnionitis
	Forceps delivery
	Cesarean section
	General anesthesia
	Mismanagement of third stage of labor
	Acute coagulation defect

From Cavanaugh D et al: Obstetric Emergencies, 3rd ed. Philadelphia, Harper & Row, 1982.

ASSESSMENT
TOOL

Shock

Perineum: obvious bleeding
Fundus: firm vs. boggy, fundal height
Vital signs
  Respirations: tachypnea, shallow, irregular, air hunger
  Pulse: tachycardia, weak, thready, irregular
  Blood pressure: hypotensive, dizziness, faintness
Skin: cool, moist, pale, cold, clammy, cyanosis of lips and fingernails, capillar
  refill
Urinary output: decreasing, <30 ml/hr
Level of consciousness: oriented, mental cloudiness, increasing restlessness,
  lethargy
Psychologic status: anxious
Laboratory values
  CBC
  Electrolytes (including blood urea nitrogen and creatinine)
  Blood gases
  Coagulation profile
  Urinalysis
  Type and crossmatch

Sample Narrative Charting: Complains of being dizzy. "I feel like I'm going to faint." Lying on stretcher in pool of blood, which has soaked through two maxi sanitary pads as well as underpad. Fundus is boggy and does not firm with massage. Asked another nurse to get physician STAT. Blood pressure is 60/0, pulse is 120, weak, and thready, respirations are 28 and shallow. Skin is cold and clammy and diaphoretic. Placed in Trendelenburg position and intravenous of Ringer's lactate started in left forearm. Oxygen at 8 L per mask started. Bleeding still profuse. Methergine 0.2 mg given IV push as ordered.

Cardiac output is adequate until approximately 15% of the total blood volume is lost (approximately 750 ml). When blood loss is greater than 15% of the total blood volume, cardiac output decreases, causing an increased degree of shock. The heart is unable to pump enough blood to supply the cardiac muscle, resulting in weakening of the heart muscle, which further decreases cardiac output. Blood flow to the brain is also decreased, causing damage to vasomotor and respiratory centers.

TABLE 25-2

Signs and Symptoms of Shock

Factor	Presenting Signs and Symptoms	
	Hypovolemic Shock	Septic Shock
Pulse	Tachycardia: weak, thready pulse	Tachycardia: rebounding pulse, palpitations
Blood pressure	Hypotension: anxious, restless	Hypotension: faint, dizzy
Tissue perfusion	Decreased: cold clammy skin, pale, cyanotic nail beds, flat neck veins	Cerebral ischemia: anxiety, apprehension, disorientation, stupor
Urinary output	Oliguria: 50 ml/hr; urinary sodium—80 mEq/L	Polyuria: 125 ml/hr; urinary sodium—10mEq/L

Assessment

Hemorrhage can be a dramatic sudden rush of blood from the vagina, or it can be steady vaginal bleeding that continues for hours before creating hypovolemia. A steady vaginal blood flow that adds up to an excessive amount may not be immediately recognized as hemorrhage. How rapidly the signs and symptoms of hypovolemia present depends on the client's blood volume before pregnancy, the percentage of blood volume increase during pregnancy, and the amount of blood volume and hemoglobin lost. Signs and symptoms appear and become more pronounced as the blood loss increases (see Assessment Tool: Degree of Hemorrhage). Pulse and blood pressure may not become abnormal until a large volume of blood has been lost; then they will change suddenly.

During the initial stage of hypovolemia a mother with normal blood pressure can respond with a higher than usual blood pressure, whereas the hypertensive mother can appear normotensive. However, both may be hypovolemic but not recognized as such until they are in difficulty. No change may occur when the client's blood pressure and pulse are taken with her in the supine position, but when she is placed in a sitting position, she may exhibit signs of hypovolemia such as dizziness, hypotension, and tachycardia. Clients with pregnancy-induced hypertension (PIH) develop symptoms of hypovolemia earlier because the PIH causes

---

Degree of Hemorrhage

Severity	Signs and Symptoms	Reduction in Blood Volume
Mild	Uterine consistency firm or boggy Bleeding from vaginal or cervical lacerations Slight or no decrease in blood pressure (1500 ml of blood can be lost before significant drop in blood pressure occurs Minimum tachycardia Mild evidence of vasoconstriction, with cool hands and feet	15%-20% (750-1250 ml)
Moderate	Atonic uterus Decreased pulse pressure Systolic pressure 90-100 mm Hg Tachycardia (100-120 bpm) Restlessness Sweating Pallor Oliguria	25%-35% (1250-1750 ml)
Severe	Atonic uterus Systolic pressure decreased to 60 mm Hg and frequently unobtainable by cuff Tachycardia >120 bpm Mental stupor Extreme pallor Cold extremities Anuria	Up to 50% (2500 ml)

an intravascular-to-interstitial fluid shift that rapidly produces hypovolemia.

Because of the potential for very rapid and dramatic onset of signs and symptoms of hypovolemia, it is imperative that blood loss be frequently assessed and the amount determined to identify the degree of hemorrhage (see Assessment Tool).

Nursing Diagnosis

Potential nursing diagnoses for the client with hemorrhage relate to tissue perfusion, anxiety, and knowledge deficit (see below).

Planning and Intervention

Shock is an emergency situation. Postpartum hemorrhage and shock are managed with intravenous (IV) fluids to replace volume, oxytocin (Pitocin) to contract the uterus, and oxygen administration. Oxytocin (10 U) may be ordered to be added to the IV fluid to stimulate the uterus to contract. In addition, if the client is normotensive, methylergonovine maleate or ergonovine maleate may be administered (see drug guides for methylergonovine maleate and ergonovine maleate p. 700). Whenever placental fragments are retained, curettage is usually indicated, and antibiotics may be ordered to prevent puerperal infection.

During the acute phase of bleeding IV fluids (usually lactated Ringer's solution) are ordered to provide a quick and available route for administration of IV medications. The nurse anticipates an order for an oxytocin to assist in restoration of hemostasis. Nursing care includes placing the client in the Trendelenburg position or elevating her legs to increase venous blood return to her heart and maximize cardiac output. Oxygen at 6 to 8 L/min is initiated by face mask, and the client's color, capillary refill, and skin temperature are reevaluated every 5 minutes.

The nurse monitors the client's vital signs every 5 minutes. If the client's fundus is palpable, the nurse massages it as frequently as necessary to ensure firmness. The amount of vaginal blood loss is evaluated by describing its color, amount, consistency and noting if blood clots are present. After their removal, the nurse weighs the perineal pads to determine blood loss further.

☐ POTENTIAL NURSING DIAGNOSES

Postpartum Hemorrhage

Fluid Volume Deficit: Immediate—related to excessive blood loss secondary to uterine atony

Fluid Volume Deficit: Delayed—related to excessive blood loss secondary to retained placental fragments

Decreased Cardiac Output—related to hypovolemia secondary to excessive blood loss

Altered General Tissue Perfusion—related to diminished circulating blood volume and shock

Pain—related to uterine contractions secondary to administration of oxytocic medications

Potential for Infection—related to bacterial invasion of uterus secondary to endometrial trauma and curettage

Knowledge Deficit—regarding surgical procedure and postoperative management

Anxiety—related to necessary separation from infant; need to receive blood and blood products; risk of contracting AIDS and hepatitis

Focus Assessment

Biophysical Aspects

Review prenatal record for history of risk factors.
    Grand multiparity
    Uterine overdistention (e.g., multiple gestation, hydramnios, fetal macrosomia)
    Placenta previa
    Pregnancy-induced hypertension
    Abruptio placentae
Review labor and delivery record for history of risk factors.
    Traumatic labor or delivery (e.g., forceps rotation or delivery)
    General anesthesia
    Precipitate labor
    Prolonged or obstructed labor (e.g., fetal malposition)
    Manual removal of placenta
Estimate time elapsed since delivery.
Assess for signs of hemorrhage and infection.
    Monitor vital signs closely.
    Monitor level of consciousness.
    Monitor fundal height, consistency, and tenderness.
    Monitor character and amount of lochia (e.g., pad count; saturation; return of rubra after progression to alba; odor).
    Monitor intake and output.
Evaluate diagnostic studies (e.g., hemoglobin, hematocrit, complete blood count).

Psychosocial Aspects

Explore nonverbal indicators of emotional status (e.g., irritability, inability to concentrate, withdrawal).
Explore individual concerns.
Identify current level of knowledge regarding the following:
    Surgical procedure
    Preoperative and postoperative medical and nursing management.
Determine current learning needs.

>> EMERGENCY NURSING INTERVENTION

The ORDER of Priorities in Managing the Client in Shock

O   **Oxygenate**

    Assure an airway
    8–10/min by closed mask, nasal catheter, or endotracheal tube

R   **Restore circulating volume**

    One or more IV lines
    Initially crystalloids or colloids
    Where possible, blood for blood, but remember clotting factors
    Initial monitoring by central venous pressure

D   **Drug therapy**

    Avoid vasopressors as a general rule
    Digitalize if in cardiac failure
    Specific drugs for condition

E   **Evaluate**

    Response to therapy
    Basic cause
    Fetal condition if appropriate

R   **Remedy the basic problem**

    Surgery if appropriate
    Specific antibiotics if organism identified

From Cavanaugh D, Marsden DE: In Quilligan EJ (ed): Current Therapy in Obstetrics and Gynecology, 2nd ed. Philadelphia, WB Saunders, 1983.

DRUG
GUIDE

Methylergonovine maleate (Methergine): Ergot alkaloid that stimulates contraction of smooth muscle.

Obstetric Action: Stimulates uterus to contract, thus clamping uterine blood vessels to prevent hemorrhage; also has vasconstrictive effect on all blood vessels (especially larger arteries), causing elevation of blood pressure.

Postpartum Administration: Usual dose is 0.2 mg (PO) after delivery and every 4 hr times six doses; dose may be repeated every 2-4 hr if necessary.

Special note: This drug usually is not given IV if client has elevated blood pressure. If it is administered to a hypertensive woman, her blood pressure must be monitored continuously.

Maternal Contraindications: Pregnancy, induction of labor, hepatic or renal disease, threatened spontaneous abortion, uterine sepsis, cardiac disease, hypertension, and obliterative vascular disease.

Potential Side Effects and Complications: Hypertension (particularly if given IV), nausea, vomiting, headache, bradycardia, dizziness, tinnitus, abdominal cramps, palpitations, dyspnea, chest pain, and allergic reactions.

Nursing Implications:
1. Assess client's medical and prenatal history to identify contraindications to administration.
2. Monitor uterine fundus for height, consistency, and lochial amount, character, and odor.
3. Assess blood pressure before administration.
4. Assess blood pressure after administration and every 15 min if client is hypotensive or hypertensive.
5. Observe for adverse effects or symptoms of ergot toxicity (nausea, vomiting, diarrhea, changes in blood pressure, chest pain, numb and cold extremities, dyspnea, weak pulse, excitability, convulsions, delirium, hallucinations).
6. Instruct client that uterine cramping is expected and that an analgesia order can be obtained from the physician if needed.

DRUG
GUIDE

Ergonovine maleate (Ergotrate): Principal oxytocic alkaloid of ergot, a fungus that grows on rye and other grains.

Obstetric Action: Induces uterine muscle contractions and exerts an effect that lasts for hours. After its administration, contraction of uterine muscle occurs rapidly and is sustained; valuable aid in control of postpartum bleeding.

Postpartum Administration: May be administered orally or parenterally. It is available in tablet form in doses of 0.2 mg to be given orally and in 1 ml ampules containing 0.2 mg (1/320 gr) for intramuscular (IM) or IV administration. Usual dose is 0.2 mg (1/320 gr).

Maternal Contraindications: Generally contraindicated in women who have hypertension, particularly PIH.

Potential Side Effects and Complications: Dizziness, headache, tinnitus, dysrhythmias, chest pain, palpitations, hypertension (if given IV), dyspnea.

Nursing Implications:
1. Assess client's medical and prenatal history to identify contraindications to administration.
2. Monitor uterine fundal height and consistency; monitor lochia for bleeding, amount, character, and odor.
3. Assess blood pressure before and after drug administration and every 15 min if client is hypotensive or hypertensive.
4. Observe for adverse effects or symptoms of ergot toxicity: nausea, vomiting, diarrhea, changes in blood pressure, chest pain, numb and cold extremities, dyspnea, weak pulse, excitability to convulsions, delirium, hallucinations.
5. Instruct client that uterine cramping is expected and that an analgesia order can be obtained from the physician if needed.

Throughout the care the nurse talks calmly to the client to assess her mental status and provide reassurance. Both the client and her family are updated about her condition. The family should be permitted to remain at her bedside as much as possible. Intervention also includes addressing anxieties that could affect parenting by encouraging the mother and the family to ask questions and to express their concerns. The nurse can assist the family in obtaining needed information from the doctor about the causes and treatment of the bleeding. If the hemorrhage occurred after the mother was discharged from the hospital, the family may need assistance planning for infant care during the mother's hospitalization. Measures to support breast-feeding (if appropriate) such as having the mother empty her breasts and providing the breast milk to family members for infant feeding at home can be instituted. It is important the client be taught before discharge that if lochia fails to follow expected progression from rubra to alba or if excessive bleeding occurs, she must call her physician immediately so treatment is prompt.

Evaluation

The mother will be anxious to return home as quickly as possible. During the hospitalization the nurse assists the client and her family to put this emergency in perspective. If she is provided with sensitive teaching and counseling, she can resolve her feelings of anxiety and cope effectively with this complication.

NURSING
CARE
PLAN

Client With the Complications of Hemorrhage and Shock

Goals (Expected Outcomes)	Interventions	Rationale	Evaluation
Alteration in Cardiac Output—Related to Hypovolemia			
Alteration in Tissue Perfusion—Related to Decreased Blood Volume Secondary to Hemorrhage and Shock			
Client will maintain adequate cardiac output and tissue perfusion.	Maintain bed rest in modified Trendelenburg position.	Increases venous blood return to heart.	Blood pressure is stable and comparable to values occurring before bleeding.
	Record vital signs every 15 min or more (often depending on severity of blood loss and shock); report significant changes promptly.	Assists in determining physiologic response to blood loss.	All vital signs are in range established before bleeding.
	Evaluate amount of blood loss by counting and weighing pads and linen. Contact primary health care provider immediately in case of hemorrhage.	Provides more objective information than visual evaluation.	Blood loss is minimal.

Continued

NURSING
CARE
PLAN

Client With the Complications of Hemorrhage and Shock—continued

Goals (Expected Outcomes)	Interventions	Rationale	Evaluation
Alteration in Tissue Perfusion—Related to Decreased Blood Volume Secondary to Hemorrhage and Shock—continued			
	Ensure IV is patent or get order for placement of an IV line. Use lactated Ringer's solution or normal saline solution to replace volume initially.	Orders should be received and implemented quickly to prevent further complications.	Fluid volume is maintained.
	Ensure bladder emptying; if unsure, request order for indwelling catheter.	Hypovolemia reduces kidney perfusion and decreases urinary output.	Kidney perfusion is stable as evidenced by 50-100 ml urinary output hourly.
	Check for central vs. peripheral cyanosis, paleness, skin tugor, and diaphoresis.	Determines general perfusion status, i.e., central to peripheral.	Skin is pink centrally and peripherally and is warm and dry.
	Administer blood plasma or volume expander as ordered.	Replaces circulating volume, increases blood return to heart, and increases perfusion to all organs.	Blood pressure and other vital signs are within normal limits, and urinary output is 50-100 ml/hr.
	Keep client and family informed.	Allays some anxiety.	Client and family verbalize they are no longer anxious.
	Administer oxygen by face mask at 6-8 L/min.	Increases oxygenation.	Client's color is pink, she reports no dizziness, and no other signs of shock are present.
Anxiety—Related to the Physiologic Crisis of Hemorrhage			
Client will express concerns and fears instead of holding them in and becoming very anxious.	Convey attitude of confidence and calm.	Client needs to feel nurse and physician are confident about her care (they are in control of the situation at hand).	Client verbalizes confidence in her care.
	Explain all care.	Helps decrease some anxiety; increases confidence in care.	Client understands much of what is being done for her and conveys confidence in her care.
	Maintain atmosphere of quiet and calm.	Helps maintain calmness in client.	Client and family remain calm.
	Keep client informed of status. Give realistic, factual information about her status.	Directs worry at reality instead of fantasized problems. Helps maintain client's calmness and confidence.	Worry is properly directed at what is real.
	Allow support person(s) to stay with client as much as possible.	Allays some worries and fears of support person(s).	Support person(s) is calm and cooperative.
	Administer medications as ordered for pain.	Maintains comfort.	Client states she is comfortable.
	Remain with client.	Provides supportive care and builds relationship.	Client responds to nursing assurance and support.

NURSING
CARE
PLAN

Client With the Complications of Hemorrhage and Shock—*continued*

Goals (Expected Outcomes)	Interventions	Rationale	Evaluation
Anxiety—Related to the Physiologic Crisis of Hemorrhage—*continued*			
	Encourage expression of feelings, asking of questions.	Helps nurse to anticipate client's worries and fears and to allay them when possible.	Atmosphere is conducive to open communication and assistance.
	Support positive coping mechanisms of client, family, or support person(s).	Facilitates effective coping with stress.	Client and support person are coping effectively.
	Provide information about infant.	Promotes bonding.	Client talks about infant.
Knowledge Deficit—Regarding Cause of Postpartum Hemorrhage and Its Management			
Client will verbalize understanding of postpartum hemorrhage, how it is managed, and follow-up care.	Explain why postpartum hemorrhage occurs.	Increases understanding of the process.	Client asks questions and discusses how postpartum hemorrhage affects unfulfilled birth plans.
	Encourage questions about care, procedures, and overall management.	Increases understanding of care given.	Client is compliant with care, asks questions easily.
	Explain effects of oxytocic drugs, particularly stimulation of contractions, which may cause cramping, and involution (to decrease bleeding).	Promotes understanding of drug effects so there is no concern or worry about stimulated contractions.	Client verbalizes understanding of effects of oxytocic medications.
	Explain need for continued observation and assessment to ensure normal involution vs. further bleeding.	Ensures risk of bleeding is diminishing.	Client experiences normal involution.

Vulvar Hematoma

Etiology and Pathophysiology

If blood escapes into the connective tissue beneath the skin covering the external genitalia or beneath the vaginal mucosa, it forms a **vulvar** or vaginal **hematoma** (Fig. 25-1). Hematoma formation usually follows injury to a blood vessel without laceration of the superficial tissues. Occasionally the hemorrhage is delayed and results from sloughing of a vessel that has become necrotic from prolonged pressure. Hematomas can be absorbed spontaneously, or pressure from the hematoma can cause tissue necrosis. The necrotic tissue can tear open as a result of the internal pressure and profuse hemorrhage occurs.

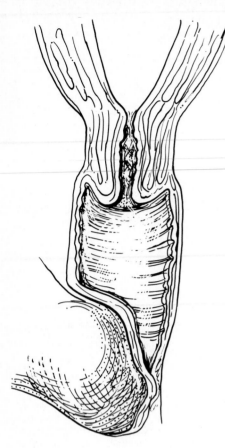

FIGURE 25-1

Vulvar Hematoma. A hematoma can contain a large amount of blood, which exerts pressure on surrounding tissues. Tissue necrosis can result from the excessive pressure.

Therapeutic and Nursing Management

The most prominent symptom of vulvar hematoma is severe perineal pain. When hematoma formation develops rapidly, the pain can be excruciating. As the tissues become more distended, the client also complains of perineal, bladder, vaginal, or rectal pressure that is not relieved by analgesia. The nurse is alert for client complaints of pain that are out of proportion to the expected. Sometimes performing a vaginal examination is necessary to diagnose a vulvar hematoma.

Visible inspection of the perineum reveals an area that is tense and swollen and bluish or blue-black in color. The area feels warm and firm.

When hematomas cause severe pain and continue to enlarge, they are treated by incision and evacuation of the blood, and bleeding vessels are ligated. After hematoma evacuation the nurse continues to assess lochia for color, amount, and odor. The perineum and incision area are checked twice each shift for recurrence of hematoma. The client is instructed to notify the nurse of any changes in sensations she notes in the hematoma area. Client teaching emphasizes good feminine hygiene and frequent changing of perineal pads. Cold and warm sitz baths are beneficial for relief of pain; however, cold to the perineum works better to decrease swelling caused by edema.[1] Using cold on the perineum for the first 24 hours after hematoma evacuation to reduce swelling and then warm sitz baths to increase circulation and promote healing may be beneficial.

Postpartum Genital Tract Infection

Etiology and Pathophysiology

Puerperal genital tract infection is one of the leading complications post partum. It results from bacterial infection originating in the genital tract during labor or the puerperium (Table 25-3). Multiple bacterial pathogens are present in the cervix and lower uterine segment during pregnancy and for a short time after delivery. Generally these organisms harbored in the female genital tract do not cause infections. However, the trauma of birth, alteration of immunologic function, and lowered resistance caused by fatigue, stress, or hemorrhage make the postpartum woman more susceptible to infection.

After placental delivery the site of attachment is raw and provides an excellent culture medium for bacteria. Lochia is another excellent culture medium for bacterial growth. During labor and delivery lacerations of the cervix, vagina, and perineum also offer access for bacterial invasion (Fig. 25-2). If a cesarean section is done, more tissue trauma and foreign bodies (sutures) are present, providing other potential sites for contamination and infection.

Puerperal infection may be caused by many kinds of bacteria, either singly or in various combinations. The most common organisms causing postpartum infections are anaerobic nonhemolytic streptococci, coliform bacteria, *Bacteroides,* and staphylococci.

Since fever is the chief sign of infection, most women with temperature elevation in the first 24 hours after delivery do have genital tract infections. Most postpartum infections are nosocomial, meaning they are acquired while in the hospital. The source of infection is an infected individual or a breech in infection control techniques. Risk factors are included in Table 25-4.

TABLE 25-3

Types of Postpartum Genital Tract Infections

Type of Infection	Etiology	Signs and Symptoms	Treatment
Perineal and vulvar lesions	Bacterial invasion of episiotomy, laceration, traumatized tissue	Fever, localized pain Edema, erythema; seropurulent discharge from lesion; usually occurs after day 5	Antibiotics Removal of stitches and promotion of drainage, sitz baths, perineal heat lamp, analgesics
Endometritis	Bacterial invasion of placental site or entire endometrium	Fever of approximately 38.4°C (101°F), chills, rapid pulse, usually occurs within 48 hr of delivery Malaise, headache, backache, loss of appetite, cramps Relaxed, tender uterus with foul-smelling discharge, dark or profuse lochia	Antibiotics, ergonovine Fowler's position to promote drainage, hydration
Pelvic cellulitis or parametritis	Bacterial invasion by way of lymphatics to tissue surrounding uterus (often following endometritis)	Fever, chills Pain and tenderness of lower abdomen, edema Signs of endometritis may be present also	Antibiotics Hydration, blood transfusion for dropping hemoglobin Bed rest, analgesics
Peritonitis	Spread of infection to peritoneum, local or generalized	High fever, rapid pulse Severe abdominal pain Vomiting, restlessness Distention	Antibiotics, analgesics, sedatives Bed rest, hydration, blood transfusion, oxygen, IV fluids
Salpingitis and oophoritis	Spread of infection to fallopian tubes and ovaries	Lower abdominal pain Temperature elevation, tachycardia Nausea and vomiting	Antibiotics, analgesics, sedatives, antipyretics Hydration, IV fluids

Continued

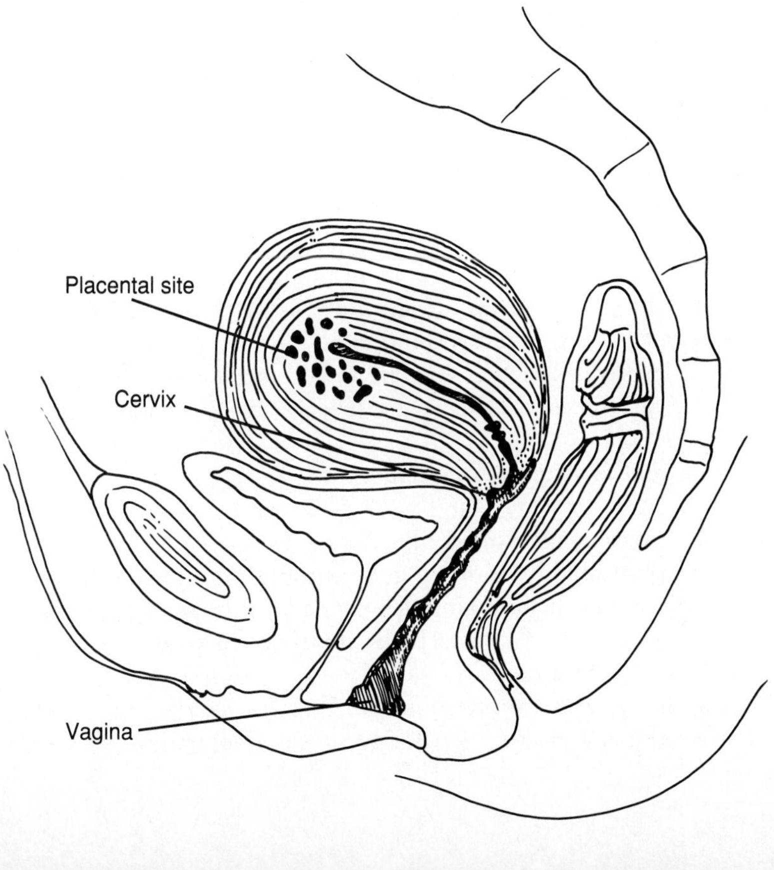

FIGURE 25-2

Postpartum Infection Sites. Common postpartum infection sites are the area of placental separation, the cervix, and the vagina. After placental separation the site is a raw wound with gaping veins occluded by thrombi. These blood clots provide a good culture medium for bacterial growth. During delivery the cervix is almost always torn. The vagina is also often torn or involved in an episiotomy. Any of these injuries provide barrier breaks that permit bacterial invasion and potential for infection.

Placental site

Cervix

Vagina

TABLE 25-4

*Risk Factors for Developing
Postpartum Infections*

Related to General Infection Risk	Related to Labor Events	Related to Vaginal and Cesarean Delivery
Lack of prenatal care	Prolonged rupture of membranes	Cesarean section
Poor nutrition		Urgency of operation
Obesity	Intrauterine fetal monitoring	Breaks in operative technique
Low socioeconomic status		Manual placental removal
	Number of examinations during labor	Hemorrhage
Sexual intercourse after rupture of membranes		Forceps delivery
	Traumatic labor	Episiotomy
	Prolonged labor	Lacerations
	Transfer of feces to vagina (in second stage)	Retention of placental tissue
		Retained blood clots

Prevention of Infection

For many days after delivery the surface of the birth canal is vulnerable to pathogenic bacterial invasion. Because of this potential for infection, nursing care includes teaching the client as soon as possible after delivery the importance of handwashing before and after caring for herself or her infant. This teaching also includes principles of personal hygiene: how to care for her perineum without using her fingers to separate the labia, avoiding touching the inner side of the peripad, and applying and removing the pad from front to back (Fig. 25-3). Each client should have her own personal hygiene equipment.

The nurse instructs breast-feeding clients about techniques for avoiding skin breakdown, which is another source of infection. They learn to assess their nipples and breasts after each nursing period and learn the signs of infection for themselves and their infants so that if a problem arises, prompt recognition and reporting to the primary health care provider will ensure prompt treatment and management.

Infections of the Perineum and Vulva

Etiology and Pathophysiology

Localized infections are less severe complications of the puerperium and involve the episiotomy or lacerations of the perineum, vagina, or vulva. Another localized wound infection involves the abdominal incision site of a cesarean delivery. These wound infections are characterized by reddened, swollen skin edges that separate and drain a seropurulent discharge. The client experiences localized pain, fever (<101°F), and dysuria.

Therapeutic and Nursing Management

An initial treatment of wound infection is to facilitate drainage. Good drainage is established by removing the sutures and opening the wound. The nurse places the client in a high-Fowler's position to promote drainage and encourages her to take sitz baths for relief of pain and to increase circulation to the perineum.

The nurse evaluates wound drainage for color, consistency, and odor. Signs of wound healing vs. redness, presence of edema or excessive pain

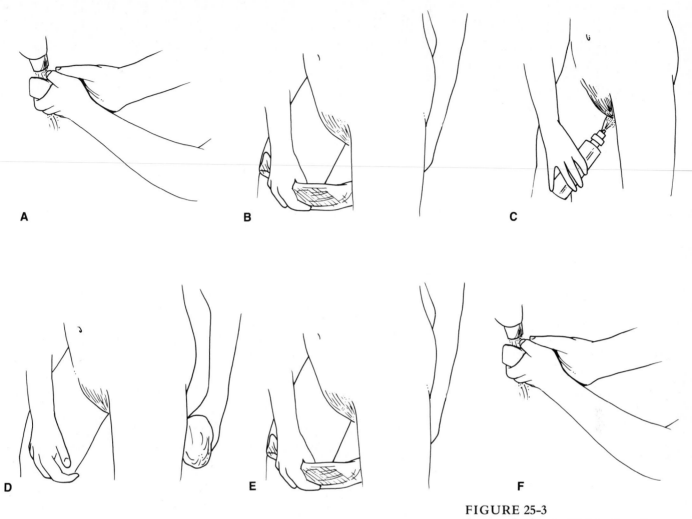

A

B

C

D

E

F

FIGURE 25-3

Bottom Basics. **A,** Wash hands well. **B,** Remove pad from front to back. Start and stop urinary flow. This exercise tones muscles and helps speed healing. **C,** Spray perineum with warm water. **D** Wipe dry from front to back. **E,** Put on new pad from front to back. **F,** Wash hands well.

at the wound site, inadequate approximation of wound edges, the presence of purulent drainage, fever, anorexia or malaise are charted.

Additional oral fluid intake (2000 ml/day) is encouraged to maintain hydration. If there is urinary retention, an indwelling catheter is inserted. Temperature, pulse, and respirations are monitored every 4 hours.

The nurse instructs the client how to perform perineal care correctly to remove irritating drainage and about the importance of handwashing before and after care. The nurse always washes hands before and after caring for the mother or the infant. Nursing care includes encouraging the mother to feed her infant and reassuring her that the newborn is not likely to become infected if good hygiene measures are followed.

Endometritis

Etiology and Pathophysiology

After delivery the placental site provides an excellent portal for bacterial entry. Infection may spread to involve the entire endometrium (see Fig. 25-2). Lacerations of the cervix also provide a focal point for bacterial entry and proliferation. If the infection is mild, the client will usually

FIGURE 25-4

Febrile Pattern in Endometritis. The four classic signs of postpartum endometritis are temperature elevation to 101° F (38.4° C), increase in pulse rate (100 to 120), delayed involution with fundal height not decreasing, and lochia remaining red with foul odor. Lochia will have foul odor unless the infection is caused by β-hemolytic streptococcus. (*R* = red; *B* = brown)

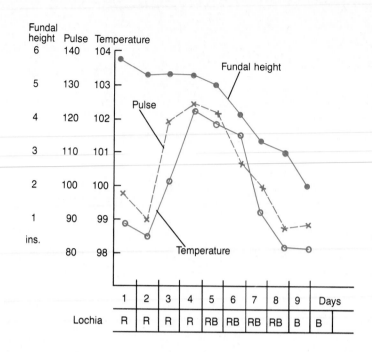

have either scant or profuse foul-smelling lochia. However, lochia may be odorless if the infection is caused by a β-hemolytic streptococcus. In severe infection there is uterine tenderness and irregular spikes of temperature, usually from 101°F to 104°F (Fig. 25-4). Tachycardia, chills, and **subinvolution** may also occur.

Therapeutic and Nursing Management

If the **endometritis** is mild, with temperatures <100°F and no chills, the nurse encourages the client to maintain a Fowler's position to facilitate lochial drainage. Administering oxytocic medication (ergonovine or methylergonovine) aids lochial flow by contracting the uterus. The nurse performs routine postpartum checks of fundal firmness, location, and tenderness and of lochial color, amount, consistency, and odor. A lochial specimen is usually ordered for culture and sensitivity.

Often clients with mild endometritis are discharged after 2 to 3 days of hospitalization. Discharge teaching includes encouraging the client to get as much rest as possible, to take all medications as ordered, to drink 8 to 10 glasses of fluids per day, to maintain a dietary intake high in protein and vitamins, and to keep the follow-up appointment with the primary health care provider.

If endometritis is severe, bed rest in a semi-Fowler's position is maintained to ensure lochial drainage. The nurse assesses the client for hydration. Fluid intake should be 3000 to 4000 ml/day. Temperature, pulse, respirations, and blood pressure are taken every 4 hours. The nurse changes the perineal pads frequently and assesses lochia for amount and odor. If there is no odor, the infection is anaerobic, usually β-hemolytic streptococcus. The nurse assesses the client's perineum for evidence of hematoma or abscess.

The nurse encourages the client to express her feelings and ask questions to help her cope. The mother may continue to breast-feed unless she is too exhausted or ill.

Pelvic Cellulitis (Parametritis) and Peritonitis

Etiology and Pathophysiology

Pelvic cellulitis (parametritis) refers to infection that involves the loose connective tissue of the broad ligament or, if more severe, the connective tissue of all the pelvic structures (Fig. 25-5). It spreads via the lymphatics in the uterine wall or with bacteria that invade a cervical laceration and extend upward into the broad ligament's connective tissue.

Pelvic cellulitis is characterized by high temperature (102° to 104°F), chills, malaise, lethargy, abdominal tenderness and pain, subinvolution of the uterus, and tachycardia. Pelvic abscess occurs if pelvic cellulitis is unresolved (Fig. 25-6). **Peritonitis** occurs when the infection involves the peritoneum. If peritonitis develops (Fig. 25-7), the client will be acutely ill and have high fever, severe pain, restlessness and anxiety, rapid, shallow respirations, tachycardia, excessive thirst, abdominal distention, and nausea and vomiting.

Therapeutic and Nursing Management

Broad-spectrum antibiotics are given to combat infection, an analgesic is prescribed for discomfort, and mild sedative drugs may be ordered to relieve the client's restlessness and apprehension. If there is intestinal involvement, food and oral fluids are withheld until intestinal function is normal. The nurse initiates and monitors IV fluids, provides a restful environment, provides physical care to promote comfort, monitors intake and output, and administers antibiotics and analgesics as ordered.

FIGURE 25-5
Pelvic Cellulitis (Parametritis). Pelvic cellulitis is an infection that extends along the lymphatics to connective tissue. As the process develops, the swelling becomes hard and may result in an abscess.

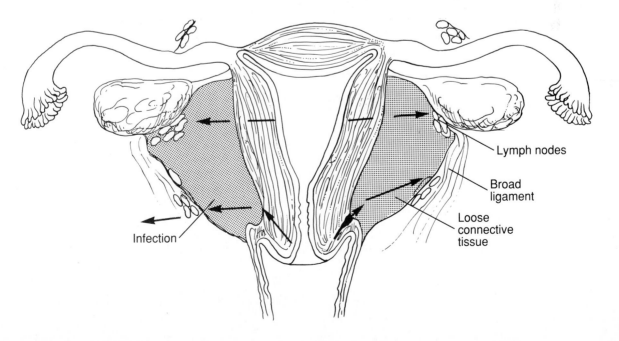

Lymph nodes

Broad ligament

Loose connective tissue

Infection

FIGURE 25-6

Pelvic Abscess. Pelvic abscess results from unresolved pelvic cellulitis and occurs on one or both sides of the abdomen. Continued swelling causes the skin to redden and become edematous and tender. Recovery is prompt after incision and drainage.

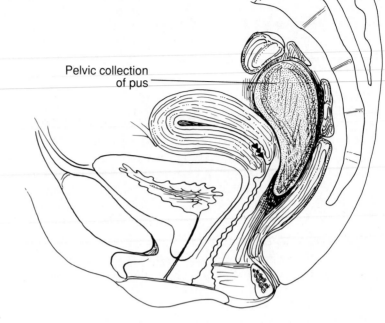

Pelvic collection of pus

FIGURE 25-7

Postpartum Peritonitis. The pelvic peritoneum may become infected in the same way as the parametrium. Generalized peritonitis may occur with development of paralytic ileus. Although uncommon, peritonitis can be severe and life-threatening.

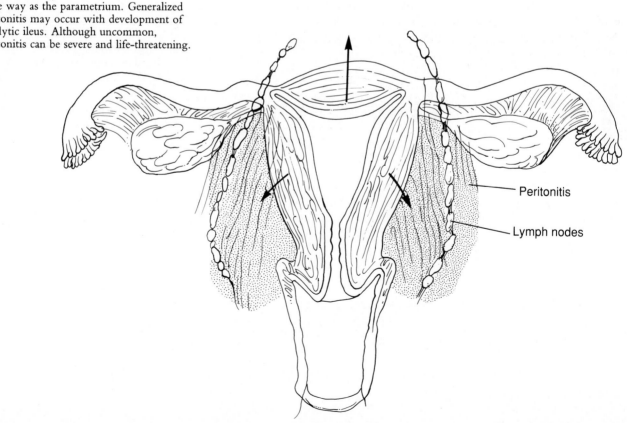

Peritonitis

Lymph nodes

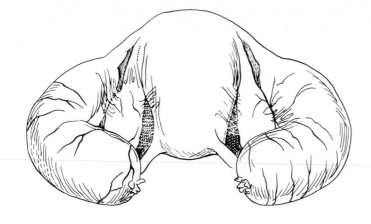

FIGURE 25-8
Postpartum Salpingitis. Salpingitis is an infection of the fallopian tubes that leads to hyperemia, edema, and purulent discharge into the tubal lumina. The tubes are enlarged, swollen, and tender. Tubal abscesses may occur, creating tender adnexal masses.

Salpingitis and Oophoritis

Etiology and Pathophysiology

When bacteria spreads into the fallopian tubes and infection occurs, it is called **salpingitis** (Fig. 25-8); if the infection extends to the ovaries, it becomes oophoritis. The infection is caused most frequently by gonorrhea, and tubal patency may be affected, causing sterility. Infection becomes apparent between postpartum days 9 and 15. Symptoms include lower abdominal pain, high temperature, tachycardia, and nausea and vomiting.

Therapeutic and Nursing Management

Treatment is with antibiotics, analgesics, and sedatives.

Nursing care for clients with these genital tract infections includes monitoring and recording vital signs (TPR) every 4 hours and assisting with physical care as needed. The nurse administers analgesics as ordered to provide comfort and antipyretics as indicated by temperature elevation to decrease fever. The nurse monitors intake and output, encourages intake of oral fluids, and checks the IV site for redness and warmth and to ensure that it is not infiltrated. Antibiotics are usually ordered for administration per IV route.

Client teaching includes the importance of handwashing before and after care and taking medications as prescribed. The nurse inquires if the client has any questions or concerns about the home care of herself or her newborn. The client is encouraged to ask questions and express concerns as they arise.

During the time the client is hospitalized, she is anxious because of her separation from her infant. The nurse provides support as indicated.

Genital Tract Infection After Cesarean Delivery

Etiology and Pathophysiology

The incidence of genital tract infection is significantly increased when delivery is cesarean. This is frequently related to several factors such as duration of ruptured membranes, number of vaginal examinations, length

---

Risk Factors for Postcesarean Section Genital Tract Infection

Obesity
Diabetes
Prolonged rupture of membranes
Chorioamnionitis
Prolonged labor
Frequent vaginal examinations
Need for invasive procedures
Placement of wound drains
Prolonged hospitalization before cesarean section
Emergency cesarean section

---

of labor, various complications, and the need for invasive procedures. However, the operative trauma itself increases infectious morbidity, generally caused by a mixed anaerobic and aerobic infection by organisms present in the genital tract at the time of labor and delivery. Surgical trauma, with devitalization of tissue and collection of blood and serum in the myometrium or endometrium, which have become infected with organisms that have ascended from the lower genital tract to the amniotic fluid, plays a key role in the development of postpartum endometritis, myometritis, incisional wound abscesses, and pelvic abscesses (see display above)

Therapeutic and Nursing Management

Treatment is by antimicrobial therapy and drainage of abscesses; the antibiotics commonly used include penicillin, tetracycline, kanamycin, and clindamycin. The organisms most frequently causing infections after cesarean section are anaerobic streptococci, aerobic streptococci, *Bacteroides* species, *Escherichia coli,* and, less often, *Clostridium* species and staphylococci. A particularly strong relationship has been found between membranes ruptured for longer than 6 hours and postcesarean-section infection (myometritis). Early treatment of endometritis with agents having both gram-negative aerobic and anaerobic spectra can be very effective.

Assessment

Each type of puerperal infection presents a very characteristic set of signs and symptoms. The nurse must recognize and report early any signs and symptoms of infection (see Deviations from Expected Patterns) so appropriate treatment can be instituted without delay. One of the first clinical signs of infection is temperature elevation. If the infection is severe, chills occur with the fever. The affected area is usually painful, reddened, edematous, and the source of profuse discharge. The client may complain of malaise, headache, and general discomfort (see Assessment Tool: Postpartum Infection).

The nurse also assesses for risk factors and signs and symptoms of infection.

Clients are at risk for **thrombophlebitis** if they cannot ambulate soon after delivery and if they have a previous history of embolic disorders. Laboratory data is also reviewed.

Deviations from Expected Patterns

The following findings should be reported to the primary care provider.

Objective Findings

Purulent drainage from wound (episiotomy or cesarean incision)
Fever (100.4°F or 38°C with or without chills)
Vomiting
Foul lochial odor
Reddened edematous lesions
Failure of skin edges to approximate (dehiscence)

Subjective Findings

Complaints of pain or discomforts in lower abdomen
Nausea
Costovertebral angle pain (kidney pain)

Postpartum Infection

1. Vital signs: temperature elevation, increased pulse or respirations
2. Incision: episiotomy, cesarean; redness, swelling, intactness, discharge
3. Lochial discharge: abnormal progression, return to rubra or purulent drainage and/or offensive odor
4. Cesarean section incision: redness, dehiscence, drainage, odor
5. General status: malaise, achy, general discomfort
6. Pain: incisional, episiotomy, breasts, abdominal extremities, headache, costovertebral angle
7. Color: flushed or pale
8. Urine: character, amount, dysuria
9. Abdomen: softness, distention, masses
10. Bowels: flatus, bowel sounds, constipation, diarrhea
11. Breasts: nipples intact vs. trauma, bruised, cracked, change in consistency with area of induration, redness, tender

Nursing Diagnosis

Nursing diagnoses for clients who have genital tract infections are related to knowledge deficit and pain (see Potential Nursing Diagnoses: Postpartum Infections).

Planning and Intervention

The curative treatment is antibiotic therapy, but good nursing care is also essential. A detailed nursing care plan is included to provide information

POTENTIAL NURSING DIAGNOSES

Postpartum Infection

Pain—related to inflammation secondary to infection
Altered Body Temperature—related to general body response secondary to infection, i.e., fever
Anxiety—related to postpartum complications and their effect on family
Knowledge Deficit—regarding cause, care, and cure of specific infection
Altered Parenting—related to separation from infant

Focus Assessment

Monitor vital signs, general appearance, intake and output.
Observe for nonverbal signs of pain and response to analgesic.
Explore nonverbal indicators of emotional status, e.g., irritability, inability to concentrate, withdrawal.
Explore individual concerns.
Determine individual learning needs.

about nursing interventions. A third element of care is client teaching to decrease the risk of infection (see Client Self-Care Education: Decreasing Risk of Infection p. 717).

Evaluation

The goal is to have infections resolved and wounds healing normally, with the client's temperature normal, lochia normal, and fundal size appropriate. She should also be able to manage self-care and infant care.

NURSING CARE PLAN

Client With a Genital Tract Infection

Goals (Expected Outcomes)	Interventions	Rationale	Evaluation
Infection—Related to Bacterial Invasion of Genital Tract as Manifested by Abdominal Pain, Fever, Malaise, Tachycardia			
Client will recover from infection and express understanding of infection and its treatment.	Record and report signs and symptoms, including pain, fever, malaise, and purulent drainage.	Early reporting allows prompt initiation of therapy.	Pain, fever, and malaise are decreasing; client has no purulent vaginal drainage.
	Keep family informed.	Information decreases anxiety and allows for increase in coping.	Family verbalizes decrease in anxiety.
	Administer antibiotics.	Treats infection.	Client states she is beginning to feel better.
	Administer other drugs as ordered (antipyretics, analgesics).	Increases client's comfort.	Client states she is more comfortable.
	Monitor fluids and hydration (intake and output).	Ensures fluid balance.	Fluid intake and output ratio is adequate.
	Collect specimens: culture of infection site; blood culture when temperature spikes.	Cultures ensure specificity of antibiotics.	Specificity of antibiotic is assured.
Pain—Related to Infection			
Client will be comfortable.	Provide physical care. Keep client clean and dry. Change dressings and pads as needed.	Mother will be more comfortable and therefore feel better.	Mother rests well and is comfortable.
	Assist client to position of comfort (semi-Fowler). Bathe client; give back-rubs.	Position encourages drainage.	
	Perform treatments. Change dressings or pads. Provide sitz baths. Provide heat or ice packs.	Provides mother more comfort.	Mother states she is more comfortable.
	Administer analgesics.	Reduces or prevents pain.	Mother reports relief from pain.
	Keep family informed of progress.	Information decreases anxiety.	Family expresses a decrease in anxiety.

NURSING
CARE
PLAN

Client With a Genital Tract Infection—continued

Goals (Expected Outcomes)	Interventions	Rationale	Evaluation
Altered Body Temperature—Related to General Body Response to Infection			
Client will respond to medical and nursing management.	Record vital signs (TPR every 4 hr).	Evaluates client's condition.	Client's vital signs are normal; she is afebrile, with no tachycardia or tachypnea.
Knowledge Deficit—Regarding Cause, Progress, and Care of Genital Tract Infection			
Client will verbalize and demonstrate care for herself and her infant, using principles to prevent infection.	Teach parents about signs and symptoms of her infection. Course of infection Treatment plans Self-care (perineal care, breast care) Principles of handwashing How to protect infant	Understanding infectious process increases compliance and decreases risk of reinfection.	Mother is recovering from infection; verbalizes understanding of infection and how to care for self and infant.
	Encourage questions.	Facilitates communication, understanding, and teaching.	Client is comfortable and able to ask questions to clarify her understanding of her care and infant's care.
	Demonstrate careful handwashing and body fluid precautions when caring for client.	Prevents cross-contamination of client and personnel.	No cross-contamination occurs.
	Change dressings and pads and place in appropriate containers.	Isolates used materials to prevent bacterial spread.	No nosocomial infection occurs.
	Instruct client to Wash hands before handling infant Perform perineal care after each voiding Remove and apply pads front to back Not touch inside of pad before applying Wash hands after voiding and completing perineal care	Prevents spread of infection and decreases risk for future infections.	Client performs perineal care correctly, washes hands after using bathroom and before and after handling infant.
	Discuss home plans for client and infant care.	Helps client plan her home care of self and infant.	Client verbalizes how she will manage herself and her infant when discharged.
	Identify resources to assist in home care or adjustment.	May need community resources.	Client verbalizes confidence in self-care and infant care at home.

Continued

NURSING
CARE
PLAN

Client With a Genital Tract Infection—*continued*

Goals (Expected Outcomes)	Interventions	Rationale	Evaluation
Altered Parenting—Related to Separation from Infant Secondary to Client's Infection			
Client will be well, and couple can devote themselves to becoming a family as they get acquainted with their infant and as they learn to care for the infant.	Bring parents and infant together as soon as possible.	Promotes strong family bond.	Family members interact well with each other.
	Encourage client to feed and care for her infant.	The more the client handles, feeds, and cares for her infant, the more confident she will be when discharged.	Client verbalizes her increasing confidence in her mothering and caretaking skills.
	Teach client good handwashing to protect infant.	Infant should be protected from all infection.	Infant has no signs of infection.
	Promote breast-feeding.	Breast-feeding provides infant with nutritional needs and causes uterine contractions to assist involution.	Client is breast-feeding successfully.
	Encourage father to give some bottles if infant is bottle-fed.	The more father is involved, the more attached he is to infant.	Father expresses interest in helping with infant care.
	Encourage father to stay with the client as much as he desires.	Family can interact as a family from beginning.	Family interacts well together.

Other Types of Infections
Mastitis
Etiology and Pathophysiology

Postpartum **mastitis** is caused by an acute infection in the glandular tissue of the breast. The most common organism causing mastitis is *Staphylococcus aureus*. Symptoms include fever, tachycardia, chills, malaise, localized pain, tenderness, and local erythema. The bacteria gains entry to the subcutaneous lymphatics through nipple fissures or erosions, or a plugged duct can precipitate the infectious process. The infection source can sometimes be traced to the infant, who may acquire the pathogen orally from the mother's skin or from a health care provider in the nursery.

The onset of postpartum mastitis can occur at any time during lactation. The client notes a tender area in the breast that is warm to touch. When the breast is inspected, a hard red area is noted. She may note some engorgement, followed by severe pain, malaise, chills, and then fever that can reach 40.5°C (105°F).

Usually only one breast is involved. Inflammation may be generalized or confined to a lobe or local area of the breast.

Therapeutic and Nursing Management

If signs indicative of possible mastitis occur, breast tenderness and erythemia are assessed and noted (see display on p. 717). The physician is

Decreasing Risk of Infection

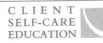

Action

1. Wash hands before and after perineal care.
2. Do not touch stitch area with fingers.
3. Do not touch inner side of perineal pad. Apply and remove from front to back.
4. Apply perineal pad snugly to prevent its sliding back and forth.
5. Use sprays and ointments no more than four times per day to avoid chemical burn or irritation.
6. Use sitz baths for episiotomy pain. Use of cold is preferable for 24-48 hr to decrease edema; then use warm sitz baths to increase circulation to tissues and promote healing.[1]
7. Wash hands before breast-feeding.
8. Inspect nipples for trauma or damage after each nursing period.
9. Drink 6-8 glasses of fluid daily.
10. Rest when infant rests.
11. Report signs of infection to the primary care provider.
    Fever or chills
    Increased bleeding
    Pain (abdominal)
    Severely lumpy, painful breast
    Calf pain or heat
    Urinary frequency, dysuria

Rationale

1. Prevents transmission of infective organisms.
2. Same as above.
3. Prevents contamination of pad from rectal area.
4. A pad sliding back and forth can introduce contamination from rectal area.
5. Many sprays and ointments have an alcohol base that can cause local irritation and impairment of skin integrity and can predispose area to infection.
6. Cold sitz baths decrease edema in first 24-48 hr then warm sitz baths increase blood circulation and promote healing.
7. Prevents introduction of bacteria from hands to newborn.
8. Ensures skin integrity is not compromised since broken skin provides portal for bacteria.
9. Ensures hydration and aids in diuresis.
10. Assists with recovery.
11. Early recognition and reporting can influence timely management should infection occur.

notified of the findings. If the mastitis is diagnosed early and broad-spectrum antibiotics (oxacillin or cephalothin) are started promptly, infection often can be controlled in 24 hours. If treatment is delayed, a breast abscess can occur. Breast-feeding education initiated in the antepartum period can reduce the risk of mastitis.

Medical opinion conflicts about continuing or discontinuing breast-feeding when mastitis occurs. Some believe it is necessary to continue breast-feeding to prevent engorgement and that continuation benefits both the mother and her infant. Others believe the infection is cured more quickly if breast-feeding is discontinued, and they express concern about the possible recurrence of mastitis when breast-feeding is resumed. Some physicians believe it is wise to discontinue breast-feeding while the client's fever is high. If the decision is made to discontinue breast-feeding, heat is applied to the breast to encourage milk flow, and a breast pump is used to remove some of the milk to decrease engorgement.

Deviations from Expected Patterns

Swelling and heat: localized area that is red, hot, and swollen
Fever: >38.4°C; occurs suddenly after approximately 10 days
Pain: intense but localized (usually unilateral)
Systemic symptoms: generalized malaise, sometimes nausea and vomiting

CLIENT SELF-CARE EDUCATION

Mastitis

Action

1. Rest is important; rest when infant sleeps.
2. Wear a good supportive nursing bra (it should be changed daily).
3. Apply moist heat to breast (stand in shower with back to spray of water or apply warm wet towel).

4. Breast-feed or use breast pump frequently (every 2-3 hr).

5. Massage breast before breast-feeding or using pump (Fig. 25-9).

   Technique
   a. Support breast with one hand.

   b. Use other hand to massage breast thoroughly in a stroking manner. Begin at outer limits of breast and stroke toward nipple.
   c. Overlap massage strokes until entire breast has been covered (always begin at the outer edge and massage toward nipple). Massage entire breast in this manner 10 times.

Rationale

1. Facilitates restorative process.
2. Enlarged breasts need support.

3. Increases circulation and comfort, reduces congestion, and encourages milk flow. Helps empty breasts if performed just before breast-feeding or pumping.
4. Frequent emptying relieves stasis and increases comfort; ensures emptying of breast and maintains milk supply. The more the breast is stimulated the greater the milk production.
5. Improves circulation, reduces swelling, and encourages milk flow.

   a. Breasts enlarged because of nursing need support.
   b. Keeps ducts open so milk will flow (massage can help prevent mastitis).

   c. Facilitates emptying the breast.

Nursing care includes teaching the mother when to wash her hands to avoid contaminating the breasts and how to massage the breasts to prevent kinking and plugging of the ducts (see Client Self-Care Education: Mastitis). She is taught how to inspect the breasts and note any changes.

Analgesics are given as ordered for pain. If concern is expressed about the effect of the drug on the infant, the drug can be given at the beginning of a nursing period.

FIGURE 25-9
Breast Massage.

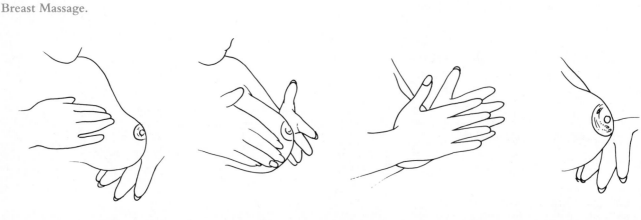

Cystitis and Pyelonephritis

Etiology and Pathophysiology

Urinary retention is a common postpartum occurrence caused by increased bladder capacity, decreased bladder tone, and decreased perception of the urge to void as a result of birth trauma. If the client is unable to empty her bladder, the retained urine serves as a culture medium that encourages bacterial growth and can result in cystitis. Cystitis can develop into **pyelonephritis** if the infection ascends the ueters and the kidneys become involved (see Assessment Tool: Urinary Tract Infection: Cystitis and Pyelonephritis). Approximately 2% to 4% of maternity clients develop postpartum urinary tract infection.

In many clients preexisting asymptomatic bacteriuria or chronic urinary tract infection contribute to urinary tract infections.

Symptoms of urinary tract infections include urinary frequency, low-grade fever with spikes, dysuria, costovertebral angle (CVA) tenderness, flank pain, urgency, and lower abdominal pain.

Therapeutic and Nursing Management

Definitive diagnosis of a urinary tract infection is based on the culture report of a clean-catch urine specimen. Continuing care includes monitoring vital signs and administering antibiotics and analgesics as ordered. The nurse encourages the mother to increase fluid intake and monitors intake and output. If pyelonephritis develops, the mother must lie on the side opposite the pain so the affected ureter can drain. Additional urine specimens may be ordered for urinalysis and culture to verify complete recovery.

Interventions should render the mother free of pain so she can be actively involved in self-care and the care of her infant. The nurse instructs her about methods to minimize the risk of infection for both herself and her infant and about signs and symptoms of infection. Discharge teaching includes the signs and symptoms of urinary tract infection that must be reported to the primary care provider (see Client Self-Care Education: Postpartum Cystitis and Pyelonephritis p. 720).

Urinary Tract Infection: Cystitis and Pyelonephritis

ASSESSMENT
TOOL

Dysuria
Frequency
Urgency
Urinary retention; inability to empty bladder completely
Marked tenderness and discomfort over bladder area
Low-grade fever
Leukocytosis noted in catheterized urine specimen

Specific to Pyelonephritis

Chills
Elevated temperature
Flank pain (on side of affected kidney)

CLIENT
SELF-CARE
EDUCATION

Postpartum Cystitis and Pyelonephritis

Action

1. Empty bladder as soon as possible after delivery (within 6-8 hr).

2. Use helpful tips to encourage voiding:
   a. Straddle toilet instead of sitting.
   b. Run water in sink.
   c. Squirt warm water over perineum with peri-bottle.
   d. Take an analgesic a few minutes before trying to void.
   e. Sit in sitz bath to void.
3. Spend time after each voiding to make sure bladder is empty.
4. Wash hands after voiding.
5. Drink plenty of fluids even if no voiding problems exist.
6. Measure urine during first few voidings.

7. If the following symptoms occur, report them to primary care provider:
   a. Pain with urination
   b. Frequency
   c. Urgency
   d. Inability to empty bladder
   e. Tenderness or discomfort over bladder area
   f. Low-grade fever
8. Report chills, fever, and flank pain *immediately* to primary care provider.
9. Take all prescribed medications *exactly* as instructed.
10. Keep follow-up health care appointments.

Rationale

1. Retention of residual urine, bladder trauma during delivery, and catheterization (if done) increase risk for bladder infection.
2. Promotes relaxation and reduces discomfort of voiding.

3. Ensures bladder emptying and prevents urinary retention and bladder distention.
4. Decreases contamination from hands.
5. Promotes diuresis of increased circulatory volume.
6. Ensures bladder is emptying and prevents urinary retention.

7. Symptoms require laboratory follow-up study so treatment can be initiated.

8. Prompt reporting initiates prompt intervention.
9. Antibiotics are ineffective unless the full course is taken.
10. Ensures that treatment is promptly rendered.

Thromboembolic Conditions

A thromboembolic condition occurs in fewer than 1% of all postpartum clients. Stasis is probably the greatest single predisposing event for deep vein thrombosis. Venous thrombosis refers to clot formation in a superficial or deep vein. There is risk for a portion of the clot to break off, causing **pulmonary embolism.** When a **thrombus** is present along with inflammation in a vessel wall, the condition is called thrombophlebitis.

The two major types of postpartum thromboembolic disease are femoral thrombophlebitis, which involves the femoral, popliteal, or saphenous veins (Fig. 25-10), and postpartum pulmonary embolism. Pelvic thrombophlebitis occurs in some clients.

Femoral Thrombophlebitis

Etiology and Pathophysiology

Femoral thrombophlebitis is characterized by fever, skin that is warm to touch over the affected area, pain, and swelling in the affected leg, which

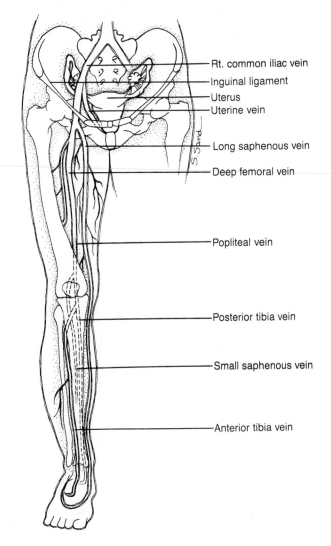

Rt. common iliac vein
Inguinal ligament
Uterus
Uterine vein

Long saphenous vein

Deep femoral vein

Popliteal vein

Posterior tibia vein

Small saphenous vein

Anterior tibia vein

FIGURE 25-10
Postpartum Thrombophlebitis.
Superficial thrombophlebitis involves the femoral, popliteal, and saphenous veins. It may develop into venous thrombosis (in the deep veins of the legs), which could develop into pulmonary emboli if not treated.

are caused by clot formation in the veins of the leg that interferes with return circulation of blood to the heart. Signs and symptoms usually occur 10 to 20 days after delivery and include malaise, chills, and fever, followed by stiffness and pain in the affected part. If the leg is affected, the pain occurs in the groin or hip and extends downward, or it may occur in the calf and extend upward. Within 24 hours the leg swells, and the skin over the swollen area is white. Acute symptoms last up to 1 week, after which the pain decreases and the client slowly improves. The process lasts 4 to 6 weeks, and the affected leg is slow to return to normal size and may remain enlarged and troublesome.

Therapeutic and Nursing Management

Treatment of femoral thrombophlebitis includes rest, elevation of the affected leg, and taking analgesics for pain. The primary care provider prescribes an anticoagulant such as heparin to prevent further thrombi formation and antimicrobials to treat generalized infection.

Nursing care includes the use of a bed cradle to keep pressure off the affected leg and may include the application of heat or ice bags along the affected vessel. The affected part is *never* rubbed or massaged. The nurse

TABLE 25-5

*Postpartum Client Care Summary for Deep Vein Thrombosis**

Interventions	Frequency
BP, P, R	On admission to recovery room (RR): then q 15 min × 4; then q 30 min × 2; then q 1 hr until stable; then q 4 hr post partum (PP)
T	On admission to RR; then q 4 hr
Contractions	Fundal checks on admission to RR: then q 15 min × 4; then q 30 min × 2; then q 1 hr until stable; then q 4 hr
	Lochia: Same as above
Bed rest	Yes
Support hose	Yes
Laboratory studies	Every month until therapy discontinued
PT	
PTT	
Fibrinogen	
CBC with platelets	
Assessment of thrombosis site	q 1 hr in RR q 4 hr on PP floor

Adapted from Knuppel RA, Drukker JE: High-Risk Pregnancy: A Team Approach. Philadelphia, WB Saunders, 1986.
*Nurse-client ratio = 1 : 6-8.

handles the leg with care to avoid trauma and possible dislodgment of the clot. Table 25-5 presents a client care summary.

Pelvic Thrombophlebitis

Etiology and Pathophysiology

Pelvic thrombophlebitis is a severe complication that usually occurs approximately the second week after delivery. The client experiences chills and temperature spikes. The infection results from bacterial infection of the placental site that causes thrombosed myometrial veins that support anaerobic bacterial proliferation. This process occurs more frequently on the right side. Chills, fever, and malaise are present.

Therapeutic and Nursing Management

Antimicrobial and anticoagulant therapy is used. These clients are often depressed and discouraged but feel physically well. The nurse assesses, observes, records, and reports any signs or symptoms of further complications.

Pulmonary Embolism

Etiology and Pathophysiology

Pulmonary embolism occurs once in every 2500 to 3000 pregnancies. It is usually caused by a thrombus fragment (**embolus**) carried by venous circulation to the right side of the heart. The thrombus usually originates

Pulmonary Embolism

Respiratory System

Chest pain
Dyspnea, tachypnea
Decreased breath sounds
Rales
Continuous clearing of throat or cough
Air hunger
Hemoptysis

Vital Signs

Temperature: elevation
Pulse: tachycardia, regularity
Blood pressure

Neurologic System

Restlessness
Headache
Lethargy or confusion
Apprehension
Anxiety
Inability to relax

Cardiovascular System

Pallor and cyanosis
Capillary refill time
Diaphoresis

in a uterine or pelvic vein. When the embolus occludes the pulmonary artery, it obstructs circulation to the lungs, either wholly or in part, and the client may die of asphxyia within a few minutes. If the clot is small, the initial episode may not be fatal, but recurrent emboli increase the risk of mortality. Emboli may follow infection, thrombosis, severe hemorrhage, or shock. A symptom associated with smaller emboli (see Assessment Tool: Pulmonary Embolism) is the sudden onset of chest pain, which may be accompanied by blood-streaked mucus from the respiratory tract and a dry cough. The signs and symptoms of large pulmonary emboli are sudden intense chest pain, severe dyspnea, apprehension, syncope, fever, irregular or imperceptible pulse, pallor, cyanosis, and air hunger.

Therapeutic and Nursing Management

Clients with large emboli may require cardiopulmonary resuscitation. Diagnosis of pulmonary emboli is based on a chest x-ray study, electrocardiogram (ECG), arterial blood gas analysis, lung scan, and pulmonary angiography. Acid-base abnormalities and shock are treated, and heparin therapy may be initiated. The use of IV morphine may allay apprehension and chest pain, and aminophylline is used if there are bronchospasms.

During the crisis phase the nurse monitors blood pressure, pulse, and respirations every 5 minutes. The nurse assists the laboratory personnel when arterial blood is drawn for blood gas analysis to assess for shock and determine oxygen needs and initiates an IV line for heparin therapy.

TABLE 25-6

*Postpartum Client Care Summary for Pulmonary Embolism**

Interventions	Frequency
BP, P, R	q 15 min until stable; then q 30 min × 2; then q 1 hr; then q 4 hr on postpartum (PP) floor
T	On admission; then q 4 hr
Contractions	Fundal checks on admission; then q 15 min × 4; then q 30 min × 2; then q 1 hr until stable; then q 4 hr on PP floor
	Lochia: Same as above
Input and output	q 1 hr until stable; then q 8 hr
Central venous pressure	Yes
ECG	Yes
O₂ therapy	1 to 2 L/min nasal prong

Adapted from Knuppel RA, Drukker JE: High-Risk Pregnancy: A Team Approach. Philadelphia, WB Saunders, 1986.
*Nurse–client ratio = 1 : 1.

The nurse monitors the client's skin color and pallor and complaints of weakness and observes for shortness of breath. He or she notes and reports the degree of neck vein engorgement and auscultates the chest for friction rub or atelectasis. Nursing care includes giving support to the client to assist in allaying her anxiety and restlessness. Both she and her family are informed and updated about the treatment progress.

Once the crisis has passed, the nurse provides leg elevation, bed rest, and local heat to a client with deep vein thrombosis, monitors the client's vital signs as ordered, and assesses her for signs of respiratory distress. Again the client and her family are kept informed about her progress.

The occurrence of emboli, whether in the hospital before discharge or at home after discharge, disrupts the mother–infant relationship. Nursing measures also include providing information to reduce knowledge deficit, to allay anxiety, and to minimize alterations in parenting. Table 25-6 provides a client care summary.

Assessment

On her admission to the postpartum unit the client's history is reviewed to identify risk factors for thromboembolic conditions (see below). Thrombi often occur bilaterally, although only one calf may appear affected. The nurse assesses the client's legs for signs of thrombosis (pain, warmth, tenderness, swollen red areas over veins that feel hard or solid to touch) on admission and once each shift.

Pregnancy Risk Factors for Thromboembolic Conditions

Maternal age greater than 35 yr
Obesity
Immobilization
Cardiopulmonary disease
Diabetes mellitus
Previous history of thromboembolism
Traumatic delivery

Focus Assessment

Examine for Homan's sign, tenderness over involved vein.

Monitor vital signs closely.

Inspect for signs of complications of therapy (e.g., bleeding gums, easy bruising, return of lochial rubra).

Be alert to signs of pulmonary embolus (e.g., severe chest pain, dyspnea, diaphoresis).

Review diagnostic studies (e.g., Lee-White clotting time, prothrombin time [PT], partial thromboplastin time [PTT]).

Explore client's nonverbal indicators of emotional stress and coping (e.g., irritability, inability to concentrate, withdrawal).

Explore individual concerns.

Determine client's current level of knowledge regarding disorder, implications, and therapy.

Identify individual learning needs.

Pedal and popliteal pulses are assessed to assure adequate circulation. The nurse assesses for the presence of Homan's sign. If the sign is present, the client may complain of calf muscle pain when the foot is dorsiflexed because of compression of the tibial veins if thrombosis is present. The nurse also is alert for client complaint of aching deep vein tenderness or muscle spasm of the calf, which could indicate a thrombosis has formed. Nursing care includes monitoring vital signs every 4 hours, giving particular attention to temperature elevation, which could indicate infection (see above).

Nursing Diagnosis

Nursing diagnoses formulated from assessment findings address pain, tissue perfusion, knowledge deficit, and injury potential.

Planning and Intervention

The nurse takes and records the client's vital signs on her admission to the postpartum floor and then every 4 hours. Nursing care includes encouraging the client at risk for or with a thromboembolic condition to wear support hose even when confined to bed for longer than 8 hours

---

POTENTIAL NURSING DIAGNOSES

Thromboembolic Condition

Potential for Injury—related to thrombus formation secondary to hypercoagulability and immobility

Potential for Injury—related to embolus secondary to thrombophlebitis

Potential for Injury—related to excessive bleeding secondary to side effects of anticoagulant or fibrinolytic therapy

Pain—related to local inflammation secondary to venous thrombosis

Altered Local Tissue Perfusion—related to occlusion secondary to venous thrombosis

Anxiety—related to implications of the disorder and effect of extended hospitalization on family

Knowledge Deficit—regarding venous thrombosis, thrombophlebitis, and medical and nursing management of the disorder

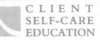

CLIENT
SELF-CARE
EDUCATION

Thromboembolic Condition

Action

1. Avoid long periods of sitting; avoid pressure under the knees such as occurs with propping with pillows.
2. Elevate foot of bed and elevate legs when sitting.
3. Do not cross legs when sitting.

4. Wear support hose; lie flat with legs elevated and roll on stockings.
5. Wear loose clothing; do not wear garters or other tight restrictions around legs.
6. Take daily dose of anticoagulant by dividing it or taking it with food.
7. Do not shave legs with safety razor.

8. If bed rest is required, the following exercises are taught:
    a. Flex and extend each foot several times.
    b. Rotate feet.
    c. Alternately flex and extend each leg.
    d. Press back of knee to bed surface; relax.
    e. Do straight leg raises.

Rationale

1. Getting up and walking every ½ hr minimizes stasis (pooling of blood in legs) by increasing circulatory blood volume to heart.
2. Increases venous return of blood to heart.

3. Decreases pressure on popliteal space behind knee to increase venous return of blood to heart.
4. Increases venous return of blood to heart.

5. Increases venous return of blood to heart.

6. Reduces gastric distress from taking anticoagulants without food.
7. Use of electric razor or dipilatories prohibits nicking or scraping.
8. Promotes circulation in legs.

and teaching her to perform low-extremity exercises to promote circulation. When the client is permitted out of bed, the nurse encourages her to ambulate frequently and discourages standing and sitting (see Client Self-Care Education: Thromboembolic Condition). If thrombus formation is suspected, the nurse notifies the primary care provider immediately and places the client on bed rest with the affected limb elevated on pillows. The primary care provider usually orders the use of warm moist packs, which the nurse applies to the affected limb several times each day to dilate blood vessels and decrease lymphatic congestion.

The nurse reviews laboratory results and reports them to the primary care provider as ordered or indicated. Heparin therapy is begun (see Drug Guide: Heparin p. 727) and continued for approximately 6 weeks. Discharge teaching includes instructing the client to report any hemotologic phenomenon that occur such as bleeding gums, hematuria, epistaxis, and occult blood in her stool.

Evaluation

Reviewing the client's history to identify risk factors, assessment for signs and symptoms of a thromboembolic condition, early therapeutic management, and nursing care should result in minimizing major complications. Client teaching includes instruction about what to expect during the time of an active thromboembolic condition and about self-care. Discharge teaching includes the importance of identifying potential problems resulting from therapeutic treatment with heparin and the necessity of reporting them to her primary health care provider.

Heparin sodium injection: Sterile solution derived from porcine intestinal mucosa, standardized for use as anticoagulant.

Obstetric Action: Inhibits reactions that lead to clotting of blood and formation of fibrin clots; acts at multiple sites in the normal coagulation systems; prolongs clotting time; has no effect on existing clots but prevents extension of old clots and formation of new ones.

Postpartum Administration: IV or subcutaneous (SC), 5000 to 30,000 U; may be ordered as a drip over 24 hr. Prophylactic dose: 5000 U SC every 12 hr.

Maternal Contraindications: Sensitivity to heparin.

Potential Side Effects and Complications: Hemorrhage (chief complication); hypersensitivity reactions with chills, fever and urticaria; possible local irritation, mild pain, and hematoma formation with intramuscular injection; acute thrombocytopenia purpura, alopecia; long-term use during pregnancy associated with maternal osteopenia, possibly from low vitamin D.

Nursing Implications:
1. Do not administer heparin intramuscularly.
2. Order laboratory tests (coagulation time) as ordered by primary health care provider (usually every 4 hr).
3. Report results of coagulation tests of prothrombin activity before start of therapy.
4. Monitor closely for hemorrhage.
5. Rotate administration site.
6. Do not massage administration site.
7. Mother may continue to breast-feed.

NURSING
◣ CARE
◢ PLAN

Client With Thromboembolic Condition

**Goals
(Expected Outcomes)**

Goals (Expected Outcomes)	Interventions	Rationale	Evaluation
Potential for Pain—Related to Venous Thrombosis or Superficial Thrombophlebitis			
Client will regain health, be free from complications (pulmonary embolism) of thromboembolic condition, and express understanding of disease process and ways to minimize future development.	Maintain bed rest for client, with affected leg elevated for 5-7 days or until symptoms are clear.	Reduces tension on vein, increases venous return of blood to heart, and decreases edema.	Edema is decreasing; leg is warm and color is good.
	Apply proper fitting antiembolic stocking and apply continuous moist heat to leg.	Speeds resolution of inflammation and pain.	Client states has less pain; redness and warmth (heat) of skin have lessened.
	Measure thighs and calves daily.	Assesses resolution of edema by measuring calf circumference (2 cm difference is significant).	Edema is decreasing with <2 cm difference in circumferences of calves and thighs.
	Provide analgesia for pain.	Decreases pain.	Client verbalizes that pain has lessened.
	Instruct client to report all pain, especially chest pain, and shortness of breath.	Symptoms may indicate presence of embolus that may lodge in heart or lungs.	Client states no chest pain or shortness of breath is experienced.

Continued

NURSING
CARE
PLAN

Client With Thromboembolic Condition—continued

Goals (Expected Outcomes)	Interventions	Rationale	Evaluation
Alteration in Tissue Perfusion: Peripheral—Related to Venous Thrombosis			
Client will maintain adequate peripheral circulation.	Assess peripheral circulation every 4 hr (palpable pulse, skin temperature, color, and edema); may check Homan's sign (calf pain when leg extended and foot dorsiflexed).	Ensures peripheral circulation is maintained.	Client has strong palpable pulses in all extremities and maintains good skin color.
	Instruct client to avoid use of knee gatch on bed and pillow under knees.	Avoids further pressure on vessels, which would inhibit venous return to heart.	Venous circulation is maintained as evidenced by strong palpable pulses and good skin color.
	Instruct client to avoid massaging and rubbing legs.	Avoids risk of dislodging thrombus.	Client states she understands importance of avoiding massage, rubbing legs.
	Change client's position every 2 hr and instruct her about and assist her with active and passive range of joint motion exercises as ordered.	Increases circulation and avoids excessive pressure on dependent areas.	Client changes position at least every 2 hr. Her skin color is good; no dependent areas are reddened or broken down.
	Apply antiembolic stockings	Increases circulation.	Circulation is maintained as evidenced by palpable peripheral pulses.
	Remove antiembolic stockings once every 8 hr for 15 min; assess skin carefully for signs of breakdown.	Ensures that all skin surfaces are intact.	All skin surfaces are intact, with no visible breakdown or loss of skin integrity.
	Encourage intake of nutritional diet and fluids.	Provides cellular nutrition and circulating blood volume.	All skin surfaces have good color and are intact; all peripheral pulses are strong by palpation.
Potential for Injury (Bleeding)—Related to Side Effects of Fibrinolytic or Anticoagulant Therapy			
Client will maintain all coagulation studies within acceptable limits and display no signs of bleeding.	Administer anticoagulants as ordered.	Prevents development of thrombosis and dissolves formed emboli.	Client's coagulation studies reveal improvement.
	Check client for bleeding gums, hematuria, epistaxis, petechiae, gastrointestinal or rectal bleeding.	Use of anticoagulants may cause bleeding at any vulnerable body site.	No bleeding is noted at any body site.
	Check laboratory results for prolonged prothrombin and clotting times.	Determines from laboratory results if bleeding is anticipated.	Coagulation studies are in acceptable limits.

NURSING
CARE
PLAN

Client With Thromboembolic Condition—*continued*

Goals (Expected Outcomes)	Interventions	Rationale	Evaluation
Knowledge Deficit—Regarding Thromboembolic Condition, Its Management, and Avoidance of Its Recurrence			
Client will be compliant with all care and will ask questions and verbalize knowledge about her care and medication, about precautionary measures to avoid venous stasis and bleeding, about exercises, and about signs and symptoms that would require reporting to and seeing the primary health care provider.	Teach client about venous stasis and its relationship to potential embolus formation (e.g., sitting with legs crossed, massaging legs, immobility, pressure on popliteal areas; tight hose, straps, or bands around thighs, knees, calves, or ankles.	Avoids measures that cause stasis and thrombus formation.	Client verbalizes understanding of stasis and how to avoid it.
	Teach client how to apply elastic (antiembolic) stockings (be sure she knows to avoid all constrictive clothing) and how to perform range of joint motion exercises.	Increases circulation and avoids stasis.	Client demonstrates application of elastic stockings and performance of range of motion exercises.
	Teach early signs of thrombosis and thrombophlebitis (stiffness, soreness, swelling, redness over affected area).	Increases understanding of signs and symptoms of thromboembolic condition and complications.	Client verbalizes signs and symptoms to monitor and to report to primary health care provider.
	Explain schedule, dosage, action, and side effects of prescribed medications.	Enhances understanding of drug therapy (especially anticoagulant therapy).	Client verbalizes schedule, dosage, actions, and side effects of drugs.
	Suggest guidelines (e.g., use soft toothbrush, avoid going barefoot, wear gloves to do cleaning) to avoid hazards that could cause bleeding during anticoagulant therapy in hospital and after discharge.	Avoids side effects of bleeding during anticoagulant therapy.	Client begins practices that will avoid injury that could cause bleeding.
	Instruct client to tell all other health care providers (e.g., dentist), she is receiving anticoagulant therapy.	Ensures avoidance of risks that could cause bleeding.	Client notes other health care providers who may be used during time of anticoagulant therapy.
	Teach client about stasis, thromboembolic condition, and managment at times when significant others are available to receive teaching and ask questions.	Increases understanding of venous stasis, thromboemblic condition, and its management.	Client and her family verbalize understanding of thromboembolic condition; their responses to questions verify their knowledge.

REFERENCE

1. LaFoy J, Geden EA. Postepisiotomy pain: Warm versus cold sitz bath. JOGN (September/October): 399-403, 1989

SUGGESTED READINGS

Cunningham FG, MacDonald PC, Gant NF: Willams Obstetrics, 18th ed. Norwalk, Conn, Appleton & Lange, 1989

Gibbs RS, Sweet RL: Maternal and fetal infections. In Creasy RL, Resnik R (eds): Maternal-Fetal Medicine: Principles and Practice. Philadelphia, WB Saunders, 1989

Gonik B: Intensive care monitoring of the critically ill pregnant patient. In Creasy RL, Resnik R (eds): Maternal-Fetal Medicine: Principles and Practice. Philadelphia, WB Saunders, 1989

Gulanick M, Klopp A, Galanes S: Nursing Care Plans: Nursing Diagnosis and Interventions, 2nd ed. St. Louis, CV Mosby, 1990

Hanson-Smith B: Nursing Care Planning Guides for Childbearing Families. Baltimore, Williams & Wilkins, 1989

Kapernick PS: Postpartum hemorrhage and the abnormal puerperium. In Pernoll ML, Bensen, RC (eds): Current Obstetric and Gynecologic Disorders. Norwalk Conn, Appleton & Lange, 1987

Lee MF: Perinatal infections and prematurity: Is there a relationship? J Perinat Neonat Nurs 2(1):10-20, July 1988

Mead PB: When your patient has postpartum endometritis. Contemp OB/GYN (May):38-39, 1984

Novy MJ: The normal puerperium. In Pernoll ML, Benson RC (eds): Current Obstetric and Gynecologic Disorders. Norwalk, Conn, Appleton & Lange, 1989

Roberts J: Emergency birth. J Emerg Nurs 11(3):125-131, May/June 1985

Varney H: Nurse Midwifery. London, Blackwell Scientific Publications, 1987

Weingold AB: Meeting the challenge of postpartum hemorrhage. Contemp OB/GYN (May):31-38, 1984

Williams C: Emergency childbirth. Emergency Med Serv (May/June):100-104, 1985

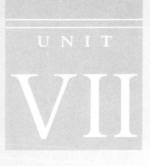

Neonatal Disorders

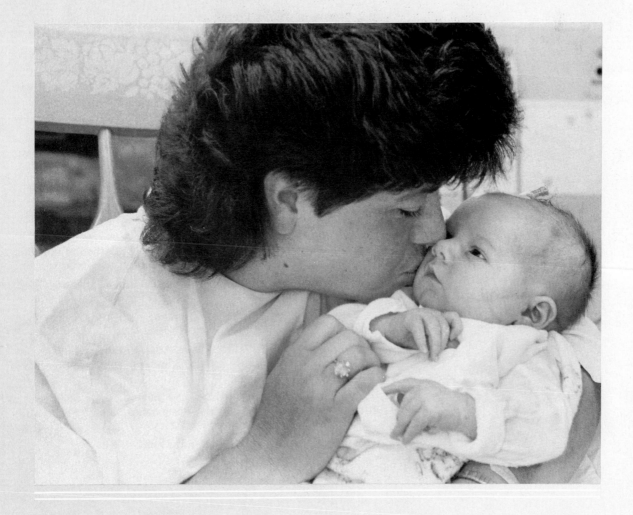

The Neonate With Developmental or Acquired Disorders

IMPORTANT TERMINOLOGY

anencephaly Congenital absence of the cerebrum, cerebellum, and flat bones of the skull

congenital anomaly Structural defects present at birth

conjugation of bilirubin Process of changing insoluble bilirubin to an excretable form

Coombs' test, direct Test used to detect maternal anti-RH antibodies coating red blood cells in cord blood of the neonate

exchange transfusion Therapy for extreme hyperbilirubinemia in which infant's blood is exchanged in small amounts for compatible blood

hemolytic disease Abnormally rapid rate of red blood cell destruction that results in severe anemia

hydrops fetalis Severe form of erythroblastosis fetalis initially seen as marked edema, cardiomegaly, and hepatomegaly

hyperbilirubinemia Excessive accumulation of bilirubin in the blood, characterized by a yellowish discoloration of the skin called jaundice or icterus

hypoglycemia Low blood sugar, <30 mg/dl for term infant and <20 mg/dl for preterm infant

kernicterus Severe brain damage resulting from deposition of unconjugated bilirubin in basal ganglia

phototherapy Use of light exposure to skin surfaces of a jaundiced infant to transform bilirubin into water-soluble molecules that can be excreted

polycythemia Increased number of circulating red blood cells causing hemoglobin level >20 g/dl and hematocrit level >65%

Rh₀ (D) immunoglobulin (Rho GAM) Anti-D immune globulin administered to the Rh-negative mother shortly after birth to prevent Rh sensitization

Rh sensitization Formation of Rh-positive antibodies in blood serum of Rh-negative woman caused by pregnancy, mismatched blood transfusion, or miscarriage beyond 6 to 8 weeks of pregnancy

sepsis Generalized bacterial infection in the bloodstream

The etiology of birth defects is not completely understood, but a multifactorial etiology is generally accepted. Because birth defects are so numerous and varied, this chapter presents selected disorders—those more commonly seen that are apparent at birth or soon thereafter and with which the maternity nurse will have to deal. The care of these infants and their parents presents a challenge to the nurse who must give competent, complex nursing care to the infants as well as help parents cope with their feelings of disappointment and despair.

Congenital Anomalies
Etiology

Congenital anomalies that cause significant alterations in structure or function occur in approximately 250,000 infants each year. When these anomalies occur, the family may experience a crisis requiring psychologic adjustment on the part of each member, and the economic and physical resources of the family may be depleted.

Feeding Newborn With Cleft Palate

CLIENT
INFANT-CARE
EDUCATION

Action

1. Feedings may be lengthy and tiring.

2. Use "preemie" nipple or soft regular nipple with large holes. Several types of nipples specific for this problem are available (Fig. 26-1).

3. Burp frequently.

4. Hold infant in sitting position with head and chest tilted slightly backward during feeding.

5. After feeding, cleanse cleft with a dropperful of water to prevent crusting.

6. If unable to nipple feed, use medicine dropper or asepto syringe with a 1½-inch soft rubber extension, or nasogastric feedings may be ordered.

7. Place on abdomen or in side-lying position between feedings with head elevated 30 degrees.

Rationale

1. Feeding must be given slowly so newborn can learn to adapt to the feeding method. Time required for feeding may tire the newborn.

2. Open palate causes difficulty in creating the suction needed to bring milk into the infant's mouth. Softer nipples with large holes allow the newborn to obtain milk without large energy output.

3. Opening in the roof of the mouth and imperfect seal during sucking cause the infant to swallow more air.

4. Sitting position enables the newborn to clear the airway more easily using the natural cough reflex. Formula may return through the nose, and episodes of coughing or gagging may occur.

5. Good mouth care reduces the potential for infection, particularly ear infection.

6. Formula flows easily with little sucking. Caregiver places the rubber piece to the back and side of the mouth and allows only a small amount at a time to flow into the mouth.

7. Position facilitates clearing of the airway.

Congenital Anomalies

The cultural background, age, and life situation of the parents affect their acceptance of the newborn's abnormality. This particular child may have special meaning to the parents, e.g., the position of the oldest male in certain cultures. The expectations of the members of the extended family are of great importance in some cultures.

Congenital deformities range from minor abnormalities, e.g., an extra finger or toe, to grave malformations incompatible with life, e.g., **an-encephaly** (the absence of portions of the brain). Some disorders such as cleft lip are highly visible at birth and may cause parents emotional distress. Other defects may not be apparent, and parents may not understand or may deny the seriousness of the problem. Grave defects are second only to accidents as a cause of death in childhood (see Cultural Implications: Congenital Anomalies).

Assessment and Nursing Interventions

Assessment characteristics and nursing interventions in the early neonatal period for selected congenital anomalies are found in Table 26-1.

Text continued on page 738.

FIGURE 26-1

Cleft Lip and Cleft Palate Nipples. These are various nipples used to feed infants with cleft lip and palate. Other commercial nipples are available. Since sucking strengthens and develops the muscles needed for speech, a nipple is used for feeding whenever possible.

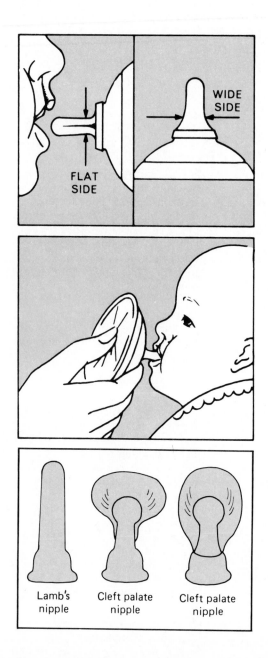

FLAT SIDE · WIDE SIDE

Lamb's nipple   Cleft palate nipple   Cleft palate nipple

TABLE 26-1

Congenital Abnormality Nursing Care Summary

Congenital Abnormality	Assessment	Nursing Interventions in the Early Neonatal Period	Therapeutic Management
Cleft lip and cleft palate (See Fig. 1 below)	May occur separately, bilaterally or unilaterally Occurs in 1:2500 births Cleft lip ranges from slight dimple to wide separation extending to the nasal structures Cleft palate may involve the soft palate alone; can extend along the hard palate and the anterior portions of the maxilla	Encourage parents to hold and touch infant. Provide information about care of infant (see Client Infant Care Education: Feeding Newborn With Cleft Palate).	Establishment of nutrition Avoiding aspiration Early referral to plastic surgeon Long-term: Orthodontic care, speech therapy, hearing evaluation
Tracheoesophageal atresia, type 3, with esophageal fistula (See Fig. 2 below)	Most common of the esophageal deformities Large amounts of oral secretions Choking on feedings Aspiration of stomach contents through the fistula into the trachea Signs of aspirating pneumonitis: tachypnea, tachycardia, pallor, cyanosis, retractions, rhonchi, decreased breath sounds	Perform frequent, careful suctioning. Avoid oral feedings. Keep infant in semi-upright position to avoid reflux of stomach contents into the trachea.	Immediate gastrostomy to reduce risk of reflux of stomach contents into trachea Intravenous (IV) fluids Antibiotics Surgical repair to close fistula and join (anastomose) esophagus; segment of colon may be used if esophagus is too short to join
Diaphragmatic hernia (See Fig. 3 below)	Severe respiratory distress shortly after birth Protrusion of abdominal contents into chest and compression of lung tissue Respiratory distress more severe as bowel fills with air during the first hours of life	Place infant in upright position. Pass nasogastric tube to remove air from stomach. Administer oxygen. Turn to affected side to permit expansion of unaffected lung.	Immediate surgical repair IV fluids Antibiotics if infection occurs

Fig. 1

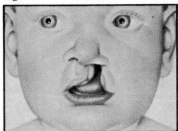

Unilateral
Complete

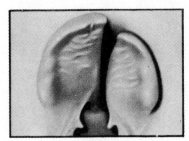

Unilateral
Complete

Fig. 2

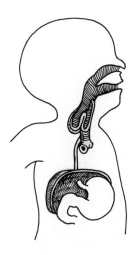

Fig. 3

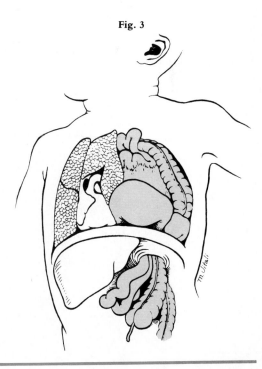

Continued

TABLE 26-1

Congenital Abnormality Nursing Care Summary—continued

Congenital Abnormality	Assessment	Nursing Interventions in the Early Neonatal Period	Therapeutic Management
Imperforate anus (See Fig. 4 below)	Inability to take rectal temperature Abdominal distention Meconium stools not present Shallow blind, rectal pouch instead of normal anal opening Possible fistula to bladder, vagina, or urethra	Observe every infant carefully for passing of first stool, abdominal distention, and failure to pass rectal thermometer. Report deviations from normal to physician.	Surgery. May need colostomy until complete repair
Omphalocele (See Fig. 5 below)	Protrusion of abdominal contents through umbilical opening Bowel covered by amniotic membrane, not skin	Immediately cover omphalocele with sterile gauze moistened with warm sterile water. Keep it moist until surgery is performed. Cover it with plastic wrap. Handle infant gently. Protect sac to prevent rupture. Prevent infection by using sterile gloves when providing care.	Nasogastric tube to prevent distention of bowel If peritoneal cavity not large enough to provide room for intestines, abdominal skin may be used to cover until complete repair Total IV alimentation may be necessary

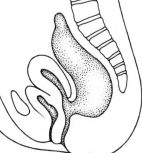 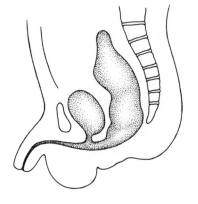

Fig. 4

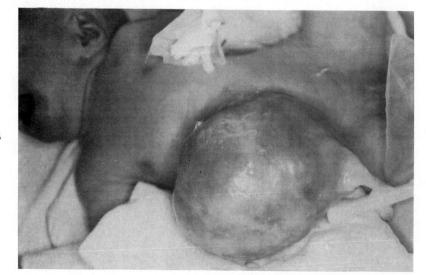

Fig. 5

TABLE 26-1

Congenital Abnormality Nursing Care Summary—continued

Congenital Abnormality	Assessment	Nursing Interventions in the Early Neonatal Period	Therapeutic Management
Myelomeningocele (See Fig. 6 below)	Saclike mass containing spinal cord, nerve roots, and meningeal covering; protrudes through bony defect in thoracic or lumbar spine (spina bifida) Level of defect determined by neurologic involvement Paralysis of extremities Poor bowel and bladder control Sensory deficits below level of defect Associated with hydrocephalus	Protect lesion from trauma and infection. Position infant on abdomen or side. Prevent fecal or urinary contamination. Use sterile dressing over sac to prevent rupture and drying. Change position frequently. Observe sac for oozing or pus.	Surgical correction early to prevent sepsis Observation for hydrocephalus IV fluids Antibiotics
Hydrocephalus (See Fig. 7 below)	Enlargement of cerebral ventricles resulting from abnormal amount of cerebral fluid Enlarging head size Wide separations of suture lines Bulging fontanels Shiny, thin-skinned appearance of forehead, with visible veins Setting-sun appearance of eyes Signs of increased intracranial pressure Lethargy High-pitched cry Irritability Vomiting Convulsions Transillumination of head indicating translucency (presence of fluid rather than cerebral tissue)	Protect head from injury. Provide support for head. Measure and record head circumference daily. Observe fontanel for bulging. Place sponge-rubber pad under head or using alternating mattress. Change position frequently.	Surgical placement of shunt to allow cerebrospinal fluid to circulate

Fig. 7

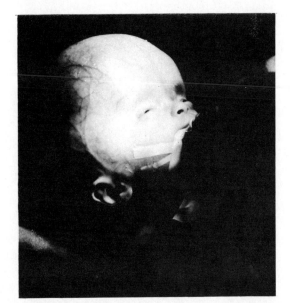

Fig. 6

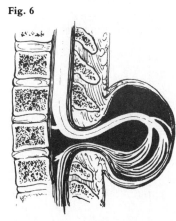

Spina bifida with meningomyelocele

Continued

TABLE 26-1

Congenital Abnormality Nursing Care Summary—continued

Congenital Abnormality	Assessment	Nursing Interventions in the Early Neonatal Period	Therapeutic Management
Down's syndrome (trisomy 21, translocation, or mosaicism) (See Fig. 8 below)	Trisomy 21 type occurs more often in children of women more than 35 years old Found in every race, color, creed Flat occiput Eyes upslanted with epicanthal folds Protruding tongue Short, broad neck Hypotonic muscles Short limbs Broad, square hands	Support parents by standing by, listening, helping them formulate questions. Call infant by name. Encourage parents to hold and feed infant. Assist parents with feedings. Contact support group.	Frequently diagnosed at birth because of obvious signs When diagnosis suspected, chromosomal analysis is ordered to determine specific cause; information is useful for genetic counseling Information about disorder and prognosis provided by physician Parents referred to appropriate community resources by physician

Fig. 8

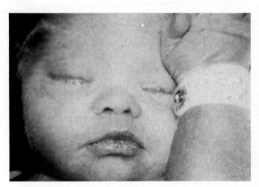

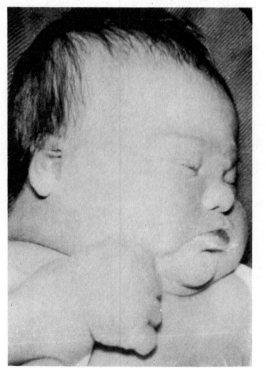

Congenital Heart Disease
Etiology

The incidence at birth of congenital heart disease is 8:1000. Cardiovascular malformations account for approximately 1.2 deaths:1000 births during infancy.

Congenital heart disease has been associated with heredity, maternal disease such as rubella and diabetes, and chromosomal abnormalities in the infant, e.g., Down's syndrome.

Pathophysiology

Structural heart defects are categorized by two features: (1) the abnormality results in cyanosis, and (2) the pulmonary blood flow is increased, normal, or decreased. Heart disease is suspected in the newborn if the child is cyanotic even in the presence of increased oxygen; the heart and respiratory rates are rapid, and heart and liver are enlarged; and a heart murmur is heard.[1]

Cyanotic heart lesions allow unoxygenated blood to mix with oxygenated blood within the heart and allow its circulation throughout the systemic circulation. The cyanotic heart lesions are tetralogy of Fallot (Fig. 26-2), transposition of the great arteries (Fig. 26-3), and hypoplastic heart syndrome (Fig. 26-4). The acyanotic heart lesions are patent ductus arteriosus (Fig. 26-5), ventricular septal defects (Fig. 26-6), atrial septal defects (Fig. 26-7), and coarctation of the aorta (Fig. 26-8). See Assessment Tool: Signs That Can Indicate Congenital Heart Defects for signs that may indicate congenital heart disease in a neonate. All of these signs are recorded and reported to the physician.

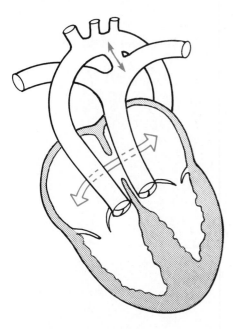

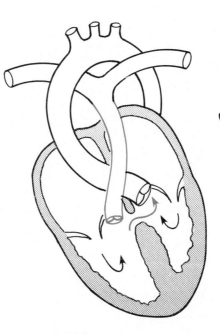

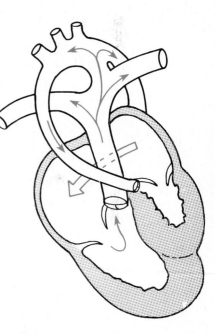

FIGURE 26-2
Tetralogy of Fallot. Tetralogy of Fallot, the most common defect causing cyanosis in children surviving beyond 2 years of age, is characterized by the combination of four defects: (1) pulmonary stenosis, (2) ventricular septal defect, (3) overriding aorta, and (4) hypertrophy of the right ventricle. The severity of symptoms depends on the degree of pulmonary stenosis, the size of the ventricular septal defect, and the degree to which the aorta overrides the septal defect.

FIGURE 26-3
Complete Transposition of Great Vessels. This anomaly is an embryologic defect caused by a straight division of the bulbar trunk without normal spiraling. As a result, the aorta originates from the right ventricle and the pulmonary artery from the left ventricle. An abnormal communication between the two circulations must be present to sustain life.

FIGURE 26-4
Hypoplastic Left Heart Syndrome. This is the most serious of the cyanotic defects because the only medical treatment available is transplantation of a new heart.

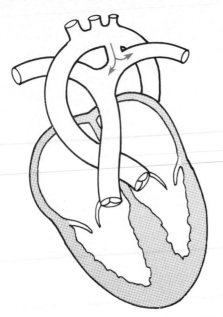

FIGURE 26-5
Patent Ductus Arteriosus (PDA). PDA is a vascular connection that, during fetal life, short-circuits the pulmonary vascular bed and directs blood from the pulmonary artery to the aorta. Functional closure of the ductus normally occurs soon after birth. If the ductus remains patent after birth, the direction of blood flow in the ductus is reversed by the higher pressure in the aorta.

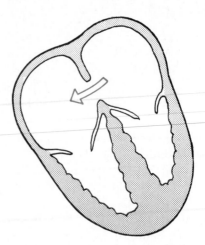

FIGURE 26-6
Ventricular Septal Defects. A ventricular septal defect is an abnormal opening between the right and left ventricle. Ventricular septal defects vary in size and may occur in either the membranous or muscular portion of the ventricular septum. Because of higher pressure in the left ventricle, shunting of blood from the left to the right ventricle occurs during systole. If pulmonary vascular resistance produces pulmonary hypertension, the shunt of blood is then reversed from the right to the left ventricle, with cyanosis resulting.

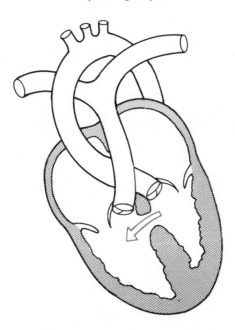

FIGURE 26-7
Atrial Septal Defects. An atrial septal defect is an abnormal opening between the right and left atria. Three types of abnormalities result from incorrect development of the atrial septum, with an incompetent foramen ovale the most common. The high ostium secundum defect results from abnormal development of the septum secundum. Improper development of the septum primum produces a basal opening known as an ostium primum defect, frequently involving the atrioventricular valves. In general, left-to-right shunting of blood occurs in all atrial septal defects.

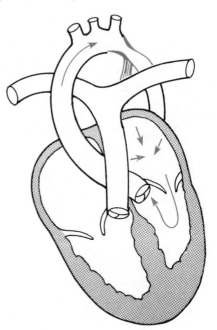

FIGURE 26-8
Coarctation of the Aorta. Coarctation of the aorta is characterized by a narrowed aortic lumen. It exists as a preductal or postductal obstruction, depending on the position of the obstruction in relation to the ductus arteriosus. Coarctations exist with great variation in anatomic features. The lesion produces an obstruction to the flow of blood through the aorta, causing increased left ventricular pressure and work load.

Signs That Can Indicate Congenital Heart Defects

Heart murmurs and dysrhythmias
Dyspnea (retractions, grunting, nasal flaring)
Tachypnea
Pulmonary edema
Tachycardia

Cyanotic episodes
Central cyanosis
Lethargy
Difficulty in feeding
Failure to gain weight
Absent or unequal pulses

Therapeutic Management

The congenital defect is diagnosed by chest x-ray examination, electrocardiography, echocardiography, and cardiac catheterization. Once the lesion is identified, the choice between medical or surgical intervention can be made. The newborn is managed by monitoring the heart rate and respirations, maintaining fluid and electrolyte status, administering oxygen, maintaining a thermoneutral environment, and administering medication. Medications most often used are digoxin, furosemide (Lasix), spironolactone (Aldactone), and morphine sulfate.

Assessment

The infant who is diagnosed with congenital heart disease is assessed for signs of congestive heart failure (see Assessment Tool: Signs of Neonatal Congestive Heart Failure).

Nursing Interventions

The nurse gathers assessment data and assists with and prepares the infant for diagnostic procedures. Because the infant may tire easily, small, frequent oral feedings are given. The use of oral-gastric tube feedings may be substituted to conserve energy. Strict records of intake and output and daily weight are kept. Oxygen is administered as needed while oxygenation status is maintained at a level of no more than 30% to 40% (Fig. 26-9). Oxygen should be kept warm and at a stable temperature. Digoxin dosage and route are checked with another nurse before its administration, and it is not administered if the apical heart rate becomes slower than normal or irregular. Potassium levels are monitored if diuretics are given.

Signs of Neonatal Congestive Heart Failure

Edema
Fatigue
Pallor

Diaphoresis
Decreased urinary output
Rales

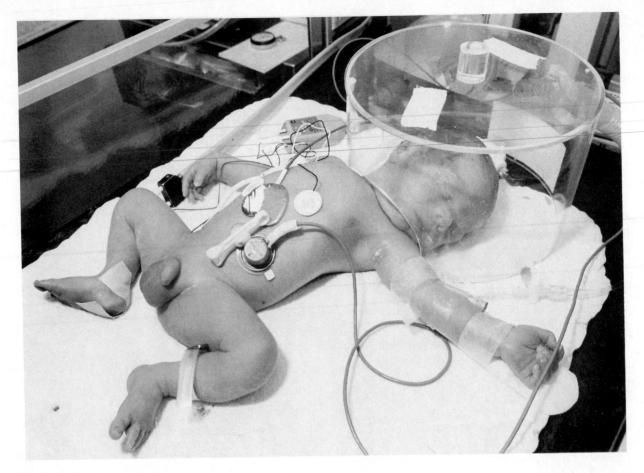

FIGURE 26-9
Oxygen Hood. The most efficient method of delivering the highest concentration of oxygen is use of the plastic oxygen hood. The nurse should position the infant and the hood to prevent oxygen's blowing directly onto the face. Cold air blowing in the infant's face can cause reflex bradycardia and shunting of blood from peripheral to central circulation.

Hyperbilirubinemia or Pathologic Jaundice in the Neonate

Etiology

Approximately 50% of newborns will develop some degree of jaundice. Jaundice is the result of bilirubin deposition in the subcutaneous fat underlying the skin. Physiologic **hyperbilirubinemia** usually results from the following:

1. Interference in the **conjugation of bilirubin**
2. Interference in elimination of bilirubin from the body
3. Decrease in the production of the liver enzyme glucuronyl transferase
4. Hemolysis of a large number of red blood cells (RBCs), coupled with the shortened life span of the newborn's RBCs

Newborns who have complications such as asphyxia, biliary obstruction, cold stress, **hypoglycemia**, **polycythemia**, sickle cell anemia, and **sepsis** are more likely to develop hyperbilirubinemia.

The most common cause of pathologic hyperbilirubinemia is incompatibility between some factor in the neonate's blood serum and maternal blood serum. The ensuing disease is called **hemolytic disease** of the newborn, and it occurs most often in the Rh-negative mother–Rh-positive

TABLE 26-2

Potential Maternal-Fetal ABO
Incompatibilities

Maternal Blood Group	Fetal Blood Group
O	A or B
B	A or AB
A	B or AB

infant or type O mother–type A or B infant pairing (Table 26-2). Ninety-eight percent of all hemolytic disease is related to either Rh or ABO incompatibilities (Fig. 26-10). Fetal hemolytic disease is markedly reduced by the injection of **Rh₀ (D) immunoglobulin (RhoGAM)** into the mother during the last trimester or in the first days after delivery or both.

Pathophysiology

Bilirubin is produced from the breakdown of RBCs. For bilirubin to be eliminated from the body, it must be transported to the liver by serum albumin for conjugation, and it must become water soluble before it can be excreted.

FIGURE 26-10

Rh Hemolytic Disease. Rh hemolytic disease is caused by an immune reaction of the mother's blood against the blood group factor on the fetal red blood cells. **A-D**, Rh-negative mother develops anti-Rh positive antibodies during one pregnancy. During subsequent pregnancy with Rh-positive fetus the maternal antibodies attach to fetal red blood cells, **E**. The fetal hemolytic response is usually mild, and mild-to-moderate hyperbilirubinemia is evident in the newborn.

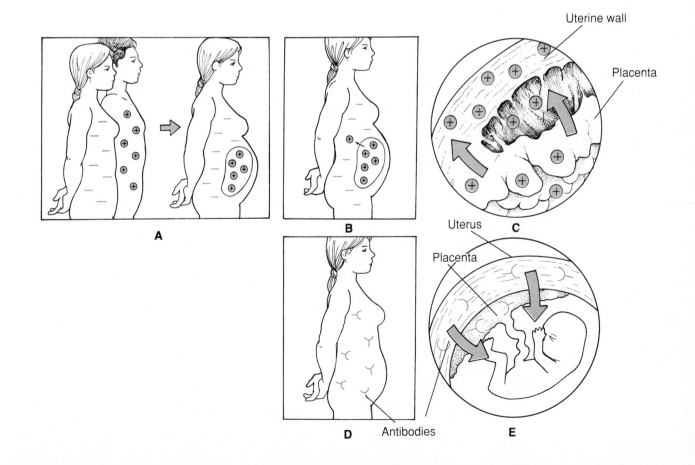

|||| LABORATORY
     VALUES

*Bilirubin Levels**

	Term Infant (mg)	Preterm Infant (mg)
Mean peak of bilirubin at 60-72 hr	6	Rises more rapidly in preterm infant; jaundice occurs at lower levels
Indication for photo-therapy	12*	10* (lower for smaller infants)
Indication for exchange transfusion	20*	15* (lower for smaller infants)

From Korones SB, Lancaster J: High-Risk Newborn Infants. St. Louis, CV Mosby, 1981.
*These values are guides. Variables such as size, age, rapidity of rise of bilirubin level, other test results, and cause of hyperbilirubinemia enter into the physician's decision to initiate therapy.

If a disturbance in the mechanisms necessary to conjugate and eliminate bilirubin from the body occurs, the free, unconjugated bilirubin may be deposited in the subcutaneous fat underlying the skin, certain other tissues, or brain cells. Conjugated bilirubin is not toxic since it does not enter body cells. However, if toxic levels of unconjugated bilirubin are reached, the baby's life may be endangered (see Laboratory Values: Bilirubin Levels).

Complications of Pathologic Hyperbilirubinemia

Hydrops fetalis, the most severe form of erythroblastosis fetalis, is the result of progressive hemolysis that causes fetal hypoxia, cardiac failure, and generalized edema. The baby will be delivered stillborn or in severe respiratory distress.

Kernicterus is the deposit of toxic, unconjugated bilirubin on the basal ganglia of the brain (see Assessment Tool: Signs of Kernicterus). Permanent neurologic damage may occur, resulting in cerebral palsy, seizure disorder, and mental retardation.

Therapeutic Management

The therapeutic management of hyperbilirubinemia is directed toward diagnosing the cause, preventing or reducing hyperbilirubinemia, and preventing anemia. **Phototherapy** and **exchange transfusion** are used. The appropriate treatment is based on the level of serum bilirubin, the birth weight, and the newborn's age in hours.

Phototherapy

A phototherapy unit containing fluorescent light tubes is placed over the crib or isolette of the undressed newborn (Fig. 26-11). The light breaks

ASSESSMENT
TOOL

Signs of Kernicterus

Lethargy	Rigidity
Hypotonia	Convulsions
High-pitched cry	Diminished
Poor feeding	reflexes
Tremors	Seizures

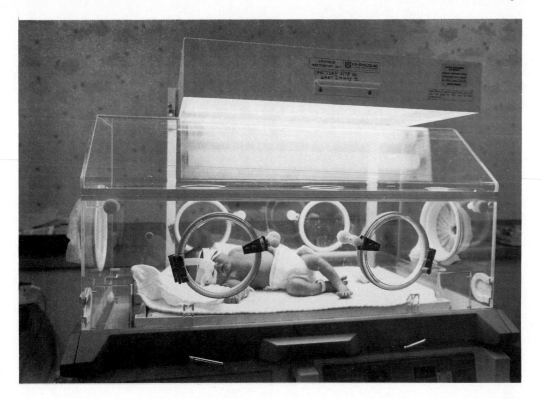

FIGURE 26-11

Phototherapy. The nude infant's skin is exposed to special high-intensity lights that break down unconjugated bilirubin in the skin. The infant is placed in an isolette for warmth, and the eyes are protected with eye patches. The phototherapy is continuous except for breaks each shift for eye assessment and for feeding.

Courtesy Air-Shield.

down the bilirubin in the skin by photooxidation into nontoxic compounds that can be excreted. Serum bilirubin levels are determined every 8 to 12 hours. While the serum is drawn, the bili-light is turned off to prevent break down of bilirubin in the sample, which would produce a false low reading.

Exchange Transfusion

The purpose of exchange transfusion in the infant with hemolytic disease is to decrease levels of bilirubin and correct anemia. An exchange transfusion alternately removes a small amount of blood from the infant and replaces it with a small amount of donor blood. The procedure is typically performed in an intensive care unit nursery.

Assessment

Every newborn is observed for jaundice at least every 8 hours (see Assessment Tool: Ongoing Assessment of the Newborn for Jaundice). The nurse presses firmly on the skin over bony prominences such as the forehead, nose, or sternum. After pressure is released, the area appears yellow when jaundice is present. The nurse checks the color of the oral mucosa and schlera of dark-skinned infants. When jaundice is present, the area will have a yellowish hue. Jaundice appears first on the face; as the serum bilirubin level rises, the color deepens and advances to the trunk and extremities.

A noninvasive screening tool called transcutaneous bilirubinometry (Fig. 26-12) may be used. This hand-held fiberoptic instrument illumines

Ongoing Assessment of the Newborn for Jaundice

1. Report jaundice that occurs in the first 24 hr of life or that continues beyond 1 week in the full-term newborn.
2. Press firmly on the skin, especially over bony prominences, i.e., forehead, nose, and sternum.
   a. Jaundice first appears on face and upper body.
   b. After pressure is released, area appears yellow.
3. Observe sclera and oral mucous membrane, especially in dark-skinned infants.
4. Jaundice deepens in color and advances to trunk and extremities as serum bilirubin level rises.
5. Assess newborn for conditions associated with jaundice, i.e., bruising, cephalohematoma, breast-feeding, Rh factor, maternal blood type O.

the skin and measures the intensity of yellow color. Phototherapy decreases the accuracy of the instrument, as does race.

Blood samples are taken. Diagnostic tests commonly ordered by the physician are determination of direct and total serum bilirubin levels, platelets, reticulocyte count, hemoglobin, serum albumin level, glucose levels, serology, blood type and Rh factor, and **direct Coombs' test** on cord blood (see Laboratory Values: Pathologic Jaundice of Newborn With Rh Sensitization).

FIGURE 26-12

Transcutaneous Bilirubinometer. The transcutaneous bilirubinometer is a device used to screen for neonatal jaundice. A small probe is applied firmly over the bony surface of the forehead or sternum. The hand-held fiberoptic instrument measures the intensity of the yellow color of the skin. The skin's degree of yellowness is displayed as a number that correlates with an estimation of serum bilirubin concentration. This instrument is not suitable for monitoring the infant treated with phototherapy or exchange transfusion.

Courtesy Air-Shield.

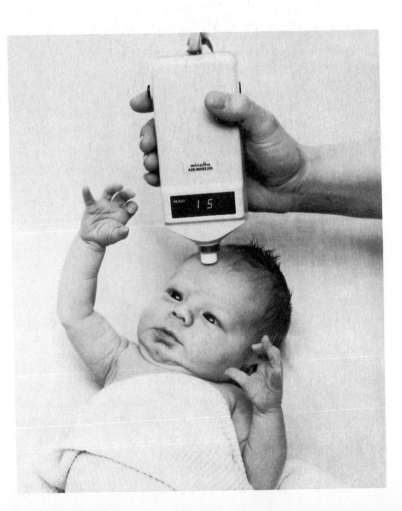

Test	Results
Rh factor	Rh positive
Direct Coombs'	Positive
Total serum bilirubin level in first 24 hr	Elevated >6 mg/dl
Direct (conjugated) serum bilirubin level	More than 1-2 mg/dl
Daily increases in total serum bilirubin level	More than 5 mg/dl/24 hr
Total serum bilirubin level (combination of direct and indirect)	More than 12 mg/dl
Reticulocytes (3%-7%)	>6% after third day of life
Hemoglobin (15-18 g/dl)	Low value suggests anemia

||| LABORATORY VALUES

Pathologic Jaundice of Newborn With Rh Sensitization

Nursing Interventions

Phototherapy

During phototherapy the eyes of the newborn are covered with eye patches. It is not known whether the bright light can injure the eyes of the newborn. Because eye patches are easily dislodged during activity and crying, the baby is frequently assessed for their placement. The nurse carefully monitors the temperature of the baby and the isolette so that temperature variations can be detected early. Neonatal position is changed every 2 to 3 hours so that all body surfaces are exposed to light. The newborn is removed from the light, the eye patches are removed, and he or she is held during feedings. The eyes are inspected for drainage or signs of infection or injury. Removing the eye patches allows eye contact with parents and visual stimulation and fosters socialization. The effects of phototherapy on the genitalia are unknown; therefore minimal covering is applied over the genitalia. Glucose water may be given between feedings to compensate for insensible fluid loss and to encourage bilirubin excretion through the urine and feces. Side effects of phototherapy are loose, green stools and transient skin rash or "bronzing of the skin," which may last for several weeks (see Nursing Care Plan: Infant With Hyperbilirubinemia).

Exchange Transfusion

Before the exchange transfusion the nurse obtains an informed consent signed by the parents and prepares the equipment and sets up the sterile exchange transfusion tray. Donor blood must be carefully checked for type, unit number, and expiration date. Blood-warming units keep the blood at an even temperature during the procedure. The infant is placed on monitors and is restrained.

During the procedure the nurse monitors and records the infant's temperature and other vital signs and records on the exchange transfer sheet the amount of blood transfused into the infant and removed. Monitoring of vital signs continues throughout the procedure.

Birth Trauma
Etiology

Injuries that happen during birth are more likely to occur when the infant is large, the mother's pelvis is disproportionate in size, the infant is preterm, the presentation is breech, or forceful extraction is used.

NURSING
CARE
PLAN

Infant With Hyperbilirubinemia

Goals (Expected Outcomes)	Interventions	Rationale	Evaluation
Fluid Volume Deficit (2)—Related to Fluid Loss			
Newborn's temperature will remain within normal parameters (36.5°-37°C) during phototherapy.	Offer feeding every 3-4 hr.	Adequate fluid intake is 140-200 ml/kg/24 hr. Feedings replace fluid losses.	Temperature within normal parametes (97°-99° F axillary) Fontanels not depressed Skin not tenting Urinary output >30 ml/kg/24 hr Six diapers moderately saturated in 24 hr Weight loss not >5% in 24 hr Newborn weighing 3200 g—intake is approximately 75-100 ml every 4 hr
Potential for Injury—Related to Hazards of Phototherapy			
Infant will exhibit no signs of redness, edema, or drainage from eyes during phototherapy.	Place eye patches securely over infant's eyes during phototherapy. Evaluate placement at least every 2 hr.	Patches protects eyes from direct, bright lights. Patches may be dislodged during activity and crying. Detects conjunctivitis early.	Eye patches securely in place while infant under phototherapy No signs of redness, edema, or discharge from eyes
Potential Impaired Skin Integrity—Related to Excoriation From Loose Stools			
Newborn's skin in genital and rectal areas will remain intact.	Cleanse genital and rectal area gently with warm water and pat dry.	Phototherapy can cause more frequent, loose, green stools as conjugated bilirubin is excreted. Stools may be irritating and cause excoriation in the rectal and genital areas.	Skin free of irritation
Altered Family Processes			
Newborn will experience periods of social contact with parents or caregiver.	Shut off bili-light and remove eye patches during parent contact and feeding. Offer explanations to parents. Encourage parents to hold and feed, stroke and touch baby. Reposition every 3-4 hr.	Provides frequent visual stimulation. Promotes parental attachment. Provides tactile stimulation.	Parents exhibit signs of bonding, e.g., eye contact, cuddling, calling by name.

Some injuries are minor and resolve spontaneously, although they may require some degree of intervention and explanation to parents. The nurse's responsibility is to observe and assess for potential injuries so that appropriate intervention may be initiated.

Head Trauma

Common head trauma birth injuries are summarized in Table 26-3.

Caput Succedaneum

Caput succedaneum (Fig. 26-13) is a commonly occurring soft, vaguely outlined edema of the scalp. The swelling occurs over the portion of the scalp that presents in a vertex delivery. No treatment is indicated.

Cephalohematoma

Cephalohematoma (Fig. 26-13) is less common and is caused by the rupture of blood vessels during a difficult labor or delivery. Usually the swelling is unilateral but may be bilateral. Hours or days may pass before the swelling becomes obvious.

TABLE 26-3

Head Trauma Birth Injuries

Birth Trauma	Assessment	Nursing Interventions in the Immediate Neonatal Period
Caput succedaneum (see Fig. 26-12)	Soft, vaguely outlined swelling of scalp May cross sagittal suture lines	Explain to parents that swelling will subside in 2 or 3 days (see Client Infant-Care Education: Caput Succedaneum and Cephalohematoma).
Cephalohematoma (see Fig. 26-12)	Bleeding between cranial bone and its covering, the periosteum May appear bluish or bruised Does not cross limits of the bone	Explain to parents that swelling will subside in few weeks to 3 months. In the first few days place infant in side-lying position opposite from injury or in a prone position; area may be sensitive if touched for first few days.
Intracranial hemorrhage	Hemorrhage in various areas of brain caused by rupture of cerebral blood vessels Low Apgar scores Irregular respirations Apneic episodes Cold, pale, clammy skin Lethargy Signs of increasing intracranial pressure	Assess for developing symptoms. Provide quiet environment, usually in isolette. Monitor temperature and respirations.
Facial paralysis (see Fig. 26-13)	Mouth drawn to one side Eye on affected side may remain open Possibly unable to blink on affected side	Administer artificial tears as prescribed by physician. Provide small, frequent feedings, using soft nipple if sucking is difficult.
Arm paralysis (Erb's palsy) (see Fig. 26-14)	Arm limp and internally rotated Grasp reflex present Moro reflex lessened or absent on affected side	Maintain proper position as prescribed. Apply intermittent splinting as prescribed. Perform daily passive range of motion exercises.
Fractures of clavicle, humerus, or femur	Decreased or absent mobility of affected arm or leg Cries in pain when arm or leg moved Local swelling	Handle gently to minimize pain. Immobilize by splinting. Maintain proper alignment. Arm on side of fractured clavicle may be held in place by pinning the shirt sleeve to the shirt.

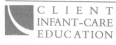

CLIENT
INFANT-CARE
EDUCATION

Caput Succedaneum and Cephalohematoma

Information	Rationale
Caput succedaneum Swelling will disappear in several days. No special care is needed.	Parents may ask questions or show concern because of the head's swelling. The swelling occurs in the area that presented at the cervical os.
Cephalohematoma Swelling may not disappear for days or weeks. Time is needed for absorption of the hematoma.	Cephalohematomas absorb spontaneously. Attempts to aspirate them may cause infection and thus are contraindicated.
Position infant on the stomach or side opposite the hematoma. Infant may be irritable and fussy if he or she lies on the swollen area. Be gentle when washing the area during the first several days.	If swelling is large, there may be pressure against the surrounding tissue, causing sensitivity.

FIGURE 26-13

Comparison of Caput Succedaneum, **A,** and Cephalohematoma, **B.**

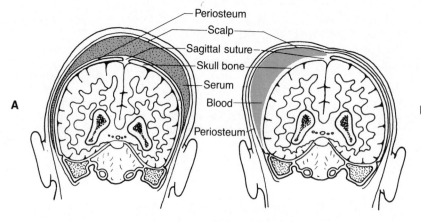

Caput Succedaneum	Cephalohematoma
Appears at birth; no increase in size	Appears several hours after birth; increases in size for 2–3 days
Disappears several days after birth; outline is vague, poorly defined	Disappears approximately 6 weeks after birth; outline is well defined
Sometimes crosses suture lines	Never crosses suture lines
Caused by diffuse, edematous swelling involving the soft tissues of the scalp	Caused by subperiosteal hemorrhage
Complications: rarely, anemia	Complications: Jaundice, underlying skull fracture, intracranial bleeding, shock

Adapted from Waechter EH, Phillips J, Holaday B: Nursing Care of Children, 10th ed. Philadelphia, JB Lippincott, 1985

Signs That May Indicate Intracranial Hemorrhage

Low Apgar scores
Irregular respirations
Apneic episodes
Cold, pale, clammy skin
Lethargy
Signs of increasing intracranial pressure
    Increasing head circumference
    Full or tense anterior fontanel
    Poor feeding or vomiting
    Irritability
    Diminishing Moro reflex
    Seizures

Intracranial Hemorrhage

Intracranial hemorrhage is often associated with difficult and very rapid deliveries, most frequently with the birth of a preterm infant. Pressure to the head and rupture of cerebral blood vessels and hypoxia cause hemorrhage in the subdural, subarachnoid, intracerebral, or intraventricular areas of the brain.

THERAPEUTIC MANAGEMENT. Ultrasound examinations and computed axial tomographic (CAT) scans are useful in determining the location and extent of the hemorrhage. Cerebrospinal fluid examination may reveal blood. Phenobarbital may be ordered to control seizures. If the neonate survives after a severe bleeding episode, there is risk of hydrocephalus, cerebral palsy, and mental and neurologic impairment.

ASSESSMENT. Signs of intracranial hemorrhage may be present at birth or develop within several days after birth. They depend on the area of the brain involved and the extent of the hemorrhage. The nurse assesses the neonate for developing signs and their increasing severity (see Assessment Tool: Signs That May Indicate Intracranial Hemorrhage).

NURSING INTERVENTIONS. Nursing interventions include placing the newborn in a quiet environment, usually in an isolette. Stressful procedures that may cause the onset of seizure activity should be avoided. Feeding methods depend on the infant's ability to suck, swallow, and retain oral feedings. The infant's temperature and respirations may be unstable and should be monitored carefully.

Birth Problems Involving the Nervous System

Facial Paralysis

Facial paralysis (Fig. 26-14) may occur as the result of a difficult vaginal delivery or the pressure of forceps on the facial nerve. Temporary paralysis of the muscles on one side of the face causes the mouth to draw to the

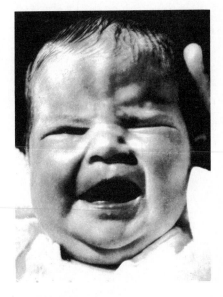

FIGURE 26-14
Facial Nerve Paralysis. Note the asymmetry of the mouth during crying. Sucking may be difficult for the baby. This birth injury is temporary, and full recovery is usual.

FIGURE 26-15

Erb's Palsy. If the brachial plexuses are traumatized during difficult delivery of the shoulders, paralysis of the arms can result. The paralysis can involve the upper or lower arm or both, depending on the nerves involved. Prognosis depends on the degree of nerve damage, and recovery can be complete, partial, or nonexistent.

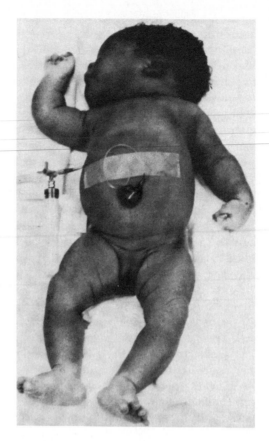

side, which is noticeable when the newborn cries. If the eye on the affected side remains open, a protective eye patch may be ordered by the physician (see Table 26-3).

Arm Paralysis

Injury to the brachial plexus (Fig. 26-15) is the most common nerve injury of the newborn. Damage to the upper brachial plexus (Erb's palsy) usually results from pulling or stretching the shoulder away from the head during breech or vertex delivery. Injury to the lower plexus causes limpness of the hand and wrist.

Treatment is directed toward preventing contractures of the affected muscles and maintaining correct placement of the humerus into the scapula. Treatment includes providing proper positioning, intermittent immobilization, and frequent full range of joint motion exercises. Immobilization may be completed by splinting or by pinning the shirt sleeve to the mattress (see Table 26-3).

Phrenic Nerve Injury

In a difficult breech delivery injury to the phrenic nerve may result in diaphragmatic paralysis. The most important symptom is respiratory distress.

Fractures

The clavicle, or collarbone, is the bone most often fractured during delivery. Fractures of the humerus and femur can occur in difficult deliveries. Because of the flexibility and molding of the neonate's head, skull fractures of the head are uncommon. Signs of fractures of the clavicle, humerus, or femur include decreased or absent mobility of the affected arm or leg, crying in pain when the arm or leg is moved, absence of the Moro reflex in the affected arm only, and local swelling. Treatment consists of gentle handling to minimize pain, immobilization, and proper alignment. The arm on the side of the fractured clavicle may be held in place by pinning the shirt sleeve to the shirt.

Neonatal Sepsis

Etiology

The newborn is at special risk for infection, and once it is acquired, the newborn is more likely to die from sepsis. A major concern in the infant with infection is that any infection can become generalized, producing sepsis or meningitis.[1] Sepsis occurs in approximately 1:1500 neonates. High-risk babies, including preterm infants, are particularly vulnerable to sepsis.

The newborn may be infected before he is born through the placenta or after rupture of the membranes. Infections may also be acquired during passage through the birth canal or during exposure to the hospital environment and caregivers (Fig. 26-16). Postnatal infections can also be

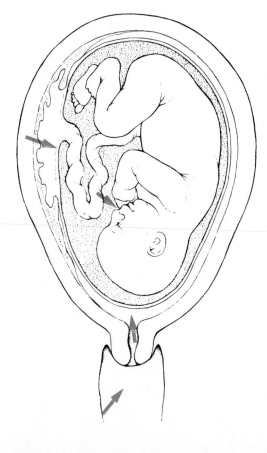

Transplacental infection
Toxoplasmosis
Rubella
Cytomegalovirus
Herpes simplex
Group B coxsackievirus
Varicella
Malaria
L. *Monocytogenes*
Group B β-hemolytic streptococcus
Gonococcus (?)
Tuberculosis (rare)
AIDS (HTLV-III)

Ascending infection and infections acquired by direct contact with birth canal
E. *coli* and other gram-negative bacilli
L. *monocytogenes*
Vibrio
C. *albicans*
M. *hominis*
Varicella
Herpes simplex
Gonococcus
Group B β-hemolytic streptococcus

FIGURE 26-16
Routes of Fetomaternal Infection.
Arrows indicate probable routes of fetomaternal infection. The neonate acquires infections from the mother's circulating blood in utero through the cord. Following rupture of the membranes or during birth, the infant is at risk for different infections if the mother is infected.

Adapted from Evans ME, Glass L: Perinatal Medicine. Hagerstown, Md, Harper & Row, 1976.

acquired by cross-contamination from other infants or from objects used in care such as mechanical ventilators.

Therapeutic Management

A series of tests useful in diagnosing the presence of infection and identifying the causative infectious agent is known as a diagnostic or septic workup. This workup may be indicated for newborns with symptoms of infections or with an increased risk factor such as premature rupture of the membranes.

The diagnostic workup may include a complete blood count, chest x-ray examinations, lumbar puncture, and suprapubic aspiration of urine. Cultures are obtained from spinal fluid, urine, blood, ear, nose, gastric aspirate, skin, umbilical cord, and rectum.

After the septic workup antibiotic therapy is generally started immediately. The antibiotic may be changed when culture and sensitivity results are returned in 24 to 72 hours.

Assessment

Because the signs of infection may be similar to those of other conditions, the nurse must be aware of slight changes in the infant's condition. The behaviors and signs of sepsis are often subtle and may be noticed only by experienced caregivers. Clinical signs of sepsis are listed in Assessment Tool: Ongoing Assessment of Clinical Signs of Sepsis in the Newborn.

ASSESSMENT
TOOL

Ongoing Assessment of Clinical Signs of Sepsis in the Newborn

Subtle, nonspecific signs

"Is not doing well"
"Does not look right"
Nonspecific respiratory problems

Respiratory signs
Tachypnea
Apnea
Grunting

Gastrointestinal signs
Diarrhea
Abdominal distention
Vomiting
Poor sucking or feeding

Skin
Pallor, cyanosis, mottling
Rashes
Jaundice

Central nervous system
Temperature instability
Full or bulging fontanel
Irritability
Seizure activity

Fever is frequently absent

TABLE 26-4

Commonly Occurring Pathogens, Transmission, Characteristics, and Nursing Considerations in Neonatal Sepsis

Pathogen	Transmission	Characteristics (Assessment)	Nursing Considerations
β-Hemolytic streptococci	In utero or after a long, difficult delivery (10% mothers are vaginal carriers) Premature rupture of membranes Exposure to adult carrier	Early onset Low Apgar scores Respiratory distress Pneumonia at birth Sepsis Meningitis	Assist with septic workup. Assess for neurologic status: bulging fontanel, irritability, seizures, high-pitched cry. Measure head circumference. Administer antibiotic therapy as ordered.
Gonococcus	Contamination of infant's eyes with infected secretions from mother's vagina	On second or third day of life, serosanguineous discharge from eye, which becomes purulent (ophthalmia neonatorum) Ulceration and scarring of cornea, leading to blindness	Apply prophylactic medication to eyes at time of birth. Obtain smears for culture as ordered. Administer antibiotic as ordered.
Escherichia coli or other enteric pathogens	Gastrointestinal route through hands of caregiver Maternal fecal contamination at birth	(Serious problem in neonate requiring careful separation and isolation) Multiple loose stools Greenish or blood-tinged watery stools Weight loss Dehydration Sepsis Shock	Carefully isolate baby; when infection is confirmed, care for in a separate area with handwashing and isolation facilities. Restrict exposure to new admissions. Administer antibiotics as ordered by the physician.

Nursing Interventions

Antibiotic therapy for neonatal sepsis is often continued for as long as 2 weeks. Since the intravenous (IV) route is most reliable for most antibiotics, the maintenance of IV access for this period is often a challenge. The IV site requires meticulous care. The nurse must know the antibiotic prescribed, its dosage and side effects, and any specific precautions.

Nursing intervention includes the assessment of changes in the neurologic status that could indicate meningitis. The parents are reminded to handle the newborn gently and are shown ways to relate to their infant that do not increase discomfort such as stroking.

Some commonly occurring pathogens, mode of transmission, assessment, and nursing considerations can be found in Table 26-4.

Infants of Drug-Dependent Mothers
Etiology

The newborn whose mother is a habitual user of narcotics such as heroin or cocaine or a barbiturate will become passively addicted to the drug. Narcotic drugs readily cross the placenta into the fetus' body. The neonate may be born with malformations or undergo withdrawal in the days following birth. Placental dysfunction, intrauterine growth retardation, prematurity, or fetal hypoxia may also occur. Cocaine use increases the incidence of abruptio placentae.

≡ LEGAL AND ETHICAL
≡ CONSIDERATIONS

At least 3 dozen pregnant women in the United States have been arrested for endangering their fetuses through use of alcohol, cocaine, cigarettes, or other substances during pregnancy. Convictions have been handed down by the court for crimes ranging from manslaughter to delivering a controlled substance to a minor.

≡ LEGAL AND ETHICAL
≡ CONSIDERATIONS

Does the government have an obligation to provide care to pregnant women who are substance abusers? If a pregnant woman is convicted of substance abuse, who is responsible for providing the necessary care to the mother and her fetus?

Signs of Withdrawal in the Neonate

Tremors
Restlessness
Sleeplessness
Frequent yawning and sneezing
Hyperactive reflexes
High-pitched, shrill cry
Irritability
Uncoordinated, ineffectual sucking and swallowing
Exaggerated rooting reflex
Increased secretions, drooling, gagging
Vomiting
Diarrhea
Fever
Flushing
Dehydration

Assessment

Symptoms of withdrawal may begin as early as 12 hours after birth if the mother is addicted to heroin or as late as 1 week if the mother has been taking methadone. Typically symptoms are most pronounced 48 to 72 hours after birth and may last 6 days to 8 weeks (see Assessment Tool: Signs of Withdrawal in the Neonate).

Nursing Interventions

Nursing interventions primarily involve recognition of the symptoms that may indicate withdrawal. The nurse can reduce the stimuli that trigger hyperactivity and irritability by using a gentle, soothing voice, handling the newborn gently, holding it close, and wrapping it snugly. Irritable and hyperactive infants respond to comforting and close contact. Stimulating procedures are kept to a minimum during the withdrawal period. If excess secretions are a problem, the infant is positioned on his or her side with the head of the bed elevated. Drugs used to relieve withdrawal signs include phenobarbital, chlorpromazine (Thorazine), paregoric, diazepam (Valium), and codeine.

Fetal Alcohol Syndrome
Etiology

In general, infants diagnosed as having fetal alcohol syndrome (FAS) have been born to mothers who are chronic alcoholics who drank heavily during pregnancy. Alcohol crosses the placenta, and the fetus has the same blood alcohol level as the mother. Infants may exhibit mild manifestations of the syndrome. It is still unclear how much alcohol is too much alcohol.

Assessment

Neonates exhibit signs of alcohol withdrawal within the first few days after delivery. These signs may include hyperactivity, tremors, seizures, and difficulties in feeding and sleeping. In addition to withdrawal signs, the infant may show anomalies or developmental problems such as the following:

Microcephaly

Craniofacial abnormalities

Mental retardation

Developmental delay apparent in 1 to 2 years

Prenatal or postnatal growth retardation

Hypotonia

Nursing Interventions

Nursing interventions for FAS are directed toward decreased stimulation during withdrawal. Feeding may be difficult and require extra time and patience because of poor sucking. Temperature stability may be a problem if the newborn is small for gestational age. The newborn is double wrapped, and a cap is used to cover his or her head if the temperature is low.

REFERENCE

1. Waechter EH, Phillips J, Holaday B: Nursing Care of Children. Philadelphia, JB Lippincott, 1985

SUGGESTED READINGS

Klaus MH, Fanaroff MB: Care of the High-Risk Neonate. Philadelphia, WB Saunders, 1986

Knuppel RA, Drukker JE: High Risk Pregnancy: A Team Approach. Philadelphia, WB Saunders, 1986

Korones SB: High-Risk Newborn Infants. St Louis, CV Mosby, 1981

Larson JW: Recognizing and treating group B strep infections. Contemp OB/GYN 19:41-42, 1982

Mead PB: Infection control in the era of AIDS. Contemp OB/GYN 32:116-118, September 1988

Reeder SJ, Martin LL: Maternity Nursing, 16th ed. Philadelphia, JB Lippincott, 1988

Sever JL: TORCH infections: The list keeps growing. Contemp OB/GYN 33:65-72, 1989

High-Risk Neonatal Care

IMPORTANT TERMINOLOGY

high-risk neonate Newborn, regardless of gestational age or birth weight, who has a greater-than-average chance of mortality or morbidity

hypoglycemia Low blood sugar; <30 mg for term infants and <20 mg/dl for low birth weight infants

intrauterine growth retardation (IUGR) Infant whose rate of intrauterine growth was slowed and who was delivered before or later than term

large-for-gestational-age (LGA) infant Infant whose birth weight falls above the 90th percentile on growth curves

meconium aspiration syndrome Condition caused by intrauterine hypoxia in which relaxation of the anal spincter permits passage of meconium into amniotic fluid; aspiration occurs before or at birth; results in obstruction of air passages, infection, or chemical pneumonitis

neutral thermal environment Permits infant to maintain a normal core temperature with minimum oxygen consumption and caloric expenditure

polycythemia Increased number of circulating red blood cells, causing hemoglobin level >20 g/dl and hematocrit rate >65%

postmature or postterm Infant born after 42 weeks of gestation, regardless of birth weight

premature or preterm Infant born before completion of 37 weeks of gestation, regardless of birth weight

small-for-gestational-age (SGA) infant Infant whose birth weight falls below the 10th percentile on growth curves

Early identification of the infant at high risk is often life-saving for the potentially compromised baby. Classification of a newborn as high risk may be the result of antepartal, intrapartal, or neonatal risk factors. Many of the factors contributing to the birth of a high-risk infant are not specific for a particular problem or condition but are generally related to increased morbidity and mortality. Others have specific associations with neonatal disorders or fetal abnormalities. This chapter presents the risk factors associated with **premature** and **postmature** infants.

Regionalization of Neonatal Care

Since 1978, most states have developed plans for regionalization of perinatal care. Purposes of regionalization of care are to (1) deliver care to most high-risk infants in any geographic area and (2) deliver skilled care most economically to a larger number of people. Three levels of hospital care, primary, intermediate, and tertiary, have been identified. After his or her identification, the newborn is transferred to a facility with the appropriate level of care. Level 1, or primary, care facilities are generally community hospitals. Care is provided for healthy term infants and the larger, healthier premature infants. Because all complications cannot be identified in advance, level one units must be able to provide emergency services until the baby can be transferred to a facility with greater capacity. Level 2, or intermediate, facilities focus on care of infants with more complex needs, premature infants with mild-to-moderate hyaline membrane disease, term infants with certain illnesses such as sepsis, and recovering infants. Initial care is provided for severely compromised infants until transport can be arranged. Level 3, or tertiary, centers provide sophisticated care. They are staffed by highly skilled, experienced nurses and doctors who are consultants to the centers within the specified region. Respiratory support and a full range of surgical and other services are available.

Neonatal Intensive Care Units

Specialized nurseries providing highly skilled care to the premature or sick newborn were introduced in the United States in the mid-1960s. Neonatal mortality is lowest and newborns who survive have the best outcome when cared for by a skilled, caring health team in a well-equipped neonatal intensive care unit (NICU) (Fig. 27-1). From the time of birth resuscitation, stabilization, possible transport, and continued care in the NICU provide the newborn with the most optimistic outcome.

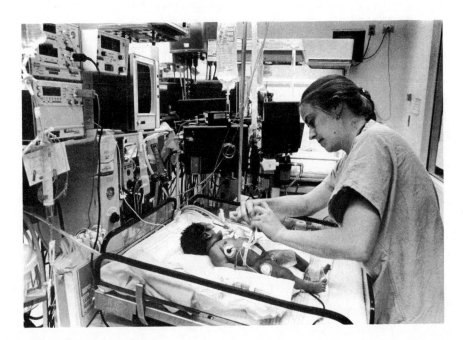

FIGURE 27-1

A Typical NICU Scene. Infant is being cared for in an open radiant warming bed that allows easy access for assessment and care. The temperature is assessed by a probe attached to the skin or by the axillary or rectal route. Note the sophisticated equipment, which includes a variety of monitoring devices and IV pump. The nurse prepares family members before they visit the NICU so they are not frightened or overwhelmed by the equipment.

The nurse who cares for critically ill neonates requires specialized knowledge and skills achieved through advanced education and experience in neonatal nursing.

The NICU must have the equipment needed for resuscitation and maintenance of respiration and for monitoring temperature, respirations, heart rate, blood pressure, blood gas values, and other factors in the newborn's health status. Thermoregulation is maintained in open radiant warmers or isolettes. One-to-one nursing care is provided when intense critical newborn care is required.

Assessment (Identification) of the High-Risk Neonate

Although the causes of prematurity and altered fetal growth are not completely understood, several associated factors have been identified that alert nurses and physicians to the possibility of these problems. Early recognition of mothers with high-risk pregnancies and careful prenatal care can often contribute to a better outcome for the infant and the mother. Factors associated with **high-risk neonates** are listed in Table 27-1.

Disorders of Gestational Age and Birth Weight

In the past all newborns weighing 2500 g or less were termed premature, and those weighing more were designated fullterm. This approach assumed that intrauterine growth rates were the same for all fetuses and that birth weight corresponded to gestational age (Fig. 27-2). A consid-

FIGURE 27-2

Intrauterine Growth Chart. This chart records intrauterine growth status for gestational ages according to appropriateness of growth. Points A, B, and C (added to original diagram) correspond to infants shown in Fig. 27-3. Not all infants are 32 weeks gestation.

From Battaglia FC, Lubchenco LO: Pediatrics 71:159, 1967.

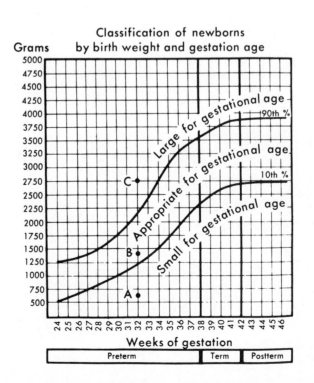

TABLE 27-1

Identification of High-Risk Infant: Associated Factors

ANTEPARTUM FACTORS

Maternal Characteristics

Age less than 15 or more than 35 yr
Low socioeconomic status
Unmarried
Family or marital conflicts
Emotional illness or family history of mental illness
Persistent ambivalence or conflicts about the pregnancy
Stature less than 5 feet
20% underweight or overweight
Malnutrition

Reproductive History

Parity greater than eight
Two or more previous abortions
Previous stillborn or neonatal death
Previous premature labor or low-birth-weight infant (<2500 g)
Previous excessively large infant (>4000 g)
Infant with isoimmunization or ABO incompatibility
Infant with congenital anomaly, genetic disorder, or birth damage
Preeclampsia or eclampsia
Uterine fibroids >5 cm or submucous
Abnormal Papanicolaou smear
Infertility
Prior cesarean section
Prior fetal malpresentations
Contracted pelvis
Ovarian masses
Genital tract abnormalities (incompetent cervix, subseptate or bicornate uterus)
Pregnancy occurring 3 mon or less after last delivery
Previous prolonged labor or significant dystocia

Substance Abuse

Drugs
Alcohol
Heavy smoking (>2 packs/day)

Medical Problems

Chronic hypertension
Renal disease (pyelonephritis, glomerulonephritis, polycystic kidney)
Diabetes mellitus (classes B to F)
Heart disease (aortic insufficiency, pulmonary hypertension, diastolic murmur, cardiac enlargement, heart failure, dysrhythmia)
Sickle cell trait or disease

Anemias with hemoglobin <9 g and hematocrit <32%
Pulmonary disease (tuberculosis, chronic obstructive pulmonary disease)
Endocrine disorders (hypothyroidism or hyperthyroidism, family history of cretinism, adrenal or pituitary problems)
Gastrointestonal or liver disease
Epilepsy
Malignancy (including leukemia and Hodgkin's disease)

Complications of Present Pregnancy

Low or excessive weight gain
Hypertension (mean arterial pressure >90, blood pressure 140/90, increase >30 mm Hg systolic or >20 mm Hg diastolic)
Recurrent glycosuria and abnormal fasting blood sugar or glucose tolerance test
Uterine size inappropriate for gestational age (either too large or too small)
Recurrent urinary tract infections
Severe varicosities or thrombophlebitis
Recurrent vaginal bleeding
Premature rupture of membranes
Multiple pregnancy
Hydramnios with a single fetus
Rh negative with a rising titer
Late or no prenatal care
Exposure to teratogens (medications, x-ray, radioactive isotopes)
Viral infections (rubella, cytomegalovirus, herpes, mumps, rubeola, chickenpox, shingles, smallpox, vaccinia, influenza, poliomyelitis, hepatitis, Western equine encephalitis, coxsackie virus B)
Syphilis, especially late pregnancy
Bacterial infections (gonorrhea, tuberculosis, listeriosis, severe acute infection)
Protozoan infections (toxoplasmosis, malaria)
Postmaturity
Anemia with hemoglobin of 9 g or less
Severe preeclampsia, eclampsia
Abnormal contraction stress test
Falling urinary estriol levels

INTRAPARTUM FACTORS

Complications of Labor and Delivery

Labor longer than 24 hr in primigravida

Labor longer than 12 hr in multigravida
Second stage longer than 1 hr
Ruptured membranes more than 24 hr
Abnormal presentation or position
Heavy sedation or injudicious anesthesia
Maternal fever or infection
Placenta previa or abruptio placentae
Cesarean section
Meconium-stained amniotic fluid
Fetal distress caused by monitoring or scalp blood sampling
Prolapsed cord
High forceps or midforceps delivery, difficult or operative delivery
Premature labor
Severe preeclampsia, eclampsia
Precipitous labor less than 3 hr
Elective induction
Oxytocin (Pitocin) augmentation

Immediate Problems of Infant

Malformation or other significant abnormality
Birth injury
Asphyxia (Apgar <6 at 5 min)

NEONATAL FACTORS

Characteristics of Infant

Preterm or premature
SGA or LGA
Birth weight <5½ pounds or >9 pounds
Low-set ears
Enlargement of one or both kidneys
Single palmar crease
Single umbilical artery
Small head size

Clinical Problems

Feeding problems
Anemia
Hyperbilirubinemia
Temperature instability
Respiratory distress
Hypoglycemia
Polycythemia
Sepsis
Rh or ABO incompatibilities
Hypocalcemia
Persistent cyanosis
Shock
Seizures
Heart murmur

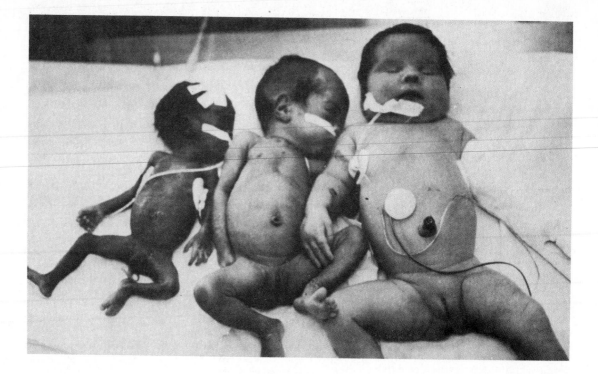

FIGURE 27-3

Variations in Infants of Identical Gestational Ages. These three infants are the same gestational age but weigh 600, 1400, and 2750 g, respectively, from left to right. They are plotted on Figure 27-2 at points A, B, and C. The smallest infant is malnourished, probably because of impaired placental function, the middle infant is premature, and the largest infant is characteristic of an infant from a diabetic mother.

From Korones S, Lancaster J: High-Risk Newborn Infant. St. Louis, CV Mosby, 1981.

erable amount of data has accumulated to demonstrate the inaccuracy of this assumption, and the two dimensions of birth weight and gestational age are now considered separately (Fig. 27-3).

The World Health Organization has designated a term birth as one occurring between 38 weeks and 42 weeks gestation, with age calculated from the date of the mother's last menstrual period. Premature are those infants born before 37 weeks gestation, and postmature are those born after 42 weeks gestation.

The most widely used growth chart gives percentiles of intrauterine growth for weight, length, and head circumference. Infants who fall below the 10th percentile are **small-for-gestational-age** (SGA), and those above the 90th percentile are **large-for-gestational-age,** (LGA).

Clinical signs, potential problems, and nursing interventions for large-for-gestational-age, small-for-gestational-age, and postmature infants are found in Table 27-2.

≡ LEGAL AND ETHICAL
≡ CONSIDERATIONS

A hospital reached a $1.86 million settlement in a lawsuit brought for the negligence of its nurses and residents that resulted in brain damage to an infant. Forceps were used during delivery of an infant whose mother had previously delivered a child with hemophilia.

The nurses, residents, and pediatrician were charged with negligence in failing to observe the increased head circumference and failing to recognize and treat the signs and symptoms of intracranial bleeding. The obstetrician was charged with negligence in performing a forceps delivery.

From Northrop CE, Kelly ME: Legal Issues in Nursing. St. Louis, CV Mosby, 1987, p. 172.

TABLE 27-2

Comparison of Nursing Interventions for Infants of Varying Gestational Age Groups

Classification	Assessment of Clinical Signs	Potential Problems	Nursing Interventions
Small for gestational age (intrauterine growth retardation [IUGR])	Loose, dry skin Vernix often decreased or absent Decrease in subcutaneous tissue and fat Sunken abdomen Thin, yellow, dull umbilical cord Sparse scalp hair Wide-eyed look	Increased risk of morbidity and mortality Related to abnormalities of fetus or pregnancy Prone to asphyxia at birth Prone to meconium aspiration Temperature instability Polycythemia Hypothermia Hypoglycemia	Nurses and doctors skilled in resuscitation present at birth Blood glucose evaluation on admission and every 2-4 hr Provision of caloric and fluid requirements Early feeding if hypoglycemic Provision of thermal environment
Large for gestational age	If infant of diabetic mother (IDM): Fat and enlarged appearance Ruddiness Puffy appearance Early lethargy Irritability, jitteriness, tremors	Often the infant of a diabetic mother Other factors: heredity; males are larger than females; occurs in second or third pregnancies Prone to birth injuries, cephalohematoma, ecchymosis Hypoglycemia Hyperbilirubinemia Polycythemia If IDM: congenital anomalies	Assessment of gestational age in relation to birth weight Assessment for complications Monitoring of temperature and respiratory status Frequent glucose assessment Provision of glucose, fluid, and caloric intake based on condition of infant
Postmature	May have symptoms of IUGR (see above) or of infant 1 to 3 wk old Lanugo absent Abundant scalp hair Long fingernails Cracked parchment or desquamating skin Long, thin appearance Worried look	Prone to uterine hypoxia related to decreasing efficiency of the placenta Meconium aspiration Hypoglycemia Polycythemia	Nurses and doctors skilled in resuscitation present at birth Blood glucose evaluation on admission

Potential Problems of the High-Risk Newborn

Asphyxia

Any newborn may be a victim of asphyxia during the labor and delivery process or immediately after birth. Some infants, e.g., SGA infants, are particularly vulnerable to asphyxia.

Primary asphyxia occurs when asphyxia has been prolonged more than 1 to 2 minutes. The newborn with asphyxia is cyanotic and has diminished reflexes, bradycardia of 60 to 100 beats/minute, and an Apgar score of 3 to 5. Gasping respirations begin approximately 2 minutes after performance of gentle suctioning and administration of oxygen.

Secondary apnea occurs with severe bradycardia of 20 to 60 beats/minute. The newborn is ashen, and the Apgar score is 1 to 3. No gasping is initiated with suctioning. The infant must be resuscitated.

Resuscitation technique includes maintaining an open airway, assisting with breathing, and maintaining circulation. All procedures should be performed under the open warmer to allow easy access and temperature monitoring. After the resuscitative measures, the newborn is transferred to the NICU.

The neonate with asphyxia is prone to acidosis, **hypoglycemia,** and cold stress. Glycogen stores may be depleted during asphyxia, and hypothermia increases glucose use.

An NICU nurse, a neonatologist, and a respiratory therapist should be present at all high-risk deliveries and should be available on call at all deliveries.

Meconium Aspiration Syndrome

Aspiration of meconium into the alveoli, occurring in utero or after birth, results from fetal hypoxia. The fetal response to hypoxia includes reflex relaxation of the anal sphincter and accelerated intestinal peristalsis, in addition to reflex gasping, which draws the meconium into the tracheobronchial system.

Meconium in the respiratory tract acts like a foreign body and blocks the flow of air into the alveoli. Increasing inflation of the alveoli distal to the obstruction can lead to their rupture and the leakage of air into the interstitial tissue. This initiates a series of complications such as pulmonary interstitial emphysema, pneumomediastinum, and pneumothorax. The asphyxia that results from these meconium effects on the lungs leads to involvement of the central nervous system, kidneys, erythropoietic system, and metabolism, which is associated with the **meconium aspiration syndrome.** The syndrome may be prevented or minimized through appropriate obstetric management of the mother in whom there is evidence of meconium-stained amniotic fluid and prompt removal of meconium from the infant's upper respiratory tract immediately after birth.[1] Direct visualization and suctioning are essential preventive measures.

Hypoglycemia

Transient hypoglycemia is a frequent occurrence in high-risk infants. All neonates have a drop in glucose after birth; however, most neonates are able to stabilize at a normal level (<40 mg/dl) within several hours. Hypoglycemia is defined as a blood glucose level <40 mg/dl using a Dextrostix test (or similar test) on capillary blood obtained from a heel stick or a level of 30 mg/dl when venous blood is used. For the small infant who weighs <2500 g, hypoglycemia is defined as a level <20 mg/dl.

Factors related to the occurrence of hypoglycemia are an SGA infant, prematurity, respiratory distress, a diabetic mother, hypothermia, and **polycythemia.** The neonate with hypoglycemia may be asymptomatic or have any of the following symptoms: apathy, jitteriness, tremors, hypotonia, high-pitched or weak cry, cyanosis, eye-rolling, or sweating.

Therapy for hypoglycemia consists of oral or intravenous administration of glucose followed by glucose determinations. Continued monitoring of glucose levels is necessary every 4 hours for 24 hours.

The Premature or Preterm Infant

It is generally recognized that the major cause of morbidity in the neonatal period is prematurity. The premature neonate is one born before the 37th week of gestation, regardless of birth weight. Most infants who weigh <2500 g at birth and almost all neonates <1500 g are born prematurely. The majority of these newborns are appropriate in size for the gestational age. However, the premature neonate of a diabetic mother may weigh >2500 g. The main criteria for prematurity is gestational age as determined by assessment.

The cause of the majority of premature births is unknown. Some conditions that have been clearly related to premature births include pregnancy-induced hypertension, cervical incompetence, diabetes, sepsis, multiple pregnancy, placenta previa, and abruptio placentae.

Kangaroo Care

A method of caring for preterm infants without the risk (or with modified use) of highly technical equipment is becoming well-known throughout the world. Once the infant is stabilized, the mother (or father) carries the newborn skin-to-skin to maintain the infant's warmth. The mother holds the diaper-clad infant upright and prone between her breasts and allows self-regulatory breast-feeding.[2] The skin-to-skin, or kangaroo, care originated in 1979 in Bogota, Columbia, because of the lack of incubators there. Infant mortality and morbidity rates were significantly reduced with this method. The method with modifications is widely used in Europe.

Assessment

The length of gestational age greatly affects the infant's chances for survival. Mortality rates increase as birth weight and gestational age decrease. Survival is unlikely in the 24- to 27-weeks gestational age range, is better in the 28- to 30-weeks range, and is good in the 31- to 36-weeks range for infants who receive appropriate therapy. Characteristics of the preterm infant are found in Assessment Tool: Characteristics of Premature Infant.

Characteristics of Premature Infant   ASSESSMENT
                                                                          TOOL

Periodic breathing with episodes of apnea
Thin, transparent skin
Abundant vernix
Fine, feathery hair
Little subcutaneous fat
Head large in relation to body
Limbs extended
Ear cartilages poorly developed
Clitoris prominent in female
Scrotum underdeveloped in male
Absent, weak, or ineffectual grasping, sucking, and swallowing
Unable to maintain body temperature

Nursing Intervention

Nursing care of the preterm newborn is directed toward maintaining major physiologic functions, preventing complications, and supporting the parents (see Nursing Care Plan: High-Risk Infant).

Common Health Problems of the Preterm Infant

Potential for Ineffective Gas Exchange

The preterm infant is at risk for respiratory problems. The lungs are not fully mature until 37 to 38 weeks gestation. Air sacs tend to collapse

---

NURSING
CARE
PLAN

High-Risk Infant

Goals (Expected Outcomes)	Interventions	Rationale	Evaluation
Ineffective Thermoregulation—Related to Immature Temperature Control, Infection, Decreased Subcutaneous Tissue			
Infant's temperature will remain within normal limits (97.7° to 98.6° F axillary).	Place infant in isolette or radiant warmer or wrap well in an open crib. Avoid chilling infant when removed from warming unit.	Preterm infant has high skin surface relative to body mass, which promotes heat loss, and has a small subcutaneous fat layer. Promotes a neutral thermal environment in which the infant's core temperature is normal and oxygen use and calorie output is minimal.	Temperature is within normal parameters (97.7° to 98.6° F axillary). Mechanical temperature of isolette or radiant warmer is within set parameters.
Altered Nutrition: Less Than Body Requirements—Related to Inability to Ingest Adequate Nutrients Because of Immature Sucking Ability, Weakness, or Fatigue			
Infant will ingest adequate formula or breast milk (specify amount). Infant will demonstrate steady weight gain (6-8 ounces/wk).	Maintain intravenous lines. Offer enteral feedings when infant is stable as evidenced by: Temperature neutral Normal breathing Good color and cry Offer amounts determined by infant's size, age, condition. Feed for 20-30 min only to avoid tiring infant. Gavage feed infants more than 32 wk old or more than 1650 g with poor sucking. Conserve neonate's energy.	Oral feedings are contraindicated if tachypnea is present because of danger of aspiration. Amount and method of feeding are ordered by the physician according to size and condition of the infant. Coordination of sucking and swallowing occurs at approximately 32 to 34 wk gestation. Intermittent gavage feeding through the mouth is a safe means of feeding for infants who are too weak to suck effectively or who become excessively tired, listless, or cyanotic during feedings.	Infant tolerates formula without vomiting, distention of abdomen, or changes in heart rate or blood pressure. Infant begins to make attempts at sucking and swallowing during gavage. Infant has steady weight gain.

NURSING
CARE
PLAN

High-Risk Infant—*continued*

Goals (Expected Outcomes)	Interventions	Rationale	Evaluation
Impairment in Skin Integrity—Related to Immature Skin Structure and Use of Tape to Fasten Monitoring Devices and Intravenous Lines			
Infant's skin remains intact without evidence of irritation or trauma.	Cleanse skin with water. Use transpore tape to secure items to skin. Apply protective covering to skin before taping. Exert great care when handling skin. Place on water pillow or fleece. Change position every 2-3 hr.	Skin of the preterm infant is thin, sensitive, and fragile and is easily damaged. Damaged skin provides an entrance for pathogens and resultant infections.	Infant's skin remains intact.
Altered Parenting—Related to Interruption of Bonding Process or Lack of Parental Knowledge			
Parents express feelings and concerns about the infant and his or her progress. Parents visit infant as frequently as possible.	Give parents adequate preparation and information when visiting infant. Answer parents' questions and allow expressions of concern. Provide photographs and emphasize specialness of newborn.	There is evidence that the physical and emotional separation of the parent(s) and infant interfere with the normal bonding and attachment processes.	Parents share their concerns and anxieties about their infant. Parents visit at times when they can become involved in infant's care.
Parents demonstrate care for infant as appropriate.	Demonstrate care of newborn when parents show readiness.	Parental involvement, assisted by the nurse, helps parents to cope with care of their infant and to assume care when infant is discharged.	Parents call their infant by name and verbalize interest in infant as an individual.
Ineffective Breathing Pattern—Related to Immature Breathing Center, Impaired Gas Exchange, Decreased Lung Expansion or Fatigue			
Infant's breathing is unlabored, and periods of apnea are within normal limits (state parameters). Infant's breathing rate is within normal limits (state parameters).	Observe, record, and report signs and symptoms of respiratory distress: Tachpnea Cyanosis Retractions Grunting Nasal flaring Diminished breath sounds Keep airway open by suctioning and positioning. Administer O_2 along with appropriate monitoring of blood gas values. Change position frequently. Gently stimulate to breathe during periods of apnea. Monitor heart and respiratory rates and number and length of apneic periods.	Without surfactant the preterm infant has difficulty keeping the lungs inflated. Atelectasis and hypoxemia may result. The preterm baby also has weak chest wall muscles. O_2 therapy provides adequate O_2 to the tissues.	Respirations are regular and the rate within normal limits.

Continued

NURSING
CARE
PLAN

High-Risk Infant

Goals (Expected Outcomes)

Goals (Expected Outcomes)	Interventions	Rationale	Evaluation
Fluid Volume Deficit—Related to Insensible Water Loss, Inadequate Fluid Intake, or Infectious Process			
Infant exhibits no symptoms of dehydration. Infant loses minimum birth weight.	Maintain intravenous lines and monitor closely for infiltration. Administer correct fluid and correct amount per hour. Record total intake per shift and daily.	Providing adequate fluids is very important for the preterm infant because his or her extracellular water content is higher than that of a fullterm infant.	Intravenous site is free of infiltration signs. Intravenous fluids are flowing at correct rates as ordered by physician.
	Observe for signs of dehydration: Skin turgor Urinary output Condition of fontanel Temperature Weight loss Mucous membrane Urinary specific gravity	The preterm infant's kidneys are underdeveloped and are very vulnerable to water loss.	Minimal weight loss. No symptoms of dehydration.

because of minimum surfactant production. Mature alveoli are not present until 34 to 36 weeks. The regulatory center for respiration in the brain is also immature.

Apnea

A pattern of periodic breathing is quite common in the preterm baby. True apneic periods last 10 to 15 seconds and are accompanied by pallor, cyanosis, hypotonia, and bradycardia. This disorder is a result of immature neurologic and pulmonary function. Nursing care is directed toward maintaining body temperature, using tactile stimulation, a rocker bed, or a water bed, and using theophylline, a respiratory stimulant and bronchodilator (see Drug Guide below).

 DRUG GUIDE

Theophylline: Used in treatment of apnea and bradycardia of prematurity.

Therapeutic Action: Relaxes bronchial smooth muscle, causing bronchodilation and increasing vital capacity that has been impaired by bronchospasm and air trapping.

Dosage: 2 mg/kg/day to maintain serum concentrations between 3 and 5 μg/ml. Special note: The initial and maintenance doses in preterm infants must be reduced because elimination of theophylline apparently is delayed.

Potential Side Effects and Complications: Tremors, dysrhythmias, tachycardia, seizures, vomiting.

Nursing Implications:
1. Monitor serum theophylline levels carefully. Report results to physician.
2. Carefully monitor infant for clinical signs of adverse effects. Monitor apical pulse, respirations, blood pressure, lung sounds, and input and output for diuresis.
3. Provide environmental control (heat, light, noise) if irritability, restlessness, or sleeplessness occurs.

Adapted from Karch A, Boyd E: Handbook of Drugs and the Nursing Process. Philadelphia, JB Lippincott, 1989.

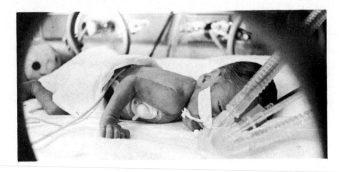

FIGURE 27-4
Continous Positive Airway Pressure
(CPAP). Nasal continuous positive airway
pressure is a method of ventilation used in
infants with respiratory distress syndrome.
The objective is to apply just enough
pressure to open and keep open the alveoli.

Respiratory Distress Syndrome

Respiratory distress syndrome is one cause of morbidity and mortality among preterm neonates. A deficiency in surfactant forces the infant to work to reexpand the lungs with each inspiration. The result is fatigue, rapid and labored respirations, and other symptoms of respiratory distress. All the infant's energy is directed toward the effort of sustaining respirations. Mechanical ventilation is frequently used to assist the infant or to breathe for him or her (Fig. 27-4). Under study is the administration of surfactant to the lungs in an effort to facilitate respiration.

Potential for Alteration in Cardiac Function

Incomplete development of the pulmonary system in the preterm infant significantly affects the change from fetal to neonatal circulation in the preterm neonate.

PATENT DUCTUS ARTERIOSUS. Functional closure of the ductus arteriosus, the bypass for the lungs that connects the pulmonary artery and the aorta, occurs in the fullterm infant in the first 24 hours of life. Anatomic closure occurs in a few days. In the preterm infant closure is delayed. Clinical manifestations of this failure to close are evident on the third or fourth day after birth. Murmurs, tachycardia, bounding pulses, and signs of pulmonary edema may be observed.

Potential for Alterations in Nutrition

Maturity of the gastrointestinal tract is established by 36 to 38 weeks gestation. Sucking, swallowing, and gag reflexes are often decreased or absent. Stomach capacity is reduced. Absorption of fat may be decreased. Infants may require an alternative route for delivery of nutrients such as gavage (Fig. 27-5), nasojejunal tube, or parenteral hyperalimentation. Infants who are able to nipple feed are easily fatigued by sucking efforts and may experience apnea, cyanosis, and pallor during feeding. Special formulas have been commercially formulated to provide sufficient calories and nutrients for growth in an amount of liquid that can be tolerated by the preterm newborn.

Necrotizing Enterocolitis

Necrotizing enterocolitis (NEC) is a serious disease of the preterm newborn in which necrosis of the bowel results from asphyxia. During an

FIGURE 27-5

Gavage Feeding. With a gavage feeding the formula or breast milk flows in by gravity. The feeding tube is placed intermittently through the mouth into the stomach by the nurse. The infant sucks on a pacifier between feedings to stimulate sucking. The nurse observes the infant for apnea, regurgitation, and distention after feeding.

From Murray EH, Phillips J, Holaday B: Waechter's Nursing Care of Children, 10th ed. Philadelphia, JB Lippincott, 1985.

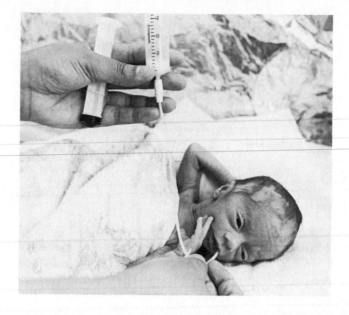

asphyxial episode blood is shunted from the intestine to the brain and heart, resulting in ischemia of the bowel. Perforation of the bowel may occur. Signs include abdominal distention, vomiting, diarrhea, and gastrointestinal bleeding. Most infants who have developed NEC were fed a cow's milk formula; few were fed only breast milk.

REFERENCES

1. Korones S, Lancaster J: High-Risk Newborn Infants, 3rd ed. St. Louis, CV Mosby, 1981

2. Anderson GA: Skin-to-skin: Kangaroo care in Western Europe. Am J Nurs 89:662-666, May 1989

SUGGESTED READINGS

Copel J et al: Contraction stress testing with nipple stimulation. J Reprod Med 30(6): 465-471, June 1985

Foster RLR, Hunsberger MM, Anderson JJT: Family-centered nursing care of children. Philadelphia, WB Saunders, 1989

Holmes J, Magiera L: Maternity Nursing. New York, Macmillan, 1987

Iyer P, Toptich BJ, Bernocchi-Losey D: Nursing Process and Nursing Diagnosis. Philadelphia, WB Saunders, 1986

Karb A, Boyd E: Handbook on Drugs and Nursing Process. Philadelphia, JB Lippincott, 1989

Klaus M, Fanaroff A: Care of the High-Risk Neonate, 3rd ed. Philadelphia, WB Saunders, 1986

Knuppel R, Drukker I: High-Risk Pregnancy. Philadelphia, WB Saunders, 1986

Murray EH, Phillips J, Holaday B: Waechter's Nursing Care of Children, 10th ed. Philadelphia, JB Lippincott, 1985

Northrop CE, Kelly ME: Legal Issues in Nursing. St. Louis, CV Mosby, 1987

Patrick M et al: Medical-Surgical Nursing. Philadelphia, JB Lippincott, 1986

Reeder S, Martin L: Maternity Nursing, 16th ed. Philadelphia, JB Lippincott, 1987

Whaley L, Wong D: Essentials of Pediatric Nursing, 3rd ed. St. Louis, CV Mosby, 1989

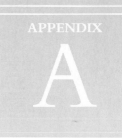

Universal Precautions for Prevention of Transmission of HIV, Hepatitis B Virus and Other Bloodborne Pathogens in Health Care Settings

Body Fluids to Which Universal Precautions Apply

Universal precautions apply to blood and to other body fluids containing visible blood. Occupational transmission of HIV and HBV to health-care workers by blood is documented. Blood is the single most important source of HIV, HBV, and other bloodborne pathogens in the occupational setting. Infection control efforts for HIV, HBV, and other bloodborne pathogens must focus on preventing exposures to blood as well as on delivering HBV immunization.

Universal precautions also apply to semen and vaginal secretions. Although both of these fluids have been implicated in the sexual transmission of HIV and HBV, they have not been implicated in occupational transmission from patient to health-care worker. This observation is not unexpected, since exposure to semen in the usual health-care setting is limited, and the routine practice of wearing gloves for performing vaginal examinations protects health-care workers from exposure to potentially infectious vaginal secretions.

Universal precautions also apply to tissues and to the following fluids: cerebrospinal fluid (CSF), synovial fluid, pleural fluid, peritoneal fluid, pericardial fluid, and amniotic fluid. The risk of transmission of HIV and HBV from these fluids is unknown; epidemiologic studies in the health-care and community setting are currently inadequate to assess the potential risk to health-care workers from occupational exposures to them. However, HIV has been isolated from CSF, synovial, and amniotic fluid, and HBsAg has been detected in synovial fluid, amniotic fluid, and peritoneal fluid.

From Centers for Disease Control: Morbidity and Mortality Weekly Report 37(24):377-388, June 24, 1988.

Body Fluids to Which Universal Precautions Do Not Apply

Universal precautions do not apply to feces, nasal secretions, sputum, sweat, tears, urine, and vomitus unless they contain visible blood. The risk of transmission of HIV and HBV from these fluids and materials is extremely low or nonexistent. HIV has been isolated and HBsAg has been demonstrated in some of these fluids; however, epidemiologic studies in the health-care and community setting have not implicated these fluids or materials in the transmission of HIV and HBV infections. Some of the above fluids and excretions represent a potential source for nosocomial and community-acquired infections with other pathogens and recommendations for preventing the transmission of nonbloodborne pathogens have been published.

Precautions for Other Body Fluids in Special Settings

Human breast milk has been implicated in perinatal transmission of HIV, and HBsAg has been found in the milk of mothers infected with HBV. However, occupational exposure to human breast milk has not been implicated in the transmission of HIV nor HBV infection to health-care workers. Moreover, the health-care worker will not have the same type of intensive exposure to breast milk as the nursing neonate. Whereas universal precautions do not apply to human breast milk, gloves may be worn by health-care workers in situations where exposures to breast milk might be frequent, for example, in breast milk banking.

Saliva of some persons infected with HBV has been shown to contain HBV-DNA at concentrations 1:1,000 to 1:10,000 of that found in the infected person's serum. HBsAg-positive saliva has been shown to be infectious when injected into experimental animals and in human bite exposures. However, HBsAg-positive saliva has not been shown to be infectious when applied to oral mucous membranes in experimental primate studies or through contamination of musical instruments or cardiopulmonary resuscitation dummies used by HBV carriers. Epidemiologic studies of nonsexual household contacts of HIV-infected patients, including several small series in which HIV transmission failed to occur after bites or after percutaneous inoculation or contamination of cuts and open wounds with saliva from HIV-infected patients, suggest that the potential for salivary transmission of HIV is remote. One case report from Germany has suggested the possibility of transmission of HIV in a household setting from an infected child to a sibling through a human bite. The bite did not break the skin or result in bleeding. Since the date of seroconversion to HIV was not known for either child in this case, evidence for the role of saliva in the transmission of virus is unclear. Another case report suggested the possibility of transmission of HIV from husband to wife by contact with saliva during kissing. However, follow-up studies did not confirm HIV infection in the wife.

Universal precautions do not apply to saliva. General infection control practices already in existence — including the use of gloves for digital examination of mucous membranes and endotracheal suctioning, and handwashing after exposure to saliva — should further minimize the minute risk, if any, for salivary transmission of HIV and HBV. Gloves need not be worn when feeding patients and when wiping saliva from skin.

Special precautions, however, are recommended for dentistry. Occupationally acquired infection with HBV in dental workers has been documented, and two possible cases of occupationally acquired HIV infection involving dentists have been reported. During dental procedures, contamination of saliva with blood is predictable, trauma to health-care workers' hands is common, and blood spattering may occur. Infection control precautions for dentistry minimize the potential for nonintact skin and mucous membrane contact of dental health-care workers to blood-contaminated saliva of patients. In addition, the use of gloves for oral examinations and treatment in the dental setting may also protect the patient's oral mucous membranes from exposures to blood, which may occur from breaks in the skin of dental workers' hands.

Use of Protective Barriers

Protective barriers reduce the risk of exposure of the health-care worker's skin or mucous membranes to potentially infective materials. For universal precautions, protective barriers reduce the risk of exposure to blood, body fluids containing visible blood, and other fluids to which universal precautions apply. Examples of protective barriers include gloves, gowns, masks, and protective eyewear. Gloves should reduce the incidence of contamination of hands, but they cannot prevent penetrating injuries due to needles or other sharp instruments. Masks and protective eyewear or face shields should reduce the incidence of contamination of mucous membranes of the mouth, nose, and eyes.

Universal precautions are intended to supplement rather than replace recommendations for routine infection control, such as handwashing and using gloves to prevent gross microbial contamination of hands. Because specifying the types of barriers needed for every possible clinical situation is impractical, some judgment must be exercised.

The risk of nosocomial transmission of HIV, HBV, and other blood-borne pathogens can be minimized if health-care workers use the following general guidelines:*

1. Take care to prevent injuries when using needles, scalpels, and other sharp instruments or devices; when handling sharp instruments after procedures; when cleaning used instruments; and when disposing of used needles. Do not recap used needles by hand; do not remove used needles from disposable syringes by hand; and do not bend, break, or otherwise manipulate used needles by hand. Place used disposable syringes and needles, scalpel blades, and other sharp items in puncture-resistant containers for disposal. Locate the puncture-resistant containers as close to the use area as is practical.
2. Use protective barriers to prevent exposure to blood, body fluids containing visible blood, and other fluids to which universal precautions apply. The type of protective barrer(s) should be appropriate for the procedure being performed and the type of exposure anticipated.
3. Immediately and thoroughly wash hands and other skin surfaces that are contaminated with blood, body fluids containing visible blood, or other body fluids to which universal precautions apply.

*The August 1987 publication should be consulted for general information and specific recommendations not addressed in this update.

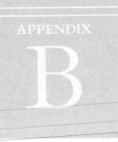

Professional Practice Standards

Standard I

THE NURSE HELPS CHILDREN AND PARENTS ATTAIN AND MAINTAIN OPTIMUM HEALTH.

Rationale

Attainment of optimum physical and psychological health by family members is the ultimate goal of health care. Nurses are in a unique position to help clients and/or families achieve this goal. Health-oriented nursing interventions include health teaching, anticipatory guidance, assistance in problem solving, and identification of actual or potential health problems and treatment and referral.

Process Criteria

The nurse—
1. Takes a health history and does a physical assessment using appropriate screening and assessment tools
2. Identifies immediate, interim, and long-term health needs of clients
3. Identifies human responses and reactions to actual and potential health problems
4. Formulates a plan of care in consultation with client and/or family and with nurse experts and other professionals as needed
5. Identifies cultural and belief systems which influence health and health practices
6. Refers health problems requiring other services to appropriate professionals
7. Helps client and/or family resolve concerns and problems in management of immediate, interim, and long-term health needs
8. Assesses client and/or family readiness for learning self-care skills
9. Teaches client and/or family essential self-care skills
10. Teaches client and/or family to detect changes in health status
11. Provides anticipatory guidance concerning changes in health and developmental status
12. Evaluates nursing interventions with the client and/or family on the basis of specific goal-oriented client outcomes

13. Reassesses and reorders priorities with the client and/or family, including setting new goals and revising care plans
14. Carries out physical interventions when indicated by the client's health and developmental needs
15. Functions as a resource person for the client and family in the transition period between health and illness and afterward.

Outcome Criteria

Knowledge—
1. The client and/or family explain a concept of health.
2. The client and/or family describe health practices which influence health status.
3. The client and/or family describe appropriate health related treatment and rationale.
4. The client describes normal developmental and physical processes.
5. The client and/or family describe significant health and illness cues which indicate current health status.

Skills—
1. The client and/or family demonstrate the ability to perform practices essential to health maintenance.
2. The client and a family member demonstrate the ability to perform treatment measures essential to management of minor illnesses.

Adaptation—
1. The client's health status is stable to improved.
2. The client and/or family demonstrate the ability to successfully treat minor disturbances in health status.
3. The client and family consistently carry out health practices essential to health maintenance.
4. The client and family recognize cues of changes in health status and take appropriate action.

Standard II

THE NURSE ASSISTS FAMILIES TO ACHIEVE AND MAINTAIN A BALANCE BETWEEN THE PERSONAL GROWTH NEEDS OF INDIVIDUAL FAMILY MEMBERS AND OPTIMUM FAMILY FUNCTIONING.

Rationale

Families seek to provide for the physical, psychological, and cultural needs of their members. Nursing assists clients and families in the attainment of optimum family relationships and family functioning. In addition, nursing helps families achieve a balance that respects the personal growth needs of all family members by carrying out nursing interventions that enhance role development.

Process Criteria

The nurse—
1. Collects data concerning role relationships and interaction patterns of family members
2. Diagnoses alterations or disturbances in family role relationships and family interaction patterns
3. Diagnoses deficits in the provision for personal growth needs of individual family members
4. Promotes understanding of the influence of family relationships on health status
5. Helps family develop a plan that provides for personal growth needs for all family members
6. Provides anticipatory guidance about role and family transitions and family interaction patterns
7. Creates opportunities and support for successful parenting behaviors
8. Participates in or provides leadership in parent and child support groups
9. Assesses adequacy of family support systems and mobilizes sources of support when indicated
10. Creates face-to-face opportunity for family members to share perceptions and feelings about illness
11. Evaluates nursing interventions on the basis of specific goal-oriented client outcomes
12. Reassesses and reorders priorities, including setting new goals and revising care plans.

Outcome Criteria

Knowledge—
1. The client and family describe own roles and personal needs and those of other family members.
2. The client and/or family members describe family relationships as a critical factor influencing health status.
3. The client and/or family verbalize potential for role conflict and role strain.
4. Parents and children point out successful parenting behavior.
5. Parents and children point out situations where they need to talk together about feelings.
6. Parents and children verbalize awareness of support groups as an option for meeting their emotional needs.

Skills—
1. The client and family demonstrate the ability to communicate within the family.

Adaptation—
1. The client and family carry out role transitions without major symptoms of family dysfunction.
2. Family members verbally demonstrate concern for and awareness of personal growth needs of each other.
3. Family members are able to express feelings and conflict to each other.

4. Each family member provides for the developmental and emotional needs of other members.
5. Parents consistently modify roles to meet the personal growth needs of self and others.
6. All family members are receiving adequate health care.

Standard III

THE NURSE INTERVENES WITH VULNERABLE CLIENTS AND FAMILIES AT RISK TO PREVENT POTENTIAL DEVELOPMENTAL AND HEALTH PROBLEMS.

Rationale

Individuals and families at risk are particularly vulnerable to potential health problems. Nursing seeks to identify individuals and families at risk. It also monitors them and provides protective intervention either independently or collaboratively.

Process Criteria

The nurse—
1. Collects data about individuals and families at risk, using appropriate assessment and screening tools
2. Uses knowledge of risk factors to identify individuals and families at risk
3. Monitors at-risk individuals and families for actual and potential developmental and health problems
4. Formulates a plan of care for at-risk management of vulnerable clients and families
5. Intervenes therapeutically with high-risk individuals or groups
6. Collaborates with other disciplines in treatment and referral of at-risk clients and families
7. Provides anticipatory guidance consistent with identified at-risk factors
8. Monitors clients' and families' reactions to at-risk status
9. Provides support to at-risk individuals and families
10. Teaches clients and families about at-risk situations and management
11. Evaluates nursing interventions on the basis of specific goal-oriented client outcomes
12. Reassesses at-risk status of clients and families and sets new goals and priorities.

Outcome Criteria

Knowledge—
1. The client describes at-risk status and potential physical, emotional, or developmental health problems.
2. The client and family explain strategies to prevent or minimize potential developmental and health problems.
3. The client and family explain the need for follow-up care.

Skills—
1. The client and family carry out strategies needed to prevent developmental or health problems.
2. The client and family demonstrate ability to work with other health professionals.

Adaptation—
1. At-risk clients receive the follow-up care needed.
2. The client and family consistently communicate physical and psychological needs at appropriate times.
3. At-risk clients and families maintain or improve health status.
4. The client and family manage activities of daily living (ADL).
5. The client and family manage therapeutic strategies successfully.
6. The client and family members solicit support in stressful situations.
7. The client and family notify appropriate health personnel when health status deteriorates.

Standard IV

THE NURSE PROMOTES AN ENVIRONMENT FREE OF HAZARDS TO REPRODUCTION, GROWTH AND DEVELOPMENT, WELLNESS, AND RECOVERY FROM ILLNESS.

Rationale

Nurses have historically been concerned with the provision of an environment which promotes health.

Hazards in the environment can jeopardize reproduction, growth and development, and health status. Nurses are often in a position to detect environmental hazards and help clients learn how to maintain a safe environment.

Process Criteria

The nurse—
1. Collects data on environmental hazards to reproduction, growth and development, and wellness in institutions, homes, and communities, using available assessment tools
2. Identifies actual and potential hazards to maintenance of health
3. Monitors legislative activity related to environment
4. Provides anticipatory guidance about environmental hazards to reproduction, growth and development, and health status
5. Monitors hazardous environments
6. Administers preventive measures, e.g., immunizations, according to protocols
7. Teaches clients and families about changes in life-style that minimize or eliminate environmental hazards
8. Teaches to personnel the practices that minimize or eliminate environmental hazards
9. Intervenes to minimize or eliminate environmental hazards to the client and family
10. Supports others in their efforts to maintain safe environments and provides positive reinforcement and feedback

11. Evaluates nursing interventions on the basis of specific goal-oriented client outcomes
12. Reassesses and reorders priorities, including setting new goals.

Outcome Criteria

Knowledge—
1. The client and family describe environmental hazards to reproduction, growth, and development.
2. The client and family describe environments which will support recovery from illness or healthy living.
3. The client and family describe measures to eliminate or control environmental hazards.
4. The client and family explain the effects of potential or actual environmental hazard on health.
5. The client and family describe changes in life-style to avoid environmental hazards.

Adaption—
1. Family members participate in maintaining a safe environment.
2. Family members carry out practices which minimize or eliminate environmental hazards.
3. The family monitors the environment for potential hazards.
4. The client has a decreased incidence of health problems due to environmental hazards.
5. The client has fewer complications due to hazards in the hospital environment.
6. The client demonstrates adequate growth and development.

Standard V

THE NURSE DETECTS CHANGES IN HEALTH STATUS AND DEVIATIONS FROM OPTIMUM DEVELOPMENT.

Rationale

Early detection of deviations in health and optimum development and changes in health status are essential to the prevention of illness. Nurses are in a unique position to detect these changes, initiate treatment, and promote development and health potential.

Process Criteria

The nurse—
1. Collects baseline data about health and developmental status
2. Detects subtle and significant changes in health and developmental status
3. Diagnoses physical and psychological responses to changes in health status and developmental status
4. Alters the plan of management collaboratively with the client and family, nurse experts, and other professionals as needed
5. Intervenes to treat physical and psychological responses to changes in health status and developmental deviations

6. Initiates treatment in collaboration with other health professionals to improve health and developmental status
7. Monitors health and developmental status following changes or provides for monitoring by others
8. Coordinates delivery of care when other health professionals are involved.

Outcome Criteria

Knowledge—
1. The client and family describe significant physical and psychological responses which indicate changes in health or developmental status.
2. The client and family explain the rationale for strategies required to treat changes and deviations in health and developmental status.
3. The client and family describe resources to meet health and developmental needs.

Skill—
1. The client and family demonstrate the ability to participate in evaluation of health and developmental status.
2. The client and family detect changes in health and developmental status.
3. The client and family are able to carry out therapeutic strategies.
4. The client and family are able to communicate about the client's health and developmental status.

Adaptation—
1. The client and family act appropriately when a change in health or developmental status is noted.
2. The family carries out the treatment indicated by a change in health or developmental status.
3. The client has decreased incidence of serious health or developmental problems.
4. The client has fewer complications from health or developmental problems.
5. The client and family consistently seek health teaching and anticipatory guidance about health and development.
6. The client and family comply with negotiated plan of care.

Standard VI

THE NURSE CARRIES OUT APPROPRIATE INTERVENTIONS AND TREATMENT TO FACILITATE SURVIVAL AND RECOVERY FROM ILLNESS.

Rationale

Acute care nursing requires assessment and diagnosis of the physiologic and psychological reactions of clients to illness and detection of changes in status. Nursing interventions in the independent practice domain are directed toward alleviation or resolution of problems such as pain, separation anxiety, self-care deficit, or alteration in body image. Nursing also provides a physical and psychological environment conducive to recovery and restoration of health. Nursing interventions in the interdependent practice domain, carried out in collaboration with physicians, are directed toward the alleviation or resolution of illness-related conditions.

Process Criteria

The nurse—
1. Uses data collected about physiologic and psychological responses of clients to illness to make nursing diagnoses
2. Identifies nursing problems related to illness in the interdependent domain
3. Formulates a plan of nursing management which supports the therapeutic regimen and prevents complications in collaboration with the client and family
4. Consults with nursing specialists and other professionals as needed
5. Carries out therapeutic interventions to facilitate physical and psychological recovery from illness and prevent complications
6. Initiates emergency interventions to facilitate survival
7. Provides for the client's basic physical needs as indicated by health status
8. Creates opportunities for clients to exercise control and move toward self-care and independence
9. Provides physical and psychological environment conducive to recovery and achievement of health
10. Creates opportunities for family members to participate in client's care and provide support
11. Provides information about illness and the therapeutic regimen and their rationales to client and family
12. Teaches clients and families skills and knowledge needed for home management
13. Functions as a resource person for clients and families during transition from hospital to home
14. Evaluates nursing interventions on the basis of specific goal-oriented client outcomes
15. Reassesses and reorders priorities, including setting new goals and revising plans of care.

Outcome Criteria

Knowledge—
1. The client and family explain illness and its effect on body functions.
2. The client and family explain the treatment and its rationale.
3. The client and family explain the psychosocial responses to illness of family members.
4. The client and family explain their own goals for health care, and purpose of the nursing care plan.
5. The client and family describe factors in the physical and psychological environment which facilitate recovery.
6. The client and family explain the importance of progressive independence in management of illness.

Skill—
1. Family members demonstrate strategies to provide physical and psychological support for the client during acute illness and recovery.
2. The client and family verbalize the need for support.
3. At least one member of the family can demonstrate emergency measures.

Adaptation—
1. Clients have increased rates of survival and recovery.
2. The client has fewer or less severe physical and psychological reactions to illness, treatment, and hospitalization.
3. The client recovers with fewer complications.
4. The client and family demonstrate progress toward independent care.
5. The client and family participate in the development, implementation, and evaluation of nursing care planning.
6. The client and family evaluate the achievement of their own goals with regard to illness management.
7. The client and family carry out therapeutic regimen.
8. The client and family take appropriate action in response to change in health status or in an emergency.
9. The client and family control environmental factors which enhance recovery and prevent further illness or disability.

Standard VII

THE NURSE ASSISTS CLIENTS AND FAMILIES TO UNDERSTAND AND COPE WITH DEVELOPMENTAL AND TRAUMATIC SITUATIONS DURING ILLNESS, CHILDBEARING, CHILDREARING, AND CHILDHOOD.

Rationale

Clients of maternal and child health nurses often experience developmental and/or situational crises. Due to the closeness of their relationships with clients, nurses are in a unique position to practice crisis intervention. Nursing interventions are designed to help clients and families reduce or manage stress and facilitate adaptive coping.

Process Criteria

The nurse—
1. Collects data about client's and family's perception of the situation, the amount and intensity of stress experienced, their responses, and strengths and weaknesses
2. Makes nursing diagnoses of adaptive and maladaptive coping patterns
3. Formulates a plan collaboratively with client and family to assist them in coping with the situation
4. Provides information to the client and family to prepare them for potential stressors and stress points
5. Assesses the ability of client and family to assimilate information
6. Provides support to the client and family in their adaptive coping efforts
7. Reduces or helps them reduce or manage stress

8. Suggests strategies for environmental support by the family and significant others
9. Practices crisis intervention with individuals and groups
10. Refers clients with maladaptive coping patterns to appropriate resources when indicated
11. Evaluates the effectiveness of nursing interventions based on specific goal-oriented client outcomes
12. Reassesses and reorders priorities, including setting new goals and revising plans of care.

Outcome Criteria

Knowledge—
1. Family members describe important aspects of a developmental or situational crisis.
2. Family members describe the support that they need to cope adaptively.
3. Family members describe strategies which may be used to cope adaptively.
4. Family members describe resources which they can use during current crisis.

Skill—
1. Each member of the family communicates his/her need for support.
2. Each member of the family communicates his/her need for crisis intervention.

Adaptation—
1. The client and family demonstrate flexibility in using coping strategies during developmental and situational crisis.
2. The client and family manage and reduce stress.
3. Each family member seeks and receives support during crisis.
4. The client and family participate in developing and evaluating nursing care plans aimed at enhancing coping strategies.
5. The client and family demonstrate the ability to seek and utilize information during crisis.
6. The client and family seek appropriate resources when maladaptive coping patterns predominate.

Standard VIII

THE NURSE ACTIVELY PURSUES STRATEGIES TO ENHANCE ACCESS TO AND UTILIZATION OF ADEQUATE HEALTH CARE SERVICES.

Rationale

The quality of health of childbearing and childrearing families depends on the availability and utilization of adequate health care services. MCH nursing assists clients to utilize appropriate health care services and resources. In addition, MCH nursing collaborates with consumers, other health disciplines, and governmental agencies in efforts to insure the availability and adequacy of health care services.

Process Criteria

The nurse—
1. Identifies available resources and their adequacy to meet the needs of clients
2. Collects data about the degree of utilization of health services by a client
3. Makes nursing diagnoses about adequacy of utilization of health care services by a client and family
4. Formulates a plan of care to facilitate use of health care services
5. Supports efforts of clients and/or family to make appropriate health care decisions and choices
6. Helps client and/or family to identify appropriate health care services and develop strategies for their utilization
7. Evaluates nursing interventions on the basis of specific goal-oriented client outcomes
8. Assesses adequacy of health care services
9. Supports or participates in appropriate action to obtain adequate health care services and resources.

Outcome Criteria

Knowledge—
1. The client and family describe community resources and services.
2. The client and family explain how their goals relate to the goals of the community resource.
3. The client and family explain how to select and use community resources.
4. The client and family identify a role for themselves in improving community resources and services.

Skill—
1. The client and family communicate own health care goals.
2. The client and family demonstrate skill in decision making.
3. The client and family demonstrate strategies for locating and contacting community resources.

Adaptation—
1. The client and family make appropriate health care decisions.
2. The client and family use community resources appropriately.
3. The incidence of kept appointments is high.
4. The rate of participation with treatment regimen is high.
5. The client and family develop meaningful goals to guide themselves in their use of community resources.
6. The client and family participate in the evaluation of community resources.
7. The client and family participate with other consumers, health professionals, and governmental agencies in the development of new resources or the improvement of existing ones.

Standard IX

THE NURSE IMPROVES MATERNAL AND CHILD HEALTH
NURSING PRACTICE THROUGH EVALUATION OF PRACTICE,
EDUCATION, AND RESEARCH.

Rationale

Improvement of the practice of maternal and child health nursing depends
upon a commitment of the nurses in this field to participate in programs
of practice evaluation, to acquire additional knowledge through informal
and formal education, to use new knowledge and research findings in
practice, to participate with others in research activities, to carry out own
nursing research, and to disseminate research findings. Outcomes are
measured in terms of behaviors of maternal and child health nurses.

Process Criteria

The nurse—
1. Critically examines and questions accepted modes of practice
2. Applies new knowledge to modify and improve accepted modes of
   practice
3. Systematically collects empirical data to address nursing problems
4. Identifies clinical nursing problems and uses the research process to
   address them
5. Uses a research approach to contribute new knowledge to maternal
   and child health nursing.

Outcome Criteria

The nurse—
1. Participates in peer review programs
2. Is involved in quality assurance programs
3. Consistently participates in continuing education programs in her
   field
4. Obtains additional formal education and certification
5. Keeps informed of and critically evaluates new knowledge in the field
6. Disseminates new knowledge and research findings among colleagues
7. Applies research findings to alter established modes of practice and
   to develop new modes
8. Participates in data collection and other research-related activities
9. Conducts or assists with research on identified clinical nursing
   problems
10. Reports own research findings at professional meetings and in re-
    se. ch publications.

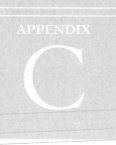

Nutritional Guidelines for the Pregnant Woman

Daily Food Plan for Pregnancy: Protein, Minerals, Vitamins, and Energy

Foods	Daily Amount	Suggested Uses
Protein-Rich Foods		
Primary protein		
Dairy products Milk, cheese	1 qt milk 2 + oz brick cheese or ½ cup + cottage cheese	Beverage, in cooking, or milk-based desserts such as ice milk, custards, puddings, cream soups; cheese in cooked dishes, salads, or snacks throughout the day
Eggs	2	Breakfast use, chopped or sliced hard eggs, in salads, custards, whole boiled eggs, deviled eggs, plain or in sandwiches
Meat	2 servings (total of 6 oz), liver frequently, 1-2 times per week	Main dish, sandwich, salad, snack
Supplementary protein		
Grains Enriched or whole grains, breads, cereals, crackers	4 to 5 slices or servings, whole grain or enriched	Bread, plain or toast, sandwiches, with meals, snacks, cereal (breakfast or snack); cooked grain as meal accompaniment (corn, rice, pasta, grits, hominy, hot breads: corn bread, biscuits, etc.)

Legumes, seeds, nuts
  Dried beans and peas
  Lentils
	Occasional servings as meat or grain substitute or in combination with meat or grains	Cooked and served alone or in combination with grains, cheese, or meat; soups, salads; nuts as snacks or in salads; peanut butter sandwich

Mineral-Rich Foods		
Calcium-rich		
Dairy products	1 qt milk (as above)	As above
Grains, whole or enriched	4-5 slices or servings (as above)	As above
Green leafy vegetables	1 serving	Cooked or raw in salads
Iron-rich		
Organ meats, especially liver	1-2 servings per week	
Grains, enriched	4-5 slices or servings	Breakfast cereals, main dish, or in combination with meats, cheese, egg, cooked grain foods, enriched breads
Egg yolk	2	As above
Green, leafy vegetables or dried fruits	1-2 servings	Cooked or stewed, raw in salads, snacks
Iodine-rich		
Iodized salt	Daily in cooking and on foods	On salads, in cooked food dishes, according to taste
Seafood	1-2 servings per week	Main dish, salad, sandwiches

From William S: Handbook of Maternal and Infant Nutrition. Berkeley, Calif, SRW Productions, 1988.

Daily Food Plan for Pregnancy: Protein, Minerals, Vitamins, and Energy—continued

Foods	Daily Amount	Suggested Uses
Vitamin-Rich Foods		
Vitamin A		
Animal sources		
Butterfat (whole milk, cream, butter)	2 tbsp butter (or fortified margarine)	In cooking or on foods
Liver	1–2 servings per week	Main dish
Egg yolk	2 (as above)	As above
Plant sources		
Dark green or deep yellow vegetables or fruits	1–2 servings	Cooked dishes, salads, snacks
Fortified margarine	2 tbsp	In cooking and on foods
Vitamin C		
Fruits		
Citrus	1 or 2 servings	Snacks, salads, juices
Other fruits—papayas, strawberries, melons	Occasional serving to substitute for one citrus portion	Salads, snacks
Vegetables		
Broccoli, potatoes, tomato, cabbage, green or chili peppers	1 serving as a substitute for 1 citrus occasionally	Cooked, snacks, salads, juices
Folic acid		
Liver, dark green vegetables, dried beans, lentils, nuts (peanuts, walnuts, filberts)	1 serving	Cooked as main dish or soups, snacks, in salads
Additional Energy Foods (as Needed)		
Carbohydrates		
Grains, breads, legumes, vegetables, fruits	Added portions (as above)	
Fats		
Butter, margarine, oil, mayonnaise, salad dressing, etc.	Moderate additions (as above), in cooking or on foods	

Ethnic Food Preferences / Sources

Grain Products	Vegetables and Fruits	Protein	Milk and Milk Products
Tortillas	Chili peppers	Tofu	Soy milk
	Refried beans		
Millet		Rice	
Polished rice		Noodles	
Corn bread	Okra	Legumes	
	Greens		
	Dried beans		
	Lentils	Soybean curd	Goat milk
Sesame, sunflower seeds		Nuts	
		Seeds	

Suggested Menus for Adequate Prenatal Vegetarian Diets

Meal Pattern	Semivegetarian Diet	Lactoovovegetarian Diet	Vegan
Breakfast			
Fruit	¾ c orange juice	Same as semivegetarian	Same
Grains	½ c granola, 1 slice whole wheat toast	Same	1 c granola, 1 slice whole grain toast
Meat group	1 scrambled egg with cheese		
Fat	1 tsp butter		1 tsp sesame butter
Milk	½ c milk		1 c soy milk
Midmorning			
Milk	1 c hot chocolate		1 c protein drink★
Lunch			
Meat group/vegetable	1 c lentil chowder (make with ground beef)	1 c lentil chowder† (no ground beef)	1½ c lentil chowder (1 tsp torula yeast, wheat germ added)
Grains	1 corn muffin	Same	2 corn muffins‡
Fat	1 tsp butter, honey		2 tsp margarine, honey
Fruit/dessert	½ peach, ½ c cottage cheese salad		½ peach, ½ c tofu salad
Tea	1 c tea		Decaffeinated or herbal tea

★Protein drink recipe is: 3 c cow's or goat's milk, ½ c nonfat soy milk powder, 2 tbsp wheat germ, 2 tbsp brewer's yeast, fruit, and vanilla. Vegans may make the drink with soy milk in place of cow's or goat's milk.
†Lentil chowder is made from lentils, celery, carrots, potatoes, onion, and tomatoes.
‡Wheat germ and soy flour are added to corn muffin mixture.

Food and Nutrition Board, National Academy of Sciences—National Research Council Recommended Dietary Allowances,[a] Revised 1989

Designed for the maintenance of good nutrition of practically all healthy people in the United States

							Fat-Soluble Vitamins			
Category	Age (Years) or Condition	Weight[b] (kg)	Weight[b] (lb)	Height[b] (cm)	Height[b] (in)	Protein (g)	Vitamin A (μg R.E.)[c]	Vitamin D (μg)[d]	Vitamin E (mg α-T.E.)[e]	Vitamin K (μg)
Females	11–14	46	101	157	62	46	800	10	8	45
	15–18	55	120	163	64	44	800	10	8	55
	19–24	58	128	164	65	46	800	10	8	60
	25–50	63	138	163	64	50	800	5	8	65
	51 +	65	143	160	63	50	800	5	8	65
Pregnant						60	800	10	10	65
Lactating	1st 6 months					65	1300	10	12	65
	2nd 6 months					62	1200	10	11	65

[a]The allowances, expressed as average daily intakes over time, are intended to provide for individual variations among most normal persons as they live in the United States under usual environmental stresses. Diets should be based on a variety of common foods in order to provide other nutrients for which human requirements have been less well defined.
[b]Weights and heights of Reference Adults are actual medians for the US population of the designated age, as reported by NHANES II. The median weights and heights of those under 19 years of age were taken from Hamill et al. The use of these figures does not imply that the height-to-weight ratios are ideal.

Suggested Menus for Adequate Prenatal Vegetarian Diets—continued

Meal Pattern	Semivegetarian Diet	Lactoovovegetarian Diet	Vegan
Midafternoon			
Milk	¾ c vanilla pudding	Same	1 c pudding (soy milk)
Fruit	¼ c sliced banana	Same	½ banana
Grain	1 graham cracker	Same	1 graham cracker with peanut butter
Dinner			
Meat group/vegetable	¾ c meat sauce (onion, celery, carrot, tomato, mushroom in sauce), parmesan cheese	¾ c tomato sauce (same vegetables as in semivegetarian diet), ¼ c cheese	Same (use tofu instead of cheese)
Grains	¾ c spaghetti, bread	1 c whole-wheat spaghetti, 1 slice French bread	Same
Vegetable	Mixed vegetable salad	Mixed vegetable salad with ¼ c sprouts, ½ egg, ½ oz cheese, ¼ c kidney beans added	(Add tofu, no egg in salad)
Fat	Oil-vinegar dressing, ½ tsp butter	Same	1 tsp margarine
Fruit	Fresh pear or baked pear half	Same	Same
Tea	1 c tea	Same	Decaffeinated or herbal tea
Bedtime			
Milk	1 c milk	Same	
Meat group/vegetable	2 tsp peanut butter on celery or on wheat crackers	Same	1 c protein drink★
Grain			corn muffins‡

	Water-Soluble Vitamins						Minerals						
Vitamin C (mg)	Thiamin (mg)	Ribo-flavin (mg)	Niacin (mg N.E.)[f]	Vitamin B_6 (mg)	Folate (μg)	Vitamin B_{12} (μg)	Calcium (mg)	Phospho-rus (mg)	Magne-sium (mg)	Iron (mg)	Zinc (mg)	Iodine (μg)	Sele-nium (μg)
50	1.1	1.3	15	1.4	150	2.0	1200	1200	280	15	12	150	45
60	1.1	1.3	15	1.5	180	2.0	1200	1200	300	15	12	150	50
60	1.1	1.3	15	1.6	180	2.0	1200	1200	280	15	12	150	55
60	1.1	1.3	15	1.6	180	2.0	800	800	280	15	12	150	55
60	1.0	1.2	13	1.6	180	2.0	800	800	280	10	12	150	55
70	1.5	1.6	17	2.2	400	2.2	1200	1200	320	30	15	175	65
95	1.6	1.8	20	2.1	280	2.6	1200	1200	355	15	19	200	75
90	1.6	1.7	20	2.1	260	2.6	1200	1200	340	15	16	200	75

[c]Retinol equivalents. 1 retinol equivalent = 1 μg retinol or 6 μg β-carotene.
[d]As cholecalciferol. 10 μg cholecalciferol = 400 I.U. of vitamin D.
[e]α-Tocopherol equivalents 1 mg d-α-tocopherol 1 α-T.E.
[f]1 N.E. (niacin equivalent) is equal to 1 mg of niacin or 60 mg of dietary tryptophan.

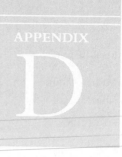

Drug Use During Breast-Feeding★

Drug or Agent	Contra-indicated	R$_x$ With Caution	No Apparent Harm	Insufficient Information	Comment
Analgesics					
Acetaminophen			X		
Aspirin			X		
Propoxyphene (Darvon)			X		
Anticoagulants					
Ethyl biscoumacetate	X				Bleeding infant
Phenindione	X				Bleeding infant
Heparin			X		No passage into milk
Warfarin Na (Coumadin)			X		
Bishydroxycoumarin (Dicumarol)		X			
Anticonvulsants					
Phenobarbital			X		Low levels in infant
Primadone (Mysoline)			X		? Drowsiness
Carbamazepine				X	Significant infant levels; no reported effects
Diphenylhydantoin (Phenytoin, Dilantin)			X		Low levels in infant, methemoglobin, 1 case
Antihistamines					
Diphenhydramine (Benadryl)			X		Small amounts excreted
Trimeprazine Temaril)			X		Small amounts excreted
Tripelennamine (Pyribenzamine)			X		Small amounts excreted
Anti-Infective Agents					
Aminoglycosides (Kanamycin, gentamicin)			X		Significant excretion in milk; not absorbed

From Avery GB (ed): Neonatology, 3rd ed. Philadelphia, JB Lippincott, 1987.
★Drug use during breast-feeding remains controversial.
†Controversy in literature, long-term effects uncertain, one case of gynecomastia.

Drug or Agent	Contra-indicated	R$_x$ With Caution	No Apparent Harm	Insufficient Information	Comment
Chloramphenicol	X				Bone marrow depression; gastrointestinal and behavioral effects
Penicillins			X		Possible sensitization
Sulfonamides		X			Hemolysis, G-6-PD deficiency, bilirubin displacement
Tetracyclines			X		Limited absorption by infant
Nalidixic acid		X			Hemolysis
Nitrofurantoin		X			Possible G-6-PD hemolysis
Metronidazole (Flagyl)		X			**Low absorption but potentially toxic**
Isoniazid		X			**High levels in milk, possible toxicity**
Pyramethamine	X				Vomiting, marrow suppression, convulsions
Chloraquine			X		Not excreted
Quinine		X			Thrombocytopenia
Anti-Inflammatory					
Aspirin			X		
Indomethacin		X			Seizures, 1 case
Phenylbutazone		X			Low levels, ? blood dyscrasia
Gold	X				Found in baby; nephritis, hepatitis, hematologic changes
Steroids				X	Low levels with prednisone and prednisolone
Antineoplastic					
Cyclophosphamide	X				Neutropenia
Methotrexate	X				Very small excretion
Antithyroid					
Radioactive iodine	X				Thyroid suppression
Propylthiouracil	X				Thyroid suppression
Bronchodilators					
Aminophylline			X		Irritability, 1 case
Iodides	X				Thyroid suppression
Sympathomimetics				X	Inhalers probably safe
Cardiovascular Agents					
Digoxin			X		Insignificant levels
Propanolol			X		Insignificant levels
Reserpine	X				Nasal stuffiness, lethargy
Guanethidine (Ismelin)			X		Insignificant levels
Cardiovascular Agents					
Methyldopa Aldomet)				X	

Continued

Drug or Agent	Contra-indicated	R$_x$ With Caution	No Apparent Harm	Insufficient Information	Comment
Cathartics					
Anthroquinones (Cascara, dan-thron)	X				Diarrhea, cramps
Aloe, senna		X			Safe in moderate dosage
Bulk agents, soften-ers			X		
Contraceptives, Oral†					
Diethylstilbestrol	X				Possible vaginal cancer
Depo-provera		X			May affect lactation
Norethisterone		X			May affect lactation
Ethinyl estradiol		X			May affect lactation
Diuretics					
Clorthalidone				X	Low levels, but may ac-cumulate
Thiazides		X			May affect lactation; low levels in milk
Spironolactone			X		Insignificant levels
Ergot Alkaloids					
Bromocriptine	X				Lactation suppressed
Ergot	X				Vomiting, diarrhea, sei-zures
Ergotamine				X	
Ergonovine	X				**Brief postpartum course may be safe**
Methylergonovine	X				**Brief postpartum course may be safe**
Hormones					
Corticosteroids				X	Low levels with short-term prednisone or prednisolone
Sex hormones (see above, Contracep-tives, Oral)					
Thyroid (T$_3$ or T$_4$)			X		Excreted in milk; may mask hypothyroid in-fant
Insulin			X		Not absorbed
ACTH			X		Not absorbed
Epinephrine			X		Not absorbed
Narcotics					
Codeine			X		In usual doses
Meperidine (Demerol)				X	
Morphine			X		Low infant levels on usual dosage
Heroin	X				Addiction withdrawal in infants
Methadone		X			Minimal levels

Drug or Agent	Contra-indicated	Rx With Caution	No Apparent Harm	Insufficient Information	Comment
Psychotherapeutic Drugs					
Lithium	X				High levels in milk
Phenothiazines		X			Drowsiness; chronic effects uncertain
Tricyclic antidepressants				X	Low levels; effects uncertain
Diazepam (Valium)	X				Lethargy, weight loss, EEG changes
Meprobamate (Equanil)	X				High levels in milk
Chlordiazepoxide (Librium)			X		Low levels in milk
Radiopharmaceuticals					
^{131}I	X				72 hr, no breast-feeding
Technetium (99M Tc)	X				48 hr, no breast-feeding
^{131}I albumin	X				10 days, no breast-feeding
Sedatives-Hypnotics					
Barbiturates		X			Short-acting, less depressant
Chloral hydrate		X			Drowsiness
Bromides	X				Depression, rash
Diazepam (Valium)	X				Depression, weight loss
Flurazepam				X	Chemically related to diazepam
Nitrazepam				X	
Social-Recreational Drugs					
Alcohol			X		Milk levels equal plasma, moderate consumption apparently safe, high levels inhibit lactation
Caffeine			X		Jitteriness with very high intakes
Nicotine			X		Low levels in milk
Marijuana			X		Minimal passage in milk
Miscellaneous					
Atropine		X			May cause constipation or inhibit lactation
Dihydrotachysterol		X			Renal calcification in animals

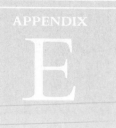
Conversion Table for Weights of Newborn

(Gram equivalents for pounds and ounces)
For example, to find weight in pounds and ounces of baby weighing 3315 grams, glance down columns to figure nearest 3315 = 3317. Refer to number at top of column for pounds and number to far left for ounces = 7 pounds, 5 ounces.

Pounds→ Ounces ↓	3	4	5	6	7	8	9	10
0	1361	1814	2268	2722	3175	3629	4082	4536
1	1389	1843	2296	2750	3203	3657	4111	4564
2	1417	1871	2325	2778	3232	3685	4139	4593
3	1446	1899	2353	2807	3260	3714	4167	4621
4	1474	1928	2381	2835	3289	3742	4196	4649
5	1503	1956	2410	2863	3317	3770	4224	4678
6	1531	1984	2438	2892	3345	3799	4252	4706
7	1559	2013	2466	2920	3374	3827	4281	4734
8	1588	2041	2495	2948	3402	3856	4309	4763
9	1616	2070	2523	2977	3430	3884	4338	4791
10	1644	2098	2551	3005	3459	3912	4366	4819
11	1673	2126	2580	3033	3487	3941	4394	4848
12	1701	2155	2608	3062	3515	3969	4423	4876
13	1729	2183	2637	3090	3544	3997	4451	4904
14	1758	2211	2665	3118	3572	4026	4479	4933
15	1786	2240	2693	3147	3600	4054	4508	4961

Or, to convert grams into pounds and *decimals* of a pound, multiply weight in grams by .0022. Thus, $3317 \times .0022 = 7.2974$ (i.e., 7.3 pounds, or 7 pounds, 5 ounces).

To convert pounds and ounces into grams, multiply the pounds by 453.6 and the ounces by 28.4 and add the two products. Thus, to convert 7 pounds, 5 ounces, $7 \times 453.6 = 3175$; $5 \times 28.4 = 142$; $3175 + 142 = 3317$ grams.

Index

Numbers followed by an f indicate a figure; t following a page number indicates tabular material.